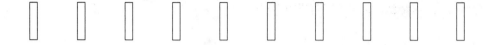

A Model of
HUMAN OCCUPATION
Theory and Application

Second Edition

A Model of
HUMAN OCCUPATION
Theory and Application

Second Edition

Gary Kielhofner, **Dr.P.H., O.T.R., F.A.O.T.A.**
Professor and Head
Department of Occupational Therapy
College of Associated Health Professions
University of Illinois at Chicago
Chicago, Illinois

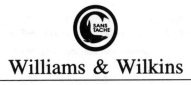

BALTIMORE • PHILADELPHIA • HONG KONG
LONDON • MUNICH • SYDNEY • TOKYO

A WAVERLY COMPANY

Editor: John P. Butler
Managing Editor: Linda S. Napora
Production Coordinator: Barbara J. Felton
Copy Editor: Bonnie Cover
Designer: Wilma Rosenberger
Illustration Planner: Wayne Hubbel
Cover Designer: Wilma Rosenberger
Typesetter: Brushwood Graphics, Inc.
Printer: Port City Press
Digitized Illustrations: Trinity Graphics
Binder: Port City Press

Copyright © 1995
Williams & Wilkins
351 West Camden Street
Baltimore, Maryland 21201-2436 USA

Rose Tree Corporate Center
1400 North Providence Road
Building II, Suite 5025
Media, Pennsylvania 19063-2043 USA

Accurate indications, adverse reactions, and dosage schedules for drugs are provided in this book, but it is possible that they may change. The reader is urged to review the package information data of the manufacturers of the medications mentioned.

Printed in the United States of America

First Edition 1985

Library of Congress Cataloging-in-Publication Data

Kielhofner, Gary, 1949–
  A model of human occupation: theory and application / Gary Kielhofner. — 2nd ed.
    p.   cm.
  Rev. ed. of: A model of human occupation / edited by Gary Kielhofner. c1985.
    Includes bibliographical references and index.
    ISBN 0-683-04601-2 (pbk.)
    1. Occupational therapy.   I. Title.
    [DNLM: 1. Occupational Therapy.   2. Models, Psychological.   WB 555 K47m 1995]
RM735.K55   1995
615.8'515—dc20
DNLM/DLC
for Library of Congress   95-7615
                                                                                CIP

The publishers have made every effort to trace the copyright holders for borrowed material. If they have inadvertently overlooked any, they will be pleased to make the necessary arrangements at the first opportunity.

To purchase additional copies of this book, call our customer service department at **(800) 638-0672** or fax orders to **(800) 447-8438**. For other book services, including chapter reprints and large quantity sales, ask for the Special Sales department.

Canadian customers should call **(800) 268-4178,** or fax **(905) 470-6780.** For all other calls originating outside of the United States, please call **(410) 528-4223** or fax us at **(410) 528-8550.**

Visit Williams & Wilkins on the Internet: http://www.wwilkins.com or contact our customer service department at **custserv@wwilkins.com.** Williams & Wilkins customer service representatives are available from 8:30 am to 6:00 pm, EST, Monday through Friday, for telephone access.

                                                                    98   99
                                                        5   6   7   8   9   10

With love for Nancy, Kim, and Kris
and in gratitude for the gift of family

Acknowledgments

This Second Edition of *A Model of Human Occupation* goes to press exactly 20 years after the whole process began in my graduate work at the University of Southern California. As I write this, I cannot help but recall the many persons and events that have been a part of the evolution of the model of human occupation. While I cannot personally acknowledge everyone, I hope that this book, in various ways, bears testimony to their contributions.

The earliest debt is, of course, owed to Mary Reilly who, over many years, led development of the occupational behavior tradition in which this model has its roots and who, along with Linda Florey, Nancy Takata, and Phillip Shannon, oversaw my first efforts to give the model shape in my master's thesis. Later, Janice Burke and Cynthia Heard Igi collaborated to refine and elaborate the model.

Uncounted hours of conversation and debate among myself, Janice, and numerous colleagues and students resulted in shaping the model as it was originally published in 1980. During the years which led to the publication of the First Edition, I had the good fortune to work with Roann Barris and see the model benefit from her sharp intellect and rhetorical skill. Anne Neville-Jan joined us midway in the process and brought a keen clinical sense and her own special brand of intellectual enthusiasm. I missed the collaboration with both of them while working on this volume. I also had the good fortune to work with a number of other gifted colleagues on the First Edition. Although time, distance, and other logistics have made it necessary or expedient for me to be working with a new configuration of co-authors, I would be remiss if I did not also acknowledge the important contributions of authors from the First Edition: Florence Clark, Sally Jackson, Jana Green, Betty Herlong Harlan, Kathy Kaplan, Ellen Kolodner, Sue Hirsch Knox, Ruth Ellen Schlemm, Mike Lyons, Jeanne Madigan, Zoe Mailloux, Carol Lee McLellan, Peggy Neville, Joan Owens, Lillian Hoyle Parent, Joan Rogers, Charlotte Brasic Royeen, Cheryl Salz, Teena Snow, Cynthia Stabenow, and Janet Hawkins Watts. Additionally, I was thrilled to be able to continue collaboration with Janice Burke, Gloria Furst, Marion Kavanaugh, Fran Oakley, and Jayne Shepherd who were part of the First Edition and whose work appears again here.

In more recent years, it has been a pleasure to work with a number of superbly talented colleagues who have contributed to the present volume. Kathi Baron, Kim Bryze, Susan Doble, Laurie Rockwell-Dylla, Carmen Gloria de Las Heras, and Jaime Muñoz have been students, colleagues, and friends and it is a pleasure to have them involved in this text. Anne Fisher has brought a refreshing and much-needed new perspective and exactness to our understanding of performance. I have learned a great deal from Anne; her contributions to this volume are important advances for the model. Trudy Mallinson has been my coauthor, colleague, crutch, confidante, critic, copy editor, and creative illustrator through the entire process of producing this volume. I could speak volumes about all she has done, but suffice to say *this volume* would not readily have come to fruition without her, nor would the journey have been as pleasant.

The reader will recognize that a number of Swedish authors have contributed to this book. I wish to express a debt of gratitude to my Swedish colleagues in general for the past decade of stimulating interaction and support. In particular, I wish to acknowledge Chris Henriksson, who first brought me to Sweden, and Inga-Britt Lindstrom, who has consistently supported the model's development in Sweden. Bengt Winbladt has been an unfailing supporter of occupational therapy and I am most grateful to him for my appointment as a foreign adjunct professor at the Karolinska Institute, which has brought me into stimulating interaction with a number of occupational therapists pursuing doctoral education. Hans Jonsson is one of the main reasons I look forward to my frequent visits to Sweden. The bedroom in his basement has become my second abode, but more importantly, he always shares with me much cherished hours of fellowship, along with the joy and love of his entire family. Lena Borell has been an unfailing friend and stimulating colleague for many years now; it has been a pleasure to see her pass from student to professorial colleague. I must also acknowledge that I have learned more than a little in working with Staffan Josephson, Louise Nygård, Kerstin Tham, and Margareta Lilja.

I have had excellent support from Roberta Croll, Jalena Blaase, Laura Barrett, Renée Moore, and Lisa Eubanks, who gave feedback, edited, proofed, typed, and in other ways helped to bring this manuscript to its final form. I also owe a debt of gratitude to those persons who reviewed part or all of the manuscript and provided very helpful feedback: Alexis Henry, Betty Herlong Harlan, Clare Hocking, Frances Oakley, Jayne Shepherd, and Louise Thibodeaux.

I want to thank John Butler, who has been a patient and understanding editor over the past decade, and I wish to express gratitude to the entire Williams & Wilkins staff who worked on the production of this volume. Graphic artists Pam Cox and Allen Levinson contributed their talents to the production of the new illustrations that appear in this volume.

For reasons of my own procrastination, this volume was produced over a very short period of time. Long hours of reading, writing, and editing have stolen me away from my wife, Nancy, and my children, Kim and Kris. They have borne my absence, preoccupation, and anxiety with more understanding than I could have hoped for. Nancy has provided moral support and placed confidence in me when I needed it to keep up the pace. To them, I have dedicated this book and promised time in both quality and quantity!

Contributors

Kathi Brenneman Baron, M.S., O.T.R./L.
Clinical Specialist
McNeil Hospital
Psychiatry Unit
Berwyn, Illinois

Birgitta Berspång, Dr.Med.Sc., O.T.
Occupational Therapy Researcher
University Hospital of Northern Sweden
Umea, Sweden

Lena Borell, Dr.Med.Sc., O.T.
Stockholm University College of Health Sciences
Solna, Sweden

Kim Bryze, M.S., O.T.R./L.
Senior Occupational Therapist, Pediatrics
Department of Occupational Therapy
University of Illinois Hospital and Clinics
Chicago, Illinois

Janice Burke, M.S., O.T.R., F.A.O.T.A.
Department of Occupational Therapy
College of Allied Health Sciences
Thomas Jefferson University
Philadelphia, Pennsylvania

Carmen Gloria de las Heras, M.S., O.T.R./L.
Occupational Therapist, Private Consultant
Private Practice
Vitaguro, Santiago, Chile

Susan Doble, M.S., O.T.Reg.
Assistant Professor
School of Occupational Therapy
Dalhousie University
Halifax, Canada

Birgitta Englund, M.S., O.T.
Senior Lecturer
College of Health and Caring Sciences
Umea, Sweden

Anne G. Fisher, Sc.D., O.T.R., F.A.O.T.A.
Professor
Department of Occupational Therapy
Colorado State University
Fort Collins, Colorado

Christine Helfrich, M.S., O.T.R./L.
Research Specialist in Behavioral Sciences
Department of Occupational Therapy
University of Illinois at Chicago
Chicago, Illinois

Gary Kielhofner, Dr.P.H., O.T.R., F.A.O.T.A.
Professor and Head
Department of Occupational Therapy
University of Illinois at Chicago
Chicago, Illinois

Trudy Mallinson, M.S., O.T.R./L., N.Z.R.O.T.
Department of Occupational Therapy
University of Illinois at Chicago
Chicago, Illinois

Jaime Muñoz, M.S., O.T.R./L.
Clinical Instructor
Department of Occupational Therapy
University of Illinois at Chicago
Chicago, Illinois

Louise Nygård
Doctoral Student, Occupational Therapy
Center for Caring Sciences (CVV South)
Huddinge Hospital
Huddinge, Sweden

Frances Oakley, M.S., O.T.R./L.
Acting Chief, Occupational Therapy Section
National Institutes of Health
Bethesda, Maryland

Laurie Rockwell-Dylla, M.S., O.T.R./L.
Clinical Instructor
Department of Occupational Therapy
University of Illinois at Chicago
Chicago, Illinois

Marcelle Salamy, M.S., O.T.R./L.
Private Practice Consultant
Western Springs, Illinois

Marion Kavanagh Scheinholtz, M.S., O.T.R./L.
Mental Health Program Manager
American Occupational Therapy Association
Bethesda, Maryland

Jayne Shepherd, M.S., O.T.R./L.
Director of Occupational Therapy
Virginia Commonwealth University
Department of Occupational Therapy
Richmond, Virginia

Sandy Simon, M.S., O.T.R.
Occupational Therapist
Private Practice
Highland Park, Illinois

Cynthia A. Stabenow, M.S., O.T.R.
Occupational Therapist
Colonnades Health Care Center
Charlottesville, Virginia

Lucy Swan Sullivan, M.S., O.T.R./L.
Senior Occupational Therapist
National Institutes of Health
Bethesda, Maryland

Contents

1/ Introduction to the Model of Human Occupation

Gary Kielhofner

As an occupational therapist assisting my patients or clients to change, as an educator training new therapists to do therapy, and as a writer trying to explain therapy, I have learned the following. Theory can never tell therapists, in advance, exactly what should be done in the context of therapy. But, if therapists understand a theory, it will help them figure out what to do at the time. Practice requires therapists to imagine how persons might find their ways out of states of dysfunction and achieve better lives. Theory which supports such therapeutic imagining cannot offer a simple plan or recipe. Rather, it must sharpen and deepen the quality of a therapist's thinking.

This book presents a conceptual model designed to be used by occupational therapists in practice; however, nowhere in this text will the reader find a set of procedures to follow or specific instructions for what to do in practice. What you should look for are ways of thinking about a person's occupational behavior and occupational difficulties that will serve as a foundation for the creative imagining that occupational therapy practice requires.

Two decades of trying to better comprehend and explain occupation has taught me that no *one* way of thinking about something is ever complete. In fact, the more one seeks to fit a single explanation to any phenomenon, the more unsympathetic become the data. Consequently, in trying to develop theory for occupational therapy, I am increasingly compelled to approach a problem and explain it from many perspectives. That is the tack taken in this book. Consequently, readers will encounter

a wide range of ideas, each one contributing to the total picture. The theoretical and practical arguments should become progressively clearer, like a picture coming into focus over time. Consequently, understanding the model of human occupation and knowing how to use it should emerge gradually as one studies this text and experiments, in practice, with the ideas it presents.

NATURE AND ROLE OF CONCEPTUAL MODELS OF PRACTICE

Since this text proposes to describe and elucidate a *model* of human occupation, it is important to first address what is meant by a model. I use the term *conceptual model of practice* in the context of a specific way of viewing the organization of knowledge in occupational therapy (Kielhofner, 1992). In this view, models have a particular place in the overall knowledge generated and used by the field.

Place of Models in the Field's Knowledge

I have argued elsewhere (Kielhofner, 1992) that the unique knowledge of occupational therapy is made up of both (1) a paradigm and (2) conceptual practice models. The paradigm refers to a broad collection of assumptions and perspectives that give coherence to the profession and that elucidate the nature and purpose of occupational therapy. Shared by members of the field, the paradigm is a collective professional culture. The paradigm is expressed as core concepts articulated in the literature and is reflected in the everyday perspectives of therapists. Occupational therapy's current paradigm emphasizes the field's concern with humans' occupational well-being and with problems of occupational dysfunction (Kielhofner, 1992). Moreover, it recognizes that the unique therapy provided by members of this profession employs the health-giving potential of participating in occupations.

While the paradigm is important to bind together members of the field, other knowledge is necessary to guide everyday practice. This is the role of conceptual practice models. Each conceptual model contains theory that serves as the rationale for some aspect of occupational therapy practice.

At any point in time the field may have a number of conceptual models of practice. I have observed previously (Kielhofner, 1992) that eight conceptual models of practice can be identified in occupational therapy. The model of human occupation is one of those eight models. Because each model has a specific focus, a single model ordinarily does not address all of the multiple factors involved in the occupational functioning of any patient or client. Therefore, therapists will typically require more than one model in practice.

Nature of Conceptual Practice Models

A conceptual practice model presents and organizes a number of theoretical concepts that are used by therapists in their therapeutic work. In occupational therapy, each model addresses some specific phenomenon or area related to occupational functioning. For example, three of occupational therapy's models address, respectively, the biomechanics of movement, perceptual and cognitive processes, and group processes involved in occupational performance. The model of human occupation focuses on *the motivation for occupation, the patterning of occupational behavior into routines and lifestyles, the nature of skilled performance, and the influence of environment on occupational behavior*. I will elaborate this focus later in this chapter.

Developers of conceptual practice models ordinarily select relevant interdisciplinary concepts, integrating them into the theoretical arguments they wish to make about the phenomena with which they are concerned. For example, in order to address the motivation for occupation we have used concepts derived from psychology, anthropology, and sociology.

The theoretical arguments of models ordinarily address three practical concerns. The first concern is to explain the organization and function (*order*) of those aspects of occupation on which the model focuses. So, for example, we will attempt to explain how people are ordinarily motivated to choose their occupational behavior. The second concern of a model is to conceptualize *disorder* or dysfunction. Since occupational therapists work with persons who have become dysfunctional in their occupational behavior, there is a need to understand this disorder. In the case of motivation, we would seek to explain what happens to motives when persons become disabled. The third concern of models is to provide theoretical explanations of how therapy can help restore order in occupational functioning. Once again, using the example of motivation, our theory will seek to explain how motives can be enhanced or changed in the course of therapy. One can see, then, that the theoretical arguments give logic and coherence to the clinical applications which emanate from a model.

Since models are intended to guide practice, they also yield a technology for application. This technology may consist of such things as methods of gathering data, principles to follow in practice, and case examples showing how the model can be applied.

Models of practice are always changing. Research findings, new theory, and insights encountered in practice may all lead to refinements and additions to the model. Consequently, developing a conceptual practice model is a dynamic process in which knowledge is continuously generated, used, tested, and refined.

NATURE OF HUMAN OCCUPATION

By virtue of its title, the model of *human occupation* promises to provide an explanation of occupation. Let us consider, then, how occupation will be conceptualized in this text.

In the broadest sense, we use the term occupation to denote the action or doing through which humans *occupy* their world (Nelson, 1988; Reilly, 1962; Rogers, 1983).[a] Human occupation refers, in part, to humans' unique capacity to manipulate and transform their physical world. Human occupation of the physical world extends from the primitive tool-using and tool-making activities of our ancestors to the space age achievements of modern technology. Moreover, as Reilly (1962) notes, occupation begins with the child's struggle against gravity and continues with the mastering of a complex world of objects.

Humans are also intensely social creatures. They coordinate their behavior together and communicate their intentions and needs. Just as occupation is directed at the physical world, it also occurs in and through a world of social relations (Rogers, 1983).

Human life is deeply cultural. Our cultures are the medium through which we make sense of ourselves and our behavior. Through culture, humans attach meaning to their occupations (Yerxa, et al., 1989). That is, the accumulated experience of a culture generates a whole range of occupations that are given shape and significance. When persons engage in occupations they are replicating ways of behaving developed in the culture. Moreover, they know what they are doing by virtue of how their culture views and makes sense of their behavior.

Temporality defines human experience; we cannot exist outside of time (Hall, 1969; Kerby, 1991). Human awareness of the past and future, of the passage of time, gives experience its particular character. Consequently, persons experience their occupations as unfolding in the course of time.

Humans occupy life in many ways. Consequently, occupational therapy has always been challenged to provide descriptions or taxonomies of those activities which comprise occupational behavior. Occupation is often described as comprising three general areas of behavior: play, daily living tasks, and work. *Play* is the earliest occupational behavior, persisting throughout life (Reilly, 1974; Robinson, 1977; Vandenberg & Kielhofner, 1982). Exploring, pretending, gaming, sporting, creating, and celebrating are all part of the human experience of play. *Daily living tasks*[b] are activities aimed at self-maintenance and maintenance of one's lifestyle. They include such diverse activities as self-care, ordering of one's life space (e.g., cleaning and paying bills), and accessing resources (e.g., traveling and shopping) (Kielhofner, 1989). *Work* refers to activities (both paid and unpaid) which provide services or commodities to others (e.g., ideas, knowledge, help, information-sharing, utilitarian or artistic objects, and protection) (Shannon, 1970; Chapple, 1970). Activities such as studying, practicing, and apprenticing improve abilities for productive performance. Thus, work, broadly defined, includes activities engaged in as a student, employee, volunteer, parent, serious hobbyist, and amateur.

Toward a Definition of Human Occupation

In the foregoing discussions I pointed out that occupation implies action or doing in the physical and social world. This action is infused with awareness or meaning provided by one's culture. It is action that unfolds in time. Finally, I pointed out that occupation takes on the forms of work, play, and daily living tasks. Thus, we can define human occupation as *doing culturally meaningful work, play or daily living tasks in the stream of time and in the contexts of one's physical and social world.* This definition should be viewed as a starting point. It should orient the reader to what, in general, the model of human occupation seeks to address. The theoretical arguments made in this book should give the reader a deeper and more thorough appreciation of occupation than any definition can hope to achieve.

---

[a]While not all of what we might wish to designate as occupation necessarily involves doing (Rowles, 1992), it is nevertheless the case that doing is a central feature of the domain of behavior we refer to as occupation.

[b]The term *activities of daily living* is also frequently used to refer to self-care and related daily life behaviors necessary for maintaining oneself and one's living environment.

BACKGROUND AND GENESIS OF THE MODEL

The model of human occupation grew out of the occupational behavior[c] tradition developed by Reilly and her colleagues. Consistent with this tradition, the goal of the model has always been to provide a deeper understanding of the nature of occupation in human life and its role in health and illness.

This model was originally articulated in my unpublished masters thesis 20 years ago (Kielhofner, 1975). We first published the model five years later after refining the concepts and experimenting with them in practice (Kielhofner, 1980a, 1980b; Kielhofner & Burke, 1980; Kielhofner, Burke, & Heard, 1980). Ten years ago, *A Model of Human Occupation: Theory and Application*, introduced an expanded theory and a wide range of clinical applications (Kielhofner, 1985). Other literature which discusses and elaborates upon the model now includes several books, book chapters, manuals, and over 160 articles. Over the course of our discussions, we will introduce much of that literature. Moreover, at the end of this book readers will find a current bibliography on the model.

This second edition of *A Model of Human Occupation* presents the most recent theory and application of this model. Since models are constantly changing and developing, this book is, in part, a progress report. As such, it tells what we have learned in 20 years since the model first began to take shape. If the ideas contained herein are truly generative, we will further alter and add to the model in the future. Since the first edition appeared a decade ago, many new concepts have evolved and

[c]Reilly coined the term *occupational behavior* to refer to that domain of behavior with which occupational therapy was concerned. During the time she was at the University of Southern California (mainly the 1960s and 1970s) she led a group of graduate students and colleagues in developing concepts which helped to explain occupational behavior in humans. The term occupational behavior was used in the field to refer to those collective theoretical efforts. Current usage of the term (and that followed in this text) parallels Reilly's original intention of circumscribing a domain of behavior of concern.

some arguments and ideas have been deleted. Some of these changes reflect research findings; others draw upon theoretical advances in related fields from which we borrow ideas. Some new ideas are the result of conceptual contributions of colleagues working on the model. Still other changes reflect the work of clinicians who have critiqued the model's utility and developed creative ways of applying the model in practice. A great deal has been learned from each of these contributions.

CONTENT AND ORGANIZATION OF THIS VOLUME

As I mentioned earlier, this book is organized to take the reader to successively deeper levels of understanding. I will begin here with an overview of the major concepts which will be discussed in the text and provide a guide as to how they will be introduced and developed in successive chapters. In so doing, I will provide some suggestions for how to read and use this book.

The model of human occupation begins with a particular way of viewing the human being. In earlier publications, the model explained the human being as an open system (Kielhofner & Burke, 1980; Kielhofner, 1985). The concepts of open systems portray the human being as complex, dynamic, and ever-changing. While open systems concepts may seem to emphasize the obvious, they represented an important and novel argument at the time the model was first introduced. Twenty years ago, occupational therapy was much more closely aligned with medicine. There were still very strong remnants of thinking about occupational therapy practice which built upon medicine's view of the human being as a mechanism which could break down and be repaired. Open systems concepts provided a way of asserting that occupational therapy was not a matter of repairing the broken or malfunctioning "human machine." Instead, these concepts allowed us to characterize therapy as a process of enabling active, living entities to change and reorganize themselves following trauma, disease, life distress or other factors which impaired everyday occupation.

This edition continues the systems' view of

human beings. Chapter 2 provides this perspective, conceptualizing the human being as a complex, dynamic system. Some older systems concepts have been eliminated or modified and a number of new systems concepts are introduced. In the decade since the last publication of the model, important and exciting new systems theory has emerged. I have drawn upon this theory to attempt a more contemporary explanation of the human system.

Chapter 2 presents abstract and challenging ideas; however, the theoretical arguments in this chapter constitute an important foundation for understanding how, where, when, and why humans engage in occupations. The subsequent chapters (3–7) build a progressively more detailed view of humans and their occupational behavior. Following the assertion that the human being is a complex, dynamic system, the model will address three critical issues in understanding occupation.

The first issue concerns how persons are motivated toward and choose the occupations that fill their lives. To explain human motives and choices for occupations a number of questions must be answered: What is the source of this motivation? Why are humans generally so active? What accounts for the individual differences in what persons want and choose to do? Why do different people experience occupations in different ways? Why is one bored by what another enjoys? Why does one person find valuable what another considers a waste of time? One of the purposes of the model is to achieve a coherent explanation of the motivation for occupation by attempting to answer such questions.

The second issue comes from the observation that much of everyday life is made up of recurrent patterns of behavior in familiar physical and social environments. People behave in similar ways over and over again, they follow similar patterns of time use, and they do things in pretty much the same way they did before. A great deal of human life simply follows a routine pattern. Questions arise as to how persons sustain these patterns of everyday life: What holds all this regularity in life together? How do people know how to find their way through the course of the day and through familiar locales? How do persons manage to

know more or less automatically how to behave as students, workers, parents, and members of organizations? As such questions indicate, the second issue requires that we explain the observed regularity of human behavior along with the ability of persons to perform more or less automatically and efficiently this regular behavior in their ordinary physical and social worlds.

The third issue is that human beings are exquisite performers. Whether it be lifting food to one's mouth or playing first violin in an orchestra, humans demonstrate fine and coordinated movements when they perform their occupations. When performing occupations, humans also anticipate, plan, observe what happens, make adjustments, decide what to do next, and so on. Whether it be getting one's clothes washed, folded, and stored away in the closet or designing and assembling an automobile, humans show an uncanny ability to figure out how to get something done. Finally, humans participate and communicate with others. From simple conversation to participation in a scientific discussion the ability to coordinate action and share information is part of everyday occupation.

The dimensions and complexity of human performance are beyond the explanatory power of current knowledge. Most certainly, they are beyond the concepts of any single discipline. Nonetheless, there are certain questions about human performance which are especially important for occupational therapy: What capacities are critical for performance in occupations? What do persons do when they perform in their occupations? How does impairment of capacity influence this performance? How can performance be restored when it has been impaired? Such questions orient us to what persons do in their everyday occupations and to how therapists can understand and support that doing.

In pursuing these three issues outlined above, the model of human occupation asserts that the human being can be thought of as being made up of three subsystems. Each of these subsystems corresponds to one of the issues. Chapter 3 provides a more detailed review of the three issues introduced here and elaborates this view of the human system as being made up of three subsystems. The first subsystem, volition, accounts for motivation. It orients persons to anticipate, experience, interpret, and choose their occupations. Chapter 4 explains this subsystem. Chapter 5 explains the second subsystem, habituation; it is responsible for maintaining the patterns of everyday behavior. The mind-brain-body performance subsystem organizes the capacities which persons draw upon in their occupational performance. This third subsystem is the subject of Chapter 6.

As noted earlier, all occupation takes place in one's environment. Chapter 7 discusses the environmental context of occupational behavior, explaining what aspects of the environment influence occupation, and how they exert this influence.

Chapter 8 provides a detailed conceptualization of the nature of occupational performance in one's environment. This chapter introduces and describes the motor, process, and communication/interaction skills that are used in everyday occupational performance. Chapter 9 views occupation over the course of development, noting how the human system changes through the life course.

These first chapters mainly present the theoretical arguments about order and change in occupational behavior. I noted earlier that the theoretical arguments of a conceptual practice model also concern disorder. Chapter 10 addresses this topic by discussing occupational dysfunction. In this chapter, the perspectives gained in the earlier chapters concerning humans and their occupational behavior are used to create an understanding of what goes wrong when persons experience problems in their occupational lives.

The remainder of the book focuses mainly on the technology for the application of this model. Chapters 11 and 12 discuss the process of gathering and reasoning with data and introduce and discuss a number of data-gathering tools developed for use with the model of human occupation. Chapter 13 discusses the process of change in therapy, introducing principles of change derived from earlier theoretical arguments. Chapter 14 presents a number of case studies to illustrate the process of gathering and reasoning with data and the im-

plementation of principles of change. Finally, Chapter 15 discusses how the model can be used in the process of program development.

Throughout this book, we have sought to amplify and clarify points through liberal use of case examples and anecdotes. Some of the chapters use tables and figures extensively to present the main points in the discussions. Many of the chapters conclude with some form of summary of the main points or concepts. However, the chapters require study in order to be properly understood. In this book we have sought to grapple with how complex occupation is. We have tried not to oversimplify our explanations in the belief that good therapy requires thorough understanding.

Readers should not be discouraged if not all is understood upon first reading. Sometimes it will be helpful to continue on and return to parts which require more careful rereading. Additionally, fair warning is served here that many chapters cannot be read all at once. Either by virtue of length, conceptual density, or both, some chapters will simply require more than one session to read. A good strategy would be to look at the table of contents and/or briefly skim each chapter to have some idea of what is contained in it. The chapter then can be tackled in manageable sections. While some chapters contain resources the reader is expected to refer to more than once, the entire book is probably best considered a resource to which one may wish to return occasionally.

We hope the reader will enjoy this book. There are many implicit and explicit voices here. They include those of theoreticians from many fields, those of colleagues who have helped to conceptualize the model, those of persons who have told their stories of struggling with disabilities, and those of therapists who have created practical means of applying the model. In the end, it is our hope that these voices have come together in an interesting, instructive, and instrumentally useful way.

References

Chapple, E. (1970). *Rehabilitation: Dynamic of change.* Ithaca, NY: Center for Research in Education, Cornell University.

Hall, E. T. (1969). *The silent language.* Greenwich, CT: Fawcett Publications.

Kerby, A. P. (1991). *Narrative and the self*. Bloomington, IN: Indiana University Press.

Kielhofner, G. (1975). *The evolution of knowledge in occupational therapy: Understanding adaptation of the chronically disabled*. Unpublished master's thesis, University of Southern California, Los Angeles.

Kielhofner, G. (1980a). A model of human occupation, part three. Benign and vicious cycles. *American Journal of Occupational Therapy, 34*, 731–737.

Kielhofner, G. (1980b). A model of human occupation, part two. Ontogenesis from the perspective of temporal adaptation. *American Journal of Occupational Therapy, 34*, 657–663.

Kielhofner, G. (1985). *A model of human occupation: Theory and application*. Baltimore: Williams & Wilkins.

Kielhofner, G. (1989). Occupation. In Willard & Spackman (Eds.), *Occupational therapy*. Philadelphia: JB Lippincott.

Kielhofner, G. (1992). *Conceptual foundations of occupational therapy*. Philadelphia: FA Davis.

Kielhofner, G., & Burke, J. (1980). A model of human occupation, part one. Conceptual framework and content. *American Journal of Occupational Therapy, 34*, 572–581.

Kielhofner, G., Burke, J., & Heard, I. C. (1980). A model of human occupation, part four. Assessment and intervention. *American Journal of Occupational Therapy, 34*, 777–788.

Nelson, D. (1988). Occupation: Form and performance. *American Journal of Occupational Therapy, 38*, 777–788.

Reilly, M. (1962). Occupational therapy can be one of the great ideas of 20th century medicine. *American Journal of Occupational Therapy, 16*, 1–9.

Reilly, M. (1974). *Play as exploratory learning*. Beverly Hills, CA: Sage Publications.

Robinson, A. (1977). Play: The arena for acquisition of rules for competent behavior. *American Journal of Occupational Therapy, 31*, 248–253.

Rogers, J. (1983). The study of human occupation. In G. Kielhofner (Ed.), *Health through occupation: Theory and practice in occupational therapy*. Philadelphia: FA Davis.

Rowles, G. D. (1992, March). *On individual experience and occupation*. Paper presented at the AOTF Research Colloquium, Houston, TX.

Shannon, P. (1970). The work-play model: A basis for occupational therapy programming. *American Journal of Occupational Therapy, 24*, 215–218.

Vandenberg, B., & Kielhofner, G. (1982). Play in evolution, culture, and individual adaptation: Implications for therapy. *American Journal of Occupational Therapy, 36*, 20–28.

Yerxa, E. J., Clark, F., Frank, G., Jackson, J., Parham, D., Pierce, D., Stein, C., & Zemke, R. (1989). An introduction to occupation science: A foundation for occupational therapy in the 21st century. *Occupational Therapy in Health Care, 6*(4), 1–17.

2/ Human System

Gary Kielhofner

INTRODUCTION TO SYSTEMS CONCEPTS

When persons work, play, and complete the tasks of daily life, a myriad of motivational, cognitive, developmental, motoric, environmental, and other factors come into play. Any coherent explanation of occupational behavior must provide some way of relating these diverse elements to each other. It must answer the question: How are persons and their occupations organized? Systems theory allows us to grapple with the problem of this organized complexity. Systems theory is represented in a wide range of literature, spanning four decades. Within systems theory, one can identify distinct areas or subfields. In this book I will draw primarily upon three areas: General Systems Theory, Open Systems Theory, and Dynamical Systems Theory. Each are briefly described in this section.

General Systems Theory (GST) proposes that we should recognize the universe as a vast, interconnected, and interdependent whole. All phenomena in the universe, therefore, belong to this larger whole and share important features. Consequently, GST aims to identify and explain properties that are found across a range of phenomena, independent of the type of system studied (von Bertalanffy, 1968a, 1968b). A *system* refers to any complex of elements which interact and together constitute a logical whole with a purpose or function. For instance, the musculoskeletal system refers to the organized complex of bones, connective tissue, and muscles which, together,

allow functional motion. Systems concepts are applied to such disparate phenomena as a solar system, a social system, a personality system, a family system, and a cardiorespiratory system. The importance of discovering universal properties across such different systems is that insights gained by examining one type of system can be useful for understanding another. What we learn about organization of the cell may serve as an analogy for understanding personality. For example, cells need to import nutrients to sustain their organization; humans need experience and information to nourish the beliefs and attitudes that make up their personalities.

Open Systems Theory was developed to explicate characteristics and processes of living phenomena. Many of its original insights came from the field of biology. Open systems theory refers to all life forms, whether they be simple cells, plants or human beings. Open systems are defined as dynamic, self-organizing entities, exhibiting ongoing interaction with their environments (Allport, 1968; von Bertalanffy, 1968a, 1968b; Brody, 1973; Koestler, 1969).

Scientists observing a wide range of physical systems have noted that when sufficient energy flows through these systems whole new states of organization emerge spontaneously. Such observations led to the conclusion that "ordered structures can arise out of formerly chaotic states" and that these emergent orders were "maintained by fluxes of energy and matter passing through the systems" (Haken, 1987, p. 419). These phenomena are called dynamical systems and the concepts used to explain them are referred to as Dynamical Systems Theory.[a]

What has fascinated scientists is that the behavior of these dynamical systems seems to arise spontaneously when sufficient energy was present. The components of a dynamical system behave in ways that cannot be predicted by their individual properties. Instead, they "cooperate together" toward achieving some higher order (Haken, 1987).

While Dynamical Systems Theory arose from observations in the physical sciences, a number of theorists and researchers have applied it to human phenomena, including motor behavior, communication, motivation, and emotional expression (Brent, 1978; Fogel & Thelen, 1987; Kamm, Thelen, & Jensen, 1990; Wolf, 1987). They have used ideas derived from dynamical systems theory to emphasize the dynamically emergent character of both behavior and change in humans.

General, Dynamical, and Open Systems theories present many similar and intersecting ideas. Throughout the rest of this book, I will not differentiate between these theories. Instead, I will interweave them to build a systems view of human occupation.[b] Consistent with the vision of GST, I will be employing concepts used to explain other phenomena as analogies for comprehending occupational behavior. As with all theory, this use of systems concepts to explain human occupation is necessarily speculative. Further scrutinization will determine how well it explains occupational function and dysfunction.

FROM A MECHANISTIC TO A SYSTEMIC WORLD VIEW

Since systems concepts are complex and challenging it is worth considering what they add to our understanding of human behavior.

To do so requires one to appreciate how systems concepts differ from the ideas and concepts which have guided much theorizing about human behavior in the 20th century.

The goal of theories is to create insights into nature. These insights are made possible because theories provide us with a metaphorical way of thinking. Theory asks, in effect, that we think of phenomena "as if" they were something already familiar or understood. Whether or not theories are explicit about their metaphors, they nonetheless evoke analogies that bring what is unknown closer to what we do know. For example, Freud's view of unconscious drives evokes the analogy of bottled-up forces pushing for expression. Emotions "boil over" or "explode" or create "pressure" that drives us to behave. Such imagery borrows its analogies from everyday physical events.

Pepper (1942) used the concept of a "root metaphor" to refer to the deepest analogies found in theories characteristic of an age. The root metaphor which has dominated science in the past two centuries has been the analogy to the machine. Prigogine and Stengers (1984) argue that western civilization was so enamored with its creation of machines that early scientists employed the machine as metaphor for understanding the physical world. Later the machine metaphor was applied to the biological and behavioral sciences as well (Koestler, 1969; von Bertalanffy, 1968a, 1968b). This perspective, called mechanistic thought, sees phenomena as exhibiting lawful properties characteristic of machines. To un-

---

[a]The term *chaos theory* is often used to refer to this same literature. As the title of Prigogine and Stenger's 1984 book, *Order out of Chaos,* indicates, the thesis of this literature is that chaos is not an aberration from the fundamental order of the universe. Rather, what appears chaotic can represent a new energy state out of which new order will emanate. Morever, what appears chaotic may reveal a deeper, underlying pattern.

[b]While not all the concepts from General Systems Theory, Open Systems Theory, and Dynamical Systems Theory are in agreement, I have sought to use the most recent and widely accepted ideas. I also have selected those concepts which best enable me to present a coherent conceptualization of the system of human occupation. In doing so, I have neglected some concepts and terminology. Moreover, since the problem to which I am addressing systems theories is unique, I have speculated in my application of these concepts to new phenomena. In this process, I have sought to be true to the best existing literature and logical in my extensions and applications of the ideas. Beyond these efforts, the test of this theorizing will be in practical utility and empirical scrutiny.

derstand how the mechanistic metaphor has led scientists to view naturally occurring phenomena, consider a simple machine, the clock. Mechanical clockworks consist of various cogs and springs (structures) which interact, impinging on each other, transferring movement along a continuum from spring to hand (function). As illustrated in Figure 2.1, a simple cause-and-effect chain of events transfers movement from one part to another. The structure of the clock (its mechanism) determines how it functions. The mechanistic model assumes that the world works according to similar principles. It begins with the observation that any phenomenon (e.g., an atom, a cell, a brain) is made up of parts. These parts are in lawful interaction with each other according to how the structure is built. To explain any phenomenon one must discover its parts, how they are put together, and how they interact.

Reductionistic Science

The mechanistic analogy generated a scientific method called reductionism. Underlying reductionism is the assumption that all phenomena, like machines, can be investigated and explained by taking them apart to discover how they are built. It is also assumed that once one knows how a system is constructed, one can predict how it will behave in the future. In fact, the test of whether one's explanation is correct is successful prediction. In reductionist research, one makes predictions of behavior or function from the theory that seeks to explain the structure or organization of the phenomenon. If the prediction is accurate, it is considered as evidence that the explanation is

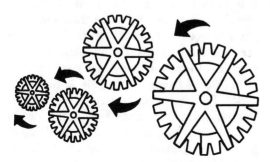

Figure 2.1. Clockworks: A simple cause-and-effect chain of events.

true. Importantly, explanation is focused on understanding how the system is put together, and its function is mainly viewed as evidence that the explanation of structure is correct.

The emphasis on prediction from structure further assumes that the laws governing the structure or organization of systems will stay the same over time (Prigogine & Stengers, 1984). It was expected that, by knowing how a system is put together, a scientist could predict how it will function in the future. This prediction is possible because the mechanism remains the same over time. It means, for example, that if the structure of oxygen, hydrogen, and carbon are known, then it is possible to predict how these elements will behave in any future circumstances. Many psychological theories have argued that if we know how a person's psyche is put together, we can predict how he or she will behave in the future. Concepts which are used to describe and explain these elements of personality structure have variously been called traits, personalities, defense mechanisms, and the like. Behind these explanations of behavior is the implicit or explicit assumption that what is being explained is an underlying structure or organization of the person's psyche which, in turn, determines how he or she will behave. Thus, a person whose personality is obsessive will behave in obsessive ways; a person who has the trait of being internally controlled accepts responsibility for and directs the course of his or her own life; and a person who is externally controlled can be expected to acquiesce and blame others for what happens in his or her life.

This way of thinking is also applied to understanding how the "building blocks" of nature contain the possibilities from which new systems can be built. For example, living cells are made of such elements as hydrogen, oxygen, and carbon. The explanation of how living cells function is to be found in the properties of these and the other elements that make up cells. Following this line of reasoning, strict reductionism claims that biological phenomena can ultimately be explained by the properties of the chemicals that make up living things. This is anticipated since chemicals are the building blocks of organic matter and therefore contain the instructions for how they can be combined in living systems. In similar fashion, reductionist thought anticipates that movement and mental processes can be explained by finding out how the nervous system is constructed. After all, if these phenomena are like machines, then we should be able to explain their behavior by knowing how their parts are put together (i.e., the underlying mechanism). As illustrated in Figure 2.2, the structure of the human system was thought to be the cause of its behavior.

Viewing the body or the mind as a machine-like system (i.e., as a miniature or giant clockwork) has been a particularly fruitful enterprise. Reductionist analysis has allowed scholars to decompose many phenomena into their constituent parts, thereby providing important insights into how they function. For example, the mechanistic approach in anatomy revealed the various organs and tissues which compose the body. Clever and influential ways of describing human behavior were also devised from this reductionist approach. For example, Freud divided the psyche by reductionistic analysis into ego, id, and superego and from this specification of the mechanism involved sought to explain much of human motivation.

However, theories that employ the mechanistic metaphor have simply come up short in helping us explain vital aspects of human behavior. One example of this process is the use of cybernetic machines as an analogy for physiological processes. Cybernetics refers to machines or processes that use feedback to modify behavior; the thermostat is an everyday example. When feedback tells the thermostat it is too cold, it starts up the furnace. When feedback says it is warm enough, the thermostat stops the furnace. By using feedback, cybernetic systems maintain conditions close to some preset value. The thermostat has been used as an analogy for understanding some aspects of human behavior. For example, behavior modification theory, which stresses the role of feedback (i.e., consequences) in modifying behavior, uses cybernetics as an analog to complex animal and human behavior. To a certain extent, animals and people do behave in ways analogous to the household thermostat, increasing or decreasing behavior according to the kind of feedback they receive. However, this theoretical analogy vastly oversimplifies all these phenomena and fails to recognize many features of animal and human behavior, such as spontaneous playfulness and persistence in the face of adversity. Cybernetic models of human behavior are, at best, only partial explanations.

Knowledge gained from reductionist analysis has also been used to guide efforts to repair malfunctioning systems, just as broken or maladjusted machines can be fixed. For example, understanding the structure and functions of the human body is basic to the practice of modern medicine, which involves adjusting, repairing, and replacing dysfunctional body parts. Thus, the mechanistic metaphor and its reductionistic scientific method have been powerful tools for science and successful frameworks for medical practice. We shall return to this topic in Chapter 12 when we explore principles of intervention which emanate from a systems view of humans.

Limits of Reductionism

While mechanistic thinking has proved to be a successful scientific root metaphor, it has also showed important limitations. For example, physicists now recognize that, while the physical world behaves like a machine under certain circumstances, the mechanistic metaphor fails to explain many important features of physical systems (Prigogine & Stengers, 1984). For example, Sameroff (1983) notes that physicists have gone beyond the idea of the atom as a miniature machine made up of parts (e.g., electrons spinning around a nucleus) for a new vision:

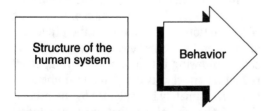

Figure 2.2.   Structure as the cause of behavior in mechanistic thought.

Instead there is the conception of a series of fields within which are embedded particle-like concentrations of energy and spin. The atom is currently conceived of as functionally interacting nuclear and electronic fields rather than the older notion of mechanically interacting parts. (p. 265)

Instead of structures, scientists discovered forces and processes at the foundation of the physical world. The very parts or building blocks out of which the physical world is built (i.e., atoms) are themselves sustained by underlying dynamic forces.

The limits of the mechanistic analogy are even more apparent in the material world of living systems. Even the most sophisticated machine cannot reproduce itself, while the simplest of living organisms does. Changes in the structure of organisms through growth and development defy mechanical analogy. The psychosocial experiences of self-awareness, emotions, and cognition defy description as being produced by underlying physiological mechanisms. Indeed what comes to fill the minds and hearts of humans is influenced not so much by the underlying human brain as the surrounding milieu (Bruner, 1990). Humans are most certainly biological systems constrained by their genetic inheritance, but what different people come to know, feel, and do as individual human beings may be radically different. The experience and behavior of a native in the South American rain forest is deeply different from that of a city-dwelling corporate attorney. The lives we lead are certainly made possible by, and sometimes constrained by, the capabilities of our bodies, but they are just as surely owed to all we have experienced in our social surroundings.

The most important human functions are too complex to be explained by the mechanistic view of behavior (Allport, 1968; von Bertalanffy, 1968a, 1968b). Human creativity, free will, innovation, and the flexibility to perform under vastly different circumstances are beyond the reach of mechanistic thought. These phenomena were conveniently ignored in reductionistic analysis (Allport, 1968; von Bertalanffy, 1968a, 1968b, 1969).

Finally, the most important challenge to mechanistic thought is the assertion that, contrary to its assumption, the laws governing systems *do change* over time. Prigogine and Stengers (1984) note that physical nature provides us with multiple examples of new behavior spontaneously emerging. Two everyday examples are a pot of boiling water and the whirlpool that occurs when we empty a bathtub. Water molecules themselves have no characteristics that determine ahead of time that they will boil or form a whirlpool. Nothing to be found in the chemical makeup of water is sufficient to predict either boiling or whirlpooling. Rather, the overall dynamics brought on by the activity of energy flowing through the water (i.e., heat and gravitational pull) recruit the water molecules to cooperate together to create a simple system. These two examples illustrate that new states of dynamic organization simply emerge when sufficient energy is present.

When an otherwise nonathletic girl becomes suddenly obsessed with the desire to take up horseback riding, when children become capable of formal operational thought, when two people fall in love and decide to share their lives together, when a former white collar criminal undergoes religious conversion, new conditions emerge that become powerful forces in their lives.

Each of us can quickly recall such emergent processes that changed the courses of our lives. Such processes are not predictable and therefore have been left out of most explanations of human behavior; however, they do have influences equally potent to the more orderly traits and personality characteristics that provide insights into our tendencies to behave in certain ways. Moreover, as therapists, we frequently encounter persons who need, or who are in the midst of, such transformations.

The course of development is also characterized by the ability of the human system to transform and create new lawfulness within its own order. As we develop, we accumulate information and experiences that reorganize our motives and behavior. The laws that govern how we are motivated at the ages of 3 and 30 are not identical. Development is an ongoing process of metamorphosis.

Thus, the history of a system—both its evolutionary history (inherited through genetics and socialization) and its personal history—represents the accumulation of new laws governing behavior. There is much we cannot predict about what the state of a child will be when he or she is an adult. Too many new laws are accumulated along the way. As Allport (1968) notes, it is the nature of the human personality to "achieve progressive levels of order through change in cognitive and motivation structure" (p. 349).

It has become apparent that those aspects of the world which behave in ways explained by mechanistic thought are best understood as special instances in a more complex world. Human behavior is, at best, partly understood by reductionism. Moreover, to use only the insights offered in the mechanistic world view leads to misunderstanding human behavior. Recognizing the limits of mechanistic thinking and reductionistic analysis has led to the search for additional conceptual tools, and consequently, to systems concepts.

Returning to the question of why we are adopting systems thinking, the answer is that it offers a more complete and integrated view of human behavior when compared with mechanistic thinking. Thus, my goal in using systems concepts as the foundation of this model is to provide a theoretical explanation for human occupation that begins to recognize and grapple with its complexity. If we can understand the systems nature of human beings, we will have gone some distance in deciphering how humans and their occupational behavior are organized.

SYSTEMS PROPERTIES OF HUMANS

I focus now on the role and nature of occupational behavior. In the following discussions, I will draw upon systems concepts to consider how humans generate occupational behavior and how that behavior, in turn, influences the human system. My purpose here is to present a series of explanations. Later, in Chapter 14, I will translate these explanations into a series of principles for change in the context of therapy.

Dynamical Assembly of Behavior

Mechanistic thought proposes that behavior is caused by an underlying structure. The function of a system is explained as the "consequence" of how it is put together. For example, the mechanistic approach sees human movement as a function of musculoskeletal structure and the hard-wiring of the nervous system (Fogel & Thelen, 1987; Kamm, Thelen, & Jensen, 1990). The mechanical metaphor also finds its expression in the computer model of the mind, which presumes cognition to be the function of appropriate hardware and software (Bruner, 1990).

One important reason that the mechanistic idea of structure causing function fails to explain human systems is that potentials for behavior exceed the actual behavior of the system. One can predict the behavior of machines because there are quite specific constraints on behavior. In a clock, each cog is connected to something else so that a specific causal chain connects all the parts and the resulting behavior of the system represents all that the system can do. Complex living systems have much more behavioral flexibility, which is referred to as degrees of freedom.[c] In human systems these degrees of freedom abound. They include, for example, the scores of movement combinations of which the body is capable and the myriad of choices the conscious organism has for behavior.

The problem of how the system selects action from so many possibilities can be exemplified by considering movement in the upper extremity. Each of the digits of the hand involve three joints which may or may not be flexed (leaving aside for the moment that they may be flexed to lesser or greater degrees and at different velocities). Between the hand and trunk three other joints provide flexion and rotation possibilities. However, in functional behavior a specific subset of these possible motions are elected. When one reaches out to grasp an ob-

---

[c]Degrees of freedom as used here should not be confused with the degrees of freedom of movement about the axis of a joint. Here, degrees of freedom refer to the unrealized potential at any point in time for a myriad of feelings, thoughts or behaviors to occur.

ject, all possible motions are suppressed into a more disciplined form. A subset of potential motions must be systematically harnessed for such functional movements as reaching, waving, pushing, pointing, grabbing, and holding. A vast amount of information is required during each movement to permit selection from among so many alternatives.

The degrees of freedom problem is further complicated by the fact that humans perform in an almost infinite variety of emotional, cognitive, and physical circumstances. This contextual variability gives a character of uniqueness to each and every performance. No two instances of performing the same action (e.g., signing one's name, hammering a nail, reaching for a cup, putting on one's clothes, typing out a word) are exactly the same (Turvey, 1990). This is true at the level of motor requirements for task performance, where "control problems become monumental in the face of the nearly infinite variability demanded by everyday tasks" (Fogel & Thelen, 1987, p. 748). It becomes even more complicated when we try to factor in other elements such as cognitive and motivational factors. The human system cannot possibly have internally coded/instructed plans for behavior sufficiently comprehensive to expect and adjust for all possible contextual conditions and variations (Turvey, 1990). When a student raises her hand in response to a question, when a gardener spies a weed and hoes it, and when a writer types out his thoughts, an incredible number of cognitive and motor behavioral potentials have been organized into a refined and purposive act.

If the human system does not possess all the instructions for how to perform beforehand, how can humans know what to do? As we will see, our earlier discussion of new laws emerging over time becomes very helpful for answering this question. Systems theorists use the concept of *soft assembly* to account for how the behavior adjusts to the changing demands of tasks as they unfold (Turvey, 1990). *In the process of soft assembly, the human system, the task, and the environment together contribute to how behavior is assembled* (see Figure 2.3). This means that movement is not merely the execution of some

motor program, nor is behavior simply caused by an underlying trait. Rather, all the components of the human system, the task, and the environment together create a network of conditions in which the performance is suspended.

Behavior has a fluid and improvisational character; it is spontaneously organized in real time and in the context of action (Fogel & Thelen, 1987). By factoring in the task and environmental conditions as contributors to how behavior is assembled, system theorists offer a viable explanation of how the human system deals with the infinite variety of conditions in which they perform. The system need not have all the instructions for performance stored within it, since much of that information is contributed by the task and environment. Fogel and Thelen (1987) explain that:

> The constraints of the task produce a dynamic cooperativity of the components . . . The nature of the cooperativity is not rigidly fixed beforehand, but is strictly a function of the status of the organism in a particular task context. (p. 749)

For example, the nervous system does not have to give centrally directed individual commands to each muscle and joint involved in every act of reaching. Rather, the individual muscles and joints become functionally linked together into the gestalt act of a particular reach. The action of reaching exerts its organizational demands on the cooperating constituents. The instructions that govern an act of reaching are not all stored ahead of time in

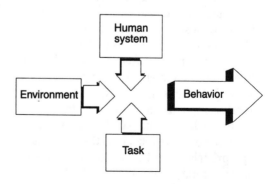

Figure 2.3. Soft assembly of behavior from conditions to which the human system, the task, and the environment contribute.

the nervous system. Rather, those instructions emerge in the context of the action itself. This is not to say that there is not some lawfulness attributable to how the nervous system is organized. It is just that this organization is not enough to account for functional movement.

In the same way, we do not need to have in advance all the instructions for how to behave socially. Rather, the social situations we encounter create much of the necessary information. We possess at best an overall map of the social terrain built up from experience. However, no amount of learning can pre-inform us about how to behave in social circumstances any more than a road map can specify all of what is necessary to drive to a given destination (e.g., when to speed up or slow down, how to steer on the road, how to recognize an intersection as the one represented on the map). Rather, the abstract map must interact with the performance situation and in the course of this interaction the "instructions" for what to do are created. This is not to imply that instructions are somehow generated and then followed in behavior. Rather, the behavior itself is evoked in the task situation; the instructions are *implicit* in the behavior. Let us consider this idea further through an example. When my children stay overnight with a friend, my wife and I invariably remind them to be thoughtful, courteous, and appreciative. We know these are not literal instructions. Rather we expect that events will take place in which it will become evident to our children how to follow these directions. Neither they nor we can know exactly what will occur and exactly how they should behave. But the circumstances themselves will provide the additional information needed and, in that regard, interact with the manners we hope we have instilled in our children. When my daughter reports that she helped clear the dishes at dinner, complimented her friend's mother on a new hairstyle, and thanked her friend's father for a ride home, we recognize that she behaved appropriately when the occasions offered her the opportunity to do so. Importantly, the occasions themselves contributed vital instructions for how to be thoughtful, courteous, and appreciative.

Self-Organization through Behavior

In machines, structure is everything. But humans are not machines. The physical and mental structures of human systems are temporary manifestations of a deeper, underlying dynamic process (Sameroff, 1983). In fact, Brent (1978) argues that the distinction between structure and process is arbitrary and depends on the time frame we use to view them. What in a shorter time frame appears to be structure in a larger time frame appears to be process. This point is made comprehensible if we consider the human being in ontogenetic and historical time frames. In the course of human development, the structure of the body takes on very different forms: fertilized ovum, fetus, infant, adolescent, and adult. Across this developmental time, psychological structures also change dramatically. Both the mental and physical structures are made possible by more basic enduring processes which belong to the species and are passed on to each individual from generation to generation. What is more definite about the human system than physique or personality is the underlying process of their development in individuals and the production of successive generations of human beings. This underlying dynamic process flows through and supports the creation of the structures we know as human bodies and psyches. Moreover, in this larger time perspective, bodies and psyches are recognizable for what they really are: dynamically changing organizations of matter and mind.

Consequently, when referring to human biological structures (such as the brain) or mental structures (such as personality), systems theory recognizes that these are highly organized states of matter and mind "maintained dynamically through interchanges with the environment" (Sameroff, 1983, p. 266). Thus the emergence, continued existence, and transformation of the human system depends on the underlying actions of the system. As Weiss (1967) notes, understanding how living systems organize themselves requires us to "reorient thinking from static *form* to formative *behavior*" (p. 808).

Many structures of human systems are built up, maintained, and changed through the very processes by which they are put to use. For example, Sameroff (1983) notes that cognitive development,

> ... is not a direct consequence of having the biological equipment for thought but rather the result of the operation of this equipment in interpreting input, in organizing that input into meaningful units based on further activity, and eventually in patterning those meaningful units into whole systems based on intellectual experience. (p. 266)

Without action, the organization and reorganization of intellectual structures cannot occur.

In effect, the human system is carried along and shaped by the nature of its behavior. To behave is to organize the various components of the system (e.g., cognitions and movements) into a particular dynamic order required by the task undertaken and afforded by the environmental conditions. By virtue of dynamically assembling behavior, the system configures or organizes itself around the task being done. Notably, this configuration is not a static "pose" but a dynamic sequence of ordered action. For example, when learning a new skill, such as riding a bicycle, one must bring into alignment a whole range of factors including the desire to achieve the feat, coordination of motor actions in order to balance self and steer the vehicle, and so on. The act of achieving this organized state in real time has the effect of predisposing the human system to achieve the same configuration again. That is, engaging in action increases the probability of the system reconfiguring itself in such a way in

the future to accomplish the same action. Once the system configures itself for a dynamic performance, it facilitates the possibility of returning to such a dynamic configuration later. Consequently, by repeatedly behaving in a particular way the system is both temporarily self-organizing and increasing its capacity to achieve such an organized state again.

Consequently, with repeated assembly, behavior begins to imprint itself on the organization of the structure (Figure 2.4). For example, repeated jogging reshapes existing physical, psychological, and social structures involved in the behavior. The aerobic capacity of the body is increased, muscles used to run are strengthened, the image of oneself as capable of jogging is reinforced, and one's public identity as a jogger may be affirmed as neighbors take note of one's repeated behavior. In all these ways, the act of jogging transforms one (physically, psychologically, and socially) into a jogger. As long as the behavior is sustained, the corresponding organization of the human system is maintained. However, if the jogger abandons the behavior for long enough, aerobic capacity diminishes, muscles weaken, and confidence and identity wane. Human systems can also un-become what they cease to do.

The process of maintaining a structure has a tendency to be self-perpetuating since each successive behavior sustains the probability of the behavior occurring again. Albeit a crude analogy, walking over the same pathway repeatedly exemplifies this process. Each traverse more clearly outlines the path in the grass. As the path is laid down, it increases the

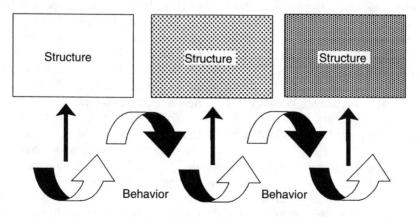

Figure 2.4.   Repeated assembly of behavior creates structure.

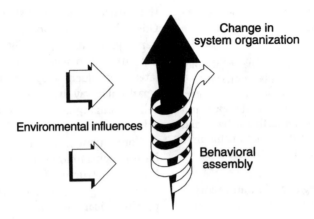

Figure 2.5.   Dynamic assembly of behavior.

probability of a similar route in the future. The process becomes self-perpetuating.

The implication of these arguments is that action imprints itself on the human system. Figure 2.5 illustrates this process. With each successive dynamic assembly of behavior, the system is pulled toward an organization which increases the system's capacity and propensity for the behavior. When human systems behave, they become, in some real measure, what they do. Persons who run become so organized as runners, persons who read become literate, persons who build houses fashion themselves into carpenters. Occupational behavior is a process of self-organizing—maintaining and becoming through doing.

Behavior as the Author of Change in the Human System

The previous discussion implies that novel assemblies of behavior emerge and, when repeated, serve to stabilize new patterns of organization in the system. Now, we need to ask: Where do new behaviors come from? The answer to this question is basic to understanding how human systems change. Without the emergence of new behaviors, the system will just go on behaving so as to maintain its current organization.

Mechanistic thought assigns change to preprogrammed alterations in the structure, such as maturation of the nervous system. Change, like behavior, is caused by the organization of the structure. Therefore, as the underlying

structure naturally matures, new behaviors become possible. The limitations of this explanation are readily apparent. We have already asserted that the building up and alteration of structures is dependent on underlying processes. If process builds structures, then process is likely responsible for changing them. Consequently, we must look to the behavior of the human system for the clues about how changes take place.

We have already noted that several factors combine to influence the assembly of any behavior. A change in one of the contributing variables can shift the system into a new assembly of behavior (Thelen & Ulrich, 1991). For example, if someone nearby tosses a ball to us, we will ordinarily respond by attempting to catch it. If the person throws it faster and faster each time, there will probably be a point at which we duck or flinch instead of trying to catch it. In this case, the speed of the oncoming ball (once it exceeds a critical threshold) shifts the system to a new assembly of behavior (i.e., from catching to ducking). As Figure 2.6 illustrates, different control parameters can shift the network of conditions, leading to a new assembly of behavior.

When a variable that contributes to the assembly of behavior changes enough to lead to the assembly of some new behavior, the variable is called a *control parameter*. This does not imply that it causes the behavior. Rather, the control parameter serves a catalytic role, creating a new set of conditions with instructions for the emergence of the new assembly of behavior. Importantly, the control parameter does not itself provide instructions for the change in behavior. It instead contributes something new to the total configuration of elements, causing them to relate to each other in a new way. Change another factor (e.g., increase distance from the person tossing the ball) and new dynamical relations emerge with consequent alteration in behavior.

Both the internal organization of the human system and external environmental factors contribute to the assembly of behavior. Consequently, changes within or outside the human system are equally capable of changing the dynamic assembly of behavior. As Thelen (1989) notes, "There is no dichotomy between organism and environment. Neither has privileged status in effecting change" (p. 85).

Thus, behavior may change as a function of changes in the internal organization of the system, such as growth, increased strength, or acquisition of a new mental or motor skill. Behavior may also change as a result of conditions in the environment. Across time, different parts of the system or environment may take their turns as control parameters creating the new conditions to initiate change in behavior. For example, the encouragement of a friend may serve as a control parameter leading one to try a new hobby. Interest, confidence, and skill change with practice. As these factors change, any one of them may take over and lead one to become much more seriously involved than the friend ever envisioned. In such a case, the motivating control parameter shifted from the external to internal. It is possible that the same behavior may be assembled as a result of different control parameters. For example, a person may choose not to do an ac-

tivity at one point because of a lack of motivation, at another point because of fatigue, and at another point because of weather. Any of us who have sustained an activity over time (such as running or walking outside) know that this can be the case.

Changes in behavior can be nonlinear even though the change in the control parameter continues to be linear (Thelen & Ulrich, 1991). Consequently, a small change in a control parameter may lead to large changes in the dynamic assembly of behavior (Haken, 1987). This is because the overall dynamic state created by all contributing factors is shifted by change beyond some critical value in the control parameter (Kelso & Tuller, 1984). The control variable serves as the proverbial straw that breaks the camel's back. As an example, I recall teaching my children to ride bicycles. Up to a certain speed, I could walk alongside, increasing my pace as my child pedaled faster, but with just a bit more speed, I had to shift into running to keep up. A small change in speed completely reorganized my locomotion. Notably, my locomotion shifted from walking to running without any conscious decision; it was demanded by the task of keeping pace with my child on the bike. The same circumstance provides an example from the domain of motivation. As both children practiced, their confidence grew, but up to a certain point they needed me along side to feel safe. However, each child reached a critical point marked by the request to change the performance: "I want to try it *by myself* now."

Within a single domain of behavior, a variety of different factors may serve as control parameters initiating change in the human system. For example, in the course of a child's

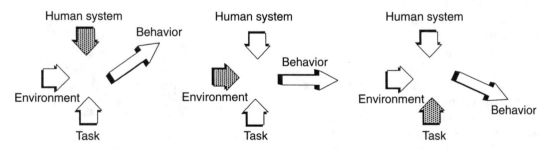

Figure 2.6. Different control parameters shift the network of conditions leading to new assembly of behavior.

school career, motivation for a topic, peer attitudes, parental approval or disapproval, relationship with a teacher, intellectual maturation, and learning may all contribute in different ways to changes in the child's study habits and rate of learning.

The potential for many factors to serve as control parameters and to create new dynamics that shift behavior may account for some important features of change. We are aware that not all change in human behavior is incremental and linear. Rather, it is sometimes dramatic and represents a transformation. Some examples include becoming a parent, changing careers, going back to school, and retiring.

In the case of dramatic change, a whole new organization of behavior cascades forward with the process of change, creating its own momentum. Imagine for a moment what happens to the world of a child when lower extremity strength increases to a critical value, permitting the child to bear the weight of her body on one leg: this change in a control variable means that she now can begin to walk. More importantly, however, a whole new world opens up. The child's visual experience changes during locomotion, new things may be reached, there is a newfound sense of personal freedom, and parents become excited over the new developmental milestone. Throughout life, change often involves analogous quantum leaps and reorganizations set off by relatively straightforward changes in one area.

If the control parameter is a temporary condition (e.g., fatigue, a time-limited change in environment), the behavioral assembly may not be repeated and therefore it will have little or no effect on the enduring organization of the system. However, if the change in a control parameter is more persistent and the new assembly of behavior is repeated, the system's organization will eventually coalesce toward a new state.

As the human system moving forward in time acquires a new lawfulness, current laws which governed its organization earlier are not necessarily binding. What the human system is at any point in time cannot determine all of what can happen in the future (von Bertalanffy, 1968a, 1968b, 1969; Prigogine &

Stengers, 1984). The organization of the human system at any point in time is a reflection of the dynamic process of life. Ongoing behavior, and its degree of stability or change, can either maintain or reorganize the system. Most often, new order emerges over time, changing the rules of how the system functions (Figure 2.7). This kind of metamorphosis, in which the system literally becomes something different than it was before, is manifested in a number of well-known developmental changes. The attainment of formal operations in cognitive thought is one. Entering marriage is another. Less dramatic transformations occur throughout life as the human system is reorganized continually. In all cases, the emergence of new order in the system is the key to change.

SYSTEMS NATURE OF HUMANS AND THEIR OCCUPATIONAL BEHAVIOR

This chapter began the process of thinking about humans as systems and about their occupational behavior as a systems process. In the previous discussions three important assertions were made:

1. Human systems are dynamic organizations of mind and matter.
2. Occupational behavior is dynamically assembled.
3. Human systems self-organize through their occupational behavior.

I will briefly revisit them now to consider more fully the view of human occupation that I have been proposing.

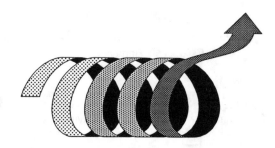

Figure 2.7. As a system moves forward in time it acquires new laws, becoming more complex.

Humans as Dynamic Organizations

When we encounter another human being, we have before us a living, breathing, thinking organism. This human organism has form or structure, most obvious as a body, but also evident as mind or personality. We cannot help but be aware of these structures. Moreover, our scientific and popular thought emphasizes all the ways in which they behave as structures. We are challenged now by emerging scientific thought to see them also as organized processes.

With reference to self-concept, Gergen and Gergen (1983) point out that mechanistic thought assumes "an internal structure governed in a mechanical fashion by external inputs . . . Thus the individual is generally imbued with a structure of self-descriptions (conceptus, schemata, prototypes) that remain stabilized . . ." (p. 255). They go on to point out that we also need to appreciate how the individual "actively constructs his or her view of self" (p. 255). In other words, we require an understanding of the relationship of structure and function in the human system which recognizes the former not as static, but as dynamically organized.

The structure of a human system is always being remade. A degree of stability in this organized structure is "essential to the continued identity of a system" (Sameroff, 1983, p. 267). But the ability to adapt to permanent environmental or systemic changes through self-reorganization is equally important. Therefore, the fact that the human system is a flexible organization rather than a rigid machine has an adaptive advantage.

We must also recognize that what it means to be human does not reside entirely "within the skin"; that is, within a bounded set of physiological and intrapsychic operations. It also includes the exchange between the human system, physical environment, and sociocultural environment. Without this constant exchange there is little we can call truly human. Moreover, since past behavior generates present structure, the individual at any point in time is the deliverance of a personal history of such exchanges.

Dynamic Assembly of Occupational Behavior

Occupational behavior emanates not from some mechanical workings, but from a dynamic process in which internal biological and psychological factors interact with the physical and sociocultural world to assemble behavior. When the human system is behaving, it creates a dynamic process: the organization of the process grows out of relations among elements. Said another way, the constituents need only be capable of participating in the new order. The instructions for how to participate are generated by the dynamic state that emerges. What comes about is *new* and could not by predicted from initial conditions; it is not completely caused by pre-existing characteristics or instructions in the human system (Thelen, 1989).

Consequently, all behavior is a form of improvisation in emergent circumstances. Moreover, the behaving individual is no more important in shaping behavior than the task being performed or the environment in which it is performed. All three elements must contribute. Stated more simply, who, what, and where are inseparable factors in behavior.

The dynamic assembly of behavior pervades every aspect of how persons pursue their everyday occupations. Factors as diverse as the cultural meaning of a task, the required skills, the tools and materials used, the motives and abilities of the person, and how the task itself proceeds, all coalesce in the "ballet" of ordinary occupational behavior. These diverse factors come together as a dynamic system in the midst of which behavior is assembled. When we behave, we participate in an unfolding process. Like all the participating elements, we are only part of what goes on. Dancers move with the rhythm of music. The child bobs up and down in the game of peek-a-boo with her father. The mechanic handles a tool according to its purposes and corresponding engine parts. The child interacts with others within the rules and actions of the game. The ways in which persons assemble their behavior to fit the contours of space, task, tool, rhythm, game, and job illustrate the eloquent orchestration of self with the environment and the occupation to achieve behavior.

Self-Organization through Occupational Behavior

Occupational behavior is a dynamic process through which we maintain the organization of our bodies and minds. When we work, play, and perform the tasks of daily life, we are not merely engaging in occupational behavior. We are organizing ourselves. We use our bodies and minds in the contexts of occupations, organizing them accordingly. We create our motor abilities, our self-concepts, our social identities in our occupations. Occupational behavior is self-making.

By playing a guitar, typing on a computer keyboard, or driving a car, persons internalize the forms of behavior maintaining themselves as guitarists, typists, and drivers. Occupational behavior expresses the human system into the potentials and constraints of the occupation performed and the environment in which it is performed. When we shift our modes of behavior, we reshape ourselves opening up new possibilities for becoming. Our behavior molds us after our new occupations. We are not born carpenters, teachers, therapists, guitarists, fishers, writers, dancers, gardeners, poets, typists, and singers. But we may become them by behaving as such. Our forms follow our functions. By taking up new occupations we reconstitute ourselves.

CONCLUSION

This chapter began articulation of the theoretical assertions of the model of human occupation. I have used systems concepts to provide a foundation for viewing human occupation. In the following chapters, we will further apply systems concepts to explain how and why persons engage in occupation. We will build on this foundation with additional concepts which are pertinent to understanding human occupation. Future discussions will also employ systems concepts to explain disability in the human system. We will examine how disease, trauma, environmental stresses, and lifestyles can produce *dis*organization in the system. Finally, this text will explore in various ways the implications of systems thought for application in the context of data gathering and intervention.

References

Allport, G. W. (1968). The open system in personality theory. In W. Buckley (Ed.), *Modern systems research for the behavioral scientist*. Chicago: Aldine.

Brent, S. B. (1978). Motivation, steady-state, and structural development. *Motivation and Emotion, 2*, 299–332.

Brody, H. (1973). The systems view of man: Implications for medicine, science and ethics. *Perspectives in Biology and Medicine*, Autumn, 71–92.

Bruner, J. (1990). *Acts of Meaning*. Cambridge, MA: Harvard University Press.

Fogel, A., & Thelen, E. (1987). Development of early expressive and communicative action: Reinterpreting the evidence from a dynamic systems perspective. *Developmental Psychology, 23*, 747–761.

Gergen, K. J., & Gergen, M. M. (1983). Narratives of the self. In T. R. Sarbin & K. E. Scheibe (Eds.), *Studies in social identity*. New York: Praeger.

Haken, H. (1987). Synergetics: An approach to self-organization. In F. E. Yates (Ed.), *Self-organizing systems: The emergence of order*. New York: Plenum.

Kamm, K., Thelen, E., & Jensen, J. (1990). A dynamical systems approach to motor development. *Physical Therapy, 70*, 763–772.

Kelso, J. A. S., & Tuller, B. (1984). A dynamical basis for action systems. In M. S. Gazzaniga (Ed.), *Handbook of cognitive neuroscience*. New York: Plenum.

Koestler, A. (1969). Beyond atomism and holism: The concept of the holon. In A. Koestler & J. R. Smithies (Eds.), *Beyond reductionism*. Boston: Beacon Press.

Pepper, S. C. (1942). *World hypotheses*. Berkeley: University of California Press.

Prigogine, I., & Stengers, I. (1984). *Order out of chaos*. New York: Bantam Books.

Sameroff, A. J. (1983). Developmental systems: Contexts and evolution. In P. H. Mussen (Ed.), *Handbook of child psychology*. New York: John Wiley & Sons.

Thelen, E. (1989). Self-organization in developmental processes: Can systems approaches work? In M. Gunnar & E. Thelen (Eds.), *Systems and development: The Minnesota symposia on child psychology* (Vol. 22). Hillsdale, NJ: Erlbaum.

Thelen, E., & Ulrich, B. D. (1991). Hidden skills: A dynamic systems analysis of treadmill stepping during the first year. *Monographs of the Society for Research in Child Development, 56* (1, Serial No. 223).

Turvey, M. T. (1990). Coordination. *American Psychologist, 45*, 938–953.

von Bertalanffy, L. (1968a). General system theory: A critical review. In W. Buckley (Ed.), *Modern systems research for the behavioral scientist*. Chicago: Aldine.

von Bertalanffy, L. (1968b). *General systems theory*. New York: George Braziller.

von Bertalanffy, L. (1969). General system theory and psychiatry. In S. Arieti (Ed.), *American handbook of psychiatry*. New York: Basic Books.

Weiss, P. S. (1967). One plus one does not equal two. In G. Quarton, T. Melnechuk, & F. Schmitt (Eds.), *The neurosciences: A study program*. New York: Rockefeller University Press.

Wolf, P. H. (1987). *The development of behavioral states and expression of emotion in early infancy*. Chicago: University of Chicago Press.

===================================== **KEY CONCEPTS** =====================================

GENERAL SYSTEMS THEORY
- universe is a vast, interconnected, and interdependent whole.
- all phenomena belong to this larger whole and share important features.
- similar properties are found across a range of phenomena.

OPEN SYSTEMS THEORY
- living phenomena are dynamic, self-organizing entities, exhibiting ongoing interaction with their environments.

DYNAMICAL SYSTEMS THEORY
- when sufficient energy flows through systems whole new states of organization emerge spontaneously.
- components of a dynamical system behave in ways that cannot be predicted by their individual properties.

Mechanistic Metaphor
- phenomena exhibit lawful properties characteristic of machines.
  - any phenomenon (e.g., an atom, a cell, a brain) is made up of parts.
  - parts are in lawful interaction with each other according to how the structure is built.
- to explain any phenomenon one must discover its parts, how they are put together, and how they interact.

Reductionistic Science
- assumes that all phenomena, like machines, can be investigated and explained by taking them apart to discover how they are built.
- assumes that, once one knows how a system is constructed, one can predict how it will behave in the future.
- assumes the laws that govern how the structure of systems stay the same over time.

Limits of Mechanistic Thought and Reductionism
- while the physical world behaves like a machine under certain circumstances, the mechanistic metaphor fails to explain many important features of physical systems.
- living systems' growth and development and experiences of self-awareness, emotions, and cognition defy reductionistic explanation.
- laws governing systems do change across time.
- those aspects of the world which behave in ways explained by mechanistic thought are best understood as special instances in a more complex world.

HUMAN SYSTEMS' BEHAVIOR
- human system, task, and environment all contribute to how behavior is assembled (soft assembly).
- behavior has a fluid and improvisational character, spontaneously organized in real time and in the context of action.
- human system need not have all the instructions for behavior stored within it, since information is contributed by the task and environment.

SELF-ORGANIZATION THROUGH BEHAVIOR
- physical and mental structures of human systems are temporary manifestations of a deeper, underlying dynamic process.
- emergence, continued existence, and transformation of the human system depend on the underlying actions of the system.
- human system is carried along and shaped by the nature of its behavior.

Key Concepts, continued

- with repeated assembly, behavior begins to appear less like a process and more like a characteristic or structure.
- process of maintaining a structure has a tendency to be self-perpetuating since each successive behavior sustains the probability of the behavior occurring again.

CONTROL PARAMETER
- variable whose change in value leads to the assembly of some new behavior.
- serves a catalytic role creating a new set of conditions with instructions for the emergence of the new assembly of behavior.
- contributes something new to the total configuration of elements causing them to relate to each other in a new way.

CHANGE IN THE HUMAN SYSTEM
- when novel assemblies of behavior are repeated, they serve to stabilize new patterns of organization in the system.
- behavior change may be a function of:
  — changes in the internal organization of the system
  — new conditions in the environment
- changes in behavior can be non-linear even though the change in the control parameter has been linear all along (i.e., a small change in a factor that serves as the control parameter may lead to large changes in the dynamic assembly of behavior).
- change is sometimes dramatic and represents a transformation resulting in a whole new organization.
- human system moving forward in time acquires a new lawfulness.

3/ Internal Organization of the Human System for Occupation

Gary Kielhofner

INTRODUCTION

Chapter 2 conceptualized humans beings as systems, highlighting occupational behavior as an organized process. That previous discussion emphasized systems properties which human beings share with other organized systems. In this chapter I will build on the systems view of the human to construct a more detailed theory of how humans are organized with regard to their occupational behavior.

PRIMACY OF ACTION

As noted in Chapter 1, occupation connotes action, activity, or doing. But where does this action come from? Why is action so basic to human life? Systems theorists address these questions by first pointing out that spontaneous activity is the most fundamental characteristic of living systems (Boulding, 1968; von Bertalanffy, 1968a, 1968b, 1969). Action, in one form or another, is the prerequisite to life. As we ascend the phylogenetic scale from simpler to more complex life forms, the basic requirement for action is greatly expanded and elaborated. This pervasive need for action is closely linked with the complex nervous system of humans. For example, von Bertalanffy (1969) notes:

Even without external stimuli, the organism is not a passive but an intrinsically active system. Reflex theory has presupposed that the primary element of behavior is response to external stimuli. In contrast, recent research shows with increasing clarity that autonomous activity of the nervous system...is to be considered primary. (p. 709)

Thus, action or activity is programmed into the very nature of living organisms and, accordingly, arises spontaneously from such systems (Weiss, 1967; Boulding, 1968; von Bertalanffy, 1968a, 1968b, 1969).

When we say that activity arises spontaneously out of the human system, we mean that humans are by nature disposed to act. Psychological theories have expressed this disposition as a drive or desire for mental and physical activity (Berlyne, 1960; DeCharms, 1968; Florey, 1969; McClelland, 1961; Reilly, 1962; Shibutani, 1968; Smith, 1969; White, 1959).

A second observation of systems theory, previously discussed in Chapter 2, is that the action or behavior of human systems is necessary to create and sustain their organization. Physical work is necessary to sustain muscle strength and weight-bearing enhances the structural integrity of bone (Trombly, 1989). The nervous system must process sensory information to self-organize (Berlyne, 1960; White, 1959). Cognitive processes are developed and sustained through interactions with the external world (Katz & Ziv, 1992). In sum, the order or organization that we find throughout the human system rests on the underlying action, or, more specifically for our purposes, the occupational behavior of the system.

This observation brings us to the next question: What is the order of the human system that is created through, and in turn contributes to, humans' occupational behavior? Each person's occupational behavior is an expression of the universal human disposition to act. However, each person's behavior is also unique. This uniqueness reflects an internal organization that contributes in three identifiable ways to the assembly of occupational behavior in everyday life. First, occupational behavior emanates from choices arising from different motives for occupations. Second, occupational behavior exhibits regularity and pattern. That is, individuals are remarkably consistent both in what they do and how they go about their occupations. Finally, occupation expresses underlying capacity. We call upon a wide range of mental and physical abilities when we produce occupational behavior.

To explain how occupational behavior is chosen, patterned, and performed, I will conceptualize the human as a system made up of three subsystems: volition, habituation, and performance. *A subsystem is an organized and interrelated collection of patterns (i.e., structures) and processes which have a coherent purpose.*

The purpose of the volition subsystem is to choose occupational behavior. The habituation subsystem serves to organize occupational behavior into patterns or routines. The mind-brain-body performance subsystem makes possible the skilled achievement of occupations. As we will discuss later, these three subsystems represent sets of structures and functions that are part of an integrated whole and which work together in an integrated fashion, along with factors in the environment, to allow human systems to assemble their occupational behavior. By conceptually unpacking the complex organization of human behavior, I am artificially separating what is naturally integrated in the human being. Thus, while I will speak of three separate subsystems, it is important to keep in mind that they are three different aspects of the total organization of the human system. In the remainder of this chapter I will further explore these subsystems and their organization in the larger human system.

CHOICES FOR OCCUPATIONS: A VOLITION SUBSYSTEM

Humans project themselves into the future, making decisions about how tomorrow is to be lived. A myriad of choices concerning what oc-

cupational activities to perform fill our hours, days, and weeks. Within the next hour or so most readers will decide to put this book down (an example, not a suggestion!). Unless that decision is determined by a need to go on to an already scheduled activity, it will be followed by the reader's decision of what to do next and, once engaged, when to terminate that activity and possibly go on to another. Throughout this text we will refer to these kinds of everyday decisions as *activity choices*. These choices are made about single occupational activities in a limited period of future time (ordinarily minutes and hours). Further examples of activity choices include having lunch with a friend, going to a movie or shopping, washing the car, mowing the lawn, going for a walk, baking a cake, playing Monopoly, and reading a newspaper. When such occupational activities flow from a conscious decision about whether and/or when to do them, they are activity choices. These choices may present themselves when we have the necessity or opportunity to make a decision about activity (e.g., when a friend invites us to join in an activity, when we anticipate free time, when we have to choose between completing a task and spending time with our spouse or children). Activity choices may also occur when we find ourselves in an emotional state (e.g., fatigue, restlessness, boredom, anxiety) that disposes us to make a choice about activity. Activity choices ordinarily require only momentary or brief deliberation. These choices are important, however, since they determine a significant amount of what we actually do. Consequently, *activity choices can be defined as short-term, deliberate decisions to enter and exit occupational activities.*

Individuals also make larger choices concerning occupations that will become an extended or permanent part of their lives. For example, most persons reading this book made a commitment at some point to become occupational therapists. This kind of resolution belongs to a class of decisions which have been called *occupational choices* (Heard, 1977; Matsutsuyu, 1971). Such decisions represent commitments to enter into a course of action or to sustain regular performance of an occupational activity over time. We recognize these decisions when someone makes a commitment to enter an occupational role such as becoming a student or a parent, or when taking a job. Moreover, occupational choices may involve making a commitment to establishing and sustaining a new activity as part of our permanent routine—for example, the decision to join a health club and exercise regularly or the decision to take up a new hobby. Finally, occupational choices may take the form of commitment to undertake personal projects[a] that require an extended series of activities to complete. As I compose this chapter, I am engaged in the personal project of writing a book. Further examples of occupational choices to undertake personal projects are the decisions to learn a foreign language, build a new fence for the yard, make a dress, or take a course for continuing education.

Occupational choices are ordinarily the result of a process of deliberation over time. They may involve information-gathering, reflection, imagining possibilities, weighing alternatives, and so on. In this way, commitment is established as a person considers the implications of a course of action over time and weighs its meaning. I refer to occupational choices as involving commitment since they are not realized in a single performance, but require a sustained series of performances. Indeed, we may or may not realize the objectives of our occupational choices depending on such factors as whether we are successful in performing the required behaviors, whether we can sustain effort over time, or whether we can establish new patterns of behavior. *Occupational choices are, thus, defined as deliberate commitments to enter an occupational role, acquire a new habit or undertake a personal project.*

Together, activity choices and occupational choices influence, to a large extent, what kinds of occupational behaviors make up our daily lives. These choices are the function of a volition subsystem.

The term *volition* connotes will or conscious choice. I have selected it to emphasize the deliberate process of willing behavior in

contrast to other concepts of motivation which deemphasize conscious choice. For example, psychoanalytic and behaviorist approaches to motivation view behavior as a function of underlying drives which are not under conscious control (DeCharms, 1968; Florey, 1969; Freud, 1937/1960; White, 1959). These drives arise from tissue states (e.g., hunger and sexual drive) and motivate the organism to seek and gain satiation. Thus, behavior relieves the tension that arises in association with these drives. It is important to point out that I do not discount the influence of such drives on human behavior. Rather, motivation must be recognized as complex and multidimensional. It may involve *both* unconscious drives and choices for behavior that cannot alone be explained by concepts of unconscious drives. Nevertheless, underlying this model is the assertion that occupation represents a unique domain of behavior which mainly emanates from activity and occupational choices. While other motives may influence or affect occupational behavior, the pervasive motivation for occupation remains a deliberate expression of the need to act.[b]

Bruner (1990) argues that "our desires and our actions on their behalf are mediated by symbolic means" (p. 22). By this he means that our awareness of past experience and future possibilities is the medium through which we choose action. Building on this argument, I propose that the choices we make to engage in

---

[a]The concept of personal projects was developed by Little (1983). He referred to them as a goal-directed and thus interrelated set of actions extending across time. The reference to personal projects here is consistent with Little's definition.

[b]In response to earlier arguments that an urge for action was the motive for occupation, Nelson (1988) pointed out that other motives (e.g., the expectation for financial rewards) may enter into the complex motivation matrix that influences, for example, the choice to work. In similar vein, we can recognize that some daily living tasks (e.g., meal preparation) are in part at the service of basic drives such as hunger. Similarly, recreational activities such as dating and dancing have a sexual dimension as well. Consequently, one cannot properly assign a single motive to all occupational activities. It is recognized that a particular sphere of motivation, at best, *dominates* a domain of activity. That is the assertion being made here. In other words, a desire for action or activity manifests itself through occupational behavior and this motive is the *dominant* source of energy for those behaviors we would label as occupational behaviors.

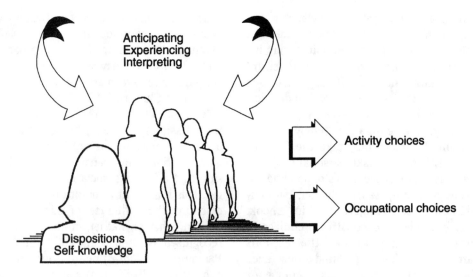

Figure 3.1.   Volition subsystem.

occupational behavior are influenced by symbolic dispositions and self-knowledge.

Dispositions refer to emotional/cognitive orientations toward occupations. These orientations are acquired from experience and they reflect an anticipation of future experience. For example, the experience of pleasure in an occupation helps create the disposition of attraction toward that occupation. Moreover, our attraction to the occupation is, in part, an anticipation of the pleasure we expect. Whenever we make an activity choice we are anticipating a particular experience or outcome. The choices to play cards with friends on Saturday night, to study for an exam, to go out for a walk, or to call up a friend are all made in anticipation of something in which we expect to partake and/or some goal we hope to reach.

Of course, we not only experience occupations as we do them, but we are able to reflect upon and interpret these experiences. The process of interpreting experience generates self-knowledge or awareness of ourselves as actors in the world. This self-awareness allows us to construct complex ideas about the future and its possibilities and therefore contributes to the more reflective process of occupational choice.

Consequently, volition is defined as *a system of dispositions and self-knowledge that predisposes and enables persons to anticipate, choose, experience, and interpret occupa-*

tional behavior. Our personal histories of experiencing and interpreting occupational behavior become organized into a set of dispositions and self-knowledge. As illustrated in Figure 3.1, volitional dispositions and self-knowledge enable the process of making activity and occupational behavior choices because they predispose us to anticipate, experience, and interpret our actions. In Chapter 4, we will examine these dispositions and self-knowledge in more detail.

PATTERNS IN OCCUPATIONS: A HABITUATION SUBSYSTEM

Much of our occupational behavior belongs to a taken-for-granted round of daily life. For example, most of us repeat the same morning scenario of getting up, grooming, and going to work or school five days a week. Such routines of daily life unfold for us with remarkable regularity and without the necessity of deliberation.

In part, these automatic routines correspond to cyclical time wherein things are repeated, familiar paths are taken, known sequences are experienced. Cyclical time is provided by the rhythms of nature (e.g., day and night and the seasons), complimented by social convention (the division of time, the recurring pattern of weeks). Interloping with these temporal cycles are other stable patterns provided by the physical and social world. The constancy of our physical environments supports the organization of redundant behavior. Similarly, social custom and the stability of social patterns of behavior also make possible the development of patterned behavior. Much of social life is marked by the familiar, the repetition of patterns of behavior and events that resemble previous ones in cyclical time (see Figure 3.2).

The sum of all our typical occupational behaviors together make up a lifestyle. While individuals' lifestyles can vary widely, each person exhibits an overall pattern and rhythm of life which constitutes a way of living (Mitchell, 1983). Lifestyles are partly the unique inventions of their owners, and partly reflect organized ways of living exemplified in the social and cultural groups of which one is a part. Indeed, we often speak of lifestyles which are characteristic of an age, such as the hippie lifestyle of the 1960s or the yuppie lifestyle of the 1980s. While lifestyles are often thought of as the province of adulthood, we can also speak of a childhood or adolescent lifestyle as well. Children and adolescents from different cultural and socioeconomic backgrounds may lead vastly different lives. Additionally, the lifestyles of children with working mothers, single parents, and blended families are different from the lifestyles of children from large extended families.

Occupational lifestyle is a person's total pattern and manner of going about occupations. Occupational lifestyle is reflected in what a person does in all social organizations (e.g., family, school, work, and other groups) to which he or she belongs, and in how a person uses time organizing the ordinary course of his or her days and weeks. While lifestyles may reflect previous occupational choices, they are held in place by forces which maintain routine and stability in the life pattern.

A curious thing about conscious decisions is that if we repeat or follow through with them enough, the need for deliberate choice goes away. Consistently chosen behavior eventually persists of its own accord. Kerby (1991) refers to this process as a sedimenting of prior choices and behaviors that accumulate and result in a "unified and unifying substrate of habitualities" (p. 20). In similar fashion, Bruner (1973) describes a process of modularization in which patterns of behavior are established. Repeated action serves to establish an internal organization that allows the same class of action to unfold semi-autonomously in the future (Koestler, 1969). Sometimes these habitualities assert their autonomy when we don't want them to. For example, we find ourselves going to the kitchen cupboard where the cereal used to be, despite our awareness that we have reorganized the kitchen and the cereal is elsewhere. Or we find ourselves relating to a new partner, boss, or coworker in ways we have in the past, despite all our intentions to behave differently.

We will use the term *habituation* to refer to the subsystem designated as responsible for this semi-autonomous patterning of behavior. Habituation is used in biological and behavioral research to refer to an organism's accommodation to some condition or stimulus in the environment to the point that it no longer impinges on the organism (Tighe & Leaton, 1976). For example, people living or working

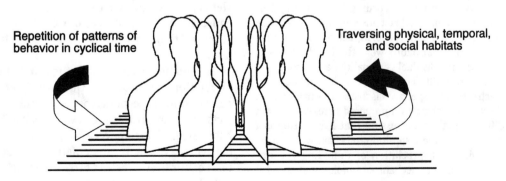

Repetition of patterns of behavior in cyclical time

Traversing physical, temporal, and social habitats

Figure 3.2.   Habituation subsystem.

near the source of a repeated noise or constant smell, in time, cease to be aware of it. However, the term will be used in a quite different manner in the present theory.[c]

Habituation refers to the subsystem which allows the human system to interact in semi-automatic ways with their environments. Given appropriate environmental conditions, we will assemble our behavior in ways which closely resemble what we have done before. Habituation refers to patterns of behavior. Thus, the organization of our patterns of daily time use and our style or manner of organizing action as influenced by culture or society are both examples of habituation.

Habituation makes recurrent behavior more probable because the system has been repeatedly organized to respond to particular tasks and to physical and sociocultural environments. Consequently, persons' habituation reflects the physical and sociocultural features of the environments in which they perform. Habituation is a particularly appropriate term since it reminds us that the habituation subsystem is organized to allow us to function automatically in our various *habitats*. The habitats or environments of occupational performance include three dimensions, temporal, physical, and social.

The habituation subsystem is organized to recognize and respond to temporal cues and time frames which repeat themselves. Thus, the rising sun or our alarm clock may serve as daily cues which contribute, along with the ha-

---

[c]The concept of habit was important in psychology early in this century. Habit was seen as evidence that environmental experiences were encoded in the nervous system. According to prevailing doctrine learned habitual responses operated much like reflexes. In the extreme form, behaviorism argued that conditional habits were the building blocks upon which individual personalities and whole societies were built. This view of habits reflects the mechanistic perspective discussed in Chapter 2. In the view of habituation proposed here, we follow a different pathway, stressing that habituation is a more generalized disposition to behave which operates with an appreciation of unfolding circumstances, not as a mechanized unfolding of encoded action.

bituation subsystem, to initiating a sequence of morning behaviors which unfold within fairly specific time frames. Each morning, I am cued by the alarm clock into a sequence of behaviors which includes, more or less in order, taking a shower and shaving, dressing, eating breakfast, saying goodbye to my family, driving to a train station in a neighboring town, taking the train into the city, and then catching a shuttle bus to my office. All this is accomplished with remarkable consistency in the first three hours of my waking day. In fact, changing the routine takes an explicit act of will on my part, or the intervention of nature (e.g., a snowstorm or a sick child). As the example illustrates, this habituated behavior also involves using and traversing a physical world of shower, shaving equipment, clothes, car, train, and bus. Moreover, while it is mostly an individual and solitary routine, it implies a background of social systems including my family and the university at which I am employed. Once at work, my routine is guided by a more formal schedule and the relationships within the social world of my workplace. The routine and recurrent features of my behavior relate specifically to the temporal, physical, and social world in which I routinely exist. That I am habituated so as to function within those specific worlds is underscored when I travel to conduct a workshop or attend a conference. At those times I must become much more aware of what I am doing, of how the hotel room is organized, of where I am heading, when I should do things, and with whom I will relate. Creating a reasonable facsimile of my typical morning requires energy and thought not required in my daily routine. Hence, one of the virtues of habituation: it conserves energy and frees our consciousness to attend to other matters while routine tasks unfold.

Habituation is also manifest in our patterns of relations with others. Our worlds are as surely worlds of people as they are worlds of objects. Behavior in this social world is similarly habituated. We assume consistent identities and behaviors as we enter the different social contexts of our lives. Whether behaving as a checkout clerk in a supermarket, a parent, a band

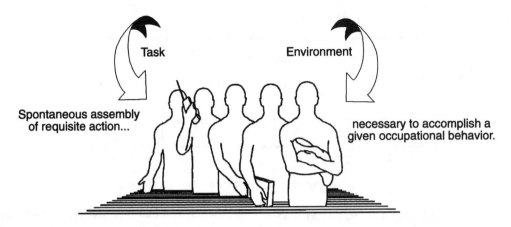

Figure 3.3. Mind-brain-body performance subsystem.

member, or a neighbor, we fall into modes of behavior which are automatic and redundant.

As illustrated in Figure 3.2, *The habituation subsystem is an internal organization of information that disposes the human system to exhibit recurrent patterns of behavior.* These behavioral patterns are fitted to the characteristics of routine tasks and temporal, physical, and social environments. They are reflected in a daily routine of behavior, in a style or manner of performance, and in our patterns of involvement in the social world.

PERFORMANCE OF OCCUPATIONS

The third problem that concerns us is that of human performance in daily occupations. By performance we mean *the spontaneous assembly of requisite actions necessary to accomplish a given occupational behavior.* As the definition indicates, to perform we must call upon latent capacities of our bodies and minds. From the simplest of performances (e.g., tying a shoe or buttoning a button) to the more complex tasks (building a house, composing a song or poem, or designing an airplane) human beings show an amazing capacity to use their own bodies to alter the external word toward the various ends which they imagine and desire.

This performance involves a complex interplay of musculoskeletal, neurological, perceptual, and cognitive phenomena. A complex organization is required to coordinate these cognitive, neurological, and musculoskeletal constituents to allow the performance to be assembled. The mind-brain-body performance subsystem refers to this organization of such components.

We recognized in the previous chapter that the assembly of such skilled performance always involves multiple contributions from factors both inside and outside the human system. The mind-brain-body performance subsystem is neither a machine that causes performance nor does it possess the detailed instructions for performance. However, it must be sufficiently organized to facilitate the assembly of competent occupational behavior.

Theory and practice in occupational therapy have always recognized the importance of underlying performance components or constituents for the ability to assemble competent performance. Traditionally, the mind (including perceptual and cognitive processes) along with the nervous system and the musculoskeletal system are recognized as critical to occupational performance. Other body systems such as the cardiopulmonary and gastrointestinal are recognized as providing necessary energy to support neuromuscular operations.

Thus, *the mind-brain-body performance subsystem refers to the organization of physical and mental constituents which together make up the capacity for occupational performance.* This subsystem supplies the internal factors which contribute, along with the task and the environment, to the assembly of skilled performance (see Figure 3.3).

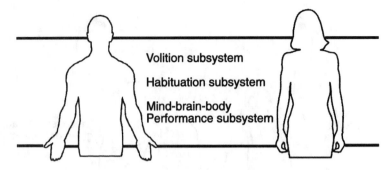

Figure 3.4.   The human system.

A HETERARCHY OF SUBSYSTEMS

I have proposed that the human system is composed of three subsystems (Figure 3.4). Each subsystem represents a coherent collection of structures and processes which are, in turn, organized into the larger system. Thus, each subsystem has its own internal organization which governs, within certain bounds, how it can function. These subsystems are tied together into the larger whole of the human system. That whole exercises its organizing functions recruiting appropriate contributions from the participating subsystems.

The three subsystems must be able to cooperate if the human system is to function in the course of daily life. These internal subsystems must be linked together into a *heterarchy*[d] of subsystems, each contributing toward the action to be performed by the person. The concept of heterarchy emphasizes that the three subsystems each contribute different but complementary functions to the operation of the whole system. It also implies that the functional relationship of the three subsystems will change across time.

When and how a subsystem contributes to the assembly of behavior depends on external circumstances and on the overall dynamic state of the total system. When a task or environmental challenge requires conscious application of problem solving, the mind-brain-body performance subsystem may be in the foreground, with habituation in the background influencing the style with which the person completes the problem solving task. On the other hand, volition may dominate one's attention consistently while one is making an important occupational choice. Following this, the commitment one has made results in the assembly of new behavior that deviates from habituated patterns. At other times, when volition is insufficient to guide our choices of action, our habituated routines carry us through our occupations. Consequently, behavior is sometimes directly motivated, sometimes simply habituated, and at other times it is simply demanded by the task at hand and guided by the mind-brain-body performance subsystem.

While one subsystem may be dominant (i.e., serve as a control parameter) at a given point in time, ordinarily the three subsystems operate in concert with each other, making simultaneous contributions to the assembly of behavior. For example, one may be taking the routine shower or making the routine drive to work, guided by habituation and performance. At the same time one may be contemplating whether or not to engage in an activity later in the day or planning for a long-term occupational goal. Much of our everyday performance has this layered quality in which simultaneous operations of the subsystems manifest themselves.

[d]In the previous edition of this book the three subsystems were proposed as a hierarchy with volition at the top and performance at the bottom. Hierarchical principles were important in earlier systems literature, but current views reject the idea of fixed hierarchies in any system. While functional hierarchies can be established when one component of a system becomes a control parameter, there is nothing permanent or necessary about this arrangement. The concept of heterarchy recognizes that systems arrange themselves according to the demands of situations in which they are performing, not according to a preordained or fixed structure.

Most commonly, we will recognize that there is a mixture of all the subsystems cocontributing to the assembly of behavior. This view of behavior as simultaneously influenced by an admixture of volitional choice, habituation, and performance provides a more balanced and holistic explanation of behavior than is available in models that stress one or another aspect of behavior.[e] Occupational behavior always reflects a complex interplay of our motives, habitualities, capacities, and context. We cannot fully understand occupational behavior without reference to all these contributing factors.

CONCLUSION

I began this chapter by noting that action was fundamental to the human system. Action, in the form of occupational behavior, emanates spontaneously from the system. Moreover, occupational behavior helps create and sustain the organization of the human system. Turning to the problem of identifying the nature of that organization, I identified motivation, organization, and performance of occupational

---

[e]Dewey (1922) recognized the complementary roles which will or volition plays in moral behavior. He pointed out that discussions of morality which focus on intentionality fail to recognize that much of human moral failing has to do with established patterns of immoral conduct which do not need current choice. More recently, Camic (1986) pointed out that social science has been so preoccupied with what is "purposive, rational, voluntary, or decisional" (p. 1040) that it has ignored the important role that the habitual plays in sustaining patterns of behavior. Similar criticisms could be made of many psychological theories of behavior which stressed the motives of behavior to such a degree that every behavior was attributed a latent or unconscious motive while there was no discussion of how the person managed to produce the behavior. On the other hand, occupational therapy could be criticized for a tendency to overemphasize performance, neglecting the role that motives play in occupational behavior. By describing occupational behavior as volitional, habituated, and performed, a wider range of issues are included in the present explanatory model. Taking this broader view presents a greater challenge for explanation and synthesis, but it nevertheless recognizes the complexity inherent in occupational behavior.

behavior as fundamental issues or problems which our theory must address.

Consequently, I proposed that we conceptualize the human system as being composed of three subsystems. The volition subsystem is an organization of dispositions and self-knowledge that influence occupational and activity choices, experiences of occupations, and interpretation of these experiences. The habituation subsystem is the organization of information from repeated performance that reflects the contexts of task and environment. It guides the performance of routine behavior. The mind-brain-body performance subsystem is the organization of mental and physical constituents that make up the capacity for occupational performance. These three subsystems constitute and collaborate together as part of the gestalt human system influencing everyday occupational behavior.

This conceptualization begins our exploration of the internal organization of the human system. In each of the subsequent three chapters we will explore in more detail how each of these subsystems is organized and functions.

References

Berlyne, D. E. (1960). *Conflict, arousal, and curiosity*. New York: McGraw-Hill.

Boulding, K. (1968). General system theory: The skeleton of science. In W. Buckley (Ed.), *Modern systems research for the behavioral scientist*. Chicago: Aldine.

Bruner, J. (1973). Organization of early skilled action. *Child Development, 44*, 1–11.

Bruner, J. (1990). *Acts of meaning*. Cambridge, MA: Harvard University Press.

Camic, C. (1986). The matter of habit. *American Journal of Sociology, 91*, 1039–1087.

DeCharms, R. E. (1968). *Personal causation: The internal affective determinants of behaviors*. New York: Academic Press.

Dewey, J. (1922). *Human nature and conduct: An introduction to social psychology*. New York: Henry Holt & Co.

Florey, L. L. (1969). Intrinsic motivation: The dynamics of occupational therapy theory. *American Journal of Occupational Therapy, 23*, 319–322.

Freud, S. (1960). *The ego and the id* (J. Riviere, Trans.). New York: WW Norton. (Original work published 1937)

Heard, C. (1977). Occupational role acquisition: A perspective on the chronically disabled. *American Journal of Occupational Therapy, 41*, 243–247.

Katz, N., & Ziv, N. (1992). Cognitive organization: A Piagetian framework for occupational therapy in mental health. In N. Katz (Ed.), *Cognitive rehabilitation: Models for intervention in occupational therapy*. Stoneham, MA: Butterworth-Heinemann.

Kerby, A. P. (1991). *Narrative and the self.* Bloomington, IN: Indiana University Press.

Koestler, A. (1969). Beyond atomism and holism: The concept of the holon. In A. Koestler & J. R. Smythies (Eds.), *Beyond reductionism.* Boston: Beacon Press.

Little, B. (1983). Personal projects. A rationale and method for investigation. *Environment and Behavior, 15,* 273–309.

Matsutsuyu, J. (1971). Occupational behavior: A perspective on work and play. *American Journal of Occupational Therapy, 25,* 291–294.

McClelland, D. (1961). *The achieving society.* New York: Free Press.

Mitchell, A. (1983). *The nine American lifestyles.* New York: Macmillan.

Nelson, D. (1988). Occupation: Form and performance. *American Journal of Occupational Therapy, 34,* 777–788.

Reilly, M. (1962). Occupational therapy can be one of the great ideas of 20th century medicine. *American Journal of Occupational Therapy, 16,* 1–9.

Shibutani, T. (1968). A cybernetic approach to motivation. In W. Buckley (Ed.), *Modern systems research for the behavioral scientist.* Chicago: Aldine.

Smith, M. B. (1969). *Social psychology and human values.* Chicago: Aldine.

Tighe, T. J., & Leaton, R. N. (1976). *Habituation: Perspectives form child development, animal behavior, and neurophysiology.* New York: John Wiley & Sons.

Trombly, C. (1989). Neurophysiological and developmental treatment approaches. In C. Trombly (Ed.), *Occupational therapy for physical dysfunction* (3rd ed.). Baltimore: Williams & Wilkins.

von Bertalanffy, L. (1968a). General system theory: A critical review. In W. Buckley (Ed.), *Modern systems research for the behavioral scientist.* Chicago: Aldine.

von Bertalanffy, L. (1968b). *General systems theory.* New York: George Braziller.

von Bertalanffy, L. (1969). General system theory and psychiatry. In S. Arieti (Ed.), *American handbook of psychiatry.* New York: Basic Books.

Weiss, P. S. (1967). One plus one does not equal two. In G. Quarton, T. Melnechuk, & F. Schmitt (Eds.), *The neurosciences: A study program.* New York: Rockefeller University Press.

White, R. W. (1959). Excerpts from motivation reconsidered: The concept of competence. *Psychological Review, 66,* 126–134.

KEY CONCEPTS

ACTION IN THE HUMAN SYSTEM
- arises spontaneously from a disposition to act.
- maintains the order or organization of the human system.

HUMAN SYSTEM IS COMPOSED OF SUBSYSTEMS
- **Subsystem:** an organized and interrelated collection of patterns (i.e., structures) and processes which have a coherent purpose.
- Volition chooses occupational behavior.
- Habituation organizes occupational behavior into patterns or routines.
- Performance makes possible the skilled achievement of occupations.

Volition Subsystem
A system of dispositions and self-knowledge that predisposes and enables persons to anticipate, choose, experience, and interpret occupational behavior.
- **Activity Choices:** short-term, deliberate decisions to enter and exit occupational activities.
- **Occupational Choices:** deliberate commitments to enter an occupational role, acquire a new habit, or undertake a personal project.

Habituation Subsystem
An internal organization of information that disposes the human system to exhibit recurrent patterns of behavior.

Mind-Brain-Body Performance Subsystem
The organization of physical and mental constituents which together make up the capacity for occupational performance.

4/ Volition Subsystem

Gary Kielhofner, Lena Borell, Janice Burke, Christine Helfrich, and Louise Nygård

INTRODUCTION

Chapter 3 defined the volition subsystem as a collection of dispositions and self-knowledge that predisposes and enables persons to anticipate, choose, experience, and interpret their occupational behavior. In this chapter we will present a more detailed conceptualization of the volition subsystem. As the definition implies, volition refers to a wide range of our feelings, thoughts, and decisions about occupational behavior. Considered together, these elements constitute the organization of motives for occupation.

Our conceptualization of volition will combine a number of perspectives which have been used to understand motivation. The original concept of the volition subsystem (Kielhofner & Burke, 1980, 1985) was primarily built upon concepts of trait theory. While this theoretical perspective is still a useful one, it has some important limitations, as we will discuss later. Therefore, we will incorporate other concepts that address some of what trait theory ignores. By incorporating these concepts, we have sought to achieve a more comprehensive way of understanding the motives for occupation.

The concept of traits refers to stable patterns of thought and/or feeling which predispose individuals to behave in related ways (Fein, 1990; Hart, 1992). A large number of traits have been conceptualized and studied; they range from compulsiveness to conformity to competitiveness. When a person is said to manifest a trait, such as low self-esteem, it means that the person tends to regard the self

as inadequate and to behave in ways consistent with thoughts and feelings of personal inadequacy. Because such patterns of thought and feeling are believed to be relatively stable over time, they are referred to as permanent traits. Such traits are considered to be latent motives for behavior inasmuch as the thoughts and feelings that made up a trait predispose one to act accordingly.

The original theory of volition contained the argument that a person's motivation for occupation was influenced by three traits: (1) interests (i.e., what they were disposed to enjoy), (2) values (i.e., what they found valuable in life), and (3) personal causation (i.e., what they felt capable of).

In the last decade, behavioral scientists have become increasingly aware of the limitations of trait theory. While research suggests that traits are relatively stable over much of the life course, studies have also shown that traits can only predict or explain a very circumscribed amount of behavior (Fein, 1990; Hart, 1992). Even the most well-researched traits only explain a relatively small percent of the variability in a person's behavior (Fein, 1990; Hart, 1992). We can examine the practical implication of this by considering interests, one of the more widely studied traits. Research shows that interests such as manual labor or artistic expression remain fairly stable from later adolescence through adulthood (Hart, 1992). Moreover, if persons have a strong interest in manual labor or artistic expression, there is some likelihood that they will enter jobs or careers consistent with those interests; however, we cannot specify exactly what work a person will choose, nor can we explain why, in many instances, persons do not choose the jobs or careers consistent with those interests. As the example illustrates, traits tell us something about the motives for occupation, but they fall short of a comprehensive explanation.

A number of studies based on the model of human occupation have examined the influence of volitional traits on adaptation in occupation (Barris, Dickie, & Baron, 1988; Barris, Kielhofner, Burch, Gelinas, Klement, & Schultz, 1986; Ebb, Coster, & Duncombe, 1989; Elliott & Barris, 1987; Gregory, 1983; Lederer, Kielhofner, & Watts, 1985; Smith, Kielhofner, & Watts, 1986; Smyntek, Barris, & Kielhofner, 1985). Like trait research in other fields, these investigations generally have found that volition traits provide some explanation for person's choices or differentiated persons who were dysfunctional from those who were not. However, the findings of these studies also suggested that volitional traits did not fully explain the motives for occupation.

Recognizing that traits only partially explain choices of occupational behavior we must seek additional explanations. One criticism of trait theory is that, by emphasizing the search for underlying or latent traits, it has ignored persons' conscious, commonsense experience of their motives for action. A number of authors argue that this common sense *is* what motivates people and should be at the core of motivational theory (Bruner, 1990b; Gergen & Gergen, 1983, 1988; Markus, 1983). In referring to everyday common sense, these authors mean the taken-for-granted perspectives that each person uses to make sense of themselves and their lives. Each person's common sense comes from his or her culture; that is, the culture provides a way of understanding and feeling about everyday life, in matters large and small. This includes what people come to know about themselves. Thus, the argument goes that persons behave as they do because their behavior makes sense to them according to the way they experience the world as members of a particular culture.

We will illustrate this cultural common sense through a simple example from our Swedish and American cultures. American culture tends to emphasize competition and individual accomplishment. Americans readily admit what they are good at. When an American has difficulty identifying something that he or she is good at, it may be interpreted as a sign of poor self-esteem. In contrast, Swedes belong to a cultural tradition in which the collectivity is stressed to a greater degree; the individual is expected not to think of him or herself as very important. In Swedish culture, a person who has difficulty identifying his or her own outstanding abilities is a person who knows his or her place. Americans and Swedes naturally interpret others' and their own behavior in these two different common sense ways. Some of us (the authors) grew up thinking we should be good at something and be proud of it while others of us grew up thinking we should keep our abilities to ourselves.

The commonsense views that persons hold about themselves, their behavior, and the contexts in which they act influence how they choose to act (Markus, 1983). This commonsense self-knowledge is not only about who one is, but also about who one might become (Markus & Nurius, 1986). Therefore, it has an anticipatory aspect—what we desire, aspire to, value, and so on. For this reason, theorists argue that self-knowledge is a particularly potent motivational force (Markus & Nurius, 1986; Markus, 1983). As Hart (1992) notes, "What people think about themselves, their goals and aspirations, has a real influence on the paths that their lives follow" (p. 18).

Consequently, in addition to the traditional concept of traits, we will incorporate newer ideas which see motivation as influenced by cultural common sense. Specifically, we will argue that volitional structure includes innate and acquired dispositions which influence how we make certain choices for action and how we experience different occupations (e.g., as enjoyable, threatening, or valuable). In that these dispositions do seem to remain stable over time, they resemble what have been called traits. We also argue that our commonsense knowledge of ourselves as actors in the world, interwoven with our dispositions, influences how we anticipate, choose, and interpret our experience in occupations.

SYSTEMS DYNAMICS OF VOLITION

Chapter 2 argued that structure and process are interrelated aspects of a system. Structure, it was noted, is an enduring state of organization that is constructed, maintained, and transformed by the process or action of the system. In this chapter we use the concept of *volitional structure* to refer to *a stable pattern of dispositions and self-knowledge generated from and sustained by experience* (Figure 4.1). Dispositions refer to cognitive/emotive orientations toward occupations, such as enjoying, valuing, and feeling competent to perform them. We purposefully refer to dispositions as having both a rational and feeling dimension. As Gergen and Gergen (1988) note, the dichotomy between rationality and emotionality is often an artificial and false one. What we think and feel is interwoven into one experience. Moreover, thought and feeling energize and direct each other. We direct our thoughts toward that which we care about and our feelings arise from how we comprehend ourselves and our world.

Consider how we readily combine thought and feeling in everyday discourse. When we ask someone what they think about a situation, we typically expect to receive an account both of what the person thinks the situation is and of what their emotional reaction to it is. Similarly, we often rely on the feeling that something is not right to activate our thoughts about what might be going wrong.

While thinking and feeling are interwoven, their processes and directions are not always in parallel with each other. We may, for example, think that we should behave in ways that we do not feel like behaving.

Self-knowledge refers to our common sense awareness of ourselves as actors in the world; it is our store of knowledge about what we experience when we perform occupations, about the quality and worth of what we do, and so on. Like volitional dispositions, self-knowledge is neither purely cognitive nor emotional. Rather, it weaves together our memory, our grasp of things, and our rational processes with our fears, hopes, and aspirations. Together, our dispositions and self-knowledge constitute our stable pattern of motives for occupations.

Volitional process refers to *the actual workings and procedures of anticipating, experiencing, choosing, and interpreting occupational behavior* (Figure 4.2). Thus, deciding to go for a walk, enjoying a game of poker, thinking about an exam grade and judging that one perhaps did not study hard enough, and imagining what it would be like to do a particular kind of work are all examples of volitional process. In each instance, the individual is involved in an ongoing process in which motives are being experienced, generated, or expressed. Building on concepts in Chapter 2, we recognize that volitional processes involve the dynamic assembly of behavior and experience. The internal organization (i.e., structure) of volition collaborates with other internal factors within the human system (e.g., physical fatigue and habits of action) and with the external context of action to contribute to how we are moved to act, experience, or reflect at any given time. Thus, while volitional dispositions

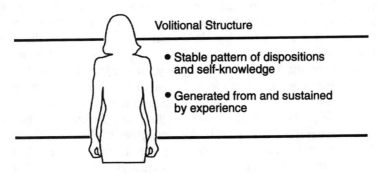

Figure 4.1. Volitional structure.

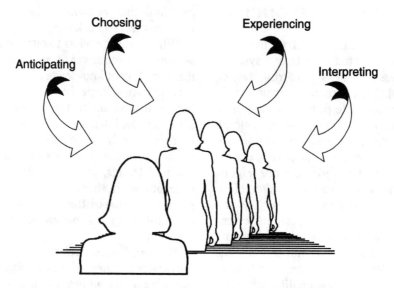

Figure 4.2.   Volitional process: Reflecting on self in action over time.

and self-knowledge do influence choices for occupational behavior, those choices are also influenced by circumstances.

PERSONAL CAUSATION, VALUES, AND INTERESTS

While each person's motives for occupations are unique and related to his or her ongoing experience, we need a way to think about volition which we can apply to a wide range of persons' choices for occupation. In the discussion so far, we have alluded to certain elements of persons' dispositions and self-knowledge. Taken together, volitional dispositions and self-knowledge can be conceptualized as comprising of three areas: *personal causation, values,* and *interests*. These pertain to what one holds as important, how effective one is in acting on the world, and what one finds enjoyable and satisfying. Personal causation, values, and interests are interrelated and together constitute the common sense content of our feelings, thoughts, and decisions about engaging in occupations. For purposes of discussion we will consider each separately. However, the reader should remember that personal causation, values, and interests are each aspects of a larger whole in which themes of competence, pleasure, and value are interwoven.

Personal Causation

One of the first discoveries of life is the connection between personal intention, action, and its consequences (Burke, 1977; Bruner, 1973; DeCharms, 1968). Throughout early development individuals become aware that they can create effects in the environment. Once the link between intention and its external consequences is established, individuals develop the personal knowledge that they can be a cause or have effects. This "subjective knowledge of actively causing things to happen in the world" (p. 259) is referred to as personal causation (DeCharms, 1968). This self-knowledge accumulates as one enters into more and more spheres of behavior and eventually represents the sum of what we know and feel ourselves to be capable of accomplishing.

A number of writers have offered similar concepts which address the phenomena of self-knowledge concerning personal ability, capacity, or control. One of the most widely researched concepts is perceived locus of control or perceived control (Rotter, 1960; Lefcourt, 1981), which refers to whether one believes outcomes in life result from personal actions (internal control) versus being the consequence of the action of others, fate, luck, or other external controls. The literature on perceived locus of control generally argues that a sense of being in control is associated with the tendency of a person to seek out opportunities, to use feedback to correct performance, and to seek to influence outcomes. In contrast, external orientation is associated with helplessness and alienation (Burke, 1977; DeCharms, 1968; Goodman, 1960). While the original concept of locus of control referred to a generic belief system believed to broadly influence behavior, recent literature suggests that locus of control is specific to different spheres of life (Connel, 1985; Lefcourt, 1981); that is, we might feel in control in certain circumstances and not in others.

A related concept is perceived competence, which refers to an individual's beliefs about areas of capacity, such as athletic prowess, scholastic ability, and social competence (Harter, 1983, 1985; Harter & Connel, 1984). In contrast to locus of control, which emphasizes self-knowledge about influencing consequences, perceived competence emphasizes awareness of specific abilities. Other writers also make this distinction between the perception that one has specific abilities or aptitudes and the belief that one can effect desired outcomes in life (Skinner, Chapman, & Baltes, 1988; Fiske & Taylor, 1985).

Based on the concepts and arguments we have identified, the following is proposed as a definition of personal causation as a component of volition: *Personal causation is a collection of dispositions and self-knowledge concerning one's capacities for and efficacy in*

occupations (Figure 4.3). As the definition implies, personal causation can be thought of as encompassing two interrelated dimensions, knowledge of capacity and sense of efficacy.[a]

---

[a] The dimensions of personal causation were first identified by Janice Burke in her Master's of Arts thesis in 1975 and her 1977 article and incorporated into the model in 1980. She identified four dimensions of locus of control: internal versus external orientation to the environment, belief in skill, sense of efficacy, and expectancy of success/failure. The goal behind such specificity was to provide a more detailed road map of personal causation. However, subsequent literature and research indicate that personal causation is a highly individual matter, imbedded in one's own particular way of construing the world. Therefore, people do not neatly organize their self-knowledge into the specific categories offered by theory. Moreover, other research (Muñoz, Lawlor, & Kielhofner, 1993) identified that experienced therapists who used the model of human occupation did not find the detailed breakdown of personal causation helpful in clinical reasoning. Rather, they tended to adapt the general concept of personal causation to the kinds of issues they routinely encountered in their patient populations. Therefore, the present formulation of personal causation (and subsequent volition concepts) employs fewer dimensions in order to achieve a more open-ended view of the concept and allow therapists to match the construct to how patients organize their own self-knowledge. This also reflects the objective stated at the beginning of this chapter to create a theory which more nearly resembled the common-sense folk psychology of everyday life.

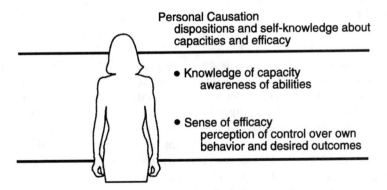

Personal Causation
dispositions and self-knowledge about
capacities and efficacy

• Knowledge of capacity
awareness of abilities

• Sense of efficacy
perception of control over own
behavior and desired outcomes

Figure 4.3. Personal causation.

Knowledge of Capacity

Knowledge of capacity refers to *awareness of present and potential abilities*. Experience teaches us what we can and cannot do well. We observe ourselves through the commonsense lens of our cultures, building up a store of knowledge about what kind of capacities we have. Moreover, as we proceed through life new experiences can alter our views of our capabilities. Sometimes experience happily shows us we have a hitherto hidden talent. Other times it reminds us that our abilities are waning.

Culture tells us what capacities we should have and why they matter. A rainforest dweller learns that he needs physical prowess and knowledge of the jungle, whereas a researcher in physics finds that she needs a swift and penetrating intelligence and a comprehension of complex math. The former is not concerned over a lack of math ability nor the latter over ignorance of rainforests. Similarly, the course of development results in changing concerns about capacity. To a ten-year-old boy, ability on the basketball court may be as important as ability to perform in the classroom; however, by the middle of college, intellectual ability may have taken a much more central place in his knowledge of capacity. Consequently, knowledge of capacity is not simply a catalogue of personal abilities, but an active awareness of one's capabilities for carrying out the life one is living or wants to live.

Knowledge of capacity engenders a disposition toward various occupations; that is, we feel confident or insecure about our physical, intellectual, or interpersonal abilities and we are predisposed to take on tasks that provide opportunities to use those capacities and to avoid tasks that are likely to overtax our capacities. Such dispositions explain why we tend to find ourselves wanting to undertake one activity with a sense of anticipation that we can perform the required behaviors and wishing to avoid others activities because we do not feel as able. The close link between our awareness of what we can and cannot do and the desire to act accordingly is underscored by Murphy (1987) in the following passage in which he describes the impact of his progressive loss of physical capacity:

> To fall quietly and slowly into paralysis is much like either returning to the womb or dying slowly, which are one and the same thing. With all bodily stimuli to movement muted and almost forgotten, one gradually loses the volition for physical activity. This growing stillness of the body invades one's apprehension of the world. I have become a receptor in physical things, and I must continually fight the tendency for this growing passivity . . . (p. 193)

Our particular knowledge of our capacities readies us to anticipate, choose, experience, and interpret occupational behavior in ways that flow from that knowledge. When we know ourselves to be capable and skilled, we are disposed to act and generate further evidence of our ability. When we know ourselves to be incapable, we feel compelled in the opposite direction.

Sense of Efficacy

Sense of efficacy is the perception of control over one's own behavior (and underlying thoughts and emotions) as well as a sense of control in achieving desired outcomes of behavior. It is one thing to know what one is capable of and quite another to realize the impact of one's abilities on what happens in life. Experience does not only teach us how able we are. It also tells us how effective we are in using our capacities and how compliant or resistant life is to our efforts. What emerges, then, is a sense of just how much we are able to bring about what we want.

Persons' beliefs about whether they can use their capacities to influence the course of events or circumstances in the external world are also powerful motivators. To be an effective agent, it is not enough to have capacity, it is also important that one is able to control and use that capacity toward desired outcomes.

Perceptions of efficacy hinge first on assessments of self-control. To effectively use one's capacities, one must be able to shape or contain one's emotions and thoughts and exercise self-discipline. One cannot have a sense of efficacy if one believes that one is at the mercy of overwhelming emotions or uncontrollable thoughts. For example, Mallinson (1994) tells of a psychiatric patient who is talented cellist. While she is aware of her musical abilities, she also sees herself as unable to apply those abilities in order to be successful. Instead, she says, "my thoughts would go around and around and around and repeat themselves and I couldn't follow through . . . on even the simplest things." In this case, her inability to exercise self-control to practice made her desire to be a professional musician seem unattainable despite her remarkable musical talent.

Conversely, a strong sense of inner control can greatly influence how persons adapt. Karen, a person with spinal cord injury, eloquently expresses how her strong sense of personal control enabled her to overcome the potentially devastating effects of quadriplegia:

> The ability to say my mind is in charge here, not this environment, not what's happening to me; it's not in charge. What determines what I will do and how I will handle things is right here (pointing to her head), and I do have control over it. That's the important thing, that events can't shake you, physical environments can't shake you as long as you are able to say, "my mind is in control here . . ." (Patsy & Kielhofner, 1989)

A sense of efficacy is also reflected in one's view of whether one's efforts outweigh other factors influencing the accomplishment of desired ends. Persons may believe that no amount of effort or skills is likely to influence an outcome because it is beyond one's sphere of control. For example, Thelma, who has a psychiatric disability, discusses her views on the efficacy of trying to re-enter the job market and discontinue disability benefits:

> I wouldn't mind going back to school if I knew it would help me, but I don't know . . . And if I ever got a job (then) I got to pay full fee for my (subsidized) apartment . . . I don't want to be making the wrong move and then I'll be stuck with nothing, you know . . . You see, you may get (a job) and then you may get sick again, or have a relapse. You're out in the cold again trying to get back on disability. You might not even get as much as you have now. (Helfrich, Kielhofner, & Mattingly, 1994, p. 316)

When the odds of ultimate success or failure appear so much beyond one's control—when illness or the vagaries of a welfare system may thwart one's efforts to achieve a better life—there is no sense of efficacy.

The sense of efficacy exerts an important influence on our motivation for occupational activities. All things being equal, we find ourselves disposed to undertake occupations for which we can expect success and to avoid those that threaten us with failure. Similarly, when we make occupational choices, we ordinarily consider the degree to which we can effectively meet the challenges posed by a project or a role.

Values

Choices for occupation are also influenced by our values, beliefs, and commitments. Fein (1990) argues that the very purpose of values is to guide choices of behavior:

> Before a person can act, he must be able to choose . . . His options need to be narrowed down to a do-able few. Internal standards help limit his alternatives. Indeed this is the very purpose of values. They are personal and/or cultural criteria used for decision-making. (Fein, 1990, p. 79)

Bruner (1990b) similarly notes that humans are "governed by shared meanings and values" (p. 20). He goes on to point out that we commit our lives to the pursuit of these values, believing "that a certain model of life merits or deserves support, even though we find it difficult to live up to it" (Bruner, 1990b, p. 22).

From earliest childhood experiences, persons interact with a coherent cultural milieu that embodies values. These values define what is good, right, and important, serving as principles to guide human conduct (Grossack & Gardner, 1970; Kalish & Collier, 1981; Klavins, 1972; Lee, 1971; Smith, 1969). Whatever else cultures may be, they are "dramatic conversations about the things that matter to their participants" (Bellah, Madsen, Sullivan, Swidler, & Tipton, 1985, p. 27). Thus, values specify for an individual what is worth doing, how one ought to perform to have merit, and what goals or aspirations deserve one's commitment.

Each person's values belong to a coherent world view provided by culture. Values are expressed in the common sense of that world and the kind of life that persons in that cultural world lead. Thus, as Bruner (1990b) notes:

> Values inhere in commitment to "ways of life," and ways of life in their complex interaction constitute a culture. We neither shoot our values from the hip, choice-situation by choice-situation, nor are they the product of isolated individuals with strong drives and compelling neuroses. Rather, they are communal and consequential in terms of our relations to a cultural community . . . They become incorporated in one's self-identity and, at the same time, they locate one in a culture. (p. 29)

Since values are commitments to performing in culturally meaningful and sanctioned ways, one experiences a sense of belonging and correctness when following values. Persons perceive value when they see a course of action as the proper way to act and all other behaviors represent improper or lesser ways of doing things (Lee, 1971). Since values emanate from our fundamental views of life, they elicit strong emotions. We strongly feel how life should be and how we should behave. Consequently, values are obligatory and one does not act contrary to one's values without a feeling of shame, guilt, failure, or inadequacy. Moreover, values determine one's view of the worth of different occupations. Therefore, they influence the sense of self-worth that one derives from succeeding at occupations. For example, in a family where academic achievement is valued, a child who does well in school is disposed to evaluate himself positively.

We define *values* as *a coherent set of convictions that assign significance or standards to occupations, creating a strong disposition to perform accordingly* (Figure 4.4). The concept of significance refers to the fact that values not only attach worth to behaviors but locate them within a world which makes sense to us. The disposition which values create is a sense of obligation to realize one's values in one's ongoing behavior.[b]

Personal Convictions

As noted above, we all acquire convictions that give significance and coherence to the world. For example, everyone develops a set of beliefs about what matters in life. These convictions both come from and imply a particular culturally-defined world. Within heterogeneous cultures, such as the American culture, the values of individuals are clustered together in ways that define a coherent lifestyle (Mitchell, 1983). For example, the following American lifestyle referred to as "Belongers" illustrates how one's convictions are embedded in a coherent view of how life should be:

> Belongers typify what is generally regarded as middle-class America. Traditional, conforming, conservative, "moral," nonexperimental, family-oriented, Belongers are mighty forces for stability in a world of tumbling change. As a group, Belongers prefer the status quo if not the ways of yesteryear. Old-fashioned values still shine bright: patriotism, home and family, sentimentality. These are people who above all cherish shared institutions such as the family, church, and loyalty to nation, job, and old associations. (Mitchell, 1983, p. 9)

From the perspective of one's personal convictions one ascribes significance to, and judges the worth of, various occupations. A variety of commonsense organizing themes may be the medium of one's convictions. For example, personal convictions may be organized around a fundamental Christian viewpoint of right and wrong that defines what is a good life. A very different set of convictions may underlie a street-smart adolescent from a broken home who learns a code of gang solidarity, territoriality, survival by aggression, and other non-mainstream views of life. While these two sets of convictions are vastly different, each represents a way that someone views the world. Moreover, each expresses what matters to that person and his or her associates. Personal convictions are based on a view of life and define what matters.

---

[b] In the first edition of this book we identified four components of values relevant to occupational behavior: temporal orientation, meaningfulness of activities, occupational goals, and personal standards. Following the same rationale as we noted for personal causation, these dimensions have been reduced to two broader concepts.

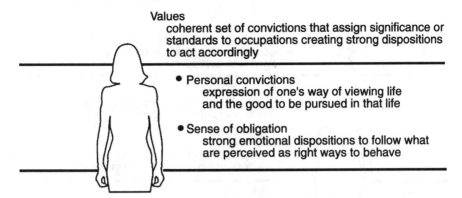

Values
coherent set of convictions that assign significance or
standards to occupations creating strong dispositions
to act accordingly

• Personal convictions
expression of one's way of viewing life
and the good to be pursued in that life

• Sense of obligation
strong emotional dispositions to follow what
are perceived as right ways to behave

Figure 4.4. Values.

Sense of Obligation

People do not simply hold views of life. They also care deeply about life as they see it. Indeed, what one thinks about life is held in place by powerful emotions. As Gergen and Gergen (1988) point out:

> Unless one cares about a given end, there is little function for reasoning powers. "Caring" is a matter of the heart—that is, the emotions. (p. 43)

Because of the powerful emotions that values evoke (e.g., feelings of importance, security, worthiness, belonging, and purpose), they create a strong disposition or sense of obligation to perform in ways consistent with those values. Thus, one is strongly compelled by values. One's sense of obligation may include convictions about how time should be spent, what aspects of performance are important, what constitutes adequate effort or outcome, and what sort of person one should be and become (Kluckholn, 1951; Hall, 1959). It may also be reflected in commitments to performing occupations in moral, excellent, efficient, or other ways made sense of by a coherent view of life. Finally, a sense of obligation often takes the form of goals that sustain behavior (Cottle, 1971). In sum, the *sense of obligation* refers to *strong emotional dispositions to follow what are perceived as right ways to behave.*

Interests

Interests are generated from the experience of pleasure and satisfaction in occupational behavior (Matsutsuyu, 1969). Occupational performance that is enjoyable to one person may

seem boring or threatening to another; hence, interests reflect highly individual tastes. Interest in an occupation arises from a variety of sources. One source is a natural proclivity to find enjoyment in a particular occupation. For example, some persons are simply taken with the game of chess while others are passionate about poker. Another source of interests are the available opportunities to experience occupations. A third influence on interests is the acquisition of tastes. Many interests require cultural instructions for how to appreciate the experience. For example, to enjoy meditation one must first learn how to reach the meditative state.

The experience and consequent self-knowledge of enjoying an occupation creates a disposition or anticipation of future pleasure. Thus, being interested in an activity means that one feels an attraction-based anticipation of positive experience. Consequently, we feel our interests as desires for participating in certain occupations (Matsutsuyu, 1969).

We define *interests* as *dispositions to find pleasure and satisfaction in occupations and the self-knowledge of our enjoyment of occupations* (Figure 4.5).

As the definition implies, interests[c] involve attraction to occupations which emerges from

---

[c] Three dimensions of interest were previously used to represent the orientation to pleasure and satisfaction in occupations: discrimination, pattern, and potency. In keeping with personal causation and values, the delineation of dimensions of the construct is simpler than the previous version.

Interests
dispositions to find pleasure and satisfaction
in occupations and the self-knowledge of our
enjoyment in occupation

• Attraction
a proclivity to enjoy certain occupations
or aspects of performance

• Preference
the propensity to enjoy particular ways
of performing or activities over others

Figure 4.5.   Interests.

the experience of pleasure and satisfaction in performance. A second dimension which we will call preference is the self-awareness of those occupations and qualities of occupational behavior which we enjoy.

Attraction

Attraction refers to *a proclivity to enjoy certain occupations or certain aspects of performance.* The feeling of enjoyment may come from a wide range of factors. These include positive feelings associated with the exercise of capacity such as physical exertion, intellectual intrigue, and the use of skill in competition. For this reason interest is closely associated with personal causation. We are more likely to enjoy what we can perform with some level of proficiency when skill is involved in the performance. Csikszentmihalyi (1990) describes a form of ultimate enjoyment in occupations which he calls *flow*. According to his research, flow involves a total absorption in the activity which occurs when a person's capacities are optimally challenged.

Other pleasures associated with the performance of occupations may emanate from sensory pleasures that arise during performance (we may enjoy how tools feel in our hands, how our cooking smells, the visual pleasure of country scenery on a hike or bicycle ride, and even the vestibular pleasure associated with such activities as snow skiing). Interest may emerge from aesthetic arousal or intellectual intrigue such as that we may gain from paint-ing or reading a book. Since many occupations produce outcomes or products, satisfaction may emanate from what we have accomplished or produced. One may find a craft particularly satisfying because of the pleasing or useful product that results. Enjoyment may come from the sense of association and fellowship experienced in occupations performed with others. Attraction to any particular occupation most likely represents a confluence of several of these factors.

Preference

Collective experiences generally result in the awareness that some performances provide one with a sense of satisfaction and pleasure while others bore, threaten, or fail to stimulate us. From such experience emerges *preference,* which is *the propensity to enjoy particular ways of performing or particular activities over others.* Implied in this concept is that persons do not experience all occupations equally. Instead, they develop preferences for certain occupations over others. Often preference is manifested as a pattern of related interests such as athletic interest or cultural interests, including theater and art. On the other hand, persons may have very diverse and seemingly unrelated preferences. Preferring certain occupations over others allows one to choose. Feeling a preference for certain activities makes it easier to know what we would like to do and, conversely, what we can readily do without.

Summary

Together, personal causation, values, and interests make up the structure of the volition subsystem. Collectively, they represent our relatively stable dispositions and self-knowledge concerning capacity, efficacy, enjoyment, and value. This volitional structure readies us to anticipate, choose, experience and interpret occupations in particular ways. Each of these latter elements make up volitional process, which we will examine next.

VOLITIONAL PROCESSES

We have just argued that volitional structure represents a stable organization of dispositions and self-knowledge which are called upon when we actively encounter the world (Figure 4.6). Our primary interest is explaining how persons choose their occupations, but the process of choice is imbedded in a cycle of anticipation, experience while doing, and subsequent evaluation or interpretation. This means that our volitional structure predisposes us to attend to the world and anticipate possibilities for action in particular ways. That is, our attraction to occupations, beliefs about capacity, and convictions about performance first and foremost influence what we notice and search out in the world. They also influence what we are likely to feel or think about prospects for involvement in the occupational opportunities we encounter. We need only observe how persons' interest (or lack thereof) in sports influences whether they pay attention to television sportscasts or the sports pages in the newspaper, whether they perk up at conversations about sports or know when upcom-

ing home teams are scheduled to play. We simply tend to be unaware of what we have no volitional investment in and, conversely, more versed in what corresponds to our competence, interests, and commitments. This means that what is "out there" in the world for persons is very much a function of how their volition is organized.

Secondly, the dispositions of volition also influence how we experience occupational activities. Over the course of time we engage in a variety of occupations which we simply find more or less enjoyable or valuable and in which we feel more or less able. For a variety of reasons, we all find ourselves in situations in which we do not share the commitment, pleasure or competence of others. Conversely, we sometimes find ourselves unable to explain to incredulous others how we manage to perform a task, why we find it fun, or why it is important to us. Volition makes us each very different appraisers of action.

Volition also influences how we interpret our behavior and experience. Our values may have an important influence on the meanings we assign to our performance (Markus & Nurius, 1986). For example, the high school senior who is committed to going to college will interpret a "C" grade differently from the one who envisions himself working as a carpenter in three months. In similar fashion, personal causation can influence how one interprets performance. An individual who does not believe he can influence his grade outcomes is more likely to assign the outcome of a good grade to luck and a bad grade to teacher bias. Experience is thus filtered through a process of sense-making that emanates from

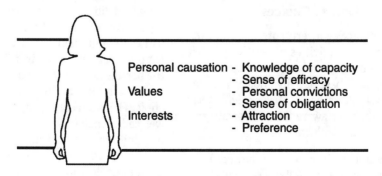

Personal causation	- Knowledge of capacity
	- Sense of efficacy
Values	- Personal convictions
	- Sense of obligation
Interests	- Attraction
	- Preference

Figure 4.6. Volition subsystem.

our particular volitional organization. Volition is more than an aggregate of feelings and thoughts about competence, values, and interests. It is an interrelated world view in which themes of personal causation, value, and interest function as commonsense apprehensions of self and the world. Hence, volition provides us a coherent framework for the interpretive process of making sense of experience.

It is important to remember that volitional structure is not only an organization of dispositions and self-knowledge influencing the assembly of experience, choice, behavior, and sense-making, but is also the product of those processes. The process of choosing, doing, and interpreting occupational behavior represents an ongoing cycle which sustains and transforms volitional structure. Volitional process provides new experiences and information which can reinforce, challenge, and elaborate upon existing dispositions and self-knowledge. Hence, volition is always under construction.

In the midst of this ongoing cycle persons make choices for action that form their everyday experience and simultaneously influence the course of life. It was argued in Chapter 3 that we make two types of choices. Activity choices refer to the occupational activities we select to perform in the course of daily life. Occupational choices refer to larger decisions which involve commitment to sustaining behavior over time. Through activity choices, we enter new roles, establish habit patterns, and undertake personal projects which involve us over time. In the remainder of this chapter we will examine these two types of volitional choices.

Activity Choices

Activity choices concern entering and exiting occupational activities of relatively short duration in our more or less immediate future. As noted above, these activity choices are embedded in a larger process. Meyer (1987) aptly points out that our awareness of capacity and feelings of efficacy influence

> . . . expectations of success and failure *before* an activity is undertaken and also affects—in choice situations—what course of action is selected or

what level of task difficulty is chosen. *While* performing a task, self-perceived ability determines the amount of effort expended and how long effort is sustained. It also affects our thoughts and feelings during the performance period. *After* a test is finished, perceived ability influences evaluations and attributions of outcome and the emotional reactions to the outcome. (Meyer, 1987, p. 74)

Thus, as the description points out, volition pervades choice, experience, and interpretation of action.

The dynamic process of choosing to do an occupational activity involves complex contributions from the components of volition and from external circumstances. For example, students reading this book will have incorporated into their volitional structure a commitment to complete a university education with the goal of embarking on a particular career. In the course of engaging in the occupational behaviors this commitment requires (e.g., doing assignments and taking exams) each student's sense of personal causation has continued to evolve around the commonsense concern of having the capacity for and utilizing the self-control necessary to receive adequate grades. Being given the dual propositions of an upcoming exam and an opportunity to join friends on a Saturday afternoon for an activity one greatly enjoys creates the necessity of an activity choice. Will one spend the afternoon studying for the exam or will one join friends? The final choice will emerge from interactions of one's feelings of efficacy, attraction to the activity, value standards for levels of performance, and so on. One may simply "feel" the collective contributions of all these elements in making the decision or one may rationally deliberate the consequences of the decision. Nonetheless, the elements of volition will exert an influence over the decision; other factors will also have their influence, including the persuasiveness of friends.

Not all activity choices are dilemmas or choices between competing dispositions. Some we readily make. When we are offered an opportunity to do something we like during discretionary time or when our values so strongly dictate the decision, there is little question or hesitation about going ahead.

The example above illustrates that activity choices may also be influenced by larger occupational choices which we previously made. Indeed, an occupational choice is a commitment to make a series of particular activity choices over time. While activity choices determine a whole range of activities which are at our immediate discretion, occupational choices are critical in setting the direction of our lives and eventually in establishing our lifestyles. Thus, we now turn our attention to the volitional process of occupational choice.

Occupational Choice

We noted above that choices are embedded in a larger process of experiencing, interpreting, and anticipating. Activity choices focus on our more or less immediate futures, but occupational choices are life choices. They have to do with the course our life stories have taken and will take. To make occupational choices we must integrate and incorporate many fragments of past experience, current circumstances, and future possibilities into a coherent whole (Schafer, 1981; Taylor, 1989). Moreover, occupational choices mean deciding who we will become (Kerby, 1991).

Occupational choices which people make are nested in an unfolding life. These choices generally reflect the subtleties of present circumstances. They reverberate with memories of past triumphs, joys, pleasures, failures, and losses. They anticipate an imagined future. This process of integrating past, present, and future selves involves the construction of personal narratives (Geertz, 1986; Gergen & Gergen, 1988; Helfrich, Kielhofner, & Mattingly, 1994; Mattingly, 1991; Mattingly & Fleming, 1993; Schafer, 1981; Spence, 1982; Taylor, 1989). Narrating some aspect of one's life means making one's experience into a story, even if that story is only for oneself. Stories may also anticipate the future by continuing what has happened in one's life into some imagined outcome. The life stories we construct carry and integrate the themes of personal causation, values, and interests. Thus, the volitional process of making occupational choices is embedded in narrating an unfolding story—a story through which we make common sense of our circumstances. When we make occupational choices we are, in effect, selecting a continuation of a story in which we see ourselves. Volitional choices therefore involve enactments of the next episodes of our life stories.

In order to illustrate this volitional process of creating personal narratives and making occupational choices within them, we will present three narratives. After presenting these narratives we will discuss them collectively. Each of these volitional narratives was told to us by a person with a disability. Hence they illustrate some of the special challenges that persons can face in making sense of their lives through their stories. In presenting these stories we have tried to remain faithful to their original telling. Each of these stories was told over a series of interviews. We subsequently condensed each set of interviews into a more manageable size, attempting to preserve the essence of how each person was making sense of his or her life. The third person, whose story is told here, chose to edit the final document himself. Although all three persons are given fictional names, they are the true authors of their stories and we are grateful for their willingness to share so much of their lives with us.

Tom

Twelve years ago, Tom[d] graduated from high school with honors. As a student he was the school newspaper editor, National Honor Society President, Quill & Scroll President, and a debate club member. He spent summers writing for a citywide student newspaper and taking advanced journalism training. He graduated as class valedictorian of a prestigious private university with a degree in journalism, having completed successful internships in two major city daily newspapers. After 16 months of work as a city reporter on a daily paper, he landed the prize—a job on a big city paper as a bureau reporter covering several beats.

Now it is six years later. Tom has been out of work for the better part of a year. He worries constantly about getting a new job. And he is palpa-

---

[d] Tom's story has been previously presented in a different format (Helfrich, C., Kielhofner, G., & Mattingly, C., 1994).

bly embarrassed about his departure from what promised to be a brilliant career. He wonders what would happen if an old professor would spy him back at his university placement office. He agonizes over how he will explain several glaring gaps of unemployment in his resume. Despite these torturous anxieties, Tom drags himself to an interview for an editing position in a monthly political newsletter. This job is admittedly several rungs below investigative journalism.

Afterwards, Tom characteristically jokes about the interview experience. All went well. He simply explained his career gaps as being due to leprosy and imprisonment. He sobers. Truth be told, he lied. He sat there and said his resume gaps were due to a recurrent eye problem. Of course, it wasn't completely fiction; he had an eye problem once in the past. Anyhow, Tom got the job! He muses:

What I am doing is about a million light years from what I originally ever thought I would be doing. I never thought I'd ever be going into the trade, the trade publications. That's what these are called. When I was in the beginning of, well, when I was towards the end of high school, I probably would have envisioned myself eventually working for the Chicago Tribune. Towards the middle of college I probably had changed that to working for a medium-sized daily paper. I really realized that with my illness you can't plan much of anything, any real long-term plans. You can't say this is the first step on the rest of my career, and in five years I plan to be in such and such a city, and in ten years I plan to be an editor of this paper. And people who don't get sick make those kind of plans. Every plan that I've made has eventually been defeated and I've had to shift to another sub-plan. I used to have—my motto in life after my first episode was—and I'd gotten this out of the newspaper—was, "What counts in life is what you do with plan B," okay? Well, I've, I've got to about plan F now. You just have to keep changing your goal. You just have to be practical, and try to be realistic, and settle for less than what you had envisioned before. You really learn to take things at, sort of, at the most, a year at a time. I was never planning more than a year ahead. Now, you know, I'm not making any plans at all. The future is, is just, a very, foggy, unclear place.

Tom has a bipolar disorder. His employment gaps and unfulfilled career hopes are due to re-

curring periods of depression and mania that usually result in hospitalization. It all began after his stellar high school experience when he had started the serious study of journalism at college:

I started panicking and really worrying a lot about my classes, thinking I was failing them. But there was no evidence for this, because I was doing really well in my classes—if you looked at test scores. Nothing could convince me that I wasn't going to fail. I couldn't figure out why this was happening to me. I tried to figure out all kind of reasons why, but I couldn't come up with anything. I was crying a lot and eventually stopped going to classes completely. It was a really, sad, sad day at the end of the quarter when my Mom and I went and we took all my stuff from the dorm room home. I went into the hospital January 2, 1982, because I had become delusional and the depression was getting worse. I was there for three months and it really messed up my academic career for a while.

Scathed but not destroyed, Tom returned to college. He graduated with highest honors. He even made it to a major city newspaper. But this and other journalism jobs have ended with exacerbations of bipolar disorder. Yet Tom struggles on:

It's awful! Its like, you know, a little ant crawling up a hill, and you just kick him down every so often, and he'll . . . he'll climb back up and continue, but its gonna take him a long time. I'm just trying to get back on any track that I can. Because once you get another job, you could just as easily lose it—like you lost the last one. Every time you lose a job it becomes harder to get another one. You have to explain the last one. You try to keep a positive attitude and think that you will find a job and that somehow, if you do go through another episode, that it won't be bad, or that you'll be able to catch it early enough that you'll cut it short, somehow. You can't predict these things. You know, you stop predicting.

Each time illness interrupts Tom's life, he reinvents his life story. Hopeful, he half-expects further setbacks. Tom eloquently bridges the distance between his adolescent dreams of greatness in journalism, his much less glamorous and less prestigious job in the trade publications, and the kind of future he expects:

One of the keys is that you realize that you don't have to move ahead—that you can stay in the same place, that it's not such a terrible thing to give up ambition to some extent. You don't have to share the same amount of ambition as your friends. I'm realizing that I have to sort of stop thinking of myself in the same peer group that I used to. My peer group was once all my college friends who are now climbing their ladders in their respective newspapers, whatever, publishing companies. I really think that if I keep comparing myself to them it's only gonna make me angry and envious and hostile. So, really, now what's emerging as my new peer group is all the other people with chronic illnesses who, like me, are just having to do the best that we can. I think you learn to scale down what you expect, but that doesn't mean that you stop enjoying life. It just means that you have to find enjoyment in other things.

Lisa

A visitor has just come to talk with Lisa who is 54, divorced, and lives by herself in her own house near her parents' home in a suburb of Stockholm. After greeting her guest, she sits down, but rises immediately, asking, "Do you want a sandwich?" "No thanks," the guest says. Then she fetches some cookies and puts them on the table. She goes to the refrigerator, opens it, and looks inside, saying something to herself about buns. Then she seems to catch herself, embarrassed. Her guest wonders aloud what she said and Lisa responds, "I was looking for the buns, but I suppose I already ate them." Lisa takes some dark bread from the refrigerator and says, matter-of-factly, "Do you want a sandwich?" The guest repeats, "No, thanks." Lisa returns to the table. She looks around. She goes to the sink, saying "What was I looking for?"

Later, after her lunch, she wipes the wash bowl then says, "I wonder where I took this from? Where do I keep it? Now I have no idea!" She looks under the sink. She turns. She looks around more. "No, I think I keep it in the laundry," she says.

In her typically Swedish, practical view of the world it is important to Lisa to remain active and be useful. She announces, "If there is laundry to do, I just start doing it." One of her favorite activities is ironing. She irons slowly and appears totally absorbed. When an observer notes that she looks so peaceful ironing, Lisa explains that when she irons, "It gets nice . . . and then I like having clean and ironed shirts in the closet . . . and then

you feel useful doing it . . ." Lisa goes on to tell about how, on good days, she becomes adventuresome and goes into the city for such things as eggs that are on sale. Being practical and useful sums up much of how life should be in Lisa's common sense view; however, she has a secret that makes this difficult.

In the autumn of 1990, Lisa's dementia first showed at work when she experienced depression, memory loss, and difficulty concentrating. Her symptoms were interpreted as depression and she began taking antidepressive medication without any benefit. Her difficulties increased instead and she was assigned to less demanding tasks. By the deep winter, she could not handle work at all and had to leave her job with disability benefits. By spring she was hospitalized.

At this time Lisa had severe memory deficits. She couldn't, for example, recall her own age. As Lisa describes it, she felt "somewhat of a chaos inside." Today, her cognition continues to deteriorate. Lisa is considered to suffer from a degeneration of the frontal cortex.

Lisa makes it clear that she must not show her disease to the world. But it is hard work to conceal her difficulties. She wonders, "Perhaps everybody can see I'm this dizzy and crazy," and then she repeats how hard she works to conceal what she is like. Even Lisa's mother, who is the person closest to her, is not entirely aware of what her problems are. Lisa considers aloud what might happen if her mother knew the facts of her dementia, "Maybe they would take my house away from me, or something like that, and believe I can't manage at all . . ." And then, there is the worry about what will happen when her mother is no longer nearby as a source of support. "I worry about the day she dies. Then I will be all by myself with this sticky mess in my head. Then I won't manage and everything will fall apart."

The impending chaos when Lisa's life will come apart hovers about her little house like a relentless enemy. It causes Lisa anxiety over all the many things that might go wrong and overwhelm her. And thus, "All small things become huge houses. I get a lot of Christmas cards, and I worry about having to first find cards to send in return, and then I have to write them out. And find addresses. And then they need stamps and I have to get out to buy stamps. And then I have to mail them and all . . ." And so go Lisa's worries about how she is going to manage.

Lisa reminisces to her guest about the frequent bus trips into Stockholm that were a part of her routine. She is very hesitant to do so on most days now. She tells how, a few weeks ago, she was going to meet her daughter in a large shopping center in the city. When the time came she couldn't imagine how to get into the city or return home so she didn't go. Today, she starts to look for her telephone books in order to call the bus company with a question about the schedule. She finds the books in the cleaning cupboard but just stares at them, apparently wondering which one she should consult. Finally, she sighs, "No, today I feel bad. I don't want to do it." Then, as if to explain, Lisa tells her guest, slowly and solemnly, "I'm not that strong anymore. I'm weak and I can't make it. It feels like I just could break down. Before this I was strong, but I'm not anymore."

Jon

I was born in 1951 on the southwest side of Chicago. My sister is older and she was married when I was nine. My father died when I was 16. I was an unremarkable student, graduating high school by the skin of my teeth. I enrolled in the local community college, but this was during the Viet Nam era. During my first year of college I joined the Air Force Reserves. I spent most of 1970 on active duty in Texas, returning to school the following spring semester. At that time I met a girl and within weeks became engaged.

I was very involved in school activities. I became editor of the college newspaper and was elected to the Student Congress. My junior year I transferred to the University of Illinois at Chicago with a major in accounting. I got married at the end of my first quarter. I took a very heavy courseload, trying to make up for lost time, but I was still not a good student. What got me though college was remembering that growing up, my parents were insistent about college, telling me, "You will go to college! You will go to college!" If I hadn't graduated from college, the sense of personal failure would have been unbearable. Nothing else, just nothing else, was more important.

It wasn't easy, but I graduated and went to work for a small accounting firm. Within a year I moved on to one of the largest CPA firms in the country. I worked there for four years. In the meantime, I bought a house and my first son was born. I left the firm in 1979 just as my second son was born and started a small accounting and tax service working with small businesses. I also began getting involved in local government, and

was appointed as a town planning commissioner and a district trustee of schools.

Within a year I purchased a small tax business to operate in addition to my primary practice. I was maintaining things, but the economy was getting worse. I found myself with more and more receivables. When an opportunity came to join a larger firm again, I took it.

Throughout my twenties I focused on my career. Most of my time went toward practice development. I loved being a dad, but my wife and I were fighting all the time. Much of the fighting had to do with my constant working. Eventually we separated. I took an apartment and tried to sort things out. I was working and seeing my boys on weekends, while evaluating both my marriage and career choices. I was feeling the pressures from the practice, the new firm, and my marriage. It was not a good time.

I was trying to work through these things when I was in a car accident on my way home from work. It was February, 1983. I was sitting at a red light when a drunken driver rear-ended my car. The car seat collapsed on impact and I was thrown head first into the back seat. I sustained a compression fracture on the C5–6 level. My only recollection of the accident spans about 30 seconds. It was about eight in the evening, a clear and cold night. I was lying on my back inside the car, and I could see the sky because the roof had been cut away. I felt light snowflakes on my face and it was very cold, yet everything else felt warm. I heard police radios and saw the reflections of flashing red lights. I heard voices, one of them was mine, but I have no idea what was being said. I was in shock.

I'm told that in the hospital I kept asking the same questions over and over, "What's going on?" and "Am I going to die?" The next morning the shock was wearing off and I began to understand about the accident and the nature of my injury. No one used the word quadriplegia. I think that would have bothered me more. They told me about loss of movement and function. I remember hoping that it was temporary, but I understood that it might be permanent.

After only seven days of intensive and acute care I was transferred to the rehabilitation hospital. I argued with the staff about transferring me so soon and told them I wasn't ready. I wanted more time to adjust and understand what was happening; however, I had no control over the transfer and the lack of control extended into the rehabilitation process.

My biggest problem going through rehabilitation was the lack of patient involvement in the decision process. I wasn't able to get a footing and it made my initial stay memorable for me, the doctors, nurses, and therapists. I was considered a problem patient because I kept asking questions until I received a satisfactory answer.

I asked, early on, if my hand function would return. I thought, if so, I could get my guitar and play all day. I had purchased a new guitar just prior to the accident. The enjoyment of playing was in developing the technique—the coordination of both hands toward a sound and a rhythm. The doctor said maybe in time, but it was a long shot. While I was in rehabilitation, one of the therapists brought me brochures for adaptable guitar equipment. The device enabled the user to construct chords on the guitar, one at a time and then strum the strings. The technique and style of playing the guitar was lost in the process. I told the therapist I could not get interested in playing the guitar in that fashion. It was a nice try though.

I knew that the Jon Smith who existed before the accident was gone. This Jon Smith was very different, at least physically. I took stock of what assets I had left, namely my mind and a certain amount of tenacity, and decided to take it from there.

I concluded that I needed to have my own agenda for the rehabilitation process. In addition to the therapy sessions which were intended to develop my abilities, I knew that the rehabilitation setting was the best place for me to test and discover my limits as well. I tried to come to grips with how things would or could be when I was out living on my own. Obvious questions, such as whether I would need 24-hour attendant care would actually be determined by less obvious questions, which unfortunately the staff was all too ready to answer for me by assumption rather than logic or deduction.

As an example, I was told I would need to turn in bed every four hours to avoid skin breakdown; however, at the time I could not turn myself. The staff response was that I would need an attendant at night to assist in turning me. I asked, "What happens if I don't get turned?" They responded that I had to be turned every four hours—they had a schedule. I suggested trying every six hours to see what would happen. "Nobody goes six hours," I was told. I argued with the doctor, the nurses, and the therapists that if I could get by without being turned then I wouldn't need an at-

tendant at night. They finally agreed to the logic and we tried no turns as an experiment, carefully checking for any signs of skin breakdown. We found none and after a few days the doctor approved a schedule with no turns at night; the prospect of a nighttime attendant was avoided.

After eight months in rehabilitation I was discharged and went to live in my mother's home. We had a large family room put on the house after my father died. I finished all of the interior carpentry and now, 16 years later, I was living in this room. There was an irony to it, but it did give me an opportunity to really get a feel for what it would take for me to live on my own. I was able to identify those skills that I needed to develop. I returned to rehabilitation three months later with very definite goals—namely to enhance certain procedures and techniques, to learn despite my disability.

I was beginning to feel more sure of myself in many ways. I accomplished the goals I had set for myself in returning to rehabilitation. I was discharged in May of 1984 after spending nearly a year in rehabilitation. Within days of my final discharge I bought a van with a lift and hand controls. I just drove all summer. It was therapeutic. I started taking the kids with me at least one day a week and they helped me a lot. They made me experiment and asked me to try new things. Because of them I stared venturing out more into public. I think nothing of it now, but it was their idea to go to a movie theater the first time. I went to a mall by myself because my son asked me to pick something up for him. I worked very hard at having our relationship work. My priorities always started with my sons. We may have a better relationship now than we would have had without the accident.

I was also realizing that I was not as helpless as I may have thought. And I was getting bored. About that time someone I knew at a Center for Independent Living suggested I apply to the center as Finance Director. Such centers work with people with disabilities to help them achieve their individual goals of personal independence despite their disability. Working at the Center I was able to experiment with different files and desk layouts to best accommodate my limited hand function. I found my way. Most important though, was my introduction to computers. Over time I found myself far more productive with computers than I had ever been before the accident.

I was still living at my mother's, but was looking for my own place. I found a local apartment complex and met with the construction people who were rehabbing six apartment buildings. We talked about making as many apartments as they could accessible. They specifically selected one building with no steps and made some minor modifications. I was getting ready to move into one of the apartments, but the day before I was supposed to sign the lease the owner of the building called, suggesting that I not come. He was vague as to his reasons, but said he didn't think the apartment was appropriate for me and that I would be happier living elsewhere. I tried to talk with the owner about the problems he saw, but I began to realize that I was being discriminated against because of my disability.

Discrimination was a new experience for me. In time I called the ACLU who referred me to the State Department of Human Rights. I obtained help from Northwestern University's law school legal aid clinic and filed a complaint. The whole process took over two years to complete. I found a different apartment in the meantime but I stayed with the case as a matter of principle. We were preparing for trial when the owner offered to settle. The owner agreed to an order of nondiscrimination, advertised the building as available to others with physical disabilities, and I won the right to the apartment with monetary damages as well.

Living on my own was an experience. I needed some help setting up the apartment; however, once I was organized I found it to be very accommodating. I felt like I was getting on with my life.

Later that year I applied to Northwestern University's graduate management program. I knew that the best way to compensate for my disability was with additional education. Graduate school was an excellent opportunity to develop skills and become more competitive in spite of my disability. I was working at the Center, attending school part-time, and feeling pretty productive.

During my second year of graduate school I learned of additional state funding available for the creation of new Centers for Independent Living. I organized a group to start a new Center providing services to people with disabilities in Suburban Chicagoland. I served as Chairman of the organizing committee. We lobbied the state legislature, played politics, and fought the government bureaucracy to establish the new center. We were frustrated at times, but overall it was a very interesting and rewarding experience. After nearly two years of effort, we were successful in securing the state funding to open the second largest Center in the midwest.

As the Center was becoming a reality, I considered taking the position of Executive Director; however, I decided it was important for me to make my career choices in spite of my disability, not because of it. I continued with the Center, but only as a volunteer, serving as Chairman of the Board of Directors. Over the six years since the Center opened we've seen it grow to a staff of 13 with a budget approaching $700,000.

I moved on to my current job, finance officer of a rapidly growing child welfare agency. In addition, I continued to focus on career development, obtaining another graduate degree and passing the CPA exam. Looking back, I may have been trying to overcompensate professionally. I wanted to keep open as many career opportunities as possible.

The accident obviously changed my life. Whatever plans I had for my life were gone. The pressures I was feeling at the time of the accident were taken out of my hands and I was forced to start over with a clean slate. I had always been a planner, but whatever I had planned for my life was gone. Whatever road I had been on, I wasn't on that road anymore.

What I was going to do with my life, my time, what my relationship with my kids would be like, who I might spend my life with . . . all of those things were unknown to me. Some still are, but I realized that I needed to start asking those questions of myself. I was making choices because life goes on. Even though I had lost so much of how I had been, I was still in a position to ask myself, "What should I do with the rest of my life?"

I think I'm stronger and more determined than before becoming disabled. I do feel a certain sense of accomplishment, although I feel I still have a lot to do. I've worked hard to maintain a strong relationship with my sons. I hope I'm more sensitive to the circumstances of other people. Before the accident, I would never have envisioned the events of my life so far.[e]

Tom's, Lisa's, and Jon's stories illustrate how they have arranged and made sense of their experiences. First of all, their knowledge

[e]We are indebted to Lisa Richter, MS, OTR, who originally interviewed Jon and supplied the transcripts of the interviews from which the final story was constructed. We also which to express our gratitude to "Jon" (who wishes to remain anonymous) for taking the time to reflect upon and ultimately write his story for this chapter.

and feelings about their lives are couched in the themes, ideas, and viewpoints provided by their everyday culture. Tom and Jon both reflect the career ambition typical of American men and they struggle, as many others do, to reconcile themselves with cultural notions of career success. Lisa reflects the Swedish idea of being useful and practical. Along with the men, Lisa reflects the Western ideal of individualism and autonomy as a guiding and organizing principle in their commonsense view of how they should live their lives.

Just as importantly, each story reflects a unique and personal journey with its own challenges and accomplishments. Woven into these stories are each person's values, personal causation, and interests. Each must make sense of his or her own competence and the issues which surround it. Each seeks to find enjoyment and satisfaction in the activities that fill their lives. And each sorts out what is important to him or her as guiding principles for action. All these issues and concerns are integrated in a natural and commonsense way in these stories. Moreover, the occupational choices made by these persons are most comprehensible within the story. Why Tom chose to leave reporting for a trade journal, why Lisa gave up her habit of taking the bus into the city, and why Jon decided to earn graduate degrees all make sense in the stories. Outside the stories these decisions would be much harder to explain. Moreover, recourse to simple trait explanations (e.g., Tom has an interest in journalism, Lisa has lost a sense of efficacy, and Jon has identified new values) lose something in the translation from the form of the story to the typically more sterile explanations for motivation we often encounter. Let us go on and consider in more detail how personal causation, values, and interest take on meaning in these stories.

Tom is on "plan F" now but, like the little ant that cannot be beaten down, he still believes in the possibilities of regrouping and taking charge of his life, hence his positive sense of efficacy. Lisa's personal causation teeters on the edge of a precipice. She fears being found out as incompetent and losing her house and her freedom as she lost her job. Her fears of in-

efficacy center on making some large mistake, such as getting lost, which she believes could bring her world crashing down on her. Jon's whole life has been radically altered. He saw his career and his family come to a halt. Forced into making a new start, he took stock of what capacities he had remaining. A tenacious planner and a fighter, he pieced together a new life of which he is proud and in which he feels a sense of control and accomplishment.

For Tom, Lisa, and Jon personal causation is interwoven with the other elements of volition. Tom had to change what was important in his story to stay in control. He learned to scale down ambition to find a new reference group, to choose a less demanding occupation. By giving up ambition he gains a measure of control; that is, he can emerge victorious over the disease and can achieve what he now desires. It is not the success story originally envisioned, but a success story nonetheless. Lisa feels out of control because the things she most values (her home, her independence, and being useful) all appear threatened. Jon gets control of his life when much of what he previously thought was important is taken away and the old Jon Smith is lost. By reinventing his sense of what matters, he experiences a renewed sense of efficacy.

Part of Tom's sense of efficacy is that he can still find enjoyment in life. While he adjusts his ambition and his sense of what is important, he remains in journalism, an area in which he has always been so passionately attracted. Jon can no longer enjoy playing the guitar because, in his view, his loss of capacities make it impossible to play the guitar the way in which he feels it should be played. He goes on to new things for a sense of satisfaction. Lisa finds some small, reassuring comfort in the midst of her anxieties by ironing. For a while, the shirts and (we suspect) life itself "gets nice."

Tom is masterful in his ability to make sense of what is important, to preserve a sense of control and enjoyment, while successfully holding at bay the devastation which his serious illness might have brought. Tom refocuses his push for achievement in a successful career to mastery of the disease process. His achievement becomes a liveable life in spite of his disease. Writing as an investigative reporter metamorphoses into writing in a trade journal. Lisa's story is one of surprise and loss. Threatened by the chaos inside and the specter of losing what little she has, Lisa hides in the shadows concealing her awful secret. The old Jon was obliterated and made anew. Out of the rubble of a life gone wrong in so many ways, Jon recreates himself, and his story is truly that of a self-made man.

These three stories should make clear that the concepts of volition index something which is alive and vibrant. Concepts give us a way to categorize and comprehend persons, but they always refer to something which is known, felt, and actively constructed by persons trying to make sense of their lives. As the stories show, these volition concepts have no meaning outside the experiences of people. And, we must know persons' stories to really know their volition and how that volition has resulted in their occupational choices.

These persons also understand themselves and choose their actions through their stories. The story works for them as a way to make sense of their experiences and to make choices. This is because each story has a form all its own and the form of the story provides a mold into which persons can pour their aspirations, actions, and experiences. Gergen and Gergen (1988) refer to this as the "forestructure" of narrative, a set of conventions about what constitutes a story, which determines how we think and talk when we use stories. Consequently, when humans engage in the volitional process of making sense of experience and making occupational choices, they draw upon the narrative mode which their culture provides as a way of making sense of experience and anticipating the future.

Stories also give a drama to our lives which makes them at once comprehensible and moving (Bruner, 1990b; Gergen & Gergen, 1983). This dramatic dimension of stories (residing, for example, in the fear that things may become worse or the hope that things will get better) gives them the power to energize and sustain the commitments we take on when we make occupational choices or, conversely, the power to overwhelm and make us unable to

choose. In the end, the story told points to where the life is headed.

CONCLUSION

This has been our argument about how persons are motivated to engage in occupations: as infants we come into the world with a need for action. Our occupational behavior begins with our attraction to objects and people and our ceaseless efforts to interact with them. As we move through life, we learn about our behavior, how it feels, how it affects the environment, and what others think of it. We learn to make sense of our action and the world in which we act as those around us do. Consequently, we acquire a commonsense knowledge of ourselves that reflects our culture and our unique experiences.

Through this ongoing process of encountering the material and human world, we create and sustain our volitional structure, a set of dispositions toward acting in the world and commonsense knowledge about self as an agent in the world. Importantly, since our volition has to do with being and acting in the world, the external world as we see it is always implicit in our volitional dispositions and self-knowledge.

Volitional dispositions and self-knowledge take on a specific form. As persons interact with their environments, they generate images about their own effectiveness. This is the view of self as a causal agent: that is, *personal causation*. They also acquire a coherent view of the world and a way of life within it which obligates them to behave accordingly. We refer to this sense of coherence and commitment as *values*. Finally, persons come to learn about the potentials for enjoyment and satisfaction in occupations. We refer to the attraction and preference they develop for occupations as *interests*. Through ongoing experience the self-knowledge and dispositions reflected as personal causation, values, and interests is maintained and reorganized. This organization of self-knowledge we refer to as volitional structure.

Volitional structure is never finished. Rather, volitional structure is the ever-chang-

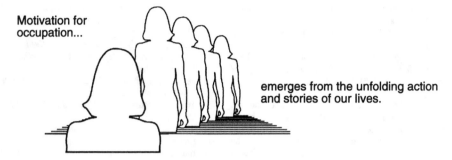

Motivation for occupation...

emerges from the unfolding action and stories of our lives.

Figure 4.7. Volitional meaning motivates us to choose our occupations.

ing product of ongoing episodes of behaving in the world and the experiences those behaviors generate for us. Each time we select and experience an occupational behavior we are rebuilding our volition.

The organization of volitional structure at any time in life influences volitional process. That is, we are energized by a need for action, but that need is only a foundation for action—a foundation that will itself be transformed as volitional dispositions and self-knowledge develop. Our choices and the interpretation of the experience of occupational behavior are influenced by what we perceive to be interesting and valuable and by what we believe ourselves capable of doing. In this way, personal causation, interests, and values build upon the need for action, shaping our choices of occupational behavior. Further, volition is a self-organizing subsystem. Choices for action are assembled with influences from past experiences; those choices in turn create new experiences to reorganize volition. Thus, the self-organizing volitional subsystem creates and recreates personal causation, values, and interests, differentiating these images throughout the course of development.

To our arguments we add one more important point. Volition represents the *meaning* that we make of ourselves acting in the world. According to Bruner, "The major activity of all human beings everywhere is to extract meaning from their encounters with the world. What is crucial about this process of creating meanings is that it affects what we do, what we believe, even how we feel" (Bruner, 1990a, p. 345). *It is this volitional meaning which*

motivates us to choose our occupations. Motives do not push themselves into the scene of action from some subterranean existence. Rather, they are made in and emerge from the unfolding action and the unfolding stories of our lives (Figure 4.7).

References

Barris, R., Dickie, V., & Baron, K. (1988). A comparison of psychiatric patients and normal subjects based on the model of human occupation. *Occupational Therapy Journal of Research, 8*, 3–37. (R) Commentary by Mann, W., & Klyczek, J., in same issue. Response to Commentary by Barris, R., & Dickie, V., in same issue.

Barris, R., Kielhofner, G., Burch, R.M., Gelinas, I., Klement, M., & Schultz, B. (1986). Occupational function and dysfunction in three groups of adolescents. *Occupational Therapy Journal of Research, 6*, 301–317.

Bellah, R., Madsen, R., Sullivan, W., Swidler, A., & Tipton, S. (1985). *Habits of the heart.* Berkeley, CA: University of California Press.

Bruner, J. (1973). Organization of early skilled action. *Child Development, 44*, 1–11.

Bruner, J. (1990a). Culture and human development: A new look. *Human Development, 33*, 344–355.

Bruner, J. (1990b). *Acts of Meaning.* Cambridge, MA: Harvard University Press.

Burke, J.P. (1977). A clinical perspective on motivation: Pawn versus origin. *American Journal of Occupational Therapy, 31*, 254–258.

Connel, J.P. (1985). A new multidimensional measure of children's perceptions of control. *Child Development, 56*, 1018–1041.

Cottle, T.J. (1971). *Time's children: Impressions of youth.* Boston: Little, Brown & Co.

Csikszentmihalyi, M. (1990). *Flow: The psychology of optimal experience.* New York: Harper & Row.

DeCharms, R.E. (1968). *Personal causation: The internal affective determinants of behaviors.* New York: Academic Press.

Ebb, E.W., Coster, W., & Duncombe, L. (1989). Comparison of normal and psychosocially dysfunctional male adolescents. *Occupational Therapy in Mental Health, 9*(2), 53–74.

Elliott, M., & Barris, R. (1987). Occupational role performance and life satisfaction in elderly persons. *Occupational Therapy Journal of Research, 7*, 215–224.

Fein, M.L. (1990). *Role change: A resocialization perspective*. New York: Praeger.

Fiske, S. & Taylor, S.E. (1985). *Social cognition*. New York: Random House.

Geertz, C. (1986). Making experiences, authoring selves. In V. Turner & E. Bruner (Eds.), *The anthropology of experience*, (pp. 373–380). Urbana, IL: University of Illinois Press.

Gergen, K. J, & Gergen, M.M. (1983). Narratives of the self. In T.R. Sarbin & K.E. Scheibe (Eds.), *Studies in social identity*. New York: Praeger.

Gergen, K.J., & Gergen, M.M. (1988). Narrative and the self as relationship. In L. Berkowitz (Ed.), *Advances in experimental social psychology*, (pp. 17–56). San Diego: Academic Press.

Goodman, P. (1960). *Growing up absurd*. New York: Vintage Books.

Gregory, M. (1983). Occupational behavior and life satisfaction among retirees. *American Journal of Occupational Therapy, 37*, 548–553.

Grossack, M., & Gardner, H. (1970). *Man and men: Social psychology as social science*. Scranton, PA: International Textbook Co.

Hall, E.T. (1959). *The silent language*. Greenwich, CT: Fawcett Publications.

Hart, D.A. (1992). *Becoming men: The development of aspirations, values and adaptational styles*. New York: Plenum.

Harter, S. (1983). The development of the self-system. In M. Hetherington (Ed.), *Handbook of child psychology: Social and personality development* (Vol. 4). New York: John Wiley & Sons.

Harter, S. (1985). Competence as a dimension of self-evaluation: Toward a comprehensive model of self-worth. In R.L. Leahy (Ed.), *The development of the self*. Orlando, FL: Academic Press.

Harter, S. & Connel, J.P. (1984). A model of relationships among children's academic achievement and self-perceptions of competence, control, and motivation. In J. Nicholls (Ed.), *The development of achievement motivation*. Greenwich, CT: JAI.

Helfrich, C. & Kielhofner, G. (1994). Volitional narratives and the meaning of therapy. *American Journal of Occupational Therapy, 48*, 318–326.

Helfrich, C., Kielhofner, G., & Mattingly, C. (1994). Volition as narrative: Understanding motivation in chronic illness. *American Journal of Occupational Therapy, 48*, 311–317.

Kalish, R.A., & Collier, K.W. (1981). *Exploring human values*. Monterey, CA: Brooks/Cole.

Kerby, A.P. (1991). *Narrative and the self*. Bloomington, IN: Indiana University Press.

Kielhofner, G., & Burke, J. (1980). A model of human occupation, part one. Conceptual framework and content. *American Journal of Occupational Therapy, 34*, 572–581.

Kielhofner, G., & Burke, J. (1985). Components and determinants of occupation. In G. Kielhofner (Ed.), *A model of human occupation: Theory and application*. Baltimore: Williams & Wilkins.

Klavins, R. (1972). Work-play behavior: Cultural influences. *American Journal of Occupational Therapy, 26*, 176–179.

Kluckholn, C. (1951). Values and value orientations in the theory of action: An exploration in definition and classification. In T. Parsons & E. Shils (Eds.), *Toward a general theory of action*. Cambridge, MA: Harvard University Press.

Lee, D. (1971). Culture and the experience of value. In A.H. Maslow (Ed.), *Neural knowledge in human values*. Chicago: Henry Regnery.

Lefcourt, H. (1981). *Research with the locus of control construct, Vol. 1: Assessment and methods*. New York: Academic Press.

Lederer, J., Kielhofner, G., & Watts, J. (1985). Values, personal causation and skills of delinquents and non-delinquents. *Occupational Therapy in Mental Health, 5*(2), 59–77.

Mallinson, T. (1994). *Narrative analysis of the occupational performance history interview*. Unpublished masters thesis, University of Illinois at Chicago.

Markus, H. (1983). Self knowledge: An expanded view. *Journal of Personality, 51*, 543–562.

Markus, H., & Nurius, P. (1986). Possible selves. *American Psychologist, 41*, 954–969.

Matsutsuyu, J. (1969). The interest checklist. *American Journal of Occupational Therapy, 23*, 323–328.

Mattingly, C. (1991). The narrative nature of clinical reasoning. *American Journal of Occupational Therapy, 45*, 998–1005.

Mattingly, C., & Fleming, M. (1993). *Clinical reasoning: Forms of inquiry in a therapeutic practice*. Philadelphia: FA Davis.

Meyer, W.U. (1987). Perceived ability and achievement-related behavior. In F. Halisch & J. Kuhl (Eds.), *Motivation, intention and volition*. Berlin: Springer-Verlag.

Mitchell, A. (1983). *The nine American lifestyles*. New York: Macmillan.

Muñoz, J., Lawlor, M., & Kielhofner, G. (1993). Use of the model of human occupation: A survey of therapists in psychiatric practice. *Occupational Therapy Journal of Research, 13*(2), 117–139.

Murphy, R. (1987). *The body silent*. New York: WW Norton.

Patsy, D., & Kielhofner, G. (1989). *An exploratory study of psychosocial adaptation to spinal cord injury*. Unpublished manuscript.

Rotter, J.B. (1960). Generalized expectancies for internal versus external control of reinforcement. *Psychological Monographs: General Applications, 80*, 1–28.

Schafer, R. (1981). Narration in the psychoanalytic dialogue. In W.J.T. Mitchell (Ed.), *On narrative* (pp. 25–49). Chicago: University of Chicago Press.

Skinner, E.A., Chapman, M., & Baltes, P.B. (1988). Control, means-end, and agency beliefs: A new conceptualization and its measurement during childhood. *Journal of Personality and Social Psychology, 54*, 117–133.

Smith, M.B. (1969). *Social psychology and human values*. Chicago: Aldine.

Smith, N., Kielhofner, G., & Watts, J. (1986). The relationship between volition, activity pattern and life satisfaction in the elderly. *American Journal of Occupational Therapy, 40*, 278–283.

Smyntek, L., Barris, R., & Kielhofner, G. (1985). The model of human occupation applied to psychosocially functional and dysfunctional adolescents. *Occupational Therapy in Mental Health, 5*(1), 21–40.

Spence, D.P. (1982). *Narrative truth and historical truth: Meaning and interpretation in psychoanalysis*. New York, NY: WW Norton.

Taylor, C. (1989). *Sources of the self: The making of the modern identity*. Cambridge, MA: Harvard University Press.

White, M. (1989). The externalizing of the problem and the re-authoring of lives and relationships. In M. White (Ed.), *Selected Papers*. Adelaide, Australia: Dulwich Centre Publications. (Reprinted from *Dulwich Centre Newsletter*. (Summer 1989).

KEY CONCEPTS

VOLITION SUBSYSTEM
- system of dispositions and self-knowledge that predisposes and enables persons to anticipate, choose, experience, and interpret occupational behavior.

VOLITIONAL STRUCTURE
- stable pattern of dispositions and self-knowledge generated from and sustained by experience.
- **Dispositions:** cognitive/emotive orientations toward occupations.
- **Self-knowledge:** commonsense awareness of ourselves as actors in the world.
- Volitional dispositions and self-knowledge can be conceptualized as being comprised of three areas: values, personal causation, and interests.

PERSONAL CAUSATION
- collection of dispositions and self-knowledge concerning one's capacities for and efficacy in occupations; encompasses knowledge of capacity and sense of efficacy.
- **Knowledge of capacity:** awareness of present and potential abilities.
- **Sense of efficacy:** the perception of control over one's own behavior (and underlying thoughts and emotions) as well as a sense of control in achieving desired outcomes of behavior.

VALUES
- coherent set of convictions that assign significance or standards to occupations, creating a strong disposition to perform accordingly; encompasses personal convictions and sense of commitments.
- **Personal convictions:** a commonsense set of beliefs about what matters in life.
- **Sense of obligation:** strong emotional dispositions to follow what are perceived as right ways to behave.

INTERESTS
- dispositions to find pleasure and satisfaction in occupations and the self-knowledge of our enjoyment of occupations; encompasses attraction and preference.
- **Attraction:** a proclivity to enjoy certain occupations or certain aspects of performance.
- **Preference:** the propensity to enjoy particular ways of performing or particular activities over others.

VOLITIONAL PROCESS
- actual workings and procedures of attending, experiencing, choosing, and interpreting occupational behavior.

Attending
- paying attention to selected aspects of the world
- anticipating possibilities for action
- reacting to prospects for occupation

Experiencing
- finding occupations enjoyable or valuable
- feeling more or less able in occupations

Choosing
- Activity choices: selecting occupational activities in the course of daily life
- Occupational choices: decisions which involve commitment to sustaining behavior over time

Interpreting
- assigning volitional significance to experiences and behavior

VOLITIONAL NARRATIVES
- persons also understand themselves and choose their actions through stories.
- stories enable us to make sense of experience and make choices because the form of the story provides a mold into which persons can pour their aspirations, actions, and experiences.
- when humans engage in the volitional process of making sense of experience and making occupational choices, they draw upon the narrative mode which their culture provides as a way of making sense of experience anticipating the future.
- stories also give drama to our lives which makes them at once comprehensible and moving.

5/ Habituation Subsystem

Gary Kielhofner

INTRODUCTION

The question to which this chapter is addressed is neatly summed up in the following words:

Why then do people repeat themselves so much? Why do they do more or less the same thing every year at Christmas, or on their own birthdays, or every day as they go about their daily rounds, getting out of bed in the morning, washing, dressing, getting breakfast, reading the paper, opening the mail, walking to the garage or the station, talking to colleagues, telephoning the same people day after day, writing letters which are much like letters written on other days, stopping themselves going into the pub with a twinge of regret, as on other days? (Young, 1988, p. 75)

In large measure, everyday occupational behavior takes on this character of being much like previous performance. We engage in redundant patterns of time use. We carry out interactions with others that mimic previous encounters. We go about completing a range of tasks pretty much as we have before. This chapter addresses these familiar, routine, and automatic aspects of daily occupational behavior.

Since we do not deliberately choose these behaviors—and sometimes would have ourselves behave otherwise than we tend to—factors other than motivation must account for their occurrence. While such performance is characterized by its similarity to previous behavior, it is never exactly the same. Consequently, as noted in Chapter 2, it is not sufficient to evoke the idea of internalized instructions which simply cause such behaviors to unfold.

How then are these automatic ways of behaving possible? What allows humans to traverse so efficiently the familiar in the physical, temporal, and social world without overt or deliberate cognition to inform action, but with sufficient flexibility to sustain familiar performances within a range of varying circumstances?

The phenomena of humans repeating familiar patterns of behavior is explained in this chapter by the concept of a habituation subsystem. I will argue that through habituation people have ways of appreciating their physical, temporal, and sociocultural ecologies so that they can cooperate with those environments to efficiently and automatically assemble routine behavior.

Like all structures, the internal organization required for habituated patterns of behavior is created and altered by ongoing action. Habituation allows persons to select from possible behaviors a subset that constitute a way of performing. Thus, habituated patterns have preselected, from all possible behavioral combinations, certain ways of doing things. Note that it is a way of doing, rather than specific actions, that are preselected in habituated structure. Consequently, the habituation subsystem structure contributes to the similarity of *ways of behaving* across time. By virtue of making a way of performing likely to be repeated again and again, habituation structure evokes the very behaviors that sustain its current organization (Figure 5.1). Habituation thus feeds off of its own redundancy.

As I noted earlier, habituated behavior is not mechanically produced according to inter-

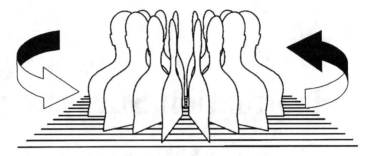

Figure 5.1.   Habituation evokes the very behaviors that sustain its current organization.

nalized instructions. Rather, habituation relies on a network of organized appreciative tendencies. These enable the human being, without deliberation or attention (to the features of behavior which are habituated), to improvise (or dynamically assemble) similar ways of behaving in similar circumstances across time.

Redundancy in the external environment is also necessary for persons to reproduce familiar behavior. People continually find themselves located in more or less the same situations. The physical environment is much the same day after day. The recurring patterns, such as day and night, work week and weekend, provide the redundant temporal structure within which we unfold our routines. Similarly, the social order around us has sufficient regularity to allow us to mostly experience "known" situations for which we have ways of responding. Because of the stability and redundancy of our environments, much of the time we find ourselves grounded in the familiar, not having to consciously calculate our moves. As Young (1988) notes, habituated performances are "generated and locked into place by recurrences" (p. 79). These recurrences are both in our contexts and in our behavior.

I will use two concepts, habits and roles, to explain habituation. Together, habits and roles weave the patterns with which we typically traverse our days, weeks, and seasons; our homes, neighborhoods, and cities; and our families, work organizations, and communities. In each of these temporal, physical, and social contexts we perform a wide range of occupations. Habits and roles give regularity, character, and order to those occupations.

HABITS

Concern with habits and their role in healthy occupation dates to the earliest occupational therapy literature. Pioneering occupational therapy writers claimed that habits are organizing and regulatory mechanisms which must be in good order for daily life to proceed effectively (Meyer, 1922; Kidner, 1924; Slagle, 1922). Early writers hypothesized that habits reflected and therefore organized behavior so as to be effective in one's environment. They also recognized that habits could be generated only by actual doing, and that in the absence of regular performance, habits atrophied much like muscles atrophy with disuse. As we will see, these basic conceptualizations of habits still appear valid.

Despite the familiarity of habit as an everyday notion (for example, the common reference we make to good and bad habits), habits are curiously complex phenomena. Moreover, habits are not well understood. As Camic (1986) argues, they are undeservedly neglected in current theorizing about human behavior. Nonetheless, a few scholars have offered conceptualizations of habit from which the present theory is constructed.

In the following words, Young (1988) describes one of the defining characteristics of habits—that they are automatic rather than deliberate:

> Once fully launched, I may have no more than a vague sense that my mind is working while I am not looking, as though my actions hardly belong to me. Who has not occasionally had to feel whether the toothbrush is damp to make sure that it has just been used? (p. 81)

Young's notion of vague awareness is an apt description of our experience of habits. Habitual behavior is not entirely unconscious. Rather, habitual performances tend to fade in and out of conscious realization. Circumstances often have a lot to do with just how conscious habitual behavior is. For example, encountering an icy road, waking up late, or the presence of a work supervisor may occasion more conscious monitoring of behaviors which otherwise unfold with much less attention. On the other hand, preoccupation with an upcoming circumstance or conversation may drive habitual aspects of behavior entirely out of awareness. When we are conscious of our habitual behavior, our awareness is different from when we encounter a new situation and must act deliberately. Rather, consciousness seems to flow along and collaborate with our habits when we are engaged in familiar routines. Habitual behavior appears to hover about the fringes of consciousness. Habits cooperate with our conscious direction when it is warranted and otherwise allow our attention to deal with different matters.

Camic (1986) describes habits as "a more or less self-actuating disposition or tendency to engage in a previously adopted or acquired form of action" (p. 1044). Consistent with this idea that habitual behavior is influenced by a latent disposition acquired from experience, Dewey (1922) defined habits as activity

which is influenced by prior activity and in that sense acquired; which contains within itself a certain ordering or systematization of minor elements of action; which is projective, dynamic in quality, ready for overt manifestation; and which

is operative in some subdued subordinate form even when not obviously dominating activity (p. 40)

Dewey's definition adds the important recognition that habits organize smaller units of behavior, which he refers to as minor elements of action. Consequently, habits exert their organizing influence at a mid-level between the smallest unit of behavior and lifestyle. Habits serve as "middlemen" between the capacities we exercise and the way of life we lead. Habits, thus, have a wide range of influence on our actions.

From the above discussion, we can construct a definition of habits as *latent tendencies acquired from previous repetitions, mainly operating at a preconscious level and influencing a wide range of behavioral patterns that correspond to familiar habitats* (Figure 5.2).

Regulated Improvisation: The Habit Map

The idea of habits being well-learned patterns of behavior that unfold without deliberation can suggest an image of habits as prepackaged behavioral strings that simply unfold in a mechanistic fashion. But as I have noted, this is not the case. While habits do regulate behavior according to some kind of broad pattern or template, habitual behavior requires improvisation to accommodate the inevitable novel elements of each new behavioral situation.

Dewey (1922) recognized that habits operate in cooperation with context: "Habits are ways of using and incorporating the environment in which the latter has its say as surely as

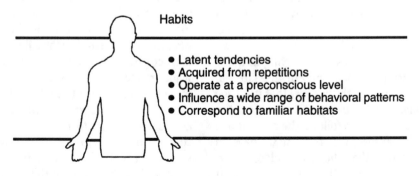

Figure 5.2. Habits.

the former" (p. 15). This means that a habit regulates behavior not by a strict set of encoded instructions for behavior, but by providing the individual with a regulated *manner* of dealing with environmental contingencies. In this regard, Dewey (1922) notes:

> The essence of habit is an acquired disposition to *ways* or modes of response, not to particular acts except as, under special conditions, these express a way of behaving. Habit means special sensitiveness or accessibility to certain classes of stimuli . . . rather than bare recurrence of specific acts. (p. 42)

Camic (1986) echoes this idea, noting that while habitual behavior may be automatic and without deliberation, it is no more mechanical than action which is guided by conscious reflection. Young (1988) points out that habits have rules that guide automatic behavior, but goes on to explain that "these rules are flexible, more like the grammar than a particular sentence" (p. 91).

Koestler (1969) also refers to habits as being regulated by rules which constrain but do not dictate behavior. According to him, they operate much like the rules of a game which keep order among players by letting them know how to play the game without dictating in advance what all their moves should be. Bourdieu (1977) makes a similar reference to habits as "a system of lasting, transposable dispositions which, integrating past experiences, functions at every moment as a *matrix of perceptions, appreciations and actions*" (p. 82).

Together Koestler and Bourdieu's ideas pave the way for understanding how habits influence and guide our behavior. Experience in the environment generates a generalized set of rules for how we can effectively traverse a period of time, a particular occupation, or a physical environment. What is internalized is a set of rules that serve as a map giving us a way to appreciate the topography of the external world. When we intuitively know that it is time for breakfast, what turn to take next on the route home, what step follows the current one in preparing a meal, it is because we have an internalized map that allows us to locate ourselves in the midst of the external world. It gives us our bearings, locating us in unfolding

events and allowing us to steer our behavior to the next occurrences which we tacitly anticipate.

Just as what one sees while driving (i.e., the road ahead, road signs, the actual terrain) is not isomorphic with the symbols on a road map, the events of everyday life do not fit perfectly with our habit maps. But we know when we are in circumstances for which we have a habit map because they have the feature of recognizability or familiarity. Indeed, so long as we experience the world as familiar, habits operate smoothly and without need of attention. It is the unfamiliarity (i.e., that for which we do not have an internalized map) that extricates us from our habitual way of doing things. The habit map provides us with a framework for appreciating or "reading" both the environment and unfolding events and for constructing behavior to achieve the purpose of the habit. Consequently, the habit map (see Figure 5.3) is defined as *internalized appreciative capacities which allow the perception of familiar events and contexts and guide the related construction of action toward accomplishing some implicit outcome or process.*

Purpose and Function of Habits

Since habits are formed from previous performances in a specific environment, they represent an accommodation to the features of that context. That is, habits *preserve a way we have learned to do* from earlier performance in the environment. It is only after a behavior proves effective in some way, and is therefore repeated over and over, that it becomes habituated. We may take the wrong turn on a journey, but with repetition such ineffective or inefficient action is weeded out. Repeated journeys incorporate and eventually put into place correct turns for reaching the destination. In a whole range of tasks, persons settle into ways of performing actions that are realized over time and that incorporate more or less successful ways of performing. This is not to say that all habits represent the most efficient ways to accomplish tasks or undertake a process, but the odds are that habits incorporate ways of doing things that have a certain

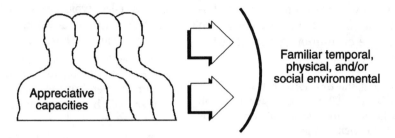

Figure 5.3. Habit map.

value within the environment in which they are performed.

Young (1988) argues that habits serve as a kind of self-perpetuating *flywheel* conserving patterns of action. Once established, habits will act as control parameters (as discussed in Chapter 2), influencing the manner of unfolding behavior. Once launched into place by the convergence of facilitating environmental factors, habits provide a momentum that allows aspects of behavior to unfold on their own. This frees up conscious attention for other purposes. In this regard James (1950) notes:

> The more of the details of our daily life we can hand over to the effortless custody of automatism, the more our higher powers of mind will be set free for their own proper work. There is no more miserable human being than one in whom nothing is habitual but indecision, and for whom the lighting of every cigar, the drinking of every cup, the time of rising and going to bed every day, and the beginning of every bit of work, are subjects of express volitional deliberations. Full half the time of such a man goes to the deciding, or regretting, of matters which ought to be so ingrained in him as practically not to exist for his consciousness at all. (p. 122)

As James alludes, habits can allow two or more behaviors to occur simultaneously. While one is performing habituated behaviors (getting dressed in the morning, driving home after work) it is possible to engage in other thoughts and behaviors (e.g., making a phone call, planning a meeting, listening to the radio).

The degree to which habits free us up in everyday life is illustrated by Murphy's (1987) description of how, with a progressive physical disability, his habitual behavior had to be replaced with conscious strategies:

> This was true of even the simplest actions. In transferring from wheelchair to toilet, bed, or armchair, I had to park in a carefully chosen position and set the brakes, lest the wheelchair fly out from under me. I next would plot my strategy for getting up, choosing my supports with care, calculating the number of steps it would take to reach my target. When I no longer was able to walk or stand, such transfers became impossible, and my movements became even more restricted, the obstacles more imposing. The house had become a battlefield, my movements well thought out strategies against a constant foe. (p. 76)

As the quote illustrates, a physical impairment can replace habit as a control parameter, shifting performance from automatic to deliberate. By serving, in ordinary life, as a web of tendencies that gather up and direct a whole range of actions, habits hold together the patterns of our behavior that give life its familiar and relatively effortless character. When some factor interferes, efficiency is lost and additional energy is required.

Habits also serve a purpose for society. Young (1988) notes that habits shared by a group of people constitute customs. These customs, in turn, guide new members of a group to develop habits that reflect the group's way of doing things. Thus, by acquiring habits, humans become carriers and messengers of the customs that make up the way of life of a particular group. The habits of each individual serve to sustain these important features of group life. Moreover, in a group one person's habitual behavior may be part of the environmental context necessary for another's habits.

For example, Rowles (1991) provided the following description of a group of elderly men engaging in the custom of gathering at the post office:

> Every morning, shortly before 10:00 a.m., Walter takes a leisurely 400-yard stroll down the hill from his house to the trailer that serves as the post office to "pick up the mail." He traces exactly the same path each day. Several male age peers from different locations within Colton embark on the same trip at about the same time . . . picking up the mail provides a rationale for an informal gathering of the elderly men of the community at the bench outside the Colton Store, which is located adjacent to the post office. The men generally linger throughout the morning. They watch the passing traffic, converse with patrons of the store, and discuss events of the day. Then, around lunch time, the group disperses and Walter wends his way home again. (p. 268)

Walter's habit of getting the mail and meeting with other older residents of Colton not only organizes his morning, but also contributes to sustaining the local custom. If Walter and others could not be counted on to show up, the custom could not exist.

By shaping behavior to correspond to features of the social environment, habits guide behavior to take advantage of, and be in harmony with, critical features of the social environment (Cardwell, 1971). Our typical behaviors are, consequently, recognizable by others in the environment. The norms and customs for behavior provided by the social environment find their ways into the habit map. For example, habits of punctuality and industri-

ousness reflect typical expectations of Western society: one is to be at work, meetings, and appointments at scheduled times and to focus on the task at hand during periods of time so designated. If a person routinely fails to be punctual or to attend to the work tasks, the habit pattern will be out of synchrony with the environment.

In sum, habits are tendencies to produce patterns of behavior which are ecologically-relevant and efficient. Moreover, habits serve efficiency by reducing the amount of conscious effort required for performance, freeing up persons for other simultaneous activity. Habits also allow a person to be integrated into the smooth functioning of society. Finally, habits make the individual a carrier of customs and thus perpetuate social groups.

Influence of Habits in Daily Occupations

The concept of habit may refer to a broad spectrum of behavioral patterning (Camic, 1986). As illustrated in Figure 5.4, habits organize occupational behavior into patterns in three ways: (a) habits influence how a particular activity is regularly performed; (b) habits regulate how time is typically used; and (c) habits generate styles of behavior that characterize a range of occupational performances.

Habits of Occupational Performance

To point out that each person has his or her own way of performing specific activities is to highlight what is painfully obvious. However, the fact that each person has a particular way of completing familiar activities is hardly triv-

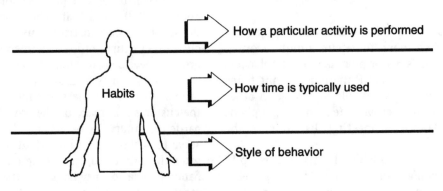

Figure 5.4.   Influence of habits on occupation.

ial. Whether these habits fit with our ideas about proper etiquette or form, represent a particular flair, recall the way a parent or mentor performed the task, or simply emanate from what is simplest and most efficient, people tend to be firmly entrenched in ways of doing familiar activities.

Camic (1986) refers to this aspect of habits as dispositions "to perform certain relatively elementary and specific activities skillfully" (p. 1045). Such habits refer to the routine of familiar actions that have become automatic: the manner of dressing oneself, the route one drives to work, the way one makes a favorite dish, and so on. Seamon (1980) eloquently refers to such habits as body ballets, noting that they are, "a set of integrated behaviors which sustain a particular task or aim" (p. 157).

Because habitual ways of performing such activities contribute to our efficiency and effectiveness, they are sometimes referred to as skill—for example, the skill of dressing oneself. In this text (see Chapter 7) we refer to skill as a more discrete feature of performance, such as being able to reach or to sequence actions. When I speak of a series of actions organized together to constitute a recognizable activity or occupational behavior, I am referring to a habit. Dewey (1922) similarly referred to habits, regarding such performances as playing a musical instrument and typewriting as habits. He noted that as such they were "passive tools waiting to be called into action" (Dewey, 1922, p. 24).

Habits of Routine

The influence of habits is also found in the rounds of behavior that characterize the routine. Chapin (1968) points out that we perform within temporal cycles of different magnitude. For example, cycles may be daily, weekly, or annual. Within these differing cycles, habitual use of time can be recognized:

> . . . cooking, eating and washing dishes during the twenty-four hour period of a day; the work, school, shopping, recreation or socializing routine during a seven day week; visiting out-of-town relatives and family vacation or other holiday outing routines during a year's time . . . (p. 13)

Such cyclical habits allow fulfillment of biological needs (e.g., needs for nourishment, exercise, and rest), of psychological needs for rhythm and alternations of modes of behavior (e.g., the rhythm of work and leisure), and social needs to coordinate action of members of a group. For example, work shifts, regular meetings, and periodic informal and formal gatherings of persons allow the coordination of collective action.

While no two days are exactly the same, most persons have and can identify a routine which is typical for a given day of the week. In industrialized societies persons generally have patterns that characterize workdays and alternate patterns that characterize weekends or days off from work or school. The optimal degree of consistency in a habit pattern depends on the individual's roles and environment. Some environments demand a fixed routine such as the grade school or factory schedule that requires persons to show up, do certain tasks, take lunch and breaks, and terminate the day at specific times. Other environments allow a much more flexible pattern of behavior.

Habits of routine can become quite fixed and important for most persons. Seamon (1980) refers to them as time-space routines and notes that they can fill a considerable portion of one's day. He offers the following description of such a routine:

> He would be up at seven-thirty, make his bed, perform his morning toilet, and be out of his house by eight. He would then walk to the corner cafe up the street, pick up the newspaper (which *had* to be the *New York Times*), order his usual fare (one scrambled egg, toast, and coffee), and stay there until around nine when he would walk to his nearby office. (p. 158)

In contrast, Murphy (1987) describes a quite different daily routine through which he and his wife accommodate his physical impairment:

> A typical day starts when [my wife] awakens me at 8 a.m. and removes my night table, along with its array of support gadgetry—phone, intercom, TV remote, bed control, light switch, and water. She then washes the lower part of my body, a procedure that requires that she roll me first on my right side, then on the left. This is not an easy job, because my body is absolute dead

weight, totally inert. After I am bathed, she rolls me back and forth again to get my pants on, following which she must roll me again to position a sling under my body. The sling is then attached to a Hoyer lift, a wheeled, hand-operated hydraulic crane that picks me up and moves me from place to place. Yolanda hoists me, then pushes the lift over to the wheelchair, and lowers me into it. Then I go into the bathroom for the next stage of my morning ablutions . . . I brush my own teeth, using a toothbrush with a special thick handle, but Yolanda first must squeeze the toothpaste tube—my grip is no longer strong enough. Since I cannot lean forward over the sink on my own, she has to push my head over it so that I can rinse my mouth afterward. She then gets my shaving equipment ready and soaps the brush; I do the rest, using a razor with a built-up handle. There will come a time, not too far away, when I will be unable to shave myself, at which point I probably will grow a beard. After shaving, a tedious chore now, Yolanda bathes my upper body and washes my hair. Total time for the morning routine is about an hour, so I usually pass up the bathing and shampoo on the mornings when I go to school. (p. 197)

Whatever our abilities or limitations, habits of routine help locate us effectively within the stream of time. They enable us to get done what we have to do, or want to do with efficiency and predictability.

Habits of Style

Dewey (1922) noted that one's habits were reflected in a typical "style of . . . being-in-the-world" (p. 20). Such characteristics as being big-picture versus detail-oriented, quick versus plodding, or prompt versus procrastinating are examples of styles of performance regulated by habits. Style is a manner of conduct which manifests itself across a whole range of activities. Camic (1986) defines such habits as:

> the durable and generalized disposition that suffuses a person's action throughout an entire domain of life or, in the extreme instance, throughout all of life—in which case the term comes to mean the whole manner, turn, cast, or mold of the personality. (p. 1045)

Indeed, the convergence of an individual's habits of style do give a unique and stable character to his or her performance.

Summary

The concept of habits has been proposed as a way of explaining how we organize patterns of time use, ways of performing occupations, and characteristic styles that typify our occupational behavior. Habits consist of an internalized map which provides one with an abstract set of rules for appreciating and constructing behavior within one's typical temporal, physical, and social ecologies. Learned from previous repetitions of behavior, habits operate on the borders of consciousness to guide the stable patterns of behavior that characterize everyday life.

INTERNALIZED ROLES

Routine occupational behavior is also influenced by the fact that each of us belongs to and behaves in social systems. Much of our occupational behavior is done *as* a spouse, parent, worker, student, and so on. The presence of these and other roles help assure that behavior has both regularity and relevance to appropriate social systems.

The phenomenon of roles in social life has been the subject of extensive theorizing in the social sciences. Role theory addresses two fundamental problems (Katz & Kahn, 1966). The first is how social systems sustain themselves. The second is how individuals learn and manage to behave as members of society. In response to the first problem, role theory views the role as a fundamental unit of social groups (Turner, 1962). That is, social organizations are conceptualized as composed of roles rather than persons. This is not to say that the person who inhabits a role has no influence on the social system. Rather, role theory asserts that the patterns of organization that make up social systems depend on a number of defined statuses and related behaviors that make up a social organization. For example, traditional families are composed of spouses, parents, and children; workplaces are composed of staff and supervisors; classrooms include teachers and students. While different persons can occupy the roles over time, most features of the social system remain stable since it is composed of enduring roles that shape new members' attitudes and behaviors.

In response to the second problem of how persons manage to produce appropriate social behavior, role theory argues that persons acquire and learn roles (Fein, 1990). The expectations that others hold for a role and the nature of the social system in which the role is located serve as guides for learning how to behave within that role. Thus, through interaction with others possibly before and as one enters the role, one learns an identity, an outlook, and a way of behaving that belongs to the role. With this learning a person internalizes the role. It is internalized roles that most concern us here, since our purpose is to explain the influence of roles on persons' patterned occupational behavior. Consequently, I will refer to an internalized role as *a broad awareness of a particular social identity and related obligations which together provide a framework for appreciating relevant situations and constructing appropriate behavior* (Figure 5.5).

Internalizing a set of roles is not an insignificant matter. As Sarbin and Scheibe (1983) note, effective behavior depends on the "correct placements of self in the world of occurrences" (p. 8). Without an understanding of one's role to provide a sense of one's relationship to others and of expected performance, it is impossible to construct competent social behavior.

Role Identification

As Sarbin and Scheibe (1983) note, "a person's identity at any time is a function of his or her validated social positions. These positions are validated through appropriate, proper, and convincing role enactments" (p. 7). We see ourselves as students, workers, parents, and so on because we recognize ourselves as occupying certain statuses or positions and also because we experience ourselves behaving *as* a person in these roles. Moreover, the process of identification of the role is abetted by the fact that we see ourselves reflected in the attitudes and behaviors of others toward us (Sarbin & Scheibe, 1983). Others (even those who do not know us personally) typically see us in terms of the roles we hold. The public identity of roles allow us to effectively locate ourselves in the humanscape of social relations. We are never total strangers to others when we have a defined role relationship. Interaction is made less problematic because we and others share fundamental expectations of what it means to be in a given role relationship. When we enter a classroom as student or professor or when we meet a potential boss in a job interview, we have a whole class of expectations for what kinds of relationships and interactions will or could occur. In essence, we know with *whom* we are dealing and *who* we should be.

It is not surprising, then, that who we are becomes intertwined with the roles we inhabit (Cardwell, 1971; Ruddock, 1976; Schein, 1971; Turner, 1962). Our public and personal identities are suffused with our roles. This is not to say that everyone who inhabits a given role experiences the same role identity. Rather, the internalized role is personal. As Fein (1990) notes, a person's "own way of understanding what she is doing defines her role. It is her intentions and understandings which make the role what it is" (p. 13). Nonetheless, we do come to see ourselves, judge our behavior, and as-

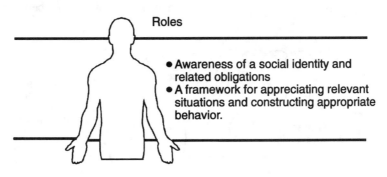

Figure 5.5. Roles.

sign worth to ourselves in terms of our own understanding of the roles we inhabit. What we believe those roles connote and how we see ourselves carrying out the roles constitute a significant measure of what we know ourselves to be. As Miller (1983) argues, personal identity is the integrated collection of our awareness of all our various roles.

Role identity is kept in place by the fact that others recognize and respond to us as occupying the role. Moreover, as we come to think of ourselves and experience ourselves acting in a role it becomes an essential part of our self-understanding. We are hard put to describe to anyone who we are without some reference to the roles we fill.

Role Scripts

While the terminology varies somewhat, role theorists generally agree that persons know how to produce appropriate role behavior because of an internalized role script. Miller (1983) defines this internal script as "a set of schemas that organize how persons perceive, communicate, make judgements, and act toward others" (p. 319). These scripts allow persons to make sense of events because the script anticipates what kind of interaction or actions should occur (Mancuso & Sarbin, 1983). Similarly, Fein (1990) notes,

> Lurking behind all roles are role scripts. These are the structures that guide people during the performance of their behavior patterns. They give role players a general idea of what is expected of them and with whom they are supposed to interact. These scripts are not explicit sets of instructions, but guidelines for how to improvise a part. (p. 18)

Role scripts, like habit maps, do not specify the details of performance, but rather provide parameters that allow the person to improvise or assemble behavior in unfolding circumstances. Role scripts (see Figure 5.6) can be defined as *a collection of appreciative capacities that guide comprehension of social situations and expectations, and the related construction of action that enacts a given role.* In interactions, role scripts allow one to appreciate that a particular kind of social event is underway, that the event is likely to have a particular course or outcome, and that one should behave in a particular way in this event. This is not to say that social actors must consciously plot all their actions. Rather, role scripts allow intuitive appreciation of situations and automatic assembly of behavior. As with habits, role behavior is often preconscious, operating with a vague awareness of what is happening and of what one is doing. More importantly, we find ourselves ordinarily performing a range of role-related interactions or behaviors without reflection, but with remarkable consistency. We more or less fall into the pattern of the role as a well-worn pathway, knowing who we are being and what we are doing at a very tacit level.

Fein (1990) also notes that, since roles are negotiated in interactions, the expectations and behaviors of others combine with the role script to guide the improvisation of behavior. Stryker (1968) highlights the improvisational nature of interactional role behavior, describing it as "a subtle, tentative, probing interchange among actors in given situations that continually reshapes both the form and the context of the interaction" (p. 559).

It is also important to remember that like habitual behavior, role behavior represents a

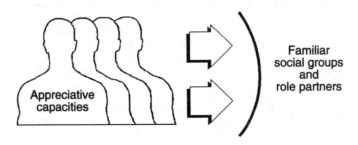

Figure 5.6.   Role scripts.

generalized way of behaving. The actual behaviors that make up any occasion of role behavior are too dependent on circumstances to be specified in advance. Nevertheless, by virtue of our role scripts we know *how* to behave. Moreover, role scripts require, call upon, and assemble smaller units of behavior into a coherent series of actions. For example, the skills we use to communicate are orchestrated together by the role script.

Purpose and Function of Roles

Roles provide a means for many individual needs to be met. Roles provide avenues of engaging in occupational behavior for the individual by giving purpose and identity to those behaviors. While roles place expectations on persons for task performance and time use, they also provide structure and regularity to life. Like habits, roles allow much of our behavior to be routine and automatic. Finally, by having a complement of roles we experience rhythm and change between these different identities and modes of doing (Shannon, 1970).

Roles also provide a means of channeling one's action into patterns and tasks required by various social systems. By engaging in role behavior, the individual satisfies social needs for individual participation. As I have noted, role performance is necessary for the functioning of social systems. Parents in the family system must provide a source of income, maintain the household, and provide instruction, guidance and authority for children. The other parent, children, relatives, neighbors, and the community at large are affected when someone in the parent role does not perform his or her share of the functions necessary for maintaining the family system. In this way, all social groups depend on expectable kinds of behaviors from persons who occupy given roles in the group. By sharing mutual expectations and by producing complementary behaviors, members of groups sustain the social order. For this reason, roles often function to constrain or direct behavior. After all, because our role behavior ordinarily affects others in complementary roles, they have a stake in our role behavior. Roles may vary in how formally they are defined. In traditional social systems roles may be very rigid and well defined; people who occupy the roles are expected to conform to a whole range of specified role behaviors. In other social systems, roles are more open or ambiguous. This is especially the case in new or changing social systems. For example, the traditional family is no longer the mode for a large percentage of families in western society. Single parent and multi-generational families, families with same-sex partners, and other arrangements are becoming more and more common. Traditional role definitions do not readily apply in such families and roles may be up for negotiation. I will examine further this aspect of changing roles in society at the end of this chapter.

Each of us ordinarily has a complement of roles which include some that are more formal and well defined and others that are more flexible. It is helpful to think of such roles as having varying degrees of resolution. Roles with high resolution are more well defined with less room for individual negotiation of the role map. Roles with low resolution may give us wide berth to establish our own role maps. In the end, however, the obligatory dimension of roles emerges because one or more people who belong to the same social system and occupy reciprocating roles have a stake in how we behave.

Types of Roles

The types of social roles that an individual may internalize have traditionally been categorized as personal-sexual, familial-social, and occupational roles (Heard, 1977; Katz & Kahn, 1966). Only the latter were originally considered to be of concern to occupational therapy (Matsutsuyu, 1971). These occupational roles were identified as player, student, homemaker, worker, and retiree. Later it was argued that a given role may have personal-sexual, familial-social, and occupational dimensions (Oakley, Kielhofner, Barris, & Reichler, 1986). A role is recognized as having an occupational dimension if it provides an avenue for expression of play or leisure, or if it requires productive behavior. For example, the role of spouse would incorporate both opportunities and expectations for familial behavior and occupational behavior. A number of roles which provide opportunities for, and which expect, occupational behavior have been delineated (Oakley, Kielhofner, Barris, & Reichler, 1986). Table 5.1 details these roles and their definitions.

Influence of Roles on Occupational Behavior

As illustrated in Figure 5.7, we can recognize that roles organize occupational behavior in three ways. First, they influence our manner and style as well as the content of our interactions with others. Second, they influence the sets of tasks or performances that become part of our role-related routine. Third, they partition our daily and weekly cycles into times when we ordinarily inhabit certain roles, creating temporal topography of our changing status and obligations across the day and week.

Style of Action

Moving from one role mode to another is often demarcated by such changes as how we dress, our manner of speech, and our way of relating to others. Persons may take on a degree of responsibility and authority and have certain concerns when they are acting as parents or supervisors versus the egalitarian air they assume when acting as spouses and colleagues. An interesting example of this is that, when my wife or I call the other at work, we more or less immediately know whether or not the other is alone. The cue that allows this inference is that our tone of voice and mode of conversation (if we are alone and thus not feeling tethered to our work role) is more intimate. Conversely, we know when the other is with a work colleague because the manner of conversing belongs to the work and not the spouse role.

The role script provides one with a subliminal awareness of being in a role and acts as a framework guiding behavior relevant to that role. As noted earlier, this does not mean that the role causes or determines the behavior. Rather, roles serve as frameworks for perceiving and acting that influence how one behaves and experiences one's own and other persons' behavior (Katz & Kahn, 1966). Awareness of being in a role colors our outlook, attitude, and behavior.

Table 5.1   Roles with Occupational Dimensions

Role	Occupational Behavior Within the Role
Student	Attending school on a part-time or full-time basis
Worker	Part-time or full-time paid employment
Volunteer	Donating services to a hospital, school, community, neighborhood, political campaign or similar benefit
Caregiver	Responsibility for the care of someone such as a child, spouse, relative, or friend
Home maintainer	Responsibility for the upkeep of a home such as house cleaning or yardwork
Friend	Visiting or doing something with a friend
Family member	Splending time or doing something with a family member such as one's partner child, or parent
Religious participant	Participation in activities sponsored by a religious organization
Hobbyist/amateur	Involvement in a hobby or amateur activity such as sewing, playing a musical instrument, woodworking, sports, theater, or participation in a club or team
Participant in an organization	Involvement in an organization such as the American Legion, National Organization for Women, Parents Without Partners, or Weight Watchers

Occupational Behaviors of Roles

Much of role theory focuses on the influence of roles on public and, in particular, interactional behavior. Nonetheless, from our concern with how internalized roles influence occupational behavior, we recognize that role obligations bind us to behaviors outside the social context of that role. For example, when I am shopping for Christmas or birthday presents for my children, or when I am grading student papers at home, I am just as surely fulfilling the parental and professorial roles as when I am interacting with my students or children. Consequently, we recognize that roles influence a whole round of occupational behavior that makes up everyday life. Within each role we encounter expectations for a range of occupational behavior. Among other

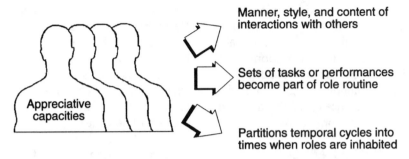

Figure 5.7. Influence of roles on occupational behavior.

things, a student is expected to attend class, take notes, ask questions, read articles or books, complete assignments, study, and take exams. A worker who is a secretary may be expected to answer the phone, take messages, type, take shorthand, and so on. Thus, every role represents a collection of occupational behaviors that become locally defined as belonging to that role. Once we have internalized the role and the expectations for occupational performance that accompany it, the role script helps orchestrate the various occupations we perform in that role.

Temporal Order of Roles

Like habits, roles are tied to cyclical time or recurrences. That is, understanding of one's roles includes the image one holds of when one is typically in a given role. The course of each day ordinarily involves a succession of roles and sometimes includes overlapping roles. By occupying parts of our daily routine, roles give regularity to our occupational behavior. They are social spaces that we enter, behave within, and exit as our days, weeks, and lives proceed.

Summary

I have used the concept of internalized roles to explain patterns of behavior which characterize our performance and correspond to features of the social environment. Roles refer to positions within social groups or organizations. The internalized role refers to the incorporation of an identity that defines one as occupying the role and the acquisition of a role script. The internalized role gives one a way of appreciating and constructing behavior for familiar social situations and for organizing one's time and task performance to fulfill role obligations.

STRUCTURE OF HABITUATION

The purpose in this chapter has been to explain that which is patterned, familiar, and routine in everyday performance. I have argued that these features of occupational behavior are influenced by a habituation subsystem. The structure of the habituation subsystem consists of two intersecting phenomena, habits and internalized roles. This habituation structure is an organization of appreciative capacities (role scripts and habit maps) which allow us to more or less automatically recognize features and situations in the environment and to construct behavior accordingly. Through our habits and roles we inhabit and belong to our physical, temporal, and social environments.

The concept of role argues that people perform within positions in a social group, exhibiting patterns of interaction, task performance, and time use which reflect expectations associated with the role. Other aspects of an individuals's routine, ways of performing occupations, and style are regulated by habits. Routine behavior within a role, but not specifically required or expected by the role, is regulated by habits. Thus, habits and roles are interwoven in daily life and reciprocally organize routine behavior.

Habits and roles are most adaptive when they are learned under recurrent conditions which have enough similarity to allow a way of doing things to emerge, but which are sufficiently different to allow flexibility in the maps or scripts that are acquired. Each time someone repeats a performance with a minor variation, the internalized habit or role becomes less literal and more flexible; that is, it is able to accommodate a range of variations while still achieving a given task or process. Thus, a well-organized but not overly rigid habituation structure allows a balance of stability and flexibility in everyday behavior.

HABITUATION PROCESS

We can conceptualize habituation as involving process in two time scales. The first, immediate time scale, is how the habit map and role script guide the assembly of behavior in everyday life. The second, extended time scale, provides a perspective of how habits and roles are formed and how they change over time. In this section, I will examine the habituation process in both ways.

Orderly Improvisation of Occupational Behavior

I have noted that the habit map and role script are not exact instructions for behavior. Rather, they are appreciative frameworks which enable one to interact with the external environment in such a way that one is facilitated to improvise within the task being performed. Moreover, roles and habits will often interrelate to guide actual improvisation of performance in daily life. For example, all of us have internalized habits of casual greetings. Greetings are so automatic that we perform them numerous times throughout the day with little or no thought. They may be very short, consisting of a mere gesture or word, or more extended, with some appropriate small talk or shop talk. When we encounter a neighbor, stranger, colleague, or friend, we appreciate the situation and can engage in an appropriate casual greeting. At the same time, our role and that of the person we encounter also influence how we participate in the greeting interaction.

When I recognize a student on campus, I need not recount to myself that I am a professor with a set of expected relationships toward students. Rather, I behave as a professor, more or less automatically engaging in what I readily and unreflectively know the student will recognize as a cordial and interested greeting. Depending on such factors as whether we are passing in the hall or sharing an elevator, on how well I know the student, and on whether either of us seems in a hurry to get somewhere, some brief conversation may also occur as part of the greeting. For example, we may chat about how the program is going, about an upcoming exam, and so on. It is not the intimate conversation I have with my children or wife, nor is it necessarily the intellectual or organized argumentation I might have with a professorial colleague in a faculty meeting or seminar. Thus, my twofold appreciation of my role as professor and of this situation as a casual greeting between a student and professor allows me to participate in the encounter and to arrange my behavior with great improvisational efficiency that is sensitive to a whole variety of relevant circumstances. All sorts of available information (e.g., knowledge of an imminent exam, awareness of a recent problem in the class, the appearance of stress on the student's face, a personal bit of information I have about the student) may come to play in how I improvise the interaction. Also important for the interaction is the student's behavior in the encounter—behavior that the student is improvising based on his or her role script and on my behaviors. Yet we engage in the behavior relatively effortlessly and both leave the interaction knowing that a casual greeting between a professor and student has taken place.

As in this example, all habituation processes involves a subtle transaction between the internalized habit and/or role, the unfolding events of moment-by-moment action, and the contingencies of context. Habituation plants us in the familiar territory of everyday life ready to interact with that physical, temporal, and social ecology in the making of our routine behavior. To the degree that our behavior flows naturally with the vagaries of our habitats, it is habituation that is guiding the process.

CHANGE IN HABITUATION

While it is a force for constancy and stability in behavior, habituation nevertheless changes over the course of the life span. In this section, I will consider how such change occurs in habits and roles. We will begin with the formation of habits and roles and look at how they are altered over the life span. As with volition, the habituation subsystem is built up, maintained, and changed over time through the system's action.

Habit Formation and Change

The early occupational therapy leader Slagle (1922) noted that habits were the products of occupation. She and other occupational therapy writers (Slagle, 1922; Meyer, 1922; Kidner, 1924; Dunton, 1945) reinforced the idea that engaging in an occupational behavior over and over was the only way to establish or alter a habit. As we saw earlier in the chapter, others echoed this theme that habits are the residuals of our earlier behaviors. I also noted that to form habits we require redundancy or stability in the environment.

A child comes into the world without internal regulators of patterned behavior save, perhaps, certain biorhythms. Soon, however, he or she is integrated into the rhythms, routines, and customs that make up the physical, social, and temporal world. Children first acquire routines through parental guidance and support. These are routines of day and night with the attending patterns of sleeping, waking, eating, bathing, and so on. Over the course of development, as routines, customs, and ways of doing things are re-experienced, the child incorporates complex habit patterns. A number of these patterns remain somewhat stable throughout life, such as sleeping and eating patterns. Others change with the attainment of developmental stages (e.g., entering the student role, the work role). Interestingly, each new environmental context has its own regular rhythms and patterns of behavior that encourage individuals to internalize a pattern of behavior like that of others in the social system. Eventually, a number of rhythms may interweave, such as the rhythms and patterns of home life and those of school or work life.

All habits serve to preserve patterns of behavior, so they are naturally resistant to change. Whenever we make alterations in our schedules or environments, we encounter the tenacity of old habits. We show up at old appointed times. We visit the wrong cabinet or office for some time after we have relocated where we keep things or where we work.

Habits resist change since they are based in certain background assumptions (Berger & Luckman, 1966); that is, they reflect our most fundamental certainties about how the world is constructed. Habits presuppose a particular order in the physical, temporal, and social world. When habits and their background assumptions are disrupted or altered it creates a feeling of disorientation or unreality. For example, when our sleep patterns are disrupted or altered we can find ourselves waking up without the usual sense of being firmly anchored in the temporal world (i.e., thinking it is dawn when it is really dusk). A similar feeling of disorientation can occur when we are in the midst of a familiar task and lose our place (e.g., suddenly realizing we do not recognize where we are on the road when driving to a familiar destination). In such cases, we are shocked into sudden consciousness with no clear footing in what is ordinarily a familiar and taken-for-granted world. Children remind us of how important this taken-for-granted background is when they react with extreme displeasure to disruptions of routines. Dewey (1922) referred to this aspect of habits, noting:

> . . . a habit, a routine habit, when interfered with generates uneasiness, sets up a protest in favor of restoration and a sense of need of some expiatory act, or else it goes off in casual reminiscence. It is the essence of routine to insist upon its own continuation . . . Breach of custom or habit is the source of sympathetic resentment . . . (p. 76)

Dewey also notes there is often a "union of habit with desire and with propulsive power" (p. 24) as in the case of all those bad habits we perform in spite of ourselves. Such unwelcome habits nonetheless provide either satisfactions or freedom from the displeasure which breaching the habit occasions. In this regard, a curious feature of habits must be noted. They are not always in accord with volition. When aspects of our volition change (e.g., when we embrace new values) they may clash with habits chosen under older motives that are still in place. Habits generated by factors outside of volition (e.g., unconscious motives, restrictions imposed by the social system) may also counter what we would otherwise chose to do. Old habits may recall previous volitional states. We are slow to act confidently in a situation which evokes old fears of failure, despite our more recently developed volitional awareness of our ability to succeed. We find it difficult to substitute exercise for eating a bag of potato chips on the couch in front of the television despite our value of a more healthy lifestyle. The force of habits is such that volitional commitment and a period of practicing contrary behaviors is required to alter them.

Socialization and Role Change

Beginning in childhood, we perceive that others in the social surroundings fill positions that nearly everyone seems to take for granted. Moreover, the people who occupy these positions (mothers, teachers, babysitters) tend to behave in predictable ways. As time goes on, we discover that we have been assigned roles as well. We learn that we and others are expected to behave in certain ways because of the statuses we and others occupy (Grossack & Gardner, 1970; Katz & Kahn, 1966; Turner, 1962).

The process of communicating role expectations to the individual is referred to as socialization (Brim & Wheeler, 1966). As children develop, parents begin to give them expectations for being a family member. These expectations involve where and how the child plays, the emergence of helping behavior and self-care, and conformity to family routines. These expectations for performance as a family member are much more informal and loosely constructed than the role expectations that come later in life. Thus, there is a developmental progression from informal to formal roles. This role progression parallels the child's ability to internalize role expectations as role scripts and to use them as guides for behavior. Later in development, socialization may be much more formal, including education, practicing or apprenticing in the role, credentialing, and supervision. For many roles society goes to great lengths to socialize and regulate those who fill the role.

Socialization is not entirely a one-way process. Persons entering a new role typically negotiate with those affected by the role behavior (Heard, 1977; Schein, 1971). This is a give-and-take process. Each person who enters a role does it differently than any other person in that role. What is most at stake in such negotiations is how the individual expresses preferences and meets needs in the role and how others are affected by the way the individual fills the role. If an individual continues to enact a role in ways that others consider improper or that negatively affect the experience and behaviors of others in the social system, it is likely they will seek to influence how the person fills the role. Different roles have different audiences and thus the negotiations over role behavior may vary widely depending on the social system in question. In work roles one may have a large number of persons in reciprocal roles who are affected by one's performance. However, family roles have a much smaller audience.

Roles change as one progresses through the course of life. Persons choose to enter and leave roles. Moreover, society expects and structures role transitions at various life stages (i.e., entering and exiting the student role, beginning work and retiring). In a less formal way, roles such as that of spouse and parent are expected of persons by a certain age in many social groups. The constraints and expectations given by society, interwoven with occupational choices, determine the succession of roles that make up a person's life.

Role change is complex, involving alterations of one's identity, one's relationships to others, the tasks one is expected to perform, and how one's lifestyle is organized. An example of the complexity of role change is the experience of family members when aging parents or grandparents require children to take care of them:

This requires a whole series of role redefinitions as people grow more frail and become progressively less capable of caring for themselves. It entails a clear reversal of roles as the older generation loses power, and the authority to make the most personal kinds of decisions gravitates into the hands of their children. This marks a difficult transition for everyone. Roles need to be thoroughly redefined, often in the face of stiff resistance and understandable resentment. And we have not broached the question of changing relationships between grandparents and grandchildren, or between parents and children when a grandparent needing attention has been introduced to the family. Complex families must develop collective solutions if they are to stay together. (Hage & Powers, 1992, p. 118)

Thus, while role change is part and parcel of human development, it is often the occasion of significant reorganization not only within the individual but also in the external social system.

HABITUATION AND HABITAT

This chapter has emphasized the fact that habits and roles organize us to routinely navigate and negotiate our habitats. It should also be emphasized that the process of occupying our habitats involves an interaction in which we also shape, through our efforts and patterns of behavior, the environments in which we function. Rowles (1991) points out that repetition of behaviors in a familiar environment can also involve an arrangement of that environment to support our routine behavior. As an example, he describes an elderly couple, Walter and Beatrice, who have lived in the same house for more than half a century:

Walter did not have to think about the location of the throw rugs or about the camber on the porch steps that made them particularly treacherous following a rainstorm. Intimate familiarity with the layout of his home had served him well as he had grown increasingly constrained by failing vision. Beatrice's use of this environment was also facilitated by her bodily awareness of the placement of furniture. The configuration of furniture had gradually evolved over the years in a manner that provided places for her to hold on should she experience one of the dizzy spells to which she had become prone. (p. 268)

As Rowle's description illustrates, habits can become particularly effective ways for persons to maintain harmony with their environments in the face of personal limitations.

Habits are equally capable of creating inefficiencies or problems for performance. A habit learned in one environment may produce behavior that is not relevant or effective in another environment. Over a century ago, Durkheim (1893, cited in Young, 1988) cautioned that habits could enslave individuals and society at large since they are not easily eradicated once in place.

Similar criticism of traditional roles exist. It is argued that roles may unfairly stereotype and constrain those who inhabit them. Along these lines, it appears that contemporary society is ushering in different kinds of roles. In the future, roles are likely to be much more flexible and organic. Sarbin and Sheibe (1983) see the role script as becoming increasingly negotiable as the pace of change and the increasing complexity of society reduces the utility of traditional role scripts.

Hage and Powers (1992) note that in contemporary society "roles must be reconstructed or remade periodically" (p. 112). By this they are not promoting ambiguity or constant flux in roles, but rather they point to the need for periodic rethinking and renegotiating of the role. They note that role "commitment can only be sustained if people creatively redesign their roles in light of shifting conditions, sometimes by borrowing ideas from others and sometimes by independently inventing change" (Hage & Powers, 1992, p. 114). They view role redefinition as necessitated by current patterns of technological change, which make social roles more complex and leave their definitions, duties, and obligations more open. They note that, while this is liberating, it can be destabilizing:

. . . being able to redesign and reconstruct our relationships requires well-developed interaction skills, constant effort, the will to sustain a certain amount of emotional oscillations, and a great deal of cooperation from role partners. (p. 133)

Our lives hover between the possibilities of too much confinement or constriction and too much uncertainty. Habituation provides a means of providing stability and consistency in our everyday lives. Life overly structured is not to be desired. On the other hand, we can take some measure of comfort that in a changing world at least some part of our tomorrows will be as yesterday and today.

References

Berger, P. L., & Luckman, T. (1966). *The social construction of reality.*. New York: Doubleday/Anchor.

Bourdieu, P. (1977). *Outline of a theory of practice* (R. Nice, Trans.). London: Cambridge University Press.

Brim, O. J., & Wheeler, S. (1966). *Socialization after childhood: Two essays.* New York: John Wiley & Sons.

Camic, C. (1986). The matter of habit. *American Journal of Sociology, 91,* 1039–1087.

Cardwell, J. D. (1971). *Social psychology: A symbolic interaction perspective.* Philadelphia: FA Davis.

Chapin, F. S. (1968). Activity systems and urban structure: A working schema. *Journal of the American Institute of Planners, 34,* 11–18.

Dewey, J. (1922). *Human nature and conduct.* New York: Henry Holt & Company.

Dunton, W. R. (1945). *Prescribing occupational therapy.* Springfield, IL: Charles C Thomas.

Fein, M. L. (1990). *Role change: A resocialization perspective.* New York: Praeger.

Grossack, M., & Gardner, H. (1970). *Man and men: Social psychology as social science.* Scranton, PA: International Textbook Co.

Hage, G., & Powers, C. H. (1992). *Post-Industrial lives: Roles & relationships in the 21st century.* Newbury Park, NJ: Sage.

Heard, C. (1977). Occupational role acquisition: A perspective on the chronically disabled. *American Journal of Occupational Therapy, 41,* 243–247.

James, W. (1950). *The principles of psychology.* New York: Dover.

Katz, D., & Kahn, R. L. (1966). *The social psychology of organizations.* New York: John Wiley & Sons.

Kidner, T. B. (1924). Work for the tuberculosis patient during and after cure: Part II. *Archives of Occupational Therapy, 3*(3), 169–193.

Koestler, A. (1969). Beyond atomism and holism: The concept of the holon. In A. Koestler & J. R. Smythies (Eds.), *Beyond reductionism.* Boston, MA: Beacon Press.

Mancuso, J. C., & Sarbin, T. R. (1983). The self-narrative in the enactment of roles. In T. R. Sarbin & K. E. Scheibe (Eds.), *Studies in social identity.* New York: Praeger.

Matsutsuyu, J. (1971). Occupational behavior: A perspective on work and play. *American Journal of Occupational Therapy, 25,* 291–294.

Meyer, A. (1922). The philosophy of the occupational worker. *Archives of Occupational Therapy, 1,* 1–11.

Miller, D. R. (1983). Self, symptom and social control. In T. R. Sarbin & K. E. Scheibe (Eds.), *Studies in social identity.* New York: Praeger.

Murphy, R. (1987). *The body silent.* New York: WW Norton.

Oakley, F., Kielhofner, G., Barris, R., & Reichler, R. K. (1986). The Role Checklist: Development and empirical assessment of reliability. *Occupational Therapy Journal of Research, 6,* 157–170.

Rowles, G. D. (1991). Beyond performance: Being in place as a component of occupational therapy. *American Journal of Occupational Therapy, 45,* 265–272.

Ruddock, R. (1976). *Roles and relationships.* London: Routledge & Kegan Paul.

Sarbin, T. R., & Scheibe, K. E. (1983). A model of social identity. In T. R. Sarbin & K. E. Scheibe (Eds.), *Studies in social identity.* New York: Praeger.

Schein, E. H. (1971). The individual, the organization, and the career: A conceptual scheme. *Journal of Applied Behavioral Science, 7,* 401–426.

Seamon, D. (1980). Body-subject, time-space routines, and place-ballets. In A. Buttimer & D. Seamon (Eds.), *The human experience of space and place.* London: Croom Helm Ltd.

Shannon, P. D. (1970). The work-play model: A basis for occupational therapy programming in psychiatry. *American Journal of Occupational Therapy, 24,* 215–218.

Slagle, E. C. (1922). Training aides for mental patients. *Archives of Occupational Therapy, 1*(1), 11–17.

Stryker, S. (1968). Identity salience and role performance: The reliance of symbolic interaction theory for family research. *Journal of Marriage and the Family, November,* 558–564.

Turner, R. (1962). Role-taking, process versus conformity. In M. Rose (Ed.), *Human behavior and social processes.* Boston: Houghton Mifflin.

Young, M. (1988). *The metronomic society: Natural rhythms and human timetables.* Cambridge, MA: Harvard University Press.

KEY CONCEPTS

HABITUATION SUBSYSTEM
- an internal organization of information that disposes the system to exhibit recurrent patterns of behavior.

HABITUATION STRUCTURE
- an organization of appreciative capacities (role scripts and habit maps) which allow us to more or less automatically recognize features and situations in the environment and to construct behavior accordingly.
- **Habit:** Latent tendencies acquired from previous repetitions mainly operating at a preconscious level and influencing a wide range of behavioral patterns that correspond to familiar habitats.
- **Habit Map:** An internalized appreciative capacity which guides the perception of familiar events and the related construction of action toward accomplishing some implicit outcome or process.
- **Internalized Roles:** A broad awareness of a particular social identity and related obligations which together provide a framework for appreciating relevant situations and constructing appropriate behavior.
- **Role Scripts:** A collection of latent appreciative capacities that guide comprehension of social situations and expectations, and the related construction of action that enacts a given role.
- **Influence of habits on occupational behavior:**
  — Habits of style
  — Habits of routine
  — Habits of occupational behavior
- **Influence of roles on occupational behavior:**
  — Style of action
  — Occupational forms of roles
  — Temporal order of roles

HABITUATION PROCESS
- occurs on two time scales, habit map and role scripts guiding the assembly of behavior in everyday life and the change in roles and habits over time.
- The orderly improvisation of occupational behavior is a transaction between:
  — internalized role and/or habit
  — events of moment-by-moment action
  — contingencies of the context
- **Habit formation and change:**
  — habits serve to preserve patterns of behavior
  — habits resist change
  — habits are not always in accord with volition
- **Socialization and role change**
  — developmental progression of roles from informal to formal
  — involves negotiation with those affected by role change
  — roles change as one progresses through life

6/ Mind-Brain-Body Performance Subsystem

Anne Fisher and Gary Kielhofner

INTRODUCTION

We have seen in the previous two chapters that the volition subsystem guides the choices for occupational behavior and the habituation subsystem organizes occupational behavior into stable patterns. Underlying all occupational behavior is the capacity to perform. Whether it be simply going for a walk or executing a pirouette in ballet, balancing a checkbook or deriving a mathematical theorem, stacking blocks or building a house, the human capacity for performance is both astounding and complex.

In this chapter, we will conceptualize the mind-brain-body performance subsystem. We will argue that this subsystem provides the capacity for effective performance. In the simplest language, the mind-brain-body performance subsystem constitutes "what we have to perform with." The mind-brain-body performance subsystem complements volition in that merely having the desire to perform a task is not sufficient; the individual must also have the underlying capacity needed to perform. In a similar manner, the mind-brain-body performance and habituation subsystems support each other. Internalized habit maps and role scripts organize occupational performance into recognizable roles and habits, and the mind-brain-body performance subsystem is needed to contribute to the assembly of the required behaviors.

EXISTING CONCEPTS OF PERFORMANCE CAPACITY

A number of occupational therapy conceptual models seek to explain capacities that make possible occupational performance. Each of these models provides a detailed framework for understanding a limited area of behavioral concern in clinical practice. For example, the biomechanical model seeks to explain human movement as the function of a complex organization of muscles, connective tissue, and bones within the musculoskeletal system (Trombly, 1989). This model uses concepts of strength, range of motion, and endurance to describe the capacity of the musculoskeletal system for movement. Similarly, the sensory integration model (Ayres, 1972, 1979, 1986; Fisher, Murray, & Bundy, 1991) has been developed in an attempt to explain various aspects of the mind-brain process and its influence on performance. More specifically, that model seeks to explain how the brain organizes sensory information and uses that information in learning and executing skilled movement.

Models of practice that focus on such limited areas of concern can provide the occupational therapist with important detailed information needed in practice. The unfortunate consequence, however, is a fragmentation of processes known to be interdependent. Indeed, it is now universally recognized that the musculoskeletal and neurological components of the body are best conceptualized as complementary parts of a single neuromuscular system. Moreover, while traditional thought separated mental processes (e.g., cognition, memory, emotion) from brain processes (e.g., neurochemical events), more recent thinking has begun to see them as complementary aspects of a single unitary process (Pibram, 1986; Sperry, 1970). Finally, a number of interdisciplinary theories recognize that mental processes, brain processes, and neuromuscular processes are interrelated and interdependent (Bernstein, 1967; Brooks, 1986; Kelso, 1982; Keogh & Sugden, 1985; MacKay, 1987; Schmidt, 1988). This literature stresses the interrelationship among mental, brain, and neuromuscular (body) structures and processes and has paved the way for conceptualizing them as a single, coherent mind-brain-body performance subsystem.

Mind, brain, and body each are recognized throughout occupational therapy literature as essential parts of the underlying capacity for performance. Our purpose in conceptualizing them as comprising a unitary mind-brain-body performance subsystem is to enhance and unify, not repeat nor supplant, the detailed information provided by existing theories and conceptual models of practice used in occupational therapy. Occupational therapists using the model of human occupation as a guide to practice will need to consult and are encouraged to use other conceptual models when detail is needed concerning the operation of the various components that compromise the mind-brain-body performance subsystem. Our view is that conceptual models often are complementary in practice and, when appropriately linked, give a more complete picture of the occupational status of any individual. Our purpose in proposing a new way of conceptualizing the range of capacities explained in these other practice models is two-fold. First, we will place this mind-brain-body performance subsystem within the context of the human system. Second, we will discuss how the mind-brain-body performance subsystem, along with the habituation and volition subsystems, contributes to occupational behavior. Viewing the mind-brain-body performance subsystem

within the context of the human system provides an important basis for understanding the uniqueness of occupational therapy practice.

CONSTITUENTS OF THE MIND-BRAIN-BODY PERFORMANCE SUBSYSTEM

The mind-brain-body performance subsystem is an organization of constituents which together make up the capacity for occupational performance. The constituents of this mind-brain-body performance subsystem are (a) *musculoskeletal*, or the muscles, joints, and bones that make up functional biomechanical units; (b) *neurological*, or the central and peripheral nervous systems that organize and carry sensory and motor messages; (c) *cardiopulmonary*, or the cardiovascular and pulmonary systems (that directly support the functioning of the neurological and musculoskeletal component), and (d) *symbolic* images that guide the system in the planning, interpretation, and production of behavior. As with habit maps and role scripts, the images of action that guide performance are not specific instructions. Rather, these images of action are abstract rules that constrain behavior (Brooks, 1986; Bruner, 1970, 1973; Hayek, 1969; Robinson, 1977; Schmidt, 1988). Like the role scripts and habit maps, the images of action underlying performance provide a tacit way of appreciating how to perform within the emergent circumstances and inevitable variability of each new performance. They provide a way of knowing how to do something that is best described as "feel" or appreciation of how to perform a given act (Brooks, 1986). Like behavior guided by habit maps and role scripts, the degree of conscious attention may vary. In some occupational performances we are only vaguely aware of our actions. At other times we are actively planning, problem solving, or otherwise focusing on the task at hand. For this reason, the terms *cognition* or *cognitive images*, which imply conscious thought, can be misleading. While conscious thought or cognition plays a major role in informing occupational behavior, there is also a more automatic or tacit dimension to performance which is guided by images of action.

The musculoskeletal, neurological, cardio-pulmonary, and symbolic images of action constituents that comprise the mind-brain-body performance subsystem contribute organized capacities to the assembly of occupational performance (Figure 6.1). This subsystem is an integrated whole. The constituents are interdependent and work together to contribute to performance; that is, the assembly of effective occupational performance is the result of the unified action of all constituents of the mind-brain-body performance subsystem as they work in collaboration with unfolding circumstances and environmental conditions.

ORGANIZATION OF THE MIND-BRAIN-BODY PERFORMANCE SUBSYSTEM

The mind-brain-body performance subsystem is organized for efficient information processing necessary for appreciating and acting effectively on the environment. The musculoskeletal, cardiopulmonary, neurological, and symbolic constituents are organized so as to effectively communicate together and to process information for making sense of experience and effecting action.

Within the mind-brain-body performance subsystem, the flow of information between constituents and the exchange of action and information with the environment together create an informational network.

Each of the constituents of the subsystem acts within the information flow that is created in this process. In this way, the mind and brain are not executive systems commanding motor action. Rather, they are collaborating constituents, contributing their particular mode of processing information to the total network. Performance emerges out of this dynamic network of information. For example, in the act of moving one's body, sensation and perception, which depend on a flow of information to the central nervous system, influence the flow of information to muscles which, in turn, respond and effect movement. Simultaneously, the movement itself is influenced by forces and objects in the environment and the movement provides sensory information about the dynamic state of the body moving in space.

The process, as Reed (1982) notes, is too complex to be explained simply by ideas of in-

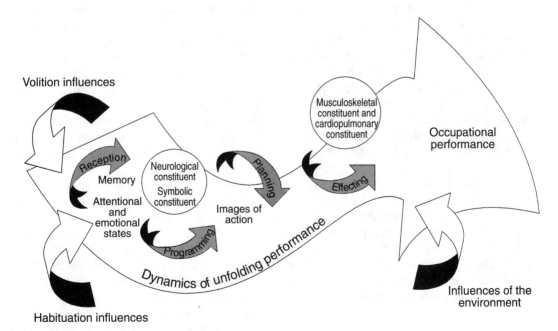

Figure 6.1.   The contribution of mind-brain-body performance subsystem, volition subsystem, habituation subsystem, environment and task dynamics to the assembly of occupational performance.

formation flow from one constituent to another. Rather, performance must be the result of a larger dynamic state. While this process is as yet not well understood, one important lesson can be taken. No specification of a single constituent of the mind-brain-body performance subsystem can be fully understood by examining only that part and its function. To attempt to do so would be like trying to explain what the roots of a plant do without reference to any other part of the plant or to what a plant as a whole is like. As illustrated in Figure 6.1, we emphasize that the informational events of this subsystem are simultaneous and belong to a dynamic network of information as just described.[a] Moreover, the mind-brain-body performance subsystem is one among several influences on the assembly of occupational performance.

Perception, planning, and effecting action represent an ongoing, mutually-influencing process in which the total informational network in the mind-brain-body performance subsystem is more important than any particular sequence of information flow. Nonetheless, it is impossible to discuss this subsystem without some reference to how information flows through the subsystem as it is processed.

The mind-brain-body performance subsystem (Figure 6.1) processes information in the following ways: (a) reception (i.e., the perception and integration of sensory information it receives from the body and the environment), (b) planning (including motor planning), (c) programming of plans of action, and (d) effecting the action through the body. Influencing information processing within the mind-brain-body performance subsystem are attentional and emotional states. Also influencing the processing of information are memory and images of action or neuronal memories of "how it feels" to perform and "what is accomplished" by performance (Brooks, 1986; Schmidt, 1988; Fisher, Murray, & Bundy, 1991). The process is also affected by volition and habituation. Information is fed forward from the mind-brain component via neuro-

chemical signals to the body (i.e., musculoskeletal and supporting cardiopulmonary constituents) which effects the action emanating from the workings of this mind-brain-body performance subsystem. Feedback to the mind-brain component also occurs as performance unfolds.

Impairment of any of the underlying constituents of the mind-brain-body performance subsystem (i.e., musculoskeletal, neurological, cardiopulmonary, and symbolic) can have an impact on the capacity of the subsystem for information processing and effecting action. For example, brain damage can have diverse influences that may affect memory, motor planning, or attention. Similarly, impairment of the musculoskeletal constituents may place limits on the force, range of motion, or stamina with which the person can act.

Both external and internal sensory information are processed within the mind-brain-body performance subsystem. External sensory information (i.e., that which informs us about our environment) includes visual, tactile, and auditory sensory information as well as the ongoing stream of information about the effect of our actions in the environment. Simultaneously, internal information provides feedback about our bodies and includes sensory information related to the movement and position of the body in space (vestibular-proprioception) (Fisher, 1991). The mind-brain-body performance subsystem registers sensory information by converting various forms of energy (e.g., light and sound waves, gravitational pull, proprioception) into neurochemical messages which are relayed to the brain and are simultaneously perceived and apprehended in the mind.

Perception and planning of action are interlinked elements of the information processing within this subsystem. When we perceive, we do so as systems acting or poised for the next action. Our planning and programming of action are realized when the body effects action. This information processing is an integrated, simultaneous process in which the human system is, at once, an acting, perceiving, planning, and reacting organism. Moreover, information processing is a proactive process. We *make* sense of sensory experience and *make*

---

[a]See Kielhofner and Fisher (1991) for a discussion of the concept of simultaneous causation.

plans of action just as surely as we *make* things happen when we act on the environment.

Interwoven with the processes of the mind-brain-body performance subsystem are influences from the volition and habituation subsystems. Volition influences include such factors as the perceived match between a person's abilities and performance requirements, the attraction the individual has toward the occupation, and the value the occupation holds for the individual. The volition subsystem can have a positive organizing influence by evoking affective or cognitive states in response to challenges, meanings, and attractions that enhance performance. Conversely, volition can contribute to states of anxiety over whether one can effectively perform, boredom due to lack of interest, or a feeling that the performance has no meaning or value. Such states may diminish performance. Therefore, occupational behavior is enhanced when the individual is performing with positive volition—that is, when the performance is experienced as interesting, and challenging, but within one's capacity, and/or as significant to one's life and social milieu.

The habituation subsystem similarly has an influence on performance. As noted in the previous chapter, habit maps and role scripts organize our use of time, and thereby determine which performance capacities we will call upon in the course of our normal routines. Habit maps and role scripts also influence the way in which we organize our performance capacities to accomplish a given occupation. Finally, habits interject our characteristic style into the way we assemble performance.

The complexity of this process can be illustrated by considering the example of a mechanic working on an engine. Armed with memory (such as the knowledge that a particular sound is diagnostic of a given engine problem) and images of what the sound is like, that mechanic actively listens for the information which will lead him or her toward a tentative diagnosis of the engine trouble. The sound enters the human system as mechanical vibration, is translated into neurological signals and thereafter to the conscious recognition of a tell-tale squeak of a fan belt. When the mechanic "hears" the squeaky fan belt, it is the result of an active process of knowing what to listen for and information processing that receives, integrates, and interprets the incoming sensory data. Enfolded within the perceptual act are the planning and programming of the motor act of tightening the belt. Memory of the correct tightness of a fan belt, an image of how it feels to push the wrench to tighten the mechanism, and the recognition of the changing sound as the tension increases, are sources of information the mechanic uses to guide (plan and program) the necessary motor behavior. The mechanic's motor movements and their effects on the environment (e.g., fan belt tension, sound of the fan belt) also create internal and external sensory feedback that allows the mechanic to continue to "feel" his or her way through the act of tightening the belt. Throughout this process, the sense of efficacy and attraction to the task, and its value as a means of livelihood provide the motives that give the mechanic a sense of satisfaction and that maintain positive emotion and attention, enhancing the ability to perform. All these and other processes are so thoroughly integrated into a whole system that the performance of the occupation of repairing the engine is fluent. Behavior is assembled with all the features we refer to as skill, from the interaction between the human system, the occupation of repairing an engine, and the engine worked upon as well as the tools and materials used.

PERFORMANCE PROCESS

Throughout this text, the improvisational nature of human conduct has been emphasized. Following systems principles, we recognize that the human system provides some of the necessary components for assembling behavior. In actual performance, however, the unfolding task is a dynamic process, and environmental conditions interact with the human system to assemble the behavior. The human system, the occupation being done, and the environment together create a web of relationships in which the actual behavior emerges.

As with other subsystems, occupational performance is also the process which maintains and changes the structure or organization of the mind-brain-body performance system.

That exercise helps to sustain the capacity of the musculoskeletal and supporting cardiopulmonary systems for action is well documented (Trombly, 1989). Similarly, images of action are built up through complex interactions with the environment in which sensory integration and motor learning take place and in which the images supporting memory and knowledge of how to perform a wide range of occupational behavior are developed and sustained (Fisher, Murray, & Bundy, 1991).

CONCLUSION

This chapter presented a conceptualization of the mind-brain-body performance subsystem. We have argued that this subsystem contributes its capacities toward the assembly of behavior by processing information and effecting action in a manner which allows for the dynamic assembly of behavior in concert with the other subsystems, and as constrained by the occupational behavior itself, and the context of performance. Our conceptualization of the mind-brain-body performance subsystem mainly aims at providing a coherent way of thinking about the unified underlying capacities for performance and their relationships to volition and habituation. As we noted earlier, other conceptual models (e.g., biomechanical and sensory integration) provide more detailed explanations of the constituents and underlying processes of performance. When linked with the explanations provided here, a more complete explanation of the factors influencing performance can be achieved. None of the conceptual models (including the model of human occupation) provides an adequate conceptualization of all factors that influence performance, hence the need to link compatible models in order to achieve more complete explanations.

Recognizing that all performance is assembled through interaction of the task and the environment, we conceptualize the mind-brain-body performance subsystem as being the organizer of capacity with which the human system engages in occupation. The mind-brain-body performance subsystem is organized to provide that capacity which is contributed to the assembly of occupational performance. Incorporating musculoskeletal, neurological, cardiopulmonary, and cognitive symbolic constituents into an integrated whole, the mind-brain-body performance subsystem processes information and effects action in the environment. This subsystem is interrelated with the volition and habituation subsystems, and with them contributes to the occupational behavior of the human system.

The underlying capacities represented by the mind-brain-body performance subsystem cannot be observed directly.[b] Rather, we must observe performance in order to make inferences about the state of constituents and/or of the information processing capacity of the mind-brain-body performance subsystem. For example, the observation of how much force an individual generates in muscle testing is used to make inferences about underlying capacity we refer to as strength. In similar fashion, the Sensory Integration and Praxis Tests (Ayres & Marr, 1991) are used to discover the status of sensory integrative capacities. When a therapist wishes to make inferences about the organization of the underlying components of the mind-brain-body performance subsystem, other models of practice and their assessment procedures should be used.

There is often value in understanding the nature of particular kinds of dysfunction in a constituent or in determining whether dysfunction in the mind-brain-body performance subsystem is contributing to problems in performance. One limit of such approaches, however, is that deficits in the underlying mind-brain-body performance subsystem do not translate in a linear fashion to specific and predictable performance deficits.

In Chapter 8, we will present an approach which examines the actual skills which are manifest in occupational behavior. This ap-

---

[b]Medical and other diagnostic procedures can be used to probe and discern the status of biological constituents of the mind-brain-body performance subsystem, so in this regard it is possible to observe some aspects of this subsystem. However, occupational therapy procedures for ascertaining performance capacity are concerned with making inferences about inherent capacity from observations of occupational behavior.

proach focuses on the performance as an action or behavior contributing to the completion of an occupational form. The approach thus enables one to locate skill deficits rather than rely solely on locating problems in the underlying mind-brain-body performance subsystem. This approach is consistent with our understanding of how the human system assembles behavior in the dynamic process of interacting with the environment.

References

Ayres, A. J. (1972). *Sensory integration and learning disorders*. Los Angeles: Western Psychological Services.

Ayres, A. J. (1979). *Sensory integration and the child*. Los Angeles: Western Psychological Services.

Ayres, A. J. (1986). *Developmental dyspraxia and adult onset apraxia*. Torrance, CA: Sensory Integration International.

Ayres, A. J., & Marr, D. B. (1991). Sensory integration and praxis texts. In A. G. Fisher, E. A. Murray, & A. C. Bundy (Eds.), *Sensory integration: Theory and practice*. Philadelphia: FA Davis.

Bernstein, N. A. (1967). *The coordination and regulation of movements*. Oxford, England: Pergamon Press.

Brooks, V. B. (1986). *The neural basis of motor control*. New York: Oxford University Press.

Bruner, J. (1970, April). The skill of relevance or the relevance of skills. *Saturday Review*, pp. 66–73.

Bruner, J. (1973). Organization of early skilled action. *Child Development, 44*, 1–11.

Fisher, A. G. (1991) Vestibular-proprioceptive processing and bilateral integration and sequencing deficits. In A. G. Fisher, E. A. Murray, & A. C. Bundy (Eds.), *Sensory integration: Theory and practice*. Philadelphia: FA Davis.

Fisher, A. G., Murray, E. A., & Bundy, A. C. (Eds.). (1991). *Sensory integration: Theory and practice*. Philadelphia: FA Davis.

Hayek, F. A. (1969). The primacy of the abstract. In A. Koestler & R. J. Smythies (Eds.), *Beyond reductionism*. Boston: Beacon Press.

Kelso, J. A. S. (Ed.). (1982). *Human motor behavior: An introduction*. Hillside, NJ: Erlbaum.

Keogh, J., & Sugden, D. (1985). *Movement skill development*. New York: Macmillan.

Kielhofner, G., & Fisher, A. (1991). Mind-Brain-Body relationships. In A. G. Fisher, E. A. Murray, & A. C. Bundy (Eds.), *Sensory integration: Theory and practice*. Philadelphia: FA Davis.

MacKay, D. J. (1987). *The organization and perception of action: A theory for language and other cognitive skills*. New York: Springer-Verlag.

Pibram, K. H. (1986). The cognitive revolution and mind/brain issues. *American Psychologist, 41*, 507–520

Reed, E. (1982). An outline of a theory of action systems. *Journal of Motor Behavior, 14*, 98–134.

Robinson, A. (1977). Play: The arena for the acquisition of rules of competent behavior. *American Journal of Occupational Therapy, 31*, 248–253.

Schmidt, R. A. (1988). *Motor control and learning: A behavioral emphasis*. (2nd ed.). Champaign, IL: Human Kinetics Publishers.

Sperry, R. W. (1970). An objective approach to subjective experience: Further explanation of a hypothesis. *Psychological Review, 77*, 585–590.

Trombly, C. A. (1989). *Occupational therapy for physical dysfunction*. Baltimore: Williams & Wilkins

===== *KEY CONCEPTS* =====

MIND-BRAIN-BODY PERFORMANCE SUBSYSTEM
- refers to the organization of physical and mental constituents which together make up the capacity for occupational performance.

Constituents of the Performance Subsystem
- musculoskeletal: muscles, joints, and bones that make up functional biomechanical units.
- neurological: central and peripheral nervous systems that organize and carry sensory and motor messages.
- cardiopulmonary: the cardiovascular and pulmonary systems.
- symbolic images: guide the system in the planning, interpretation, and production of behavior.

ORGANIZATION OF THE MIND-BRAIN-BODY PERFORMANCE SUBSYSTEM
- the flow of information between constituents and the exchange of action and information with the environment together create an informational network.
- performance emerges out of this dynamic network of information.
- the mind-brain-body performance subsystem processes information in the following ways: reception, planning, programming plans of action; effecting the action through the body.

7/ Environmental Influences on Occupational Behavior

Gary Kielhofner

INTRODUCTION

Previous chapters have emphasized that occupational behavior is dynamically assembled with contributions from both the human system and the ecology in which the performance takes place. The mutual contributions of the person and the environment to performance are described by Thelen and Ulrich (1991) when they note that

> behavior emerges strictly as a cooperative function of the subsystems within particular environmental and task contexts. There is no single element that contains the prior instructions for the behavioral performance. The task and the context recruit and assemble the cooperative system, but the essence of the behavior lies in neither the organism nor the environmental alone. (p. 24)

The environment is so intimately linked with how the human system is organized and behaves that some theorists see it as "part of the organism" (Sameroff, 1983, p. 242). Consequently, the view of the person-environment relation that is emerging in a number of fields stresses that the human being is not simply a matter of what is "under the skin." We owe our very humanness and our most essential selves to our environments. As Eisenberg (1977) argues,

> What determines the similarity between my behavior last year and what it is likely to be during the next is not nearly so much a matter of that which is "I" as it is of the social fields of force in which that "I" moves. That is, having acquired a repertoire of behaviors, I maximize their adaptive utility by seeking out the familiar and avoiding the strange in the social world around me. The apparent consistency in the self is the result, not merely of what has gone before, but of the continuation into the future of the same social forces that have given rise to it. (p. 233)

As the quote implies, the relationship between humans and their environments is a dialectical one. Human beings constantly seek out congenial environments and seek to change those environments toward their ends. In turn, the environments persons select and create influence how they perform and what they become.

The purpose of this chapter is to provide a way of conceptualizing the environmental influences and contributions to occupational behavior. To accomplish this, I will first propose a way of thinking about how environments influence behavior. I will then proceed to offer a way of thinking about those features of environments that permit and shape occupational behavior. My aim in this chapter will be to explain how the environment shapes occupational behavior in the course of ordinary daily life. As we will see in the later chapters, understanding how the environment contributes to the way we choose, organize, and enact our occupations is important for how we view and gather data on a person's occupational functioning; that is, if we want to understand any person's occupational behavior, we must also understand the environments in which that behavior takes place. A second and critical application of the concepts presented in this chapter is in the implementation of therapy. As I will argue in Chapter 13, all occupational therapy involves environmentally-based strategies that elicit, support, or influence the occupational behavior of those persons for whom we are providing therapy. Consequently, if we wish to understand our patients or clients and help them to function more fully in their occupations, we must learn about and use their environments.

ENVIRONMENTAL INFLUENCES ON OCCUPATIONAL BEHAVIOR

The first question that arises concerning environmental influences on occupational behavior is: How does the environment influence our behavior? In response, I propose that we think of the environment as having two broad influences on occupational behavior. First, the environment *affords* opportunities for performance. Second, the environment *presses* for certain types of behavior. Together the concepts of affording and pressing explain the influence of environment on occupational behavior.

Affording Occupational Behavior

Gibson (1979) developed the concept that motor action is the realization of opportunities that the environment *afforded*. Underlying this view of environmental influences on behavior is the concept that behavior consists of learned *strategies* for achieving a goal rather than specific learned motor behavior sequences. Throughout this text we have emphasized a similar view stressing that occupational behavior emanates from appreciations of situations and that it has a thoroughly improvisational character guided, in part, by the unfolding circumstances of performance. The role of the environment in the process of behavioral assembly is by no means small. According to Reed (1982), the action of behaving systems is "more directly a function of the objects and circumstances of their environs than of the proximal stimulation underlying the behavior" (p. 108).

This view places a large portion of the guiding factors for behavior outside the human system into the context in which the behavior is taking place. Further, it means that a behaving human system perceives that "an object or event in the environment offers the possibility of performing some action" (Reed, 1982, p. 124). All behavior consists of the system maintaining itself in an unfolding relationship with the environment—a relationship that achieves some objective afforded by the environment.

Although the concept of the environment affording opportunities emerged in the study of perceptual motor behavior, I will use the concept more broadly here to refer to a whole range of possibilities the environment offers for occupational behavior. Moreover, when I speak of what the environment affords I am referring to the possibility or potential for undertaking various occupational behaviors that characteristics of the environment make possible for humans.[a] Since the environment provides potentials for behaviors, it gives certain freedoms to choose and act. As an example, a mountain affords one the opportunity to simply enjoy the view, to photograph the scene, or to go hiking. What one actually does is a matter of choice. Consequently, I argue that characteristics of the *environment afford a range of opportunities for occupational behavior because they represent specific potentials for action.*

Pressing for Occupational Behavior

The concept of pressing emerged from the study of how environments shaped the behavior of their inhabitants (Lawton, 1980). Press refers to what the environment expects or de-

---

[a]The concept of environments affording action as used in traditional perceptual motor literature includes not only the idea of opportunity for action but also implies that the environment constrains (or provides limitations of opportunity at the same time) and that both opportunity and constraint influence how behavior is assembled. In this chapter, I have partitioned these two notions, emphasizing that the environment affords opportunity and using the concept of press to explain how environments constrain or direct behavior. Opportunity and constraint are always intertwined and mutually implied in the environment, but for our purposes it is useful to separate and consider them as two complementary influences of the environment on occupational behavior.

mands of the individual. Consequently, when *environments press, they strongly recruit or require particular behaviors*. For example, in an airport, the counters and agents, roped areas, security checkpoints and guards, gates, schedule of flights, and so on, strongly influence and, in part, dictate when we arrive, where we go, and the sequence of behaviors in which we engage (e.g., standing in line, obtaining a boarding pass and checking luggage, going to the gate, boarding the plane). As the example illustrates, press refers to the way the physical and human environment tends to shape behavior. We feel press by virtue both of how the physical setting is arranged and what others expect us to do. In fact, physical environments are often arranged as they are precisely because the designer wanted or expected people to behave in certain ways.

When environments press for (i.e., demand or constrain) behavior, they can evoke a range of experiences and responses. Environments which press for behavior which is at the upper end of a persons' capacities tend to evoke involvement, attentiveness, and maximal performance (Lawton & Nahemow, 1973; Kiernat, 1983). On the other hand when environments press for behavior well below capacity, they can evoke boredom and disinterest. As noted in Chapter 3, human systems are organized for action and naturally seek opportunities to use their capacity. Csikszentmihalyi (1990) points out that optimal states of pleasure in action, which he calls "flow," occur when the individual is challenged, when the environment demands that the person perform at his or her highest level. It is only when demands become too great (i.e., too far beyond capacity) that a person may feel anxious, overwhelmed, or hopeless. On the other hand, as Kiernat (1983, p. 6) notes, "lack of environmental press results in the type of negative affect and behavior seen in sensory deprivation." Thus, press should be understood as a continuum of demand for performance. If the demand is too low, it may evoke boredom; if it is too high, press can evoke anxiety. However, optimal press is a necessary condition for persons to be challenged, to be invested in performance, and to experience a positive sense of efficacy. Maladaptive performance can result from too little

or too much press for behaviors relative to an individual's level of competence (Lawton, 1980; Schultz & Hanusa, 1979).

While it is useful to think of press as high or low relative to a person's capacity, press is not a unidimensional feature of the environment. Rather, environments press for a rich variety of behaviors, and generally the press of an environment will be for a coherent set of behaviors that respond to the nature, organization, and purpose of the environment. For example, the press of a street gang is likely to be for toughness and aggression; the press of a support group will be for sensitivity and emotional openness; and the press of a business meeting is for strategic information sharing and negotiation. These different modes of behavior are recruited from participants by virtue of the different contexts.

Press may be felt for varying behaviors and in varying degrees of strength. Some environments are relatively nonspecific in their press and we may choose from among a range of behaviors. For example, at a professional conference we experience press to attend presentations, but we may choose which ones we will attend; the press in a supermarket is to move our carts along without blocking others, but which aisles we traverse and what items we stop to examine or take is up to us. Other environments press for much more specific behavior. For example, when we obtain a drivers license we have to go to a specific line, take a series of written, visual, and practical exams, fill out certain forms, and pay a set fee. Everyone who wishes to obtain a license must do the same thing.

Over time, press influences which skills and habits one will develop, and affects one's organization of them into coherent patterns of behavior or roles. Thus, for example, when we enter school, specific courses must be taken, we must go to designated rooms to attend those courses, certain public and private behaviors are expected (e.g., joining class discussions, dressing a certain way by virtue of school code or peer pressure, studying, using the library, taking exams, and completing papers). The press of a school environment is represented in the organization of the school's settings, rules and requirements, and the perceptions by teachers, peers, and parents of the student role and its obligatory behaviors. It funnels and shapes the behavior of those who would be and remain students such that their role scripts and habit maps eventually conform to the contours of the school environment.

Complementary Environmental Influences

Each environment, of course, both affords and presses for certain occupational behaviors. A mountain may offer an opportunity to hike. Its terrain and its trails constrain where we can hike. The steepness of the terrain and the state of the trail constrain how fast and far we can go. Similarly, in addition to the ways airports direct behavior, places in the airport (bookstore, bar, or restaurant) and the presence of other people afford us opportunities to purchase reading material, to eat, or to strike up a conversation.

Moreover, because environments both press and afford, they create a synergy of influences that channel our behavior in the midst of unfolding circumstances; that is, the environment, by simultaneously providing opportunity and constraint, creates behavioral pathways. As with any pathway, certain directions are easier to follow. However, pathways also imply that alternative routes are constrained, not as easy to traverse, or not accessible at all. By affording and pressing, environments invite and instruct behavior to go in particular directions.

Individuality of Environmental Influences

Throughout this chapter I will speak of the various influences the environment may have on an individual. However, it is important to remember that what the environment affords and presses for depends very much on the eye of the beholder. Imagine for a moment a game of checkers placed on a coffee table. I have watched a number of very different reactions to this environmental situation. Some persons totally ignore it; they apparently have no interest in checkers. Others have played the game. One small child who apparently had not been introduced to its purpose stacked the checkers up like blocks and made a slide for the checkers from the playing board. Later she sorted them into black and red checkers. As the example illustrates, how something in the environment influences behavior may have, in part, to do with its intrinsic properties, and in part, with social convention about its use. What someone actually does with it (if anything) depends on the person. As illustrated in Figure 7.1, the influence of the environment

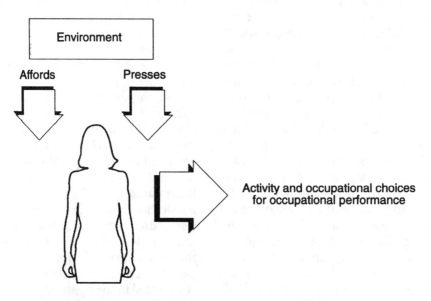

Figure 7.1. Unique influence of the environment on each person.

on the person will depend on that person's current values, interests, personal causation, roles, habits, and performance capacities. Consequently, when I speak of what the environment affords and presses for, I am speaking of potential influences. One will have to watch any environment carefully to see on whom it tends to exact its influence and what range of influences it might have.

PHYSICAL AND SOCIAL ENVIRONMENT

I have argued that the environment influences behavior by affording and pressing for certain types of performance. Our next question is, what are the features of environments that afford and press? To answer this question we must begin by having some way to conceptualize the dimensions of the environment.

The environment may be thought of as having physical and social dimensions. The former refers to the material environment including natural and fabricated spaces and objects. The social environment refers to the world of interacting people and the things they do. In everyday life we ordinarily encounter an interwoven physical and social environment. The places we go and the objects we encounter are, in large measure, the artifacts of human fabrication. Moreover, we encounter others in physical places, share objects with them, and find our interactions with them shaped and facilitated by the material world we share.

Role of Culture

Both the physical and social environment are interpreted and shaped by culture (Altman & Chemers, 1980). Culture consists of the beliefs and perceptions, values and norms, customs and behaviors that are shared by a group or society, and are passed from one generation to the next through both formal and informal education (Altman & Chemers, 1980; Rapoport, 1980). Two implications are embedded in this definition. First, one's culture is a characteristic way of perceiving and acting in the physical and social world (Rapoport, 1980). Second, because of this characteristic way of acting, a culture results in particular representative lifestyles that embody taken-for-granted ways of behaving in the physical and social world (Brake, 1980; Ogbu, 1981; Rapoport, 1980).

Within most cultures there are also a variety of subcultures. For example, in American society, there may be urban, rural, ethnic, and other subcultural groups. These subcultures show important differences from the dominant culture and, in particular, influence the organization of various groups. We need only consider the differences between the beliefs and behaviors of members of an affluent social club in New York and members of a Southern Baptist Church or between the work life of Washington politicians and that of migrant farm workers in California to appreciate vast differences in subcultural groups within the larger American culture.

The impact of culture is not necessarily a single homogeneous force. It may represent the composite of several different sources of cultural influence, depending on the range of environments in which any person behaves. For example, I live in a farming community in rural southern Wisconsin, commute to urban Chicago to work, am responsible for educational and clinical programs that have a mission of serving minority populations which brings me into contact with Hispanic and African American subcultures. In addition, I am a foreign adjunct professor at the Karolinska Institute in Stockholm. I travel there regularly and have several close Swedish friends with whom I communicate frequently. All these experiences expose me to a variety of environments and circumstances which present a significant range of cultural influences. While my experience is more diverse than that of many people, it is increasingly probable that persons will experience an array of cultural influences in a world with increasing resources for communication and mobility. The insulated and homogeneous cultural experiences of persons who lived a century ago are less and less likely in today's world (Gergen, 1991).

We can readily see how the social world, the world of human relationships and activities, is shaped by culture, but there is an equally important influence of culture on the physical environment. On the one hand, culture determines how our physical context is organized and what artifacts we are likely to encounter within it. On the other hand, culture gives us a way of seeing and encountering the physical environment, even the world of nature. In this chapter, I will not refer to culture as one of the parts of the environment, since culture influences, and is implicit in, any aspect of the environment we can describe.

Since culture is a pervasive force in the environment, I will repeatedly refer to its role in the following discussion of the physical and social environment. Moreover, it is important to recognize that culture not only pervades the environment, but it is also internalized in the organization of the human system. A person's values, sense of competence, interests, internalized roles and habits are all reflections of that person's belonging to a particular culture and subcultures (represented in the workplace, neighborhood, and other settings). Thus, culture is ubiquitous in both the environment and the person.

Physical Environment

We are material beings in a physical world. All that we experience and can do is in some measure a function of our placement in the physical world. As illustrated in Figure 7.2, the physical environment consists of the natural and human-made ecologies (Lawton, 1983), and the objects within those ecologies (Csikszentmihalyi & Rochberg-Halton, 1981).

Natural Environments

Natural ecologies are those elements of the physical world which are largely unmodified by humans or, if constructed, are organized to use and imitate nature. Thus, countryside, mountains, the sky, lakes, streams and, parks are features of the natural ecology. The natural environment also includes processes such as the change of seasons and weather (e.g., rain, snow, wind). Natural environments, while not as specialized as built environments, nevertheless afford and press for specific behaviors. We need only recall the different possibilities and demands of a warm sunny beach and the snowy cold of a winter woodland to recognize that nature has a not-so-subtle way of recruiting different occupational behaviors.

Built Environments

Built environments result from human fabrication. They are buildings and connecting structures organized to contain humans, their activities, and their possessions; to separate them from the natural environment; and to get people from one part of the built ecology to another. Examples of built ecologies are houses, barns, stadiums, stores, school buildings, libraries, shopping malls, factory buildings, and the various walkways, streets, and highways that connect them. Just as natural ecologies includes processes, so built ecologies include processes such as traffic flow, the

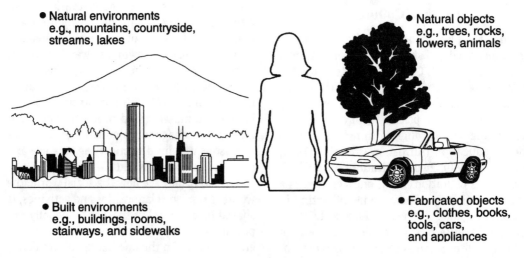

- Natural environments
  e.g., mountains, countryside, streams, lakes

- Natural objects
  e.g., trees, rocks, flowers, animals

- Built environments
  e.g., buildings, rooms, stairways, and sidewalks

- Fabricated objects
  e.g., clothes, books, tools, cars, and appliances

Figure 7.2. Physical environment.

movement of escalators and elevators, and the workings of all manner of machines.

Built environments are generally compartmentalized ecologies consisting of rooms or other specified spaces such as courts and bleachers, stages, balconies, atriums, garages, closets, and lobbies. These spaces are interconnected by hallways, stairways, elevators, escalators, and the like. The spaces within built ecologies usually have designated purposes such as sleeping, eating, congregating, watching forms of entertainment, studying, playing, and so on. By virtue of their physical organization, they naturally afford and press for behavior. For example, stairs require us to ascend or descend; a gymnasium affords an opportunity to run, whereas a closet is too small.

In complex societies there is an almost endless variety of such spaces: offices, bedrooms, classrooms, dining rooms, lecture halls, clinics, operating rooms, auditoriums, waiting rooms, laboratories, show rooms, playrooms, kitchens, lounges, chapels and the like. These spaces emanate from and are instrumental to a cultural way of life. Such built spaces are more or less readily recognized by members of the culture as having a designated purpose and as intended for certain persons' use. Hence, they readily afford and press for specific occupational behavior. In a church we are invited to pray and are restrained from disturbing others. The nature of the structure and cultural convention about its use convey solemnity and invite appropriate behavior by those properly socialized to recognize what a church is for. Upon entering a large train station we experience an altogether different press for behavior, both because it is organized in a physically different way and because social convention calls for different behavior. Ordinarily, social convention for use of space is readily illustrated by the behavior of its occupants and by their reactions to behavior that violates those conventions.

Objects

Within the physical environment, we encounter both naturally occurring and fabricated or processed objects. Within natural ecologies we find trees, flowers, and other plants; animals and insects; as well as stones, soil, water, snow, and other inanimate and animate objects.[b] Built environments include such things as furniture, food, appliances, books, plants, clothes, art, tools, pets, machines, and so on. While objects in natural environments occur according to the scheme of nature, those in built environments are placed there by human design. Which objects are present and how they are organized generally depends on the purpose of the space and cultural convention. Rubinstein (1989) notes,

> Culture suggests general rules for ordering and arranging space . . . Notions of where things should go in a dwelling vary cross-culturally and across class lines . . . The individual reproduces basic ideas about cultural order through the act of ordering domestic space and also interprets ideas about the cultural order. (p. 47)

Thus, we expect to find toilets, basins, showers, towels, toothpaste, and razors in domestic bathrooms and cars, lawnmowers, shovels, hoses, and bicycles in typical suburban garages.

Objects can make an environment arousing, comfortable, practical, safe, interesting, and aesthetically pleasing. Although people vary in the extent to which they have and relate to objects, everyone's surroundings include some artifacts that are the objects of their attention and action (Csikszentmihalyi & Rochberg-Halton, 1981).

The nature of objects present in any one space contributes to how it affords or presses for occupational behavior. Children, for instance, will engage in more solitary play when toys and play equipment are available, unless the toys are specifically designed for social play (Johnson, 1935; Quilitch & Risley, 1973). Raw materials can afford a range of behavior with less press due to the variety of ways in which they can be used. For example, objects that are important to children are often "raw" materi-

---

[b] I have included animate and inanimate objects together, thus creating a very diverse category. It is recognized that animals, in particular, may represent an altogether different class of influences and meanings for people than nonliving objects. This is an issue which bears further consideration including whether they should be considered a separate class of environmental features influencing occupation.

als (boxes, sand, tires) that lend themselves to active exploration and involvement. What they are is not as important as what one can do with them (Csikszentmihalyi & Rochberg-Halton, 1981). On the other hand, the fixed equipment found in many playgrounds may afford fewer opportunities for behavior if it can be used only in certain ways (i.e., presses for specific behaviors) (Haywood, Rothenberg, & Beasley, 1974). It should be of no surprise that children often abandon the neat structural playground designed by adults for the local woods, back lot, or storm drain where there lurks all the possibilities of the unknown.

As the previous example suggests, objects can influence behavior simply by virtue of intrinsic properties (Hocking, 1994). The weight, size, pliability, texture, and other physical attributes of objects influence what can be done with them. For example, whether we toss, carry, or bend an object is influenced by its intrinsic properties.

Objects vary in complexity—that is, the amount of skill and learning required for their use. Therefore, the complexity of an object may greatly affect how it affords and presses. Simple and familiar objects may give comfort and invite relaxing behavior, while complex objects tend to demand specialized and skilled behavior. The presence of certain objects in an environment will not always lead to their use if no one present knows what to do with them (Fietelson, 1977; Yi-Fu, 1978) or if they are not relevant to the person's lifestyle. An example of the latter is that one ordinarily will not use parking meters if one does not drive a car. At the same time, objects may be used for purposes other than those for which they were intended. For example, bicycle riders often use parking meters as objects to which they can lock their bicycles.

As adults, we tend to surround ourselves with objects that reflect our established patterns of interest and activity. Thus, we prefer objects that reflect who we are and what we do. Moreover, we imbue objects with meaning so that they become symbols of power, prestige, independence, and connection to others. For example, objects that become symbols of wealth and status typically are rare or unusual in some respect. As society has become more technologically sophisticated, operating or manipulating complex machines frequently brings more status to certain jobs.

The potential of objects to be used or manipulated to achieve particular goals also contributes to their symbolic meaning. Adolescents, for example, frequently mention musical instruments, journals, and stereo equipment as being their most prized possessions because they allow them to express their feelings and values in a socially competent manner (Csikszentmihalyi & Rochberg-Halton, 1981). In adulthood, possessions are often a manifestation of power and independence. Adults prize certain objects because they make possible some activity; they enhance one's options within the environment (Furby, 1978). In a rural setting, a large pick-up truck may be valued because it enhances the owner's potential to haul wood or to traverse mountain roads.

Objects also symbolize interests and values, thereby communicating important messages about one's identity. Adults use objects to identify their "trade," in both work and leisure (Csikszentmihalyi & Rochberg-Halton, 1981). Religious icons and artifacts in one's house can indicate a commitment to religious values, while tapestries and the presence of a floor loom can communicate that one is a weaver. Objects may also convey the "sense of having roots or of belonging in a particular setting" (Ljungström, 1989). For example, many persons keep antiques handed down from their ancestors. Such objects convey a sense of continuity with one's past and show that one belongs to a particular heritage or cultural group.

Since an object's meaning is a matter of social convention, an object may have several potential meanings that vary with context. Tilley (1989) provides an example of how the meaning of a safety pin changes depending on whether it is worn by "an infant, a grandmother or a 'punk'" (p. 185).

The symbolic meaning of objects affords and presses for ways of using them. For example, when a car is a symbol of independence and responsibility, the young adult owner may feel increased demands for competence in understanding its maintenance. The sentimental value of an object as a reminder of family or past events may become so powerful that the object is retired from use to avoid its becoming damaged or destroyed.

Objects can vary tremendously in their meaning. Some objects may have only utilitarian value; that is, their absence would make life less convenient or prevent us from doing something. For example, appliances such as a clothes washer or toaster are good candidates for this category of relatively low meaning objects in societies where they are common. Other objects may have more moderate levels of meaning. Rubinstein (1989) gives an example of an elderly woman's collection of figurines:

> She did not express much intense emotional involvement with these objects, but they marked and filled her space, gave her sensory pleasure, had a story and gave her stories to tell, and added texture to her rooms. (p. 49)

Objects seem to take on the most value when they signify something very personal about one's experiences or accomplishments and/or about one's connections to others (Csikszentmihalyi & Rochberg-Halton, 1981). One of my most prized possessions is a rocking horse I carved for my children from oak beams retrieved from a dilapidated barn on the farm where my wife was reared. Objects such as this give our lives texture and depth.

Beyond the influence that individual objects have on behavior, the collection and organization of objects in a space can create an overall aura that affords and presses in a coherent way. For example, bedrooms have traditionally been designed to afford opportunity for rest, sleeping, and intimacy. The objects (i.e., the typical bed, chest of drawers, dressing table, and perhaps a television and a lamp) creates a low arousal setting that demands very little. A recent social phenomenon, however, is the transformation of the bedroom into "the place to hang out" (Dullea, 1980, p. C-8). A trend toward keeping exercise equipment, home computers, small refrigerators, and other accoutrements in the bedroom has made this room no longer a place to unwind but, instead, a place that maintains the same press as the other environments that make up extremely active lifestyles. As this example illustrates, the objects in a setting both reflect and elicit a particular set of behaviors.

Objects may have very pervasive influences on one's way of life. For example, Hardyment (1988) argues that the widespread availability of such appliances as refrigerators and washers and driers during this past century has resulted in vastly changed patterns of work and social interaction for women who were housewives. These women stayed at home to perform many household tasks that were previously done in public places and in association with others.

SOCIAL ENVIRONMENT

The social environment can be thought of being made up of two elements (Figure 7.3): the gatherings or groups of persons that one joins and the occupational forms that persons perform. Both of these are contexts that afford opportunities for behavior and that press for certain kinds of performances.

Social Groups

Groups afford and press for occupational behavior in two ways. First, they provide for and assign occupational roles to individuals within them. Second, they create a behavioral context or social space in which those roles are acted out according to group ambience, norms, and climate, thereby allowing and prescribing the kinds of occupational behavior that members can or should perform. Social groups are collections of persons that occur with regularity. Thus, it is in the nature of most social groups that they endure over time. As such, they come to have an internal organization which makes them recognizable entities within a culture.

As noted in Chapter 5, social groups are composed of the roles of their members. These roles provide both avenues for action and constraints on how persons can act. People ordinarily belong to, and interact with, many types of social groups and organizations throughout their lives. These collections of individuals range from informal social groupings, such as a routine gathering of acquaintances at a local bar, to enduring and close knit groups (e.g.,

● Social groups
  e.g., families, church groups,
  coworkers

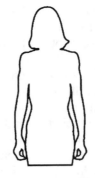

● Occupational forms
  e.g., biking, dressing,
  mowing the lawn, fishing

Figure 7.3.   Social environment.

the family), to formalized organizations developed for the explicit purpose of achieving some goal (Etzioni, 1964; Katz & Kahn, 1966). While a range of groups can occur in any society, some groups are fundamental. Each society has some version of a family group. Many traditional societies have large extended, multi-generational families. In modern society, single parent families and blended families that incorporate children from previous marriages are common. Society is beginning to recognize families made up of same-sex partners, although their rights and legal status are not yet fully recognized.

School provides natural groupings of classmates and affords the possibility of forming smaller groups such as cliques; the workplace is another source of groups. Depending on one's work, relevant groups may be the work team, the larger professional group to which one belongs, unions, committees, and so on. Within communities, groups such as clubs, lodges, church groups, and informal groups based on common interests exist.

To understand how groups influence occupational behavior, it is first important to recognize that "groups are real and have important influences that cannot be understood entirely in terms of the individual members" (Knowles, 1982, p. 19). These influences are the function of group dynamics which emanate from the group as a whole. Because a group has a dynamic property of its own it can be thought of as creating a *social space*, within which members act (Knowles, 1982). The social space of the group has boundaries, a climate, an identifiable structure, and other features which

press and afford opportunities for occupational behavior.

Group structure can press for how centrally involved members will become and how specialized their roles will be. For example, in a complex, hierarchically organized group such as a company, there may be a wide range of roles. Roles higher on the hierarchy are afforded to only a few people, whereas roles lower on the hierarchy may be more readily accessible. The structure of the group may influence with whom persons in a given role interact and what occupational performance is required by a given role.

An enduring climate of values and interests is characteristic of most groups (Moos, 1974). Therefore, people who perceive a large disparity between the values of a setting and their own will tend to leave or avoid such an environment. However, if they do not or cannot leave, they are prone to shift toward greater congruency with the setting's prevalent values (Newcomb, 1943; Pervin, 1968). This shift toward congruency enables cohesiveness to develop among users of the environment and sustains the setting's characteristic climate of values and interests.

Depending on their climates, groups press for differing levels of commitment and role internalization. If the press for involvement is low, members are afforded opportunity to choose how involved they want to become. When an organization requires substantial involvement, members must make a greater effort to internalize their roles, frequently through special training or initiation of some sort. Fraternal lodges, for example, are often closely-knit groups that carefully screen, admit, socialize, and rarely lose their members.

Groups that consist of loosely linked networks of individuals may afford members the opportunity to settle into relatively peripheral and unthreatening roles. Individuals have the opportunity to move in and out of a variety of positions and interrelationships with other members, as well as the freedom to leave the group with ease.

Whatever kind of social space they provide, social groups have a major impact on the development of role behavior. Because roles are learned in the context of groups (Versluys, 1980), the groups that are available to a person will determine the roles available to that person as well. An infant's role repertoire is limited primarily to family-derived roles in dyadic or small group relationships—daughter, son, niece, nephew, sister, brother. When they enter school, children are afforded opportunities to participate in more groups such as clubs, chorus, band, and sports teams. Throughout life the range of groups open to a person may expand or narrow. For example, going away to college may open up possibilities to participate in a number of new groups.

By adulthood, individuals in modern societies are generally involved in a complex of groups. As Allen, Wilder, & Atkinson (1983) note,

> An industrialized society produces social fragmentation, division of labor, and a heterogeneity of interests; as a consequence social identity is determined by membership in many different types of groups. Not only are there kinship, ethnic, and religious groups in complex societies, but a variety of political, economic and recreational groups exist as well. (p. 97)

An interesting example of how group membership influences development of roles and related behaviors is provided by a study of the culture of an African-American urban ghetto (Pervin, 1968). Because conventional employment opportunities for the African-American adults in this study were either menial jobs or nonexistent, work roles that are considered deviant by white middle-class American culture were deemed normal and successful. Hustlers, pimps, preacher-hustlers, and entertainers were all models of competent occupational performance. This cultural influence extended downward to affect the ghetto child's approach to the traditional pre-work role of student. By the time children had entered school, many had already begun imitating and internalizing behaviors that would lead to success in the urban ghetto culture but which were antithetical to the student role: verbal manipulativeness, resourcefulness, self-reliance, and mistrust of authorities. In doing so, these adolescents were assuming more culturally relevant pre-work roles (Ogbu, 1981).

As this example illustrates, the influence of groups on occupational behavior represents the effects of a coherent social system with its own structure and values. Members are influenced by groups because groups are meaningful gestalt contexts that represent a very real life space experienced by those in the group. It is this quality of being in a coherent life space that gives groups the power to afford and press for occupational behavior.

Occupational Forms

In the first edition of this book the concept of an occupational task was introduced (Barris, Kielhofner, Levine, & Neville, 1985). Tasks were defined as sequences of actions in which persons engaged to satisfy either external societal requirements or internal motives. It was recognized that task complexity pressed for certain occupational behavior, the conventions for how they should be performed, and their social meanings. Tasks were viewed as existing independent of any instances of actual performance; that is, tasks were sustained in the environment as defined by cultural convention.

Nelson (1988) introduced a related concept of *occupational form,* which he defined as "the preexisting structure that elicits, guides, or structures subsequent human performance" (p. 633). He also proposed that an occupational form is "an objective set of circumstances, independent of and external to a person" (Nelson, 1988, p. 633).

Nelson (1988) argues that each occupational form has two dimensions. The first dimension consists of immediate stimuli or factors which influence how the occupational form is done. These include such things as the materials used, the immediate and relevant context in which it is done, and the necessary temporal order of actions involved in completing the occupational form. The second dimension is the social context which influences how the occupational form is organized through symbolic means (e.g., values, norms, and practical guidelines for judging the performance of the occupational form). Nelson's (1988) argument and the previous, related concept of tasks provides a basis for proposing the concept of occupational forms as part of the social environment. While I will follow much of Nelson's argument, I will propose a definition of occupational forms that differs in some respects and elaborates upon his original concept.[c]

Let us first consider the origins of occupational forms in culture. Cultures are, in large measure, the ways that humans groups have come to adapt to the world (Hall, 1966). Each culture has a technology for meeting the most basic human needs as well as for undertaking the way of life represented in the culture. For example, each culture develops means for acquiring and preparing food. Over time these means become well-organized and sometimes ritualized ways of doing things. Generations of trial and error, creative refinement, and invention of new techniques and tools result in conventional ways of performing identifiable and purposive behaviors related to getting and preparing food. These conventionalized modes are occupational forms. Cultures have ways of going about hunting, raising domesticated animals that provide food, gardening, and so on. In primitive societies where hunting is a source of food, members learn to make hunting tools (e.g., bows, boomerangs, and blowguns). The way of making these implements becomes refined into an occupational form.

Thus, cultures evolve clusters of occupational forms that together make up a way of life.

It is important to note that the occupational form exists outside of, but is realized in, any single performance of the occupational form; that is, the occupational form is a *way of doing* something that is generated and stored in the cultural collective. It can be transmitted to new members; it is given a name; it is readily recognized by members of the culture as a thing some members do. Occupational forms can also come to have special significance within the cultural group. For example, Native Americans have viewed hunting or fishing as a sacred act of taking something which nature willingly provided. Thus, the occupational form of hunting or fishing required the hunter or fisher to give thanks to the animals' spirit for giving itself up.

In modern societies occupational forms are legion. Many are common to all adult members (such as dressing oneself) and others are the pursuit of a privileged and sanctioned few (e.g., only a priest, minister, rabbi, or shaman may conduct certain sacred rituals). Still, the occupational forms belong to some larger group. They are recognizable by members of the culture or subculture who do not perform, but are audience to, their performance.

Given these considerations, occupational forms can be defined as *rule-bound sequences of action which are at once coherent, oriented to a purpose, sustained in collective knowledge, culturally recognizable, and named.* Occupational forms are rule bound in that, by cultural convention, there is a typical or correct way of doing them. Culture provides the rules of an occupational form by specifying procedures, outcomes, and standards for its performance. These rules are always a matter of convention. The conventions are sustained in human collectives and passed on to those who wish to learn an occupational form. Occupational forms can vary widely on the clarity and flexibility of their rules. In some occupational forms, the rules are readily apparent. Taking an exam, for instance, requires someone to be in a particular place at a particular time and to answer a previously prepared set of questions. Success is contingent upon answering correctly a preestablished percentage of

---

[c]One important difference in the concept of occupational form as used here is that I do not include the materials or the actual circumstances of a given performance as part of what is meant by an occupational form. Rather, I am emphasizing the social conventions by which the form is generated, sustained, taught and learned, named and given meaning.

these questions. In other cases, the rules are more vague and the subject of varying opinion, such as how to best fish for trout. Generally, occupational forms done with others or in the presence of others are more rule bound. Other occupational forms, such as gardening or cooking, are more individually determined. Nonetheless, even these latter occupational forms conform to recognizable parameters that make them clearly gardening or cooking.

Creative endeavors generally have more flexible rules. Sometimes the rigidity with which an occupational form must be performed changes as the person becomes more competent and knowledgeable of the rules. Using a potter's wheel initially requires that one conform to certain rules regarding the properties of clay, the mechanics of the wheel, and laws of gravity and balance. With mastery, these rules still pertain but can be elaborated upon by the artist's creativity and imagination. Indeed, the creativity of a performance may generate new rules (i.e., new ways of doing) that become part of the cultural convention for how one does the occupational form.

Many occupational forms are so customary that their rules do not become evident until they are broken. One ordinarily does not think of a conversation as being a rule-bound occupational form. Yet we all recognize when persons break the taken-for-granted conventions underlying how to engage in a conversation. Depending on the culture and who the participants are, these conventions may include making eye contact, taking turns speaking, sticking to appropriate subject matter, and so on. Not following these rules can unnerve others and disrupt a conversation. Interestingly, most games have strict rules that must be followed by players. The person who refuses to play by the rules spoils the sport. Thus, even seemingly simple and common occupational forms have rules to which one must adhere.

Coherence refers to the fact that occupational forms represent a whole to which a number of action sequences may belong. Preparing soil, planting seeds, weeding, and picking vegetables all belong to gardening. Singing, conversing with a neighbor, and playing fetch with one's dog do not belong to the occupational form of gardening, although they may all occur while one is gardening. We may whistle while we work, but unless one is whistling instrumentally, such as when giving commands to a sheepdog while herding, whistling is not part of the work.

Occupational forms are always directed at some recognizable end even if the end is simply to experience the behavior, as in dancing or going for a walk. Indeed, it is the purposiveness of occupational forms that guarantees their maintenance as culturally recognizable acts.

By creating and sustaining occupational forms and their meanings, cultures provide the possibility of a range of occupational behaviors. The occupations we perform have a shape and identity which existed long before we learned to do them. Moreover, the occupational form itself exerts a specific influence on us each time we undertake to perform it. The culturally prescribed rules that make up the occupational form, along with the unfolding dynamics of performance which must be brought into conformity with the form, recruit the appropriate behavior.

It is very easy to see how occupational forms afford and press for behavior. The availability of occupational forms in a culture provide opportunities for performance. We learn to do those things that are part of the culture's way of life. Moreover, conventions for who should do certain forms, as well as the rules of the form themselves, press for what things we do and how we do them.

Occupational forms are performed in a discrete unit of time. However, some occupational forms are by nature repetitive, such as gardening, personal grooming, and driving to work. Sometimes a number of occupational forms are grouped together into personal projects (as discussed in Chapter 4), such as the plastering, stripping, painting, and wallpapering which are necessary for restoring an old house. Occupational forms may be bound to certain times of the day or to certain seasons, or they may be performed at an individual's discretion. Preparing a departmental annual report is both time-limited and seasonal; ongoing supervisory activities are somewhat more discretionary. In places with marked seasonal change, mowing the lawn and shoveling snow alternate in winter and summer as occupational forms.

Occupational forms may also vary in their customary degree of seriousness or playfulness. In this regard, they press for the kind of attitude a person should have when doing them. How seriously an occupational form is to be taken may reflect the context in which it is performed as well as the consequences that are contingent upon successful performance. If an occupational form belongs to work, it is likely to be more serious; if it is done for leisure, then it may be playful. For example, woodworking as a hobby will generally be performed more playfully than the woodworking of a professional carpenter; singing in a concert will be more serious than singing at a party. Further, although many activities generally fall into the domain of either work or play, people can still take their play tasks seriously or carry out their work tasks playfully.

Occupational forms may involve the measurement of one's performance against another person or some recognized standard, and the degree to which two or more people must work together to accomplish some goal. Competition and cooperation can coexist in an occupational form, as when one team competes against another. When public competitive standards must be met in an occupational form, it presses for greater effort.

Summary

I have argued that the influences of the social environment on occupational behavior come from two sources, social groups and occupational forms. In everyday life these two aspects of the social world are tightly interwoven and infused with the elements of culture. As noted, culture determines the groups that are available to, and valued by, the person as well as the occupational forms that people will perform when they become members. For example, in Chillum, a Washington, DC suburb with a large Fiumedinisi Italian community, membership in the Fiumedinisi Lodge is an important means of providing cultural continuity for these families. Certain occupational forms such as dances occur at the lodge on a regular basis (Valente, 1984).

The family is another highly valued social group in this community. Occupational forms that are commonly shared by the Fiumedinisi families include listening to a weekly radio show broadcast from Italy and an annual wine-making and tasting party. In addition, these families have held onto and passed down certain occupational forms that were practiced in Italy such as shoemaking and cabinetry. Thus, children who develop skill in these occupational forms do so partly because of their membership in a family group that is part of a culture which values them (Valente, 1984).

As this example illustrates, the social ecology is a coherent and integrated milieu which affords its members ways of thinking, feeling, and appreciating the world and which presses them toward some level of participation and conformity in that world. The social system is, at once, a fountain of possibilities and a strong current which carries its participants along.

OCCUPATIONAL BEHAVIOR SETTINGS

The physical and social are intertwined in the environments we encounter. Together they constitute what I will call occupational behavior settings. *The occupational behavior setting is a composite of spaces, objects, occupational forms, and/or social groups that cohere and constitute a meaningful context for performance.* Occupational behavior settings are not merely collections of people, objects, and forms in places where we perform. They are, after Buttimer (1976), life worlds which resonate with meaning, life, and action in configurations that make up coherent wholes. Whether it be the hot, vibrant light-sound-people atmosphere of a night spot; the peaceful shade of gold and crimson autumn woods; the monotonous movement of machinery in long lines where factory workers perform in synchrony; the quiet low light, soft music, furniture-and-rug atmosphere of a family room shared with a lover, child, or parent; or the bright lit, neat, clean, orderly, long rows of packaged food in a supermarket occupied by people meticulously pushing metal carts, each occupational behavior setting has a life world texture, organization, and rhythm. These life world features afford and press for occupational behavior. We naturally tend to become excited, aroused, relaxed, engaged, or alienated by these life worlds. And once within them, we feel the persuasion of their features to behave along certain lines.

Occupational behavior settings are places of being and acting in life, and they envelop us and become part of whatever we are doing. As Rowles (1991) and Rockwell-Dylla (1992) caution, the environment should not be seen as sterile categories that focus on mere physical structure or task requirements. Rather, it is the life world nature of occupational behavior settings that makes them so powerful in their influence on our experience and behavior.

A Taxonomy of Occupational Behavior Settings

Categorizing occupational behavior settings is a potentially complex undertaking. One factor which complicates the problem is that we can recognize smaller behavior settings within larger ones. For example, one's home (be it a house, apartment, dormitory, or other group living situation) can be considered an occupational behavior setting. However, we can subdivide most homes into smaller behavior settings such as the bedroom, kitchen, garage, and so on. Moreover, many children could further subdivide their bedrooms into the bed where they relax, read, carry on phone conversations, the desk where they do homework, and perhaps another space where hobbies are carried out or pets are kept.

In this section I will identify the coherent occupational behavior settings that most persons encounter in everyday life, recognizing that each of these behavior settings may be a composite of even smaller and more specific behavior settings. As illustrated in Figure 7.4, typical occupational behavior settings that make up the course of daily life are the home, the neighborhood, the workplace, and gathering/recreation/resource sites (e.g., theaters, churches, temples, beaches, clubs, libraries, galleries, ski lodges, restaurants, health clubs, and stores).

Readers will readily recognize that how a behavior setting is classified for any individual depends on what one does in it. Thus, for example, a restaurant is a workplace for the waiters, cook, and others who labor in it, but a gathering and recreation site for those who frequent it for a meal with family or friends.

Home

The home, of course, serves as a location where the most basic needs of persons are met. It is a source of shelter from the environment. It is a place where people can eat and sleep. It is often the setting where one cohabitates with those most intimate in one's life (e.g., with family or a lover). One's home is likely to be a place one interacts with those who become part of one's ongoing social network. Finally, home is often the place where one carries out a whole range of occupational forms. These include self-care, leisure, amateur/hobby pursuits, and interactions with friends and family.

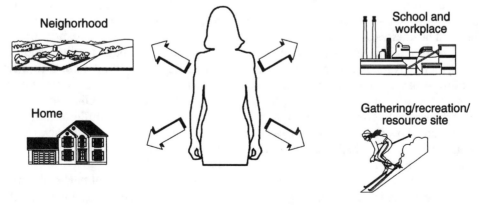

Figure 7.4. Occupational behavior settings.

The home itself is often the object of occupational performance since persons clean, decorate, and repair their homes.

Home is also an important source of meaning, comfort, security, and identity for many persons. Rowles (1987) observes that for elderly persons home can maximize a sense of person's competence since intimate familiarity allows one to function despite sensory and other limitations associated with aging. Thus, for many, home is a place of safety and refuge. Indeed, home typically becomes the central point of reference for existence (Rowles, 1987). It is the place from which all other excursions into occupational behavior settings takes place. Home can come to have a feature of *insideness* which includes physical or bodily awareness of the physical details of the home, a social sense of belonging, and an autobiographical sense of personal events which have taken place there (Rowles, 1987). While the concept of insideness emerged from the study of elderly persons who have occupied homes for a length of time, the very fact that persons spend so much of their times in their home, and that their more intimate events ordinarily take place there, insideness would appear to develop rather quickly even for new settings, though, of course, it deepens with time.

Neighborhood

Whether it be a pastoral setting, the bustling streets of urban life, a suburban subdivision, a small town, or an ethnic section of a large city, persons encounter an immediate surround to their homes typically referred to as one's neighborhood. By neighborhoods I mean both the out-of-doors and the other homes and businesses surrounding one's own home. Urban neighborhoods thus consist of sidewalks and streets, bus stops, subway entrances, newspaper stands, parks, neighbors' homes and yards, and local stores. Rural neighborhoods are less dense and, for that reason, may extend over a much larger area than we would consider to constitute a neighborhood in a large city. Occupational forms in the neighborhood depend, of course, on its character. They may range from jogging or going for a walk to visiting with neighbors or going to picnics or block parties. The neighborhood and its surroundings is also where we most frequently purchase goods, make economic and other transactions, get our possessions cleaned or repaired, and seek services such as haircuts. In meeting these personal needs, we encounter a range of neighborhood businesses. These include banks, filling stations, supermarkets, cleaners, clothing stores, hardware stores, and so on.

A number of social groups may inhabit neighborhoods. Most obvious is the local community of one's neighbors. Neighbors may associate in groups for a variety of purposes. Thus, for example, a neighborhood group may be a tenants association or an association of homeowners in a subdivision. It maybe a closely-knit ethnic community or simply a collection of families who are long-time residents of the neighborhood. Indeed, the neighborhood can be synonymous with one's dominant community and culture. As such, it is where friends and associates, if not relatives, live and it is the focus of one's public life. Some neighborhoods in both urban and rural settings still function this way, particularly when they are composed of more homogeneous groups of people with common heritage or common ties to a kind of work such as mining, forestry, or farming.

For others, especially those in today's cities, the neighborhood can mainly be a transitional setting where one catches the bus to work, does one's banking and necessary shopping for food, and encounters an occasional acquaintance. For such persons, there may be no deep ties to the neighborhood and, indeed, few inhabitants may be long-term residents of the neighborhood. For example, suburban neighborhoods are sometimes temporary repositories for highly mobile families who feel little connection to anything more than their home (Oldenburg, 1991). In contrast, some urban neighborhoods have become inhospitable due to deterioration of buildings, littered and wasted open spaces, and extensive crime which threatens inhabitants who feel uneasy in the neighborhood.

Consequently, neighborhoods may mean many different things depending on their nature and the relationship of the inhabitant to the larger area. Nonetheless, neighborhoods are our immediate surround and we cannot avoid them if we wish to go anywhere. More importantly, the kind of neighborhood which one inhabits may have a strong influence on how frequently and with what purpose one goes out, and what occupations one pursues in the neighborhood.

School and Workplace

Members of society are all expected to learn to shoulder responsibility and be productive. While persons learn to, and perform, in productive ways in a number of settings, the progression from school into work is a dominant influence on occupational life for most members of industrial societies. Schools are readily recognized by the organization of space and the objects in them. Classrooms and their requisite blackboards, audiovisual equipment and desks, labs and their specialized equipment, libraries and books are all part of the school spaces and objects. For many people, from childhood into early adulthood, a significant period of time is spent outside the home in school. Until the transition to adult work, school is the dominant institution of occupational life where individuals are socialized, educated, and otherwise prepared for all walks of adult life. The student role and the occupational forms of school are fairly standardized. Students attend class, take exams, complete assignments, and so on. School is also a primary locus of the increasingly important peer group and culture and the occupational forms that accompany it, including such things as sports, bake sales, and dances.

A majority of adults find that the workplace is the dominate setting of occupational life for many of their adult years. Given a standard five-day work week, most adults spend a large portion of their lives in the workplace. Places of work are as many and varied as the institutions and occupations of human invention. Farms, factories, schools, restaurants, subways, offices, hospitals, stores, libraries, boats, airplanes, trains, and buses are all potential workplaces.

Workplaces are characterized by the objects which must be used in the course of work (e.g., tractors, machines, books, computers, blackboards, file cabinets, desks, counters, cash registers, goods-for-sale, and the like). All these objects and their arrangement within any workplace afford and press for certain work behaviors.

Each type of work is characterized by the occupational forms which comprise it. Thus, for example, bus drivers take tickets or tokens, announce stops, and drive the bus. Carpenters frame up walls and rafters by measuring, cutting, and nailing lumber; teachers lecture, and give and grade exams.

Workplaces are also the locus of social groups and social roles. Depending on the workplace, one may encounter students, customers, patients, clients, and so on. Each workplace has its own organization and social life which makes possible the orderly production of goods or services that are the object of the workplace. The worker role locates one in a variety of social groups such as a work team, professional group, labor union, company, and so on.

Gathering/Recreation/Resource Sites

The routines of occupational life typically take persons to a number of public places that serve as resources for a range of needs. These places can include sources of information and inspiration such as museums, libraries, and churches or temples. While one may go to such a site alone and remain so (e.g., going to a library to study), they are most often places of fellowship.

Many of the behavioral settings which make up this category are what Oldenburg (1991) refers to as "third places." Noting that most persons' lives include home and work as first and second places, he designates the third place as "public places that host the regular, voluntary, informal, and happily anticipated gatherings of individuals beyond the realms of home and work" (p. 16). Examples of third places are taverns, coffeehouses, and restaurants. Ready accessibility, familiarity, and comfort are traits of the third place. As the location of informal public life where one can be renewed, escape life's pressures, enjoy light fellowship, and renew connection to the larger community, Oldenburg (1991) considers third places as essential.

This category of occupational behavior settings also includes specialized recreation sites. They may be built environments such as skating rinks, bowling alleys, theaters, health clubs. They may be the sites of clubs or groups such as the Lions Club, Shriners, or Knights of Columbus. Finally, they may be natural settings such as beaches and forest preserves.

The organization, objects, and forms of these occupational behavior settings can vary tremendously depending on their purpose. Moreover, the gathering/recreation/resource sites which make up a regular part of anyone's life vary from person to person. Nonetheless, they are important influences on occupational behavior.

Cultural Influences on Occupational Behavior Settings

Each of the occupational behavior settings discussed above involve a collation of physical spaces, objects, social groups, and occupational forms. When these features come together they collectively afford and press for the occupational behaviors we expect to encounter within them.

Each culture provides a range of occupational behavior settings which are typical for an individual given his or her age, roles, etc. Occupational behavior settings are always a function of culture and thereby a matter of convention. Today, in modern societies we generally have separate spaces for work, play, family life, spiritual activities, and so on. In preindustrial times, work and home life were more likely to be carried out in the same setting. With the advent of factories, people began to go to work in a place outside their home, a pattern that eventually gave rise to the middle-class lifestyle of commuting to the office, carrying out one's job, and then commuting home again to resume the rest of one's life. Today, however, occupational roles such as investment counselor, psychotherapist, and professor may blend home and work settings. Such technological trends as the growth of satellite media capacities and increasing ownership of home computers are making the set-ting of the centralized office less necessary (Toffler, 1980).

Cultural differences can also be found in the extent to which the play setting is separate from home life. In rural subcultures, for instance, the home is likely to be the setting for many leisure activities, whereas in large urban areas, people are more likely to leave their homes in search of leisure (Giovanninni, 1983). Away from home, play may be carried out in settings that exist solely for that purpose (e.g., health spas, tennis clubs, bowling alleys). The occupational behavior settings in which persons perform are always changing as a function of new cultural influences.

PHYSICAL AND SOCIAL GEOGRAPHY OF OCCUPATIONAL LIFE

Any persons's occupational life involves rounds of occupational performance in a number of occupational behavior settings. For example, I go to work in a setting called the occupational therapy department. The department is located in a larger medical center which is part of a university. While some of my occupational performance at work also involves settings beyond the department which are part of the larger university and medical center, I'll confine my discussion to the department. The department consists of a built environment: offices, classrooms, labs, restrooms, and storage closets connected to each other by a corridor. In each of the department's spaces are objects which members of the department readily recognize and, in fact, expect. One large classroom has blackboards, desks, projectors, chalk, a pointer, a microphone, and so on. In that room several occupational forms routinely take place: lectures, discussions, meetings. My office contains a desk, chairs, bookshelves with books, a computer, pictures of my family, a telephone, a few decorations and personal mementos of professional life, degrees and awards framed and hung on the wall, and so on. In my office a number of other occupational forms take place: small conferences and discussions with faculty and students, job interviews, writing papers and books, grading student papers, and so on.

In the course of the day I encounter, become part of, or interact with social groups (e.g., the faculty in a meeting, the student group in a lecture). Within those groups, I encounter expectations for a number of occupational forms (leading a meeting, giving a lecture, or making a budget request). In each case, what I do, when I do it, with whom I do it, and what objects I use are both afforded and constrained by the occupational forms, objects, spaces, and social groups that make up my environment.

The course of my week is characterized by movement through a number of occupational behavior settings via elevators, steps, hallways, streets, train tracks, and country roads: my house and the rooms in it; the department; restaurants; the fields, lake, or the barn on the farm where I live; the dean's office at the university; and the occupational therapy clinics in the medical center. This movement through environments is largely a function of my activity choices and of my roles and habits which are the products of previous occupational choices. When I am in each of these environments they afford and press for a range of occupational behavior. What I do in them is, in large measure, a function of those environments, their organization, the people and/or objects in them, and the occupational forms they afford to or require of me.

One of the most telling examples of our need for environment as context for our behavior is how we will rearrange the same environment so as to allow them to serve as different occupational behavior settings. Rubinstein (1989) gives a poignant example of this in telling the story of an elderly woman who lives in a studio apartment and conducts most of her occupational life there. As her day progresses she meticulously rearranges that environment:

In the daytime, her small home displayed its most public look; her big room, filled with comfortable wing chairs and "lovely things," was warm and inviting. She did her entertaining there. The largest item in her room was a sofa bed; her son had made and installed a wall-length enclosure that contained bookcases and a built-in sofa which she opened up at night. At nighttime, when the bed was pulled open, the sitting room became a bedroom . . . In her small space, the public area was now maintained between the time she made her bed in the morning, about 8:30, until about 3:00, when she pulled back the sofa cover and took her nap. Upon waking she moved the furniture so that she could dine and watch TV for the evening. She changed, too, from the clothes she wore for public appearance to more informal clothes. Finally, around 11, she got into her bedclothes and rearranged the furniture yet again for her fully private time. (pp. 47–48)

The very act of modifying one's environment to make it suitable for occupations illustrates vividly how much we depend on context for our experience and behavior. The influence of environment on occupation can perhaps be best appreciated if we consider that occupation is, above all else, action which occupies a particular social and physical space.

References

Allen, V. L., Wilder, D. A., & Atkinson, M. L. (1983). Multiple group membership and social identity. In T. R. Sarbin & K. E. Scheibe (Eds.), *Studies in social identity*. New York: Praeger.

Altman, I., & Chemers, M. (1980). *Culture and environment*. Monterey, CA: Brooks/Cole.

Barris, R., Kielhofner, G., Levine, R. E., & Neville, A. M. (1985). Occupation as interaction with the environment. In G. Kielhofner (Ed.), *A Model of human occupation*. Baltimore: Williams & Wilkins.

Brake, M. (1980). *The sociology of youth culture and youth cultures*. London: Routledge & Kegan Paul.

Buttimer, A. (1976) Grasping the dynamism of the life-world. *Annals of the Association of American Geographers, 66*, 277–292

Csikszentmihalyi, M. (1990). *Flow: The psychology of optimal experience*. New York: Harper & Row.

Csikszentmihalyi, M., & Rochberg-Halton, E. (1981). *The meaning of things*. Cambridge, MA: Cambridge University Press.

Dullea, G. (1980, July 10). The busy bedroom. *The New York Times*, pp. C-1, C-8.

Eisenberg, L. (1977). Development as a unifying concept in psychiatry. *British Journal of Psychiatry, 131*, 225–237.

Etzioni, A. (1964). *Modern organizations*. Englewood Cliffs, NJ: Prentice-Hall.

Fietelson, D. (1977). Cross-cultural studies of representational play. In B. Tizard & D. Harvey (Eds.), *Biology of play*. London: William Heinemann Medical Books.

Furby, L. (1978). Possessions: Toward a theory of their meaning and function throughout the life cycle. In P. B. Baltes (Ed.), *Life-Span development and behavior* (Vol. 1). New York: Academic Press.

Gergen, K. J. (1991). *The saturated self: Dilemmas of identity in contemporary life*. Philadelphia: Basic Books.

Gibson, J. J. (1979). *The ecological approach to visual perception*. Boston: Houghton Mifflin.

Giovanninni, J. (1983, September 11). I love New York and L.A., too. *The New York Times Sunday Magazine*, pp. 144–148.

Hall, E. (1966). *The hidden dimension*. Garden City, NY: Anchor Books.

Hardyment, C. (1988). *From mangle to microwave. The mechanism of household work*. New York: Polity Press.

Haywood, D. G., Rothenberg, M., & Beasley, R. R. (1974). Children's play and urban playground environments. *Environmental Behavior, 6*, 131–168.

Hocking, C. (1994, April). *Objects in the environment: A critique of the model of human occupation dimensions*. Paper presented at World Federation of Occupational Therapy, Symposium, International Perspectives on the Model of Human Occupation, London, England.

Johnson, M. W. (1935). The effect on behavior of variations in the amount of play equipment. *Child Development, 6*, 56–68.

Katz, D., & Kahn, R. L. (1966). *The social psychology of organizations*. New York: John Wiley & Sons.

Kiernat, J. M. (1983). Environment: The hidden modality. *Physical & Occupational Therapy in Geriatrics, 2*, 1, 3–12.

Knowles, E. S. (1982). From individuals to group members: A dialectic for the social sciences. In W. Ickes & E.S. Knowles (Eds.), *Personality, roles and social behavior*. New York: Springer-Verlag.

Lawton, M. P. (1980). *Environment and aging*. Monterey, CA: Brooks/Cole.

Lawton, M. P. (1983). Environment and other detriments of well-being in older people. *Gerontologist, 23*, 349–357.

Lawton, M. P., & Nahemow, L. (1973). Ecology and the aging process. In C. Eisdorfer & M.P. Lawton (Eds.), *Psychology of adult development and aging*. Washington, DC: American Psychological Association.

Ljungström, Å. (1989). Craft artefacts: Keys to the past. Narratives from a craft documentation project in Sweden. *Journal of Ethnological Studies, 28*, 75–87.

Moos, R. H. (1974). *Evaluating treatment environments: A social ecological approach*. New York: John Wiley & Sons.

Nelson, D. (1988). Occupation: Form and performance. *American Journal of Occupational Therapy, 42*, 633–641.

Newcomb, T. M. (1943). *Personality and social change*. New York: Dryden Press.

Ogbu, J. U. (1981). Origins of human competence: A cultural-ecological perspective. *Child Development, 52*, 413–429.

Oldenburg, R. (1991). *The great good place*. New York: Pergamon Press.

Pervin, L. A. (1968). Performance and satisfaction as a function of individual-environment fit. *Pyschological Bulletin, 69*, 56–68.

Quilitch, H. R., & Risley, T. R. (1973). The effects of play materials on social play. *Journal of Applied Behavioral Analysis, 6*, 573–578.

Rapoport, A. (1980). Cross-cultural aspects of environmental design. In I. Altman, A. Rapoport, & J. F. Wohlwill (Eds.), *Human behavior and environment* (Vol 4). New York: Plenum.

Reed, E. S. (1982). An outline of a theory of action systems. *Journal of Motor Behavior, 14*, 98–134.

Rockwell-Dylla, L. (1992). *Older adults meaning of environment: Hospital and home*. Unpublished master's thesis, University of Illinois at Chicago.

Rowles, G. (1987). A place to call home. In L. Carstensen & B. Edelstein (Eds.), *Handbook of clinical gerontology*. New York: Pergamon.

Rowles, G. (1991). Beyond performance: Being in place as a component of occupational therapy, *American Journal of Occupational Therapy, 45*, 265–271.

Rubinstein, R. L. (1989). The home environments of older people: a description of the psychosocial processes linking person to place. *Journal of Gerontology, 44*, 45–53.

Sameroff, A. J. (1983). Developmental systems: Contexts and evolution. In P.H. Mussen (Ed.), *Handbook of child psychology*. New York: John Wiley & Sons.

Schultz, R., & Hanusa, B. H. (1979). Environmental influences on the effectiveness of control- and competence-enhancing interventions. In L. C. Perlmutter & R. A. Monte (Eds.), *Choice and perceived control*. Hillsdale, NJ: Erlbaum.

Thelen, E., & Ulrich, B. D. (1991). Hidden skills: A dynamic systems analysis of treadmill stepping during the first year. *Monographs of the Society for Research in Child Development, 56*, (1, Serial No. 223).

Tilley, C. (1989). Interpreting material culture. In I. Hodder (Ed.), *The meaning of things. Material culture and symbolic expression*. London: Unwin Hyman.

Toffler, A. (1980). *The third wave*. New York: William Morrow.

Valente, J. (1984, January 3). A piece of home. *The Washington Post*, pp. A-1, A-6.

Versluys, H. P. (1980). The remediation of role disorders through focused groupwork. *American Journal of Occupational Therapy, 34*, 609–614.

Yi-Fu, Tuan (1978). Children and the natural environment. In I. Altman & J. F. Wohlwill (Eds.), *Human behavior and environment, Vol. 3, Children and the environment*. New York: Plenum.

KEY CONCEPTS

INFLUENCE OF ENVIRONMENT

- Environment has two broad influences on occupational behavior:
  - **Affords**: by providing potentials for behaviors, the environment gives certain freedoms to choose and act, thus providing opportunities for occupational behavior.
  - **Presses**: emphasizes what the environment expects or demands of the individual; thus, the environment may recruit or require particular occupational behaviors.

PHYSICAL ENVIRONMENTS

- **Natural Environments**: Those elements of the physical world which are largely unmodified by humans, or if constructed, are organized to use and imitate nature.
- **Built Environments**: Environments that result from human fabrication. They are building and connecting structures organized to contain humans, their activities, and their possessions; to separate them from the natural environment; to get people from one part of the built ecology to another.
- **Objects**: May be both naturally occurring and fabricated or processed. The nature of objects present in any space contributes to how it affords or presses for occupational behavior.

SOCIAL ENVIRONMENTS

- **Social Groups**: Collections of persons that occur with regularity. Provide for and assign occupational roles to individuals within the group as well as creating the behavioral context in which those roles are acted out.
- **Occupational Forms**: rule-bound sequences of action which are at once coherent, oriented to a purpose, sustained in collective knowledge, culturally recognizable, and named.

OCCUPATIONAL BEHAVIOR SETTINGS

- a composite of spaces, objects, occupational forms, and social groups that cohere and constitute a meaningful context for occupational performance.
- **Home**: Likely to be a place where one interacts with those who become part of one's ongoing social network. Often the place where one carries out a whole range of occupational forms (e.g., self-care, leisure, amateur/hobby pursuits, interactions with family and friends).
- **Neighborhood**: An immediate surround to a home including the out-of-doors surroundings and other homes and businesses.
- **School/Workplace**: Schools are readily recognized by the organization of space and objects in them. The student role and occupational forms of school are fairly standardized. Workplaces are characterized by the objects which must be used in the course of work.
- **Gathering/recreation/resource sites**: Readily accessible, familiar, and comfortable places where individuals are provided with opportunities to be renewed, escape life's pressures, enjoy light fellowship, and renew connection to the larger community.

8/ Skill in Occupational Performance

Anne Fisher and Gary Kielhofner
with Birgitta Bernspång, Kimberly Bryze, Susan Doble, Birgitta Englund, Marcelle Salamy, and Sandra Simon

INTRODUCTION

Chapters 4, 5, and 6 examined how persons choose, organize, and effect occupational behavior. In this chapter we turn our attention to a more detailed examination of what happens when persons actually engage in occupation. The main focus of this chapter is to examine the discrete elements of occupational performance. Occupational performance consists of meaningful sequences of action in which a person completes an occupational form. For example, when persons do such tasks as shining shoes, preparing a meal, playing cards, mowing the lawn, and painting a room, they are completing occupational forms. Underlying the completion of an occupational form is performance skill.

SKILLS

Within each of the occupations we perform in the course of a day are a number of discrete behavioral elements which we refer to as *skills*. Performance skills are observable elements of action which have implicit functional purposes. As illustrated in Figure 8.1, three types of skills can be observed during occupational performance: motor skills, process skills, and communication and interaction skills.

Motor skills are observable operations used to move oneself or objects. *Process skills* are the observable operations used to sensibly organize and adapt actions in time in order to complete an occupational form. *Communication and interaction skills* are the observable operations used to communicate intentions and needs and coordinate social behavior in order to interact with people. As one can readily see, we conceptualize skill not as something one *has* but as a feature of what one *does*. Skill is related to the underlying capacities of the mind-brain-body performance subsystem that we call upon and use when we perform. However, skill is conceptually distinct from underlying capacity. Skill is dynamically assembled and manifested in actual performance. Moreover, skill develops and improves with development and experience.

The taxonomies of skills presented in this chapter provide a conceptual language which allows a detailed examination of the actions of performance. This conceptualization provides a uniform, consistent language for describing what may be observed in occupational performance.

Traditional activity analysis is designed to identify the underlying capacities necessary for skilled performance. We instead focus on the observable skills that occur in a given performance. The following examples should both clarify the distinction we are making and demonstrate the merit of focusing on skills in performance.

Using traditional activity analysis, one would identify that making a sandwich requires such motions as elbow flexion and pin-

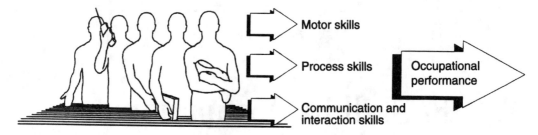

Figure 8.1.   Motor, process, and communication and interaction skills used in occupational performance.

cer grasp. While this is ordinarily true, we know that many clients, who are unable to flex their elbows or use their digits to produce a pincer grasp, still will be able to prepare a sandwich by positioning themselves, materials, and tools differently, and by using other hand movements to hold and manipulate the materials and tools. Activity analysis cannot anticipate how persons will manage to perform in spite of their limitations of underlying capacity. Likewise, attempts to break occupational forms into subroutines (often for purposes of assessment) is problematic. For example, brushing one's teeth can be broken down into components such as squeezing toothpaste, brushing, and rinsing. However, knowing that someone cannot squeeze the toothpaste onto the toothbrush is of limited value unless we know whether it is because the person is unable to grip the tube or because the person performs actions out of sequence (i.e., squeezing the tube before taking off the cap). The skills taxonomies which we will present in this chapter provide more clinically relevant descriptions since they can be used to focus occupational therapists' attention on what actually happens when one person can and another cannot complete the occupational forms of making a sandwich and brushing one's teeth successfully. Moreover, the approach allows the description of the performance to emerge from a standard language, therefore avoiding the need to create, de novo, an explanation of what happened.

Motor, process, and communication and interaction skills represent three universal taxonomies of observable actions used to complete most occupational forms. Consequently, the same conceptual language will apply not only to sandwich-making and teeth-brushing, but also to such diverse occupational forms as

bathing, washing dishes, gardening, repairing a household object, playing with toys, and operating a machine in a factory. Similarly, in the case of social situations, a standard taxonomy of skills can be applied to understanding what a person does when playing a game with others, serving as a member of a planning group, or preparing a meal with family members.

In order to create such taxonomies of skill, we first needed to consider the nature of skill in actual performance. As indicated in Chapter 2, the human system, the occupational form performed, and the environment all influence skilled performance. This means that skill is conceptualized as a function of how effectively the intended occupational form is accomplished within the contingencies of the physical, temporal, and social environments that make up the context for the performance. Consequently, skill connotes how effectively the occupational form is rendered. Occupational therapists have traditionally viewed such capacities as range of motion or strength in terms that describe the action performed (e.g., degrees of freedom, pounds of resistance generated). Such terms say nothing about how effective the action is in accomplishing some functional purpose. The concept of skill views performance in terms of its functional contribution to the completion of an occupational form, asking, in effect, how well did this action serve its purpose in this occupational form?

Consequently, we equate skill with effective instrumentality. If one's behavior achieves its objective effectively and efficiently, then it has the quality we would call skill. This view also acknowledges that there are many ways to use one's underlying abilities to accomplish an occupational form. Indeed, underlying capacities (such as range of motion, perceptual ability, and intelligence) do not predict success in performance very well because one cannot know ahead of time how one will use one's capacities in a given task and context. Returning to the example, of squeezing a tube of toothpaste, researchers could identify that a specific pinch strength is required to squeeze a tube of toothpaste. But we all know that the strength required is dependent on whether the tube is newly opened or almost empty. If it is almost empty, it also depends on whether a person tries to squeeze the remaining toothpaste using the fingertips or push the paste out using the side of the thumb or heel of the hand.

The concept of skill does not directly imply a given amount of underlying capacity. It is purposefully disinterested in underlying capacity which to a large extent cannot be observed. Instead, attention is focused on the actual doing or performance.

The taxonomies of skills are taxonomies of the motor, process, and communication/interaction actions that a person enacts in the midst of engaging in occupational behavior. Moreover, skills are not steps or sequential movements. It is possible to recognize two or more elements of skill simultaneously in a given performance. For example, while one is organizing tools together (a process skill) one must also lift and grip the tools (motor skills). These motor and process skills are integrated into a single flow of action or performance.

Development of the Taxonomies of Skills

The motor and process skills identified here were first derived from a review of information-processing, sensory integration, and motor control literature (Ayres, 1986; Brooks, 1986; Fisher, Murray, & Bundy, 1991; Kelso, 1982; Keogh & Sugden, 1985; MacKay, 1987; Martin, 1967; Radmark, 1944; Roberts, 1978; Schmidt, 1988; Trombly, 1989). This literature review resulted in the identification of underlying postural, movement, attentional/energy, knowledge, organizational, adaptive, and memory elements of performance. Doble (1991) completed the first pilot study that began the conceptualization of process skills. Subsequent studies by Fisher and colleagues (Fisher, 1993, 1994, in press; Fisher, Liu, Velozo, &

Pan, 1992, in press; Fisher & Fisher, 1993; Magalhães, Fisher, Bernspång, & Lincare, 1994) contributed to the revision of the concept of process skills, the development of the Assessment of Motor and Process Skills, and the validation of the taxonomies of motor and process skills that are included in the assessment. To date, these studies have provided substantial support for the validity of the motor and process skills identified in this chapter. A range of studies with various populations have been completed and provide further validation of the motor and process skills constructs discussed in this chapter (Bernspång & Fisher, 1994a, 1994b; Dickerson & Fisher, 1993, in press; Doble, Fisk, Fisher, Ritvo, & Murray, 1994; Doble, Fisk, MacPherson, et al., 1994; Nygård, Bernspång, Fisher, & Winblad, 1994; Pan & Fisher, 1994; Park, Fisher, & Velozo, 1994).

The conceptualization of communication and interaction skills is at an earlier stage of development. There currently exist two taxonomies related to the concept of communication and interaction skills. We will discuss here how these taxonomies are being developed and later in the chapter we will present both taxonomies.

The first taxonomy emerged from efforts to develop the Assessment of Communication/ Interaction skills. The skills that make up this assessment and taxonomy were derived from a comprehensive review of existing concepts and measures of social interaction abilities (Simon, 1989). Salamy (1993) began the work of validating communication/interaction skills taxonomy through a secondary analysis of data collected in Simon's (1989) study and by collecting and analyzing new data. Salamy's study provided provisional support for the validity of the communication/interaction skills constructs.

Concurrent to the efforts of Simon (1989) and Salamy (1993), Doble and Magill-Evans (1992) developed a conceptualization of social interaction within the context of occupational performance. In addition, they developed a preliminary taxonomy of social enactment skills that are used to communicate needs and intentions to others and to respond competently to the messages of others. Their goal was to broaden the concept of communication and interaction to consider the wide range of social enactment skills that are used in the context of self-care, productive, and play/leisure occupations. Focusing on the implied purpose or functional use of social enactment skills, they defined four domains of social enactment skills: acknowledging, sending, timing, and coordinating.

Englund and Bernspång (1994) developed the Assessment of Social Interaction based on the conceptualization developed by Doble and Magill-Evans (1992). An initial study supports the validity of the social interaction skills summarized below, as well as the ability to differentiate social interaction performances among persons of various ability levels.

Both the communication/interaction and the social interaction taxonomies (as well as the assessments related to them) will require further research and refinement. In the future, it is possible that the two taxonomies will continue to be developed and used independently. This would be the case if the two different approaches demonstrate utility in different situations or are shown to measure different constructs. Since there is some overlap between them, it is also possible that the two taxonomies of skills will be merged to produce a single taxonomy.

In the following sections, both of the approaches are presented with the definitions and descriptions of the domains and the skills within them. The first taxonomical system will be referred to as the communication/interaction skills taxonomy. The second will be referred to as the social interaction skills taxonomy. While two different terms are used to identify the two taxonomies, the reader should recognize that these represent alternative ways of approaching the single area of communication and interaction skills. They are *not* being proposed as two independent areas of skill as motor and process skills are.

MOTOR SKILLS

Our bodies are affected by the forces of a physical world (e.g., gravity). They have the same properties as do other physical objects (e.g., weight, inertia, momentum). Occupation requires us to use our bodies to traverse the geography and act upon the objects of a physical world. Humans require motor skills in order to effectively act as physical systems in dynamic interaction with a physical world. *Motor skills refer to movement of self or objects through space for the skillful execution of daily life task performance.* As illustrated in Figure 8.2, motor skills represent five domains of skilled performance: posture, mobility, coordination, strength and effort, and energy. The motor skills themselves are purposeful features of movement which allow the body to effectively encounter the physical world in occupational behavior. In what follows, we will first explain the domains and then present, define, and discuss the motor skills within each domain.

Posture

All physical action with our bodies requires that one dynamically arrange the parts of one's body with each other and with the environment to optimize performance. Postural skills relate to the ability to stabilize and align one's body (postural stability and balance) while moving, and attain and sustain an effective physical orientation of the body to the objects with which one must deal. This domain includes three skills: *stabilizes, aligns,* and *positions.*

Stabilizes

This skill refers to steadying one's body and maintaining trunk control and balance. Stabilizing occurs while sitting or standing, while performing such actions as walking and reaching, and while moving, lifting, pushing, or pulling objects. To stabilize oneself means that one maintains dynamic postural control during trunk or limb movements used in occupational performance. A lack of stability may disrupt the efficiency of such actions as reaching and make certain actions, such as walking, unsafe.

Aligns

To maintain the even distribution of one's body weight over one's base of support is to align. This skill implies that a person does not

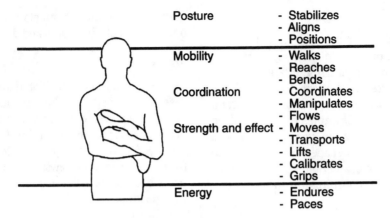

Posture	- Stabilizes
	- Aligns
	- Positions
Mobility	- Walks
	- Reaches
	- Bends
Coordination	- Coordinates
	- Manipulates
	- Flows
Strength and effect	- Moves
	- Transports
	- Lifts
	- Calibrates
	- Grips
Energy	- Endures
	- Paces

Figure 8.2. Motor domains and skills.

exhibit asymmetries, flexed or stooped posture, or excessive leaning during occupational performances. Problems with body alignment may be related to structural problems, abnormal tone, or strength limitations, but whatever its source, poor alignment diminishes the effectiveness of performance.

Positions

This skill refers to placing one's body in relation to objects in a manner that promotes efficient arm movements. Positioning requires one to use postural background movements appropriate to the task one is performing. If one's body is not positioned effectively, task performance will be awkward. Most of us have struggled to do something from the wrong angle but then experienced comparative ease when we positioned ourselves correctly.

Mobility

Occupation requires that we traverse a physical world with our bodies. Whether it be relocating our entire body or moving a body part to a new place, movement in space is necessary for effective performance of most occupations. Consequently, the domain of mobility includes those skills we exhibit when we move our bodies in space: *walks, reaches, bends.*

Walks

Walking refers to ambulating on level surfaces. It includes the ability to turn around and to change direction while walking. Unsteadi-

ness or shuffling, lurching, and ataxia are examples of difficulty in walking. Using a wheelchair or ambulating with an assistive device represent modified methods.

Reaches

One reaches when one stretches or extends the arm and, when required, the trunk in order to grasp or to place objects that are out of reach. Reaching is used, for example, to obtain and to put away objects and to take hold of railings, doorknobs, and the like.

Bends

To bend is to actively flex, rotate, or twist the body in a manner and direction required by a task that one is performing. Effective bending requires trunk mobility.

Coordination

Movement occurs simultaneously in time and space. Motion implies that each successive instant finds us somewhere new in space. To effectively interact with the environment we must move parts of our bodies in relationship to each other and to the environment. Effective movement through time and space requires that we use our body parts together effectively, that we encounter and control a variety of objects, and that the process of moving has the qualities of evenness and regularity. The domain of coordination thus pertains to the spatial-temporal organization of movements and includes the skills *coordinates, manipulates,* and *flows.*

Coordinates

To coordinate is to use different parts of the body together or to use other body parts as an assist or stabilizer during bilateral motor tasks. It includes the physical capacity to hold, support, or stabilize objects during bilateral task performance. Examples of coordination are holding a rolling pin securely with both hands, clasping a newspaper or book between one's arm and torso, and holding a shoe steady in one hand while polishing it with the other.

Manipulates

The skill Manipulates refers to using dexterous grasp and release as well as coordinated in-hand manipulation patterns. It pertains to the skillful use of isolated finger movements when handling objects. Buttoning, lacing shoes, and picking up a fork or pencil and then transferring it to the correct hand position all require manipulation.

Flows

Flows is defined as using smooth, fluid, continuous, and uninterrupted arm and hand movements. This skill pertains to the quality or refinement of motor execution, and it implies that one can isolate movements effectively. Problems with this skill can be the result of underlying problems of capacity such as dysmetria, ataxia, tremor, rigidity, or spasticity.

Strength and Effort

In order to have an effect on objects, we must be able to generate and use force. The domain of strength and effort pertains to those skills that require generation of force appropriate to effect the action a person is undertaking. These skills are: *moves, transports, lifts, calibrates,* and *grips.*

Moves

To move is to push, shove, pull, or drag objects along a supporting surface or about a weightbearing axis. Moves pertains to the displacement of objects that are not lifted, such as pushing a vacuum cleaner, shopping cart, or lawn mower; dragging a clothes basket or garbage bag; pulling blankets over a bed; and opening and closing doors and drawers.

Transports

To carry objects while ambulating or otherwise moving (e.g., crawling, scooting, cycling, or using a wheelchair) from one place to another is to transport. Carrying laundry from the dryer to the closet, groceries to the kitchen from the car, and the newspaper into the house from the mailbox are everyday examples of transporting.

Lifts

To lift means to raise or hoist objects off a supporting surface. This skill requires that one has enough strength to lift those objects used in one's occupations, whether they be a coffee pot, a bucket of paint, or a bale of hay.

Calibrates

Calibrates refers to regulating or grading the force, speed, and extent of movements executed in the context of task performance. This skill pertains to whether the force or speed of movement is appropriate to the requirements of a particular action. Applying inappropriate force or speed can result in objects or materials being broken, crushed, spilled, or knocked over. Thus calibration of force, speed, and movement is critical for acting effectively and safely in the world of objects.

Grips

To grip means to pinch or grasp in order to hold securely handles or other objects used in task performance. One must have adequate strength of pinch and grip to perform such actions as holding a knife while cutting or holding a doorknob while turning it. Gripping is also used when opening a jar, pulling a zipper, holding a razor while shaving, or grasping the handlebars of a bicycle while riding.

Energy

On the motor scale, the domain of energy refers to physical exertion and includes the skills of *endures* and *paces.* These skills connote sustained effort over time and a rate or intensity of performance which is consistent and economical over the course of completing the occupational form.

Endures

To endure is to persist and complete an activity without undue physical fatigue or without an undue need to pause, rest, or stop to "catch one's breath." This skill implies that a person can sustain sufficient effort for the occupations he or she needs to perform without overtaxing his or her capacity. Although we all have the potential to become exhausted or winded when performing an occupation, we should be able to complete occupations that comprise our daily routine without an excessive expenditure of energy.

Paces

The skill of pacing means that a rate of performance is maintained that enables one to complete the task one is doing within a reasonable amount of time. Pacing allows one to use an effective rate of performance throughout the steps of a task. Excessive sluggishness or rushing, a progressive slowing over time, or an uneven pace can result in an ineffective task performance.

Relationship of Motor Skills to Biomechanical and Motor Control Abilities

Musculoskeletal and neurological structures and processes are the major capacities of the mind-brain-body performance subsystem for the assembly of skills in actual performance. For example, joint mobility, the potential for muscle force generation, and the organization of visual-vestibular-proprioceptive mechanisms are all features of this subsystem that contribute to the assembly of movements. However, the actual movements that are created in the midst of performance also are organized by the unfolding task and by the dynamics of interacting with a physical world. These resultant motor actions are skills. Thus, motor skills are purposeful or functionally intended, and are expressed in the midst of occupational

behavior. Their character and their effectiveness are always evaluated in terms of how they contribute to the progress and outcome of occupational behavior and to the individual's safety in the midst of the performance. It should not be assumed that the biomechanical or neurological structures and processes are causal mechanisms for motor skills or that the state of the former will be perfectly correlated with the latter. Motor skills reflect how effectively the individual uses the abilities he or she has to perform an occupation.

PROCESS SKILLS

Completion of an occupational form requires that we bring together in time and space a range of events. To do so, we must manage a number of elements including time, the physical world, relevant information, and the actual process that unfolds as we perform. For example, in order for a salad to be made, a bowl, knife, and possibly other tools must make their way to a cutting board or other work surface. There they must encounter lettuce and other vegetables which have traveled to the work surface from the cupboards, drawers, or refrigerator. Interactions between the tools and the vegetables result in the latter being cut up and intermingled in a bowl. Finally, they are joined by salad dressing and served. To speak of these events without reference to human agency may sound a bit odd, but it highlights the fact that behind what happens to the objects in an occupational form are a number of human actions. These actions occur over time in a selected sequence and in particular planned places. Some of these actions we recognize as motor actions, but other aspects of action, especially the determination of what is used, how it is used, where actions occur, when actions occur, and how actions are done reflect what we mean by process skills. For example, one must decide what tools and materials are needed for the salad, which knife would be most suitable for cutting the tomato, how the tomato should be held to cut it into wedges, and whether to place the tomato wedges in the bowl before or after adding the salad dressing.

Process skills refer to how we orchestrate all these happenings in the completion of an occupational form. Process skills are those we use in managing and modifying actions en route to the completion of daily life tasks. As illustrated in Figure 8.3, these skills are conceptualized as being within *energy, knowledge, organizational* (referring to time, space, and objects) and *adaptive* domains.

Energy

On the process scale, the domain of energy refers to rate or intensity of performance that is consistent over time as well as to selective attention or allocation of attentional capacity. This domain includes two skills, *paces*, and *attends*. The skill paces (which was already discussed in the motor skill section) has been shown in research to belong to *both* the process and motor areas of skill. The overlap of paces in both the energy domain of motor skills and the energy domain of process skills points out that the energy domain represents a transition between process skills and motor skills. Conceptually, the energy domain refers to both mental processes (mental energy) and to physical processes (physical energy). Since the skill, paces, has already been defined in the previous section, only the skill attends, is discussed below.

Attends

To attend is to maintain adequate attention throughout a task sequence. For competent performance, one must attend selectively to the task to be performed and allocate appropriate attentional resources to relevant aspects of the task and environment. Problems with attending include being distracted away from the task by extraneous auditory or visual stimuli, or focusing too much on certain stimuli or aspects of the task while disregarding others. Such distractibility or over-attention interferes with the effective progression of occupational performance.

Knowledge

Knowledge processes involve the ability to use knowledge. The use of knowledge relates to the understanding or conceptualization of an occupational form and the recognition of the needed objects and actions that result in goal-directed task performance. The skills belonging to this domain are *chooses, uses, handles, heeds,* and *inquires*.

Chooses

This skill refers to selecting appropriate tools and materials. To choose effectively one must have an understanding of the kinds of tools and materials which are needed for a given occupational form. For example, when making a sandwich, one selects some form of bread, meat, or cheese, along with condiments; when serving the sandwich one selects a plate; and when cleaning up afterwards, one selects a dishcloth or sponge to wipe the counter.

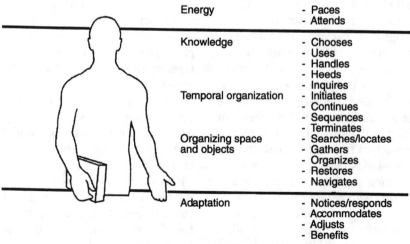

Energy	- Paces
	- Attends
Knowledge	- Chooses
	- Uses
	- Handles
	- Heeds
	- Inquires
Temporal organization	- Initiates
	- Continues
	- Sequences
	- Terminates
Organizing space and objects	- Searches/locates
	- Gathers
	- Organizes
	- Restores
	- Navigates
Adaptation	- Notices/responds
	- Accommodates
	- Adjusts
	- Benefits

Figure 8.3.   Process domains and skills.

Uses

Using means to employ tools and materials according to their intended purposes or in a reasonable (including hygienic) fashion, given their intrinsic properties and the availability (or lack of availability) of other objects. This skill requires that a person have knowledge of the intended use or purpose of the object and an understanding of the object's properties and capabilities. The person must then use that knowledge to employ tools and materials appropriately. Using, and consequently bending, a table knife when opening a paint can even though other more appropriate tools are available would be an example of poor use of skills. Other examples of inappropriate use include using a dirty counter to prepare foods or putting the wrong lid on a container.

Handles

The skill of handling means to support, stabilize, and hold tools and materials in an appropriate manner given the circumstances of the situation and abilities of the individual. To handle, one must recognize when and how to hold, stabilize, and support tools and materials so that they can be appropriately acted on and integrated into the ongoing task, as well as protected from damage. For example, when opening a vacuum-sealed food wrapper with a sharp knife, the knife should be held so that it is unlikely to slip and cut the individual handling the knife (i.e., with a firm grasp on the knife handle and not on the sharp knife edge). Other examples of handling include using two hands to transport a heavy frying pan from the stove, and using one hand to stabilize the bread on which peanut butter is being spread with a knife held in the other hand.

Heeds

Heeds refers to goal-directed task performance that is focused toward the completion of the originally intended task. This means that a person must have a basic understanding of the goal or purpose of an occupational form. Moreover, to heed the goal and purpose of a task, one's behavior must not be overly sensitive to environmental cues which can divert one from the task at hand. Consequently, the skill heeds pertains to the ability to manage one's actions and behaviors in order to accomplish the specified occupational form.

Inquires

To inquire is to seek appropriate verbal/written information by asking questions or reading directions. The skill of inquiring involves knowing what to ask in order to get necessary information such as where materials are located or how an action is performed. Inquires includes such diverse behaviors as reading a recipe or instructions on a prepared food container, consulting a map, or asking someone where a specific store is located.

Temporal Organization

Time is a universal dimension which must be managed when performing occupations. All tasks extend across a period of time (i.e., they have a beginning, followed by a series of steps arranged in order, and a point of termination or closure). Temporal organizational processes pertain to the beginning, logical ordering, continuity, and completion of the steps and action sequences of a task. Skills belonging to the dimension of temporal organization are *initiates, continues, sequences,* and *terminates.*

Initiates

To initiate means to start or begin an action or step without undue hesitation. Initiation is the observable action that is the end step of either tacit or conscious unobservable decision-making within the mind-brain-body performance subsystem. Hesitations or delays in initiation can interfere with task progression. In many occupational forms, it is important that one step follow the next readily. For example, when a stamp is wet, it must be applied to the intended surface before it dries. Once the paint is stirred and the drop cloth in place, one begins to paint the wall.

Continues

The skill of continuing refers to performing an action sequence without unnecessary interruption and as an unbroken, smooth progression. It pertains to the continuity of a series of actions such that once an action sequence is initiated, the individual continues until it is completed. For example, when watering a plant, the individual pours water from a watering can into the pot until the soil is damp; he or she does not stop halfway through watering to dust the table on which the plant sits. Similarly, one does not begin to paint one wall, stop to paint another wall, and then return to painting the first wall without disrupting the temporal continuity of the performance.

Sequences

To sequence is to perform steps in an effective or logical order for efficient use of time and energy. This skill implies an absence of random or illogical ordering or unnecessary repetition of steps. Examples of poor sequencing include turning on a faucet before one has found the container one intends to fill. Another example is putting away a toolbox before placing all the tools in it, thus making it necessary to retrieve and open the box again. Finally, repainting the same wall twice is an example of ineffective sequences that interfere with effective occupational performance.

Terminates

To terminate means to finish or bring single actions or single steps to completion without perseveration, inappropriate persistence, or premature cessation. When persons perseverate on an action (e.g., spreading butter on bread, shaking salad dressing, stirring a can of paint, sanding a piece of wood) long after the purpose has been accomplished, or when they stop an action before it has been accomplished, a terminating problem is present.

Organizing Space and Objects

We perform occupations in a world of physical objects. Each performance requires that we find and arrange the necessary materials and tools for task performance. During the performance we must negotiate our bodies among physical objects without unintended altercations. Afterwards, we leave our physical environment in order by putting away tools

and materials. The domain of organizing space and objects includes those skills necessary to achieve these ends, and includes *searches/locates, gathers, organizes, restores,* and *navigates.*

Searches/Locates

To search or locate means to look for and locate tools and materials through a process of logical searching. This skill pertains to the ability to investigate and look beyond the immediate environment in order to locate necessary or dispersed tools and materials (e.g., looking in, behind, on top of). Randomly searching through a series of drawers to find socks is an effective searching strategy.

Gathers

The skill Gathers refers to collecting together needed or misplaced tools and materials. This skill is exercised when one collects supplies into the workspace (e.g., when one brings pens or pencils, paper, and books to one's desk to make notes before writing a paper). Gathering also refers to collecting and replacing materials and tools that have been spilled (e.g., sweeping up sugar that spilled on the floor) or dispersed (e.g., picking up a garden tool that fell from a workbench).

Organizes

To organize means positioning logically, or arranging spatially, tools and materials in an orderly fashion in and between appropriate workspace(s) in order to facilitate task performance. For example, performance is enhanced when one arranges the tools and supplies on a workbench where they will be needed when repairing a small appliance. Overcrowding a workbench with tools is an example of a problem in organizing.

Restores

To restore is to return or put away tools and materials and to restore the immediate workspace to its original condition (e.g., wiping counter clean and putting dirty dishes in the sink). It includes closing and sealing opened containers and replacing coverings. For example, one restores food items to their appropriate containers or closes an opened paint can.

Navigates

To navigate is to modify the movement pattern of the arm, body, or wheelchair to avoid or maneuver around existing obstacles that are encountered in the course of moving the arm, body, or wheelchair through space. Inadvertently knocking over objects or bumping into a table are navigational problems.

Adaptation

Occupational performance requires that we anticipate, observe, and react to what happens as we progress through an occupational form. Although it is often desirable to plan one's actions so that mistakes are avoided, the reality is that all persons will make mistakes. Therefore, what is equally important is that we effectively overcome the problem as well as learn from our mistakes and avoid repeating them. The adaptive domain of process skills relates to the ability to correct for problems and benefit by learning from the consequences of errors that arise in the course of action. These skills are *notices/responds, accommodates, adjusts,* and *benefits.*

Notices/Responds

This skill refers to appropriate awareness of and reaction to nonverbal environmental/perceptual cues (e.g., sound, smell, temperature, consistency) that provide feedback about how a task is progressing. This skill implies that one first notices relevant information and, when the situation indicates, makes an appropriate response. This skill also pertains to responding appropriately to the spatial arrangement of objects to one another (e.g., noticing that the objects one is stacking are not aligned and shifting their position to restore proper alignment). Examples are turning down the stove when water is boiling over, and moving a tool that is in danger of accidentally being knocked off a workbench.

Accommodates

Accommodating means to modify one's actions or location of objects already *within* the workspace, in anticipation of, or in response to, undesirable circumstances that might arise in the course of an action or in order to avoid unwanted outcomes. The main focus of this behavior is that the individual changes his or her method of performing an action or changes the manner in which he or she interacts with tools and materials already in the workspace. This skill includes asking for assistance when appropriate or needed. An example of accommodation is beginning to apply paint or glue in a thicker coat after recognizing that a surface is being covered too sparsely.

Adjusts

To adjust is to change environmental conditions in anticipation of, or in response to, undesirable circumstances that arise in the course of action or to avoid undesirable outcomes. The main focus of this behavior is that the individual makes some change in the working environment by moving to a new workspace, bringing in or removing tools and materials from the present workspace, or changing an environmental condition such as lighting or temperature. Changing the rate of flow or temperature of water from the tap are examples of adjusting. Another example would be to go to the cupboard to get a rag and bring it to the workspace in order to clean up spilled paint.

Benefits

To benefit is to anticipate and prevent undesirable circumstances from recurring or persisting. The ability to benefit implies that the individual (a) recognizes that a problem has occurred and has the potential for recurrence or persistence; (b) learns from prior adaptations, verbal prompts, or requested information; and (c) uses prior adaptations or information from prompts or requests to alter the task progression accordingly. For example, an individual who has benefitted from his or her behaviors would realize that runs in the finish of a chair will result from applying paint too thickly, and in subsequent painting projects would instead apply two thin coats of paint.

Relationship Between Process Skills and Cognitive Abilities

It is worth noting that cognition (or mental processes) and process skills are not synonymous terms. Process skills are an observable succession of actions that are carried out in a definite manner and lead to the accomplishment of some occupational form. Cognitive skills are related to process skills, but they are by no means the same. For example, the ability to search for and locate objects used in task performance involves many basic underlying and unobservable cognitive processes, including memory, attention, problem solving, visual-spatial skills, and motor planning. However, the relative contribution of specific cognitive abilities to process skills varies across process skills and the tasks performed. For this reason, process skills should not be equated with mental processing, mental status, perceptual ability, or cognitive ability. Moreover, underlying mind-brain-body performance subsystem status cannot be assumed to cause or be correlated perfectly with process skill. Therefore, although it is likely that cognitive (as well as biomechanical and neurological) capacity represented in the mind-brain-body performance subsystem influences occupational performance, we cannot predict *whether* and *how* it will influence occupational performance. Instead, occupational performance is dependent on how the individual uses these capacities when performing tasks in various environments.

COMMUNICATION AND INTERACTION SKILLS

Occupational behavior is often social behavior. We perform many of our occupations in concert with others. Whether it be working with a team, playing cards with friends, purchasing groceries, or attending a meeting, we must be able to share information, make our needs and feelings known, ask for help, cooperate, and engage in a whole range of other behaviors that make our interactions with others effective. Whether our occupational behavior is productive or playful, much of what we do involves others. Communication and interaction skills are performance abilities for dealing with people and for receiving and sharing information. They "enable us to communicate our needs and motivations to others and to respond to the messages of others in a competent manner" (Doble & Magill-Evans, 1992, p. 146).

As noted earlier, this section will present two taxonomies which are alternate strategies for conceptualizing communication and interaction skills. Both taxonomies are illustrated in Figure 8.4. The taxonomy referred to as communication/interaction is followed by the taxonomy referred to as social interaction.

COMMUNICATION/INTERACTION TAXONOMY

These skills contained in the communication/interaction taxonomy reflect four communication and interaction domains: *physicality, language, relations,* and *information exchange*.

Physicality

This domain includes communication/interaction skills that involve physical expression or interaction with others. Physical human interaction is a social and cultural phenomenon in that social contexts and cultural expectations influence how persons use their bodies during social discourse. These physical skills are *gestures, gazes, approximates, postures,* and *contacts*.

Gestures

This skill of gesturing refers to using movements of the body to indicate, share information, or add emphasis to the communication of an idea, sentiment, or attitude. Gestures include such acts as raising one's eyebrows, smiling, or grimacing. It can involve arm and hand movements which are more literal, such as pointing, indicating numbers with the digits, or demonstrating an act such as throwing an object. It can include more abstract physical movement such as making a fist to show force or intensity or making a sweep of the arm to show inclusion. Gestures are used to signify, emphasize, or demonstrate, and as such they can supplement or complement verbal communication. The type of gestures used by individuals are differ from culture to culture.

Gazes

Gazing refers to the use of one's eyes during interaction. It refers to whether one uses eye contact to communicate and interact with others. It includes eye contact, looking away, staring, and other behaviors. In western society, we expect others to make occasional eye contact by looking at us during interaction. A person who seems to look blankly or who avoids looking at us during interactions can make us feel just as uncomfortable as a person who glares or stares at us in the absence of verbal discourse.

Approximates

Approximating refers to the distance one places oneself from others during tasks and conversation. The distance at which individuals are comfortable interacting with others is highly dependent on cultural background and the level of familiarity between persons. For effective social interaction, a person must be able to act on cues from others about "comfort zones." Thus, the distance one stands or sits from another can create comfort or discomfort, communicate intimacy or threat, or show a desire to direct interaction to a particular person. The nature of a social interaction can also determine what is considered an appropriate distance between participants. Lecturing to a group ordinarily implies some distance between the speaker and the audience, whereas dancing implies a physical closeness. The placement of one's body in relation to others in such contexts thus takes on different meanings. Persons who seem to lean too close or who place themselves apart from us send inevitable messages.

Postures

To posture is to assume various physical positions (e.g., arms and/or legs crossed, leaning forward or backward, sitting formally or comfortably, etc.) which are appropriate to the task and interaction. Posturing thus refers to the use of body language (excluding facial movements) to convey nonverbal messages. We can communicate formally or informally through more controlled versus relaxed posturing. Moreover, we can demonstrate hostility by crossing our arms and legs, or be sexually suggestive by assuming other postures.

Contacts

Contacts refers to physical contact such as touching, tapping, and shaking hands. Social and cultural norms and situational factors in-

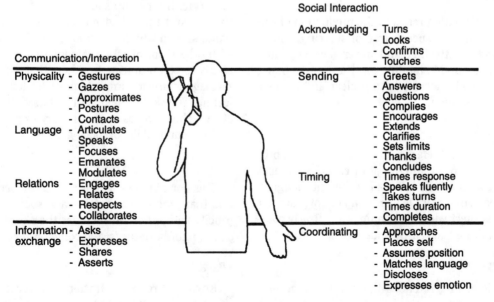

Figure 8.4.   Communication and interaction skills: Two taxonomies.

fluence what kind of physical contact persons are comfortable receiving from one another and how such contact will be interpreted. Effective use of physical contact requires that we are aware of cues from others concerning their comfort with being touched as well as the meaning that touch may have in different social situations. We ordinarily shake hands with strangers or acquaintances upon greeting, but may hug another person whom we know intimately or to whom we want to convey special concern. Other examples of social contact are tapping someone's arm to get his or her attention, giving physical assistance to someone who needs it, and patting someone on the back to show congratulations. The concept of contacts also takes into consideration the misuse and/or lack of physical contact when it affects the meaning of a social situation. Touch too forceful or minimal, too prolonged or brief can evoke discomfort or threat in another.

Language

Language pervades human interaction and communication. Complex information sharing not possible through other means is made possible through the use of language. This domain refers to the production and use of language and includes the skills *articulates, speaks, focuses, emanates,* and *modulates.*

Articulates

Articulating refers to the production of understandable speech free of slurring, mumbling, muttering, and other factors which impair understanding of the words being spoken. It refers to using clear and concise pronunciation.

Speaks

Speaking refers to the use of words appropriately in meaningful phrases and sentences to communicate internally coherent thoughts. A person's choice of words and use of grammar thus affect whether meanings are clearly communicated and easily understood.

Focuses

Focusing refers to the maintenance of a logical and meaningful progression of ideas or participation in ongoing conversation. Thus, maintaining a connection between the sentences or phrases one uses, following the topic of conversation, or relating talk to a task in which persons are involved are all examples of how one maintains focus in talking. Abrupt changes in topic, incoherent talk, or talk which strays from the conversation or task can disrupt social interaction.

Emanates

To emanate is to speak in a smooth and continuous fashion. This skill refers to the use of language in the social context and the effectiveness of language in maintaining appropriate interaction in conversation. Problems with emanating influence rate of speech (too fast to be understood or so slow as to create discomfort in conversational partners). Additionally, failure to take conversational turns, as well as prolonged hesitations, can be a problem as it can impair conversation and create discomfort in others.

Modulates

The skill of modulation refers to the use of volume, inflection, and duration of speech. Persons may have a significant effect on the meaning and consequence of language by speaking loudly, softly, briefly, or extensively, and by using speech which is animated or lethargic. If a person speaks too softly he or she cannot be heard adequately. On the other hand, speech which is too loud can interfere with others' social action. Modulation has the ability to communicate to others that a given message is private, important, or loaded with feeling. The skill of modulating is used to create a feeling, and as such it is very important to the emotional life of social groups.

Relations

This domain of skills refers to those behaviors that produce connection and social reciprocity with others. It includes the skills: *engages, relates, respects,* and *collaborates.*

Engages

Engaging refers to initiating interaction spontaneously and includes such behaviors as gaining someone's attention, entering into an ongoing interaction in which the individual is not yet a part, or re-entering a conversation. The method of entry into social interaction is often very emotionally charged since there is always the possibility that others will ignore, reject, or disapprove of the person seeking to enter.

Engaging always involves negotiating whether and how one may become part of a social exchange. It also requires sensitivity to social norms of discourse, such as waiting for a good moment to interrupt an ongoing conversation or knowing what kind of leading phrase or question can initiate interaction. Indeed, it is not surprising that a fair amount of humor exists around the "opening line" a person uses when trying to approach an unfamiliar person. How one engages another may well set the course for subsequent interactions.

Relates

To relate is to assume a manner of acting that establishes a comfortable rapport with others. Relating is what occurs once a person has successfully engaged others. It refers to a whole range of behaviors such as the use of humor, compliments, display of concern, interest, or affection, all of which connect the persons who are interacting. Relating does not imply intimacy per se, but rather a context-specific social bond which makes the interaction comfortable and connected. Problems with relating occur when a person is offensive, aloof, critical, complaining, self-absorbed, insulting, or otherwise makes others uncomfortable or creates social distance. In the end, the effectiveness of relating has its consequences in whether others prefer to remain in or leave the interaction.

Respects

To respect is to convey a sense of consideration for others' presence by following social norms. On one hand, respecting implies that one refrains from performing behaviors which are private in a public forum. Respects also implies that one follows customary behaviors (e.g., taking turns, offering others first access to resources). Respecting also suggests that a person presents him or herself in a manner that conforms with the expectations of the social setting (e.g., appearing neat and clean), displays courteous, mannerly behavior (e.g., addressing others by their preferred name). Failure to respect group norms can provoke disgust or uneasiness, and disrupt the group processes.

Collaborates

To collaborate is to cooperate with others by sharing information and objects and coordinating efforts. Effective collaboration requires ongoing participation in a given activity or interaction with awareness of appropriate group interdependence, such as receiving help or supervision, gaining reassurance, and assisting others when appropriate. Collaboration thus implies that a person is able to be interdependent appropriately (e.g., giving and seeking assistance) and is able to coordinate one's behavior with that of others toward some implicit or explicit task or interaction.

Information Exchange

This domain of information exchange includes skills with which an individual gives or obtains information. It includes the skills, *asks, expresses, shares,* and *asserts.*

Asks

To ask is to request information, assistance, or affirmation from other people. Seeking assistance, permission, validation, advice, opinions, suggestions, explanations, or clarification are all examples of asking. Asking may be posed as a query or as an entreaty. While asking is a self-directed skill, it also has the potential to affect others in a social situation. For example, asking questions that are tangential or irrelevant and making requests that impose unduly on others can be socially disruptive. Asking questions also can show interest and connection to others, such as when we seek to ascertain another's feelings or needs.

Expresses

To express is to display affect in interactions. We demonstrate our emotions through the quality of our physical and verbal actions. In addition to more dramatic expressions of emotions such as crying or laughing, persons show emotion through their tone of voice, speed of their movements, postures, and other physical and verbal indications. Persons may show a whole range of affect, and its impact on others is dependent on the interactional situation. Affection, excitement, sadness, frustration, boredom, anger, anxiety, or disappointment are examples of the types of emotions which may be expressed during interactions. Expression is also concerned with whether an individual is labile or prone to extreme outbursts of emotion (e.g., laughing hysterically or sobbing) which are incongruent with existing circumstances. The skill of expression does not refer to whether the person experiences the emotions but to observable expression of emotions in social situations.

Shares

To share is to make one's needs known and/or give personal information related to task involvement. Sharing implies that a person acts on cues from his or her own "internal state" by identifying needs, feelings, or contributing information and/or personal experiences. This includes making known whether one agrees or disagrees with others. Social situations and cultural conventions also set parameters on the kinds of sharing which are expected and which will be received comfortably by others.

Asserts

To assert is to directly, honestly, and appropriately express feelings, beliefs, and opinions without violating the rights of others. Asserting refers to a manner of interaction which indicates respect both for self and others. Overly submissive or domineering behaviors are failures of assertion. Passive behaviors fail to assert one's thoughts, needs, or desires. Aggressive behaviors disrespect the rights of others. Assertiveness requires consideration for others. Effective assertion requires awareness of social convention that may allow persons more or less assertiveness depending on age, sex, and social status. These conventions are some-

times unfairly constraining. When this is the case, asserting implies that persons are able to break such conventions effectively.

SOCIAL INTERACTION TAXONOMY

The social interaction taxonomy organizes skills under the following domains: *acknowledging, sending, timing,* and *coordinating* (Doble & Magill-Evans, 1992; Englund & Bernspång, 1994).

Acknowledging

When we are involved in social interaction, we facilitate communication when we indicate that we are listening actively to our social partner by acknowledging the other person's comments and actions. When we turn to and look at our social partner, reach out and touch our social partner, nod our head, and say "uh-huh" to convey that we are listening and comprehending what is being said, we are acknowledging our partner's contribution to the interaction. This domain includes *turns, looks, confirms,* and *touches*.

Turns

The skill of turning refers to actively positioning one's body to face one's social partner; one's attention is directed to the social partner.

Looks

Looking pertains to making visual contact by gaze with one's social partner. Looking one's social partner in the eyes in a manner that is relaxed and nonthreatening and adjusting the frequency and duration of eye contact to match that of one's social partner are important when one is sending and receiving messages.

Confirms

To confirm is to acknowledge the reception of social messages from one's partner. When one nods the head, uses encouraging words, or smiles in response to a message sent by another, one acknowledges that one is listening, and that he or she perceives and understands the message that was sent.

Touches

The skill of touching pertains to the appropriate use of touch or other physical contact during social interaction. Appropriate touch is determined by the context and level of familiarity among the persons involved (e.g., a handshake versus a hug). It also implies acting appropriately to cues conveyed by others about their comfort with being touched as well as respecting one's social partner's personal boundaries.

Sending

Sending skills are used to send messages of information and to communicate emotions to a social partner. Messages can be verbal or nonverbal and are more commonly a combination of both. Words are given meaning by such things as the pitch, tone, rate of speech, and by the use of nonverbal messages. Lack of clarity, avoidance of eye contact, or expressing statements as questions can negatively affect the meaning of a social interaction. The manner in which one greets a social partner can convey affective messages to a partner that "set the tone" for the interaction. We also use sending skills when we convey that we have not understood or need more information by asking appropriate questions, as well as by responding to the questions of others by providing requested information. Clearly expressed limits or refusals, actively entering into social interactions, and responding to offered messages are also aspects of sending skills. Sending skills include *greets, answers, questions, complies, encourages, extends, clarifies, sets limits, thanks,* and *concludes.*

Greets

To greet is to use appropriate words, phrases, and ceremonies to greet one's social partner. The greetings one uses should be appropriate to the context and level of familiarity among the social partners. Greeting includes acknowledging the arrival of one's social partner by turning to and looking at him or her, and by pronouncing or gesticulating greetings (e.g., nods, raises hand) or greeting one's social partner through the use of touch (e.g., shaking hands, embracing).

Answers

Answering pertains to giving relevant replies to questions, including providing factual information and/or personal opinions, feelings, or ideas as appropriate given the context and the person's familiarity with the social partner. Appropriately acknowledging positive feedback or an apology are also forms of answering.

Questions

To question is to ask for or request information by putting forth questions appropriate to the situation and level of familiarity among social partners and then waiting for an answer. Asking for information which is necessary if the person is to be able to complete the task at hand would be an example of appropriate questioning. Questioning includes (a) asking for clarifying information when one has not received or understood a social partner's message, and (b) showing interest in one's social partner by seeking knowledge about his or her interests, opinions, and needs as they pertain to the social context.

Complies

To comply is to agree, meet requests, and use empathy in a manner that conveys that the person is actively trying to understand and enter into his or her social partner's situation and feelings. Complying implies that the person assumes a positive, benevolent attitude toward his or her social partner.

Encourages

To encourage is to make supportive, encouraging statements or to give positive feedback. Encouraging pertains to messages that convey positive agreement and harmony with one's social partners and that focus on the positive aspects of the social partner's messages.

Extends

The skill of extending is concerned with sending messages that help to keep the conversation going. Expressing messages that are closely associated to the theme being discussed, changing the subject without causing confusion, or interrupting the conversation are methods of extending a conversation. Extending also occurs when one converses or discusses the current theme in a fluent manner that maintains one's social partner's interest.

Clarifies

To clarify is to assure that one's social partner is following the conversation or interaction by (a) recognizing the need for and then (b) sending additional and/or more precise messages in order to provide clarification for one's social partner.

Sets Limits

The skill of setting limits pertains to sending messages that express limits or refusals. Saying no, declaring one's point of view or opinion, expressing wishes, or otherwise asserting oneself in an appropriate manner are examples of setting limits. Setting limits implies an ability to stand up for one's own rights or place reasonable demands on others without offending or violating their rights.

Thanks

Thanking refers to using appropriate words, phrases, and ceremonies to acknowledge received favors, gifts, and/or compliments. Expressing gratitude for the generosity or kindness shown by a social partner or showing conventional courtesy in the context of economical transactions involving goods and services are examples of thanking.

Concludes

Concluding refers to terminating conversations or social interactions, disengaging or saying goodbyes using appropriate phrases and ceremonies concordant to the situation and level of familiarity among the social partners. Concluding includes the ability to send verbal or nonverbal signals that termination is desired, and then using appropriate strategies to carry the termination through to appropriate conclusion.

Timing

Within a context of a social interaction, we must help to maintain a smooth flow to the conversation and choose the right moments to respond to messages from our social partners. This can include responding in a manner that neither interrupts our social partner nor results in our hesitating too long before we reply. Turn-taking and tempo are timing aspects of social interactions that are influenced by a person's characteristic interactional style as well as by culture and context. Therefore, such factors must be taken into consideration when judging the appropriateness of overlapping speech and interruptions. Within the domain of timing skills are *times response, speaks fluently, takes turns, times duration,* and *completes*.

Times Response

To time a response is to react to social messages without delay or hesitation, and to initiate a response within a reasonable amount of time, without letting a social partner wait too long.

Speaks Fluently

Speaking fluently refers to the ability to speak in a fluent and continuous manner and with an even flow. An individual who speaks fluently talks without too many pauses and without awkward or long delays, but is also able to vary the tempo of his or her speech according to the content of the dialogue and the social situation or context.

Takes Turns

One takes turns by awaiting one's turn and by relinquishing it. Taking turns implies that one is able to understand others' cues and send messages, mainly nonverbal, which signal whose turn it is to send a message, as well as by taking one's own turn at an appropriate time.

Times Duration

Timing duration involves speaking for reasonable time periods that are compatible with one's social partner and the social context, as well as adjusting the length of one's turn according to the content of speech, the nature or complexity of the message conveyed, and the context of the interaction.

Completes

Completing refers to being able to stop talking when the full message has been sent or when a sequence of conversation is completed. Completing includes sending complete and comprehensive messages with distinct terminations or ending points (i.e., being able to come to a "full stop").

Coordinating

Coordinating skills are used to match one's messages with those of the social partner and with the expectations of the environment. The ability to read and interpret social cues is of vital importance for achieving social competence. Respecting the personal space of others, setting appropriate boundaries on content, choosing the right level of intimacy, and using appropriate language are examples of coordinating skills. Aspects of gender, age, social class, and culture are important determinants of what will be considered appropriate and acceptable expected behavior in different situations. For example, when a parent speaks to a child, the adult often must modify the message so that it is understandable to the child. Skills in this domain are *approaches, places self, assumes position, matches language, discloses,* and *expresses emotion.*

Approaches

Approaching pertains to the use of appropriate strategies to approach others so as to initiate interactions with a social partner. Catching the attention of a social partner through (a) stating the partner's name, (b) asking a question, or (c) making a comment to start a conversation are examples of approach methods.

Places Self

The skill of placing self refers to positioning oneself at an appropriate distance from one's social partner. This implies the ability to act on cues about personal space and to adjust oneself according to the nature of the interaction and the level of familiarity among the social partners.

Assumes Position

To assume position refers to the assumption of a physical posture that is appropriate to the type of interaction and level of familiarity among the social partners, and to vary, control, and adjust one's body posture according to the context and expectations of the situation.

Matches Language

Matching language involves using language and level of address that is appropriate to the situation and social partner's abilities and level of understanding. Matching one's level of language to that of one's social partner implies the ability to control and vary one's language according to the type and content of the interaction and social partner's parlance, and to address one's social partner appropriate to one's level of familiarity with the partner. Matching language also refers to modifying the message according to the level of understanding of one's partner.

Discloses

To disclose is to share and discuss personal information, experiences, feelings, emotions, and opinions appropriately, given the context of the interaction and level of familiarity with one's social partner. Disclosure involves revealing personal information gradually and in a manner that is compatible with the social partner's level of self-disclosure. To reveal too much too soon can disrupt effective social interaction.

Expresses Emotion

To express emotion is to display affect in a manner that is compatible with one's message and with ones' social partner's affective tone. The expectations of one's cultural group or the social context also influence or determine what is compatible affect. Expressing emotion effectively includes matching the message being sent with appropriate facial expressions and emotional tone.

Relationship of Communication and Interaction Skills to Other Skills and Capacities

Just as motor and process skills are interrelated, persons who have difficulties which are reflected in motor and/or process skills may demonstrate difficulties with communication and interaction skills. While such relationships have not yet been empirically demonstrated, the conceptualization of all three skill areas draw upon the same capacities. Nonetheless, while motor and process skills are directed at tasks and the physical world, communication and interaction skills are primarily directed at and have their consequences in the social and cultural world. Therefore, persons who do not have motor or process skill deficits may exhibit communication and interaction skill deficits, and vice versa.

Persons with cognitive deficits are among those likely to have difficulties in communication and interaction. For example, persons with memory problems may be unable to recognize acquaintances and recall previous interactions. Persons with more pronounced cognitive impairment may have difficulty recognizing social partner's needs, feelings, and communications (Doble & Magill-Evans, 1992). Because of the common observation that persons with a wide range of psychiatric diagnoses (with and without cognitive impairment) have problems in communication and interaction, it would appear that such persons may have difficulty in the rules or images of social action which they have internalized from experience or that they lack the experience to acquire such rules. For example, such persons may exhibit overly withdrawn or aggressive behavior. Early family learning no doubt may contribute to problems in the communication and interaction domain. Consequently, some communication and interaction skill problems may have their basis in learned ways of interacting. Another source of difficulty in communication and interaction for the psychologically disabled person may be the interference of emotions with performance. For example, persons who usually demonstrate effective communication and interaction skills may be less effective in their interactions when they are depressed, angry, or anxious. This, of course, illustrates that volition can have a strong influence on the communication and interaction skills that persons exhibit.

CONCLUSION

The concept of process, motor, and communication and interaction skills grew out of attempts to operationalize the concepts as originally formulated in the model.[a] However, an equally important contribution of this effort has been the development of a language which can be used by occupational therapists to conceptualize skill in occupational performance. Motor, process, and communication and interaction skill concepts provide a language for thinking about and describing the elements of skillful occupational performance. Until now, occupational therapists have been limited in their ability to describe in a clear and consistent way what they observe within the context of occupational performance.

In addition, the concepts of skills offered in this chapter present a different way of conceptualizing performance than previously available in occupational therapy. Traditionally, occupational therapists focused on underlying capacities as determinants of performance and have sought to explain performance abilities and limitations in terms of underlying capacity. The present view takes a very different approach, recognizing that, while underlying capacity contributes to the assembly of occupational behavior, it does not cause or determine it in a linear way. Actual performance represents the convergence of many factors including not only underlying capacity but also

---

[a]Originally, skills were conceptualized as innate abilities within the performance subsystem. Attempts to operationalize the concept of process skills ran into difficulties precisely because it was difficult, if not impossible, to infer from observation what internal processes are taking place. This led to an important rethinking of what we meant by skill and resulted in the current view of skill as an observable feature of actual performance. This effort to operationalize skills also led to the reconceptualization of the performance subsystem which is represented in Chapter 6.

such elements as motivation, environmental influences, and the unfolding nature of performance. By focusing on what persons do in occupational performance, the concept of skills provides a way to examine in a more detailed manner what emerges when all these factors come together.

The use of the motor, process, and communication and interaction taxonomies serves to support occupational therapists' expertise in occupational performance. Direct observation of performance in real tasks and situations is essential if we are to understand what a person can do and learn why a person may be experiencing difficulty. We have provided a language that is sufficiently detailed for occupational therapists to describe, in a meaningful way, both the strengths and difficulties demonstrated by persons when performing occupations.

References

Ayres, A. J. (1986). *Developmental dyspraxia and adult onset apraxia*. Torrance, CA: Sensory Integration International.

Bernspång, B., & Fisher, A. G. (1994a). Comparison of functional performance between persons with right or left CVA based on the Assessment of Motor and Process Skills. Manuscript submitted for publication.

Bernspång, B., & Fisher, A. G. (1994b). Validation of the Assessment of Motor and Process Skills for Use in Sweden. Manuscript submitted for publication.

Brooks, V. B. (1986). *The neural basis of motor control*. New York: Oxford University Press.

Dickerson, A. E., & Fisher, A. G. (1993). Age differences in functional performance. *American Journal of Occupational Therapy, 47*, 686–692.

Dickerson, A. E., & Fisher, A. G. (in press). Culture-relevant functional performance assessment of the Hispanic elderly. *Occupational Therapy Journal of Research*.

Doble, S. (1991). Test-retest and inter-rater reliability of a process skills assessment. *Occupational Therapy Journal of Research, 11*, 8–23.

Doble, S. E., Fisk, J. D., Fisher, A. G., Ritvo, P. G., & Murray, T. J. (1994). Evaluating the functional competence of community-dwelling persons with multiple sclerosis using the Assessment of Motor and Process Skills. *Archives of Physical Medicine and Rehabilitation, 75*, 843–851.

Doble, S. E., Fisk, J. D., MacPherson, K. M., Fisher, A. G., Bowlby, M. C., Mallery, L., & Rockwood, K. (1994). Measuring functional competence in olders persons with Alzheimer's disease. Manuscript submitted for publication.

Doble, S. E., & Magill-Evans, J. (1992). A model of social interaction to guide occupational therapy practice. *Canadian Journal of Occupational Therapy, 59*, 141–150.

Englund, B., & Bernspång, B. (1994). Development of an instrument for assessment of social interaction skills in occupational therapy. Manuscript in preparation.

Fisher, A. G. (1993). The assessment of IADL motor skills: An application of many-faceted Rasch analysis. *American Journal of Occupational Therapy, 47*, 319–338.

Fisher, A. G. (1994). *Assessment of Motor and Process Skills* (Version 8.0). Unpublished test manual, Department of Occupational Therapy, Colorado State University, Fort Collins.

Fisher, A. G. (in press). Development of a functional assessment that adjusts ability measures for task simplicity and rater leniency. In M. Wilson (Ed.), *Objective measurement: Theory into practice* (Vol 2). Norwood, NJ: Ablex.

Fisher, A. G., Liu, Y., Velozo, C. A., & Pan, A. W. (1992). Cross-cultural assessment of process skills. *American Journal of Occupational Therapy, 46*, 876–885.

Fisher, A. G., Liu, Y., Velozo, C. A., & Pan, A. W. (in press). Cross cultural assessment of process skills. *American Journal of Occupational Therapy*.

Fisher, A. G., Murray, E., & Bundy, A. C. (1991). *Sensory integration: Theory and practice*. Philadelphia: FA Davis.

Fisher, W. P., & Fisher, A. G. (1993). Applications of Rasch analysis to studies in occupational therapy. *Physical Medicine and Rehabilitation Clinics of North America: New Developments in Functional Assessment, 4*, 551–569.

Kelso, J. A. S. (Ed.). (1982). *Human motor behavior: An introduction*. Hillside, NJ: Erlbaum.

Keogh, J., & Sugden, D. (1985). *Movement skill development*. New York: Macmillan.

MacKay, D. G. (1987). *The organization of perception and action: A theory for language and other cognitive skills*. New York: Springer-Verlag.

Magalhães, L., Fisher, A. G., Bernspång, B., & Linacre, J. M. (1994). Developing the Assessment of Motor and Process Skills as a cross-cultural evaluation of IADL. Manuscript submitted for publication.

Martin, J. P. (1967). *The basal ganglia and posture*. London: Pittman Medical Publishing.

Nygård, L., Bernspång, G., Fisher, A. G., & Winblad, B. (1994). Comparing motor and process ability of persons with suspected dementia in home and clinic settings. *American Journal of Occupational Therapy, 48*, 689–696.

Pan, A. W., & Fisher, A. G. (1994). The Assessment of Motor and Process Skills of persons with psychiatric disorders. *American Journal of Occupational Therapy, 48*, 775–780.

Park, S., Fisher, A. G., & Velozo, C. A. (1994). Using the Assessment of Motor and Process Skills to compare occupational performance between clinic and home settings. *American Journal of Occupational Therapy, 48*, 697–709.

Radmark, K. (1944). Tipping reaction in cases of vertigo after head injury. *Acta Otolaryngologica, Suppl. 52*, 1–133.

Roberts, T. D. M. (1978). *Neurophysiology of posture mechanisms* (2nd ed.). Boston: Butterworth.

Salamy, M. (1993). *Construct validity of the Assessment for Communication and Interaction Skills*. Unpublished master's thesis, University of Illinois at Chicago, Chicago.

Schmidt, R. A. (1988). *Motor control and learning: A behavioral emphasis* (2nd ed.). Champaign, IL: Human Kinetics Publishers.

Simon, S. (1989). *The development of an assessment for communication and interaction skills*. Unpublished mater's thesis, University of Illinois at Chicago.

Trombly, C. A. (1989). *Occupational therapy and physical dysfunction*. Baltimore: Williams & Wilkins.

KEY CONCEPTS

MOTOR DOMAINS AND SKILLS

Posture

- relates to the stabilizing and aligning of one's body while moving in relation to objects with which one must deal.
- **Stabilizes:** Steadies one's body and maintains trunk control and balance while sitting, standing, walking, reaching, or while moving, lifting, or pulling objects.
- **Aligns:** Maintains the vertical alignment of the body over the base of support.
- **Positions:** Places one's arms and body in relation to objects in a manner that promotes efficient arm movements.

Mobility

- relates to moving the entire body or a body part in space as necessary.
- **Walks:** Ambulates on level surfaces, including turning around and changing direction while walking.
- **Reaches:** Stretches or extends the arm and, when appropriate, the trunk to grasp or place objects that are out of reach.
- **Bends:** Actively flexes, rotates, or twists the body in a manner and direction appropriate to a task.

Coordination

- relates to moving body parts in relationship to each other and to the environment; pertains to spatiotemporal organization of movements.
- **Coordinates:** Uses different parts of the body together to support or stabilize objects during bilateral motor tasks.
- **Manipulates:** Uses dexterous grasp and release as well as coordinated in-hand manipulation patterns.
- **Flows:** Uses smooth, fluid, continuous, uninterrupted arm and hand movements.

Strength and Effort

- pertains to skills that require generation of muscle force appropriate to action a person is undertaking.
- **Moves:** Pushes, shoves, pulls, or drags objects along a supporting surface or about a weightbearing axis.
- **Transports:** Carries objects while ambulating or moving from one place to another.
- **Lifts:** Raises or hoists objects off of supporting surface.
- **Calibrates:** Regulates or grades the force, speed, and extent of movements.
- **Grips:** Pinches or grasps in order to securely hold handles or other objects.

Energy

- refers to physical exertion and sustained effort over time.
- **Endures:** Persists and completes an activity without evidence of fatigue, pausing to rest, or stopping to catch one's breath.
- **Paces:** Maintains a rate or tempo of performance across an entire task.

PROCESS DOMAINS AND SKILLS

Energy

- pertains to sustained and appropriately allocated mental energy.
- **Paces:** Maintains a rate or tempo of performance across an entire task.
- **Attends:** Maintains attention focused on the task.

Knowledge

- refers to the ability to seek and use knowledge.

Key Concepts, continued

- **Chooses:** Selects appropriate tools and materials.
- **Uses:** Employs tools and materials according to their intended purposes.
- **Handles:** Supports, stabilizes, and holds tools and materials in an appropriate manner.
- **Heeds:** Uses goal-directed task performance that is focused toward the completion of the intended task.
- **Inquires:** Seeks appropriate verbal/written information by asking questions or reading directions.

Temporal Organization
- pertains to the beginning, logical ordering, continuation, and completion of the steps and action sequences of a task.
- **Initiates:** Starts or begins doing an action or step without hesitation.
- **Continues:** Performs an action sequence of a step without unnecessary interruption and as an unbroken, smooth progression.
- **Sequences:** Performs steps in an effective or logical order for efficient use of time and energy.
- **Terminates:** Finishes or brings to completion single actions or steps without perseveration, inappropriate persistence, or premature cessation.

Organizing Space and Objects
- pertains to skills for organizing space and objects.
- **Searches/Locates:** Looks for and locates tools and materials through the process of logical searching.
- **Gathers:** Collects together needed or misplaced tools and materials.
- **Organizes:** Logically positions or spatially arranges tools and materials in an orderly fashion and in between appropriate workspaces.
- **Restores:** Returns/puts away tools and materials, and restores immediate workspaces to original condition.
- **Navigates:** Modifies the movement of the arm, body, or wheelchair to avoid or maneuver around existing obstacles that are encountered in the course of moving the arm, body, or wheelchair through space.

Adaptation
- relates to the ability to anticipate, correct for, and benefit by learning from the consequences of errors that arise in the course of action.
- **Notices/Responds:** Responds appropriately to nonverbal environmental/perceptual cues that provide feedback regarding task progression.
- **Accommodates:** Modifies one's action or location of objects within the workspace in anticipation of or in response to circumstances/problems that might arise in the course of action or to avoid undesirable outcomes.
- **Adjusts:** Changes environmental conditions in anticipation of or in response to circumstances/problems that arise in the course of action or to avoid undesirable outcomes.
- **Benefits:** Anticipates and prevents undesirable circumstances/problems from recurring or persisting.

COMMUNICATION/INTERACTION DOMAINS AND SKILLS

Physicality
- refers to physical expression or interaction with others.

Key Concepts, continued

- **Gestures:** Uses movements of the body to indicate, share information, or add emphasis to the communication of an idea, sentiment, or attitude.
- **Gazes:** Uses eyes to communicate and interact with others.
- **Approximates:** Places entire body a culturally appropriate distance from others during tasks, conversations, etc.
- **Postures:** Assumes physical positions which are appropriate to the task and interaction.
- **Contacts:** Touches, taps, or makes other appropriate physical contact with others.

Language
- refers to the production and use of language.
- **Articulates:** Produces clear, understandable speech.
- **Speaks:** Uses words appropriately in meaningful phrases and sentences to communicate internally coherent thoughts.
- **Focuses:** Converses using connected sentences or phrases that are logical and directed to a conversation or task.
- **Emanates:** Speaks in a smooth and continuous fashion.
- **Modulates:** Uses volume, inflection, and duration of speech effectively.

Relations
- refers to behaviors that produce connection and social reciprocity.
- **Engages:** Spontaneously initiates interaction.
- **Relates:** Assumes a manner of acting that establishes a comfortable rapport with others.
- **Respects:** Conveys a sense of consideration for others by following social norms.
- **Collaborates:** Cooperates with others by sharing information and objects and coordinating efforts.

Information Exchange
- refers to giving or obtaining information.
- **Asks:** Requests information from other people.
- **Expresses:** Displays affect in interactions.
- **Shares:** Makes needs known and/or shares personal information related to task involvement.
- **Asserts:** Uses direct, honest, and appropriate expression of feelings, beliefs, opinions without violating the rights of others.

SOCIAL INTERACTION DOMAINS AND SKILLS

Acknowledging
- refers to actions that facilitate communication and interaction.
- **Turns:** Actively positions one's body to face one's social partner.
- **Looks:** Makes visual contact with one's social partner.
- **Confirms:** Acknowledges the reception of social messages.
- **Touches:** Appropriately uses touch or other physical contact during social interaction.

Sending
- pertains to directing messages of information and for communicating.
- **Greets:** Uses appropriate words, phrases, and ceremonies to greet one's social partner.

Key Concepts, continued

- **Answers:** Gives relevant replies to questions.
- **Questions:** Requests factual information appropriate to the situation and level of familiarity among social partners.
- **Complies:** Agrees, accepts offerings, meets requests, and uses empathy.
- **Encourages:** Makes supportive statements or gives positive feedback.
- **Extends:** Sends messages that help to keep the conversation going.
- **Clarifies:** Assures that one's social partner is following the conversation or interaction.
- **Sets limits:** Expresses limits or refusals.
- **Thanks:** Uses appropriate words, phrases, and ceremonies to acknowledge received favors.
- **Concludes:** Appropriately terminates conversations or social interactions.

Timing

- refers to maintaining a smooth flow to the conversation and choosing the right moments to respond to messages from our social partners.
- **Times response:** Reacts to social messages without delay or hesitation.
- **Speaks fluently:** Produces speech in a fluent and continuous manner.
- **Takes turns:** Awaits one's turn and relinquishes it.
- **Times duration:** Speaks for reasonable time periods compatible with one's social partner.
- **Completes:** Stops talking when the full message has been sent.

Coordinating

- refers to matching one's messages with those of the social partner and with the expectations of the environment.
- **Approaches:** Uses appropriate strategies to initiate interactions.
- **Places self:** Positions oneself at an appropriate distance from one's social partner.
- **Assumes position:** Assumes a physical posture that is appropriate to the type of interaction and level of familiarity.
- **Matches language:** Uses language and level of address that is appropriate to the situation and social partner.
- **Discloses:** Shares and discusses personal information, experiences, feelings, emotions, and opinions appropriately.
- **Expresses emotion:** Displays affect in a manner that is compatible with one's social partner's affective tone and expectations of the situation.

9/ Development of Occupation

Gary Kielhofner

INTRODUCTION

In Chapter 2 I argued that human beings can be seen as systems whose occupational behavior sustains and transforms their organization. Ongoing experience from behavior, combined with innate, biologically-based potentials, propels the human system through a trajectory of lifelong change referred to as development. For each human being that trajectory is unique, full of possibilities and stresses, and punctuated with both positive and negative events. Moreover, development is a complex process involving changes in biological, psychological, social, and other dimensions of the human being.

PROCESSES INVOLVED IN DEVELOPMENT

Throughout the developmental process, the human system's organization is constantly being transformed (Bruner, 1969, 1973; von Bertalanffy, 1966). Each period of relative stability is followed by transition to a new order. Transition from one order to the next ordinarily involves an intermediate phase of disorganization in which old patterns are broken up or relinquished and new ones are not yet realized or stabilized. For example, the child achieves a well-organized pattern of crawling, but relinquishes it for walking that is at first a less organized but eventually more efficient form of locomotion. Such successive organizational states are often referred to as stages of development.

Developmental changes result from the convergence of internal and environmental factors carried along by occupational behavior.

Changes in the mind-brain-body performance system (e.g., maturation of the nervous system and the emergence of abstract thinking) contribute to the course of development. Occupational choices guided by volition influence the life course. Across time the environment affords and presses for new behaviors thereby helping to shape the development of successive habituation patterns. These factors all contribute together to the behavior, well-established or novel, that the human system exhibits at any point in development. In the course of development one factor may become more important than others (i.e., become a control parameter) for maintaining a pattern of behavior or for recruiting novel behavior. Thus, the course of development involves a trade-off between volition, habituation, performance, and the environment as determining factors in the human system's organization and behavior.

Transformation of Work, Play, and Daily Living Tasks

Discussions of development often emphasize that particular courses or processes of development are normal. For example, most discussions of childhood development describe various attainments that, on average, have occurred by a particular age. However, great variation in the course of development occurs across persons. Too much emphasis on stages (defined by average behavior) can distract us from the more important processes which underlie observed changes. While it may produce what appear as successive stages, development is first and foremost a process by which the individual is transformed throughout life.

The most obvious outward manifestation of occupational development is that persons engage in different occupations over the course of their lives. For example, younger children play, older children and adolescents attend school, and adults work. The transformation of work, play, and daily living tasks across the life span reflects an underlying order to development. This order is realized in the individual but is sustained, in large measure, by society. Helpless at birth, children are taken care of and allowed to play as they acquire capacities necessary for survival in later life (Reilly, 1974). Later, as they mature, children are expected and taught to engage in self-care, do chores, and attend school. Adults are expected to do some form of work. The socially established and culturally defined patterns of work, play, and self-care over the life span and the ways they influence the individual to perform, to find meaning and worth, and to change are of considerable importance in development.

The following sections provide an overview of the course of development of the human system. Development is typically divided into childhood, adolescence, adulthood, and later adulthood or old age. In order to characterize the types of transformations in occupational behavior that take place throughout life these same categories will be used here. The following discussion is not meant to be an exhaustive or detailed account of developmental change. Rather, it is offered as a perspective from which to consider how persons' volition, habituation, performance, and environment contribute to and undergo change throughout the life course.

CHILDHOOD

Childhood is a period of tremendous growth and change in occupational behavior. Volition, habituation, mind-brain-body performance, and environmental factors trade off as control parameters shifting the system toward the assembly of new behavior, resulting in constant reorganization and formation of new stable orders.

Volition Subsystem

As children experience themselves performing, their personal causation, interests, and values emerge and unfold. Children become increasingly aware that their own volitional decisions lead to certain experiences. Moreover, these experiences let the child know what he or she can do, how enjoyable behaviors are, and what value they hold.

The volitional choices of early childhood are mainly activity choices. Later, children begin to make choices for personal projects take on discretionary roles (e.g., joining scouts). Occupational choices may be, at first, assisted or coached by parents who supply for children the rationale for projects, habits, and roles. The ability for narrative begins in childhood as children progress from activity to occupational choices. The increased ability to integrate past, present, and future and to imagine oneself in an unfolding story allows the child to begin to narrate parts of his or her life and to sort out meanings through stories.

Personal Causation

Play is a major vehicle through which the child first develops a sense of personal causation. As noted in Chapter 4, personal causation begins with the child's awareness that he or she can cause things to happen. Knowledge of one's capacity to affect events in the environment becomes a strong motive and manifests itself in the child's play. Children's awareness of their capacities is gained from engaging in the environment in play, in social interaction, and eventually in other occupational spheres (Sutton-Smith, 1971; Burke, 1977).

Earliest personal causation emerges around developing motor, interpersonal, and language capacities. At first, children's sense of their abilities is very general (e.g., effort and capacity are not distinguished and not always accurate (Nicholls, 1984)). Through the child's experiences of failure and success, the child's knowledge of capacity and feelings of efficiency becomes more complex and accurate.

Throughout childhood, environmental press for performance increases as the child experiences competition with peers, higher skill demands, and increased feedback from adults regarding performance. This can pose challenges to a sense of efficacy and children may go through periods of feeling inadequate.

Moreover, they come to discover that they are more effective in some circumstances than in others.

Values

Cultural messages about values influence the child early in life. Adult approval and disapproval of actions guide the child's understanding of the social value of certain behaviors. For example, norms of behavior such as taking turns and sharing are located in our commonsense understandings of manners. Growing awareness of which behaviors are negatively or positively valued by parents, siblings, and others increasingly influences activity and occupational choices. For example, as children learn the value of being productive in occupations (e.g., domestic, scholastic occupations) they increasingly assume responsibility for such behaviors and, in turn, experience the approval of others that solidifies the commitment to behave accordingly. The cultural message that one should contribute one's part is among the most crucial value lessons of childhood.

Interests

Childhood interests reflect the child's developmental process and expanding capacities. Children are at first attracted to a range of activities that allow exercise of capacity and yield new experiences. Much of the feeling of the child's pleasure comes with the mastery of new actions (Frost & Klein, 1979). As new capacities emerge, interest turns toward their utilization and expansion. For example, increased hand dexterity invites, and results from, the child engaging in play requiring fine motor control, such as constructing simple projects. Linguistic competence leads to interest in verbal humor, chanting rhymes, and so on (Takata, 1974). Children find particular interest in those activities that provide optimal arousal by challenging capacity. Preference emerges out of innate and acquired tastes for action and is shaped by the cultural surround. Early interest in objects concerns their sensory properties such as color, texture, noise, as well as the motor action they afford. Early on, interest in the social world emerges as in play-

ful social interaction in games such as peek-a-boo. Many preferences show continuity in the midst of change. For example, a preference for auditory experience may lead the child to particularly enjoy music and later to be invested in playing an instrument.

Habituation

The child's patterned behavior gradually shifts from being externally to internally regulated. Early on, internal patterns of sleeping, waking, and eating emerge followed by the acquisition of more complex habit and role patterns.

Roles

The young child's major occupational roles are player and family member. Parents and others see play as the normal business of the child and as reflective of development, ordinarily valuing the child's performance in play (Sutton-Smith, 1980). The player role has its own expectations as when parents specify where and with what objects children may play. Thus, even the player role has its own script. In addition, play is a means of trying out the scripts of other roles. That is, the child observes adult models in the environment and then enacts these roles in sociodramatic play (Lindquist, Mack, & Parham, 1982). Children also acquire and learn to use role scripts within groups through games (Mead, 1934; Reilly, 1974).

The family member role emerges as parents expect and value productive contributions of the child to the routines of family life by engaging in such occupational forms as picking up toys, doing small chores, and carrying out self-care (Shannon, 1974). As childhood progresses, the range of roles increases to include the student role and the role of friend. The child's identity may also include roles in such groups as 4-H, Brownies, Cub Scouts, or Little League.

Habits

Biological rhythms provide the child's first consistent patterns. Environmental rhythms quickly allow the child to internalize a habit map of routines such as sleeping, waking, bathing, eating, playing, and self-care. In time, the child becomes more and more able to organize behaviors in order to accomplish chores and routines of dressing, toileting, and eating. Moreover, children find repetition a source of security, predictability, and comfort (Brown, 1971). Many habits which will be essential throughout life such as regular attendance, punctuality, industry, neatness, attention, and perseverance are acquired in childhood (Bailey, 1971; Hurt, 1980; Matsutsuyu, 1971; Mauer, 1971; Shannon, 1974).

While the major influence on habits is the family routine, the child is affected by each new occupational behavior setting, such as day care and school. Habit patterns show a marked change as the child progresses through school. Setting aside increasing time necessary for homework while allowing time to play and to associate with family and friends requires the child to organize and develop more sophisticated habits.

Mind-Brain-Body Performance Subsystem

The constituents of the mind-brain-body performance subsystem undergo dramatic transformation in childhood. The potentials represented in this unfolding subsystem are activated and organized by the child's ever-changing interaction with the environment.

The course of early development is marked by the differentiation and creation of symbols and the emergence of motor, process, and communication/interaction skills. The child's capacity for these skills is organized as the child gains experience, especially from the childhood occupation of play (Reilly, 1974; Robinson, 1977).

Throughout childhood, increasing competence for interacting with the environment leads to the desire and capacity to seek out novel experiences. As the child's capacities increase (e.g., with the attainment of concrete operational thought (Piaget & Inhelder, 1969)) the child's world expands (e.g., entering formal education (Elkind, 1981)). This process results in exposure to new occupational behavior settings in which objects, occupational forms, and social groups afford and press for further development of the mind-brain-body performance subsystem.

Summary

Through the course of childhood, the extensive transformation of the three subsystems takes place. Development of performance capacity enables the child to engage the environment in increasingly complex ways. A range of habits are acquired to guide occupational behavior in an increasing number of roles. Active engagement with the environment results in the self-knowledge and dispositions of volition which enable the child to exercise activity and occupational choices reflecting interests, values, and personal causation.

Childhood provides many of the foundations for future entry into more formal occupational roles. The effectiveness of interactions and competence developed during childhood contribute to the child's ability to adapt to the occupational forms and roles of adolescence and adulthood.

ADOLESCENCE

Adolescence is typically a period of stress and turmoil due to both intrapersonal and sociocultural factors (Alissi, 1975; Goodman, 1960; Hendry, 1983; Mitchell, 1975). In addition to being a time of accelerated and dramatic biological changes, adolescence can also be an uncertain social transition from childhood to adulthood. For example, an adolescent may experience stress because he or she feels ready and wants to assume adult roles that are not yet expected or available (Hendry, 1983).

Since adolescence is both a developmental and sociocultural phenomenon, it is difficult to establish its boundaries. Most people associate the beginning of adolescence with both biological (prepuberty) and institutional (junior high school) changes (Hamburg, 1974; Muuss, 1975). The end of adolescence is also equivocal. For example, entry into the worker role is one marker of passage from adolescence to adulthood. But the timing of this can differ radically depending on whether one works directly after high school, attends college, or obtains postgraduate education (Hamburg, 1974; Muuss, 1975; Sieg, 1975). The ambiguities surrounding the beginning and end of this period are apparent in such examples as a 15-year-old mother, the 18-year-old who contributes to the family income and helps bring up younger siblings, and the 28-year-old who is still in graduate school and dependent on parental support.

Volition Subsystem

Adolescence is characterized by an increasing drive for autonomy. This urge for increased independence reaches its peak during adolescence as intellectual, cognitive, and emotional capacities allow greater depths of awareness and comprehension of the world through one's own perspective as well as that of others (Mitchell, 1975; Santrock, 1981).

At the same time, social groups, such as family, school, and other organizations afford opportunities and press the adolescent to take more initiative and responsibility for actions. Adolescents must successfully learn to make activity and occupational choices which bring personal satisfaction and meaning while meeting expectations in the social surround. Transformation of the volition subsystem of the adolescent occurs as the adolescent gains freedom to choose a lifestyle, and must define personal values and interests, and find arenas in which to feel competent. Since adolescents face more and more occupational choices, (i.e., for personal projects, habits, and roles) more complex and integrated decision making is required. Narrative organization of volitional themes serves as the foundation for this process. Adolescents begin to seriously see themselves as the authors of their own lives and to connect present actions with future outcomes and possibilities. The adolescent's need to author his or her own life culminates in several important occupational choices such as selecting a career and finding a partner.

Personal Causation

Adolescents are challenged to maintain a sense of efficacy while facing new social expectations for responsibility, having to acquire an expanding repertoire of occupational forms and performing in an expanding number of settings. For example, the adolescent encounters new peer groups: junior high, high school,

college, and/or job training, all of which afford and press for a range of new and more demanding occupational behaviors.

Adolescents' sense of efficacy is increasingly oriented to a future in which they will assume adult roles. Adolescents tend to assess their capacity in terms of expected performance in future roles. During adolescence, the sense of efficacy ordinarily shifts toward increased belief in one's ability to control life outcomes (Josslyn, 1952; Keniston, 1974). This shift enables the adolescent to move toward the responsibility and role behavior required in adulthood.

Values

Increased freedom of choice challenges adolescents to clarify and establish their values (Lambert, Rothschild, Atland, & Green, 1978; Mitchell, 1975; Morgan, 1982; Stein & Weston, 1982; Thornberg, 1975). Value commitment often entails a period of conflict and rejection of some previous or parental values leading to a more personalized world view (Morgan, 1982; Stein & Weston, 1982). Adolescent value formation reflects the movement beyond the social groups of childhood where values were prescribed and enforced (e.g., in family, in primary school). The peer group, which often holds some values at variance with mainstream adult values, contribute toward adolescent questioning or rejection of adult values. Despite the apparent conflicts over values, most adolescents still agree with their parents on most issues (Goodman, 1984; Konopka, 1976), and end up adopting the work values and even the careers of their parents (Santrock, 1981). Thus, it appears that much of the questioning of values serves mainly to confirm for adolescents that their values are their own.

Since they are about to enter into adulthood with relative freedom to choose a lifestyle, values enable the adolescent to know what kind of life to choose. Thus, values concerning productive and leisure occupations, and their personal and social significance both make sense of and shape important occupational choices. The most pressing occupational choice of adolescence is selecting a type of work (Allport, 1961). Commitment to work and building a sense of what one wants from work is a major process. Environmental influences are extremely important. If parents talk animatedly about their work and share some of its products with the adolescent, the meaning of and commitment to work is likely to be different than if the parent typically returns home exhausted and seeking solace and escape from the work day. While adolescents come to see work in a wide range of ways, most are anxious to begin work and reap the financial, social, and personal rewards of being productive.

In this regard, the lack of worthwhile work for adolescents may be the single greatest predicament of adolescence (Mitchell, 1975). Most adolescents want to be productive, and the absence of work can, for many, deny a feeling of worth. Much of the discontent of youth stems from having little of importance to do (Mitchell, 1975). This problem is even more compounded when the adolescent does not see prospects for work in the future. Adolescents whose adult models are out of work or chronically unemployed are particularly disadvantaged.

Whether an adolescent forms an image of work as personally fulfilling and socially useful, as a necessary evil unconnected to any obvious good, or as out of reach depends on the adolescent's exposure to the world of work and to cultural values and economic conditions. Social press and personal desire generally collude to lead the adolescent to see the importance of entering the world of adult productivity, either through paid labor or in a homemaker role.

In sum, adolescence is a period of important value formation. Values allow the adolescent to make occupational choices that establish early adult lifestyles. Establishing values is challenging since the sources of values in society are many and sometimes contradictory. Not surprisingly, many adolescents experiment and struggle in the process of value formation, often moving between ideal values and the realities of life (Hendry, 1983; Mitchell, 1975).

Interests

Interests undergo substantial transformation during adolescence. One of the primary influences on interest change is movement out of the family setting, where interests are often family-centered, into a peer group where new interests are espoused (Lambert, Rothschild, Atland, & Green, 1978). Interests also change because the adolescent is recognized as capable of new activities. Activities such as dating, dancing, and driving a car are newly available. Adolescents' interests also become more of an expression of self-identity (Csikszentmihalyi & Rochberg-Halton, 1981). Thus, what one enjoys becomes a kind of statement about what kind of person one is.

Interest preference is very much a function of what social context affords and for which it presses (Winch & Gordon, 1974). For example, the rural adolescent who takes a job as a laborer or begins work on a farm after high school is likely to develop interests around hunting, fishing, four-wheel drive pickups, country-western music, and the local fire rescue squad. The Ivy League college student is more likely to be attracted to intellectual games, cultural events, sports cars, and participation in social-political activities. Such preferences represent a growing personal style, an orientation to socially accepted leisure and amateur pursuits, and a maturation of interests to show social and civic concern in ways typical for the local environment.

Habituation Subsystem

Adolescence is a period of transformation in the roles and habits which regulate everyday behavior. The adolescent assumes an increasing variety of roles which are less circumscribed and less externally regulated, and more complex. Adolescence also demands a more complex set of habits.

Roles

Adolescents try out many of the roles they will hold as adults. Such role experimentation fills several needs for adolescents. It helps them to consolidate their identity (Santrock, 1981). It helps them to satisfy the desire for status and independence, to learn role scripts, and to recognize their abilities for particular roles (Mitchell, 1975).

While some roles continue from childhood into adolescence, the nature of those roles and the expectations associated with them begin to change. The student role is exemplary in this regard. The adolescent in high school and college is still a student, but now the student role is transitional. Successful completion in order to enter work is increasingly emphasized. In similar fashion, the family role becomes transformed. Parents may see adolescents as becoming more responsible for taking care of themselves (e.g., buying their own clothes, cooking meals for themselves) and contributing to the household (e.g., through part-time work). Increased expectations for productivity and responsibility within continuing roles serve as a preparation for achieving adult roles: that is, the student and family roles change in the direction of the homemaker and worker role.

There are also increasing opportunities to try on a variety of roles not available in childhood. High school provides for more self-determining groups, such as sports teams and student government, in which students can assume a variety of short-term roles. Dating allows the adolescent to explore aspects of roles that are associated with long-term relationships. The two most important roles for most adolescents are the friendship role and worker role.

For the adolescent, the peer group is a source of information about the world outside the family, and it is a testing ground for new ideas and behaviors (Santrock, 1981). The role of friend is increasingly important and may undergo several changes during adolescence (Douvan & Adelson, 1975).

The worker role is also important and valuable during adolescence, although the number of adolescents who work full-time has decreased dramatically since the turn of the century (Santrock, 1981). Nevertheless, a great many adolescents work part-time while they are going to school. Many adolescents babysit, work as waitresses or busboys, or hold other routine jobs (e.g., newspaper delivery, short-order cook, and so on) (Konopka, 1976; Santrock, 1981). Such jobs, however, may be unrelated to future vocational plans and are done primarily for spending money (Konopka, 1976; Lambert, Rothschild, Atland, & Green, 1978). However, other benefits do accrue to working

adolescents. Part-time jobs expose adolescents to the work world and afford opportunity to develop skill in getting and keeping jobs, budgeting time and money, and taking pride in accomplishments (Santrock, 1981). Volunteer work can also serve as a means for exploring future vocations (Lambert, Rothschild, Atland, & Green, 1978). Adolescence is a time of looking forward to other occupational roles. Adolescent's anticipate and in some cases enter into marriage and/or parenthood. The termination of adolescence means, in large part, the achievement of adult status through entry into adult occupational roles.

Habits

New habits are required for the changing circumstances of adolescence and for the world of work. Habits also must take over much routine behavior which was previously externally regulated. A major impact on the habits of the adolescent is the movement from grammar school to junior high and high school. No longer in a single classroom with a series of daily activities for the entire class, students have individual schedules and must be responsible for being in the right place at the right time (Moor, 1976). Adolescents also have more autonomy over their study habits, which is further accentuated when the individual goes to college, spending fewer hours in class and studying under one's own initiative.

More of adolescents' time is at their personal discretion (Lambert, Rothschild, Atland, & Green, 1978). They must use time to establish a routine which allows performance of the tasks required for the student and other roles. Adolescents must learn basic habits of industry, the ability to put aside play and to use time and energy to do some productive activity (Mauer, 1971). Habits of good workmanship, team behavior, promptness, dependability, and so on are often acquired in adolescence and facilitate the transition into productive roles of adulthood (Oakland, 1969).

Mind-Brain-Body Performance Subsystem

The adolescent continues to develop capacities for motor, process, and communication and interaction skills. A major growth in the capacity for communication and interaction occurs in adolescence. The musculoskeletal constituent completes development in adolescence; the major change is rapid growth of the long bones in association with puberty. Neurological changes during adolescence are minor, but the symbolic constituent develops substantially.

Summary

Adolescence is a time of transformation. Values, personal causation, and interests are changed, formulated, and refined; new roles and supporting habits are anticipated and developed. These changes prepare the adolescent for and lead to adult roles.

The early adolescent makes occupational choices based mainly on interest, choosing projects and roles that hold attraction. Later, the adolescent gives increasing consideration to sense of capacity and feelings of efficacy and chooses occupations according to internalized values. By late adolescence one is exploring realistic alternatives, crystallizing, and specifying major occupational choices. This process is not invariant and proceeds at different paces for different persons (Ginzberg, 1971; Perun & Del Vento, 1981; Super, 1971). In fact, because individuals and their self-concepts are continually evolving and changing with growth and experience, the process of occupational choice is continuous and dynamic (Super, 1971).

Adolescence represents the interface of various social factors with intense personal change. The major transformation of the adolescent period is the movement from the roles of childhood to adult roles. Paramount in this process is the opportunity for the adolescent to be self-determined through occupational choice supported by habits and capacities. The adolescent typically makes his or her entry into adulthood through assumption of the worker or homemaker role. When this achievement is a product of personal choice based on values, interests, and a sense of personal causation, the adolescent has a foundation for success and satisfaction in adulthood.

ADULTHOOD

The boundaries of adulthood are closely tied to one's working life. Adulthood typically begins with the assumption of a more or less permanent full-time job or other productive occupation and ends with retirement (Troll, 1975). Adulthood is the longest period of life. Contrary to popular views of adulthood as a period of stability or a state of maturity which is achieved and sustained, adults undergo considerable change. Some of these changes are externally recognizable, as the person passes through a series of steps, crises, or transitions: marriage or divorce, starting a family, changing jobs, and bidding farewell to grown children (Levinson, 1978; Sheehy, 1978; Vaillant, 1977). Other changes are internal, as the individual sorts out the various meanings, goals, and purposes that guide choice and self-evaluation in adult life.

Volition Subsystem

The refinement of personal causation, interests, and values and the ability to translate these into meaningful occupational choices typically reach their peak in adulthood. Adults have more freedom to make choices than at any other stage of life. Diverse factors such as economic constraints and obligations of parenthood affect these decisions, but for most people adulthood is the time when one truly begins to live one's own life. Adults tend to assess and reassess their own motives and choices as they experience and contemplate the unfolding of their life story (Handel, 1987). Narrative reassessment typically reflects a transformation from an early concern with competence and achievement to a later concern with value and personal satisfaction. This transformation in volition, sometimes referred to as a mid-life crisis, may lead persons to retell their stories, change work careers, or to enact similarly drastic alterations in their occupational lifestyles (Bischof, 1976; Farrell & Rosenberg, 1981; Gould, 1972; Kimmel, 1980; Levinson, 1978; Sheehy, 1978; Stevenson, 1977; Vaillant, 1977). Whatever life course they choose, adults continue the narrative process of knowing themselves, exploring the worth and meaning of their lives, and seeking to control the circumstances and direction of their lives. For some adults this struggle results in a high level of well-being. Others do their best to hang on. Still others fail to find a satisfactory and meaningful life course and, instead, live lives characterized by compromise, conflict, or catastrophe.

Personal Causation

Adulthood ordinarily is accomplished by an increasing desire to achieve and to work autonomously. For most people, this is accompanied by an increased sense of efficacy (Schlossberg, Troll, & Leibowitz, 1978). A desire for more autonomy appears to be widespread in middle-aged adults. This desire for more personal control also leads many adults to enter managerial, teaching, or other leadership roles in which they supervise or prepare new members of their field or community.

One's knowledge of capacity changes throughout adulthood. Early adulthood is generally a period of acquiring and refining abilities for one's line of work. Young workers see themselves as learning and increasing their efficacy. While they may not feel fully competent, this feeling is judged in relation to still being a novice. By middle adulthood, individuals have generally realized their peak performance and can assess how skillful they have become. Their sense of efficacy may be affected by a number of factors. In fields that require judgement and accumulated experience, older workers may feel secure in their abilities. In rapidly changing fields, they may be threatened. Young adults may have dreams of success mixed with anxiety about how they will actually perform. In some positions, one must either make the grade by moving through successive stages or levels of achievement or be considered a mediocre or failing worker (Brim, 1968). Many individuals in middle age face a sense of panic related to the realization that unless one now achieves a certain status or accomplishment, one must forego the dream of really "making it" in a career (Sheehy, 1978; Troll, 1975).

While the sense of efficacy is often dominated by work, other adult experiences such as rearing a family and maintaining a household are also areas which evoke strong feelings about one's effectiveness. Parents often find themselves facing great responsibilities with minimal preparation, sometimes questioning their capacities: facing the challenge of a newborn or confronting an adolescent's rebelliousness (Lowenthal, Thurnher, & Chiriboga, 1975). Similarly, such adult challenges as maintaining a household and managing personal finances can be sources of challenge, stress, accomplishment, and failure.

Values

During adulthood, values usually become increasingly important as a motivating force and a source of self-evaluation. Most adults have internalized a pattern of values reflective of the larger culture and/or any subculture to which they belong. While personal values related to occupation tend to remain relatively stable throughout adulthood (Troll, 1975), a generalized shift does often occur. After spending adolescence in the process of setting occupational goals and choosing a career, the young adult begins trying to fulfill these plans. The goals of early adulthood are thus focused on instrumental and material values, such as getting ahead at work, earning a satisfactory living, being able to support one's dependents, and being able to acquire the objects that signify success in contemporary society (Lowenthal, Thurnher, & Chiriboga, 1975). Middle-aged workers begin to feel that they have a limited amount of time left in which to achieve their goals. After a period of an intense "last-ditch" effort to reach their goals, they often begin to focus more on humanitarian concerns and on themes of legacy (e.g., what one will leave to the future or how one will be remembered by children) (Lowenthal, Thurnher, & Chiriboga, 1975). While this particular pattern of value change will not characterize all adults, some consideration of and shift in values are likely in the course of adult life.

Interests

Most people have well-established interests by the time they reach adulthood. In both leisure and work these interests are relatively stable. Many adults entered their work because it embodied the opportunity to channel and develop personal interests (Kimmel, 1980). However, it is not a universal phenomenon that adults find their work interesting. White-collar workers and professionals in general experience more interest in their work than assembly line workers who engage in repetitive tasks which provide minimal challenge and have little or no control over working conditions (Vroom, 1964).

In many ways adults have opportunity to shape their lives around their personal interests. Many adults do pursue interests avidly and seriously during their leisure time. Other adults use interests as a means of relaxing and regenerating themselves for work. A number of factors may shape and even redirect interests in adulthood. New couples may try to find common ground and discover new interests from their partners. Expectations and opportunities from the workplace, neighborhood, and other reference groups may also shape interests. Thus, for example, adults may attend social events with colleagues, playing golf with business associates, and belong to a work-based sports team.

Habituation Subsystem

Roles

Adulthood is characterized by a variety of socially prescribed and individually chosen roles which structure the adult's daily life and provide identity. Apart from family roles, most of these roles are enacted in community settings that exist solely for the adult age group (Barker & Wright, 1971). Typical adult role transitions include the initiation of a lasting partnership, parenthood, changes in work roles, transitions from work to homemaking or vice versa, joining civic and social organizations, and adopting major hobbies or amateur pursuits.

The one pervasive feature of adult life is work, since adults are expected to contribute productively to society if they are able to do so. Being a housewife was once the only productive expectation of adult women, but their participation in the work force has increased strikingly in recent years (Bernard, 1982). The work role is perceived by most adults to be a basic and normal condition of life and the lack of work can be stigmatizing. Nonetheless, the availability of work is subject to economic fluctuations and at one time or another many adults find themselves unemployed, which can be very stressful.

Entering work requires learning new behaviors, forming new interpersonal relationships (Brim, 1968), reapportioning one's use of time and, frequently, developing a new identity. Ultimately, identification with the work role may involve a transformation in one's outlook.

People vary in the degree to which they identify with work roles. Role identification is affected by aspirations, other role demands, priority given to work, and how the work setting affords and presses for occupational behavior. For example, executives, professors, and physicians invest long periods of time in training and are expected to give priority to the role, work long hours, continue to build competence, and incorporate a strong professional identity while moving through structured stages of credentialling, responsibility, and position.

The work role also influences other roles that are performed by the adult, especially friendship and leisure roles. Workers often share confidences and decision making with coworkers (Bischof, 1976) and may develop strong friendship ties with colleagues.

The leisure role takes several forms in adulthood, distinguished by the degree of intensity attached to them. Being a hobbyist is a typical leisure role characterized by enjoyment and enthusiasm. The amateur role, on the other hand, represents more of a middle ground between player and professional (Stebbins, 1979). Participation in organizational and social roles reaches a peak in middle adulthood (Bischof, 1976). Service groups become quite popular for people between the ages of 35 and 55 (Bischof, 1976). Volunteering and participating in religious organizations are roles that many adults pursue.

Most adults have to divide their time among work, family, community, and leisure roles. Because each of these roles can involve substantial investments of energy and time, a large number of people find inevitable conflicts in their use of time. Despite the potential for conflicts in time use, having a combination of roles appears to enhance well-being (Baruch, Barnett, & Rivers, 1980).

Habits

Habits of adulthood are necessarily concerned with the efficient allocation of time to various roles and the occupational forms they require. The division of the weekly routine into time for work, play, rest, self-care, and family is to some extent contingent upon the norms of society (e.g., the typical nine-to-five, Monday-through-Friday work week). Adult habits are influenced by the culture in other ways as well. What constitutes appropriate food at a given meal, how often one bathes, how to dress for work, and so on are all examples of cultural expectations that lead to the development of certain habits.

Adults need to autonomously regulate their own routine behavior. Different work may require vastly different routines. For example, factory and hospital work requires a rather rigid adherence to schedules, whereas farmers and university professors must develop their own routines around seasonal variations in work. Marriage, purchasing a home, and the arrival of children also place demands on persons to develop habits for home maintenance and caretaking. Previously accustomed to a routine organized around personal needs and desires, adults typically find themselves having to orient their routines to a broader set of concerns.

Mind-Brain-Body Performance Subsystem

Adulthood represents the both peaking and declining of abilities. Young adults are still acquiring new abilities for work and other areas of adult responsibility, whereas middle and later adulthood is characterized by some waning in capacity (Kimmel, 1980). A great deal of working knowledge is learned on the job such as the abilities to deal innovatively with unforeseen circumstances, to secure the cooperation of workers, and to manage workplace poli-

tics (Kusterer, 1978). Adults also find themselves newly responsible for a number of family-related tasks, including managing personal finances, home maintenance, caring for children, and communicating with a partner. These responsibilities often must be learned under "sink or swim" conditions. The ability to find the information one needs, to learn new occupational forms in the process of performing, and to problem solve in novel situations become more important than direct task performance capacities.

Physical changes do affect the occupational performance of adults. Over time, adults experience a decrease in energy and strength along with some decrement in sensory perception. For example, it is in adulthood that many people first require glasses or bifocals. Others find that they must cut back on some rigorous activities (Kimmel, 1980). Importantly habits, including the use of time, eating and drinking patterns, routine amounts of exercise, and typical levels of stress have a major impact on various abilities as well as on the incidence of diseases which may impair capacity (Kimmel, 1980; Stevenson, 1977; Troll, 1975). Consequently, the adults' responses to decreased capacities may be even more important than declines due to aging. Adults who continue to engage in physically or cognitively demanding activities sustain capacity whereas those who significantly curtail their activity may hasten decline in capacity.

Summary

Adulthood is a period of ongoing change and growth. While each individual's passage through adulthood is unique, there appears to be an early period of skill building, achievement orientation, and accomplishment followed by a period of self-examination and a search for meaning in work and other spheres of life. At the same time, it must be recognized that adulthood is an ongoing phenomenon lived anew by each new generation and its own historical experiences.

LATER ADULTHOOD

Later adulthood is defined both by biological changes and social convention. That is, aging involves a natural decline in the mind-brain-body performance subsystem and is associated with a high frequency of health conditions that affect capacity. Socially, retirement and eligibility for social benefits demarcates entry into this period of later adulthood. It is difficult to define later adulthood by chronological age. Rather, it is useful to think of later adulthood as demarked by changes in lifestyle as determined by waning capacity, personal choice, and social convention.

Volition Subsystem

Older adults' volition is important to help direct the many choices that drive or are in response to necessary changes in lifestyle. Moreover, the composition and telling of one's life story seems to gain importance. As older adults approach the end of life, the need both to make the most of the time one has and to make sense of the life one has lived become important (Karp, 1988).

Personal Causation

The fact that old age is generally accompanied by losses of capacity and of some opportunities to use abilities may lead elderly persons to experience a diminished knowledge of capacity and sense of efficacy although this appears to be quite individual rather than generally true (Bradley & Webb, 1976; Duke, Shaheen, & Nowicki, 1974; Staats, 1974; Wolk & Kurtz, 1975). Nonetheless, maintaining a sense of efficacy appears important to positive adjustment to old age (Kuypers, 1972). Since the loss of capacity may have important implications for independence and lifestyle, older adults may be especially inventive in sustaining a sense of efficacy while others may hold unrealistic views of their abilities.

Values

Values typically undergo some transformation and have a pervasive influence on occupational choices in old age. One view holds that older adults shift from instrumental values (i.e., being ambitious, intellectual, capable, and responsible (Rokeach, 1973; Ryff & Baltes, 1976)) toward terminal values such as a sense of accomplishment, freedom, equality, and comfort. While this pattern may be true of many older adults, it is most accurate to say that the nature and direction of any value change depend on past and current life circumstances. Nonetheless, for most older adults the importance of work and achievement wanes, while other values concerning family, community, and leisure become more significant (Antonovsky & Sagy, 1990).

As abilities decline, elderly persons must redefine their standards (Clark & Anderson, 1967) and revise the way in which values are satisfied. Finally, having future goals and commitments is important to maintaining morale in later life (Schonfield, 1973; Spence, 1968).

Interests

For many older adults the relative freedom from obligations in old age provides opportunity to pursue a variety of interests more seriously or fully than before. However, constrained capacity and resources in later life can prevent some persons from pursuing interests. For example, some older adults are involved in solitary and passive occupations although they preferred to be involved in social and more active occupations (McGuire, 1980). Older adults can be constrained in their activity choices by a lack of transportation, facilities, money, and companions; by fears of injury, learning new things, or disapproval; and by no longer feeling a sense of satisfaction (McAvoy, 1979; McGuire, 1983; Scott & Zoernick, 1977).

Habituation Subsystem

Roles

Role changes in later life can sometimes be involuntary and unpleasant. For example, elderly persons may lose the spouse and friend roles through death. Many lost roles are not easily replaced. Older adults who cannot replace lost or diminished roles may experience boredom, loneliness, and depression. Many older adults rely on family, community, or other institutions to provide roles. For example, Elliot & Barris (1987) found that older adults' role identification was greater in nursing homes that provided more opportunities for activity.

Some persons continue to work beyond ordinary retirement age for income, to feel satisfied, useful, and respected, and/or to have a major role in organizing their lives (Atchley, 1972; Lieberman, 1983). When it does occur, retirement can be a far-reaching event since so much of life is geared toward preparation for, entry into, and advancement in work, and since work structures a great deal of time and activity. Consequently, the transition from work to retirement is full of both possibilities and pitfalls. As Johnsson (1994) has shown, retirement is an entirely individual process. For one individual it may mean escape from arduous labor and an opportunity to devote time to occupations of a higher priority, such as family involvement, a second career, or hobbies. For another, it may mean loss of social contact and severance from a primary source of self-worth and meaning. Whatever the implications, retirement is a major life event which can be counted on to reshape an individual's occupational life.

Family roles and relationships are important and often change dramatically in the lives of older adults. Older adults often spend significant time with adult children and grandchildren. Relationships with adult children can be an important source of gratification sustained by a reciprocal exchange in the form of affection, gifts, and services (Shanas & Streib, 1963). For example, older adults often act as babysitters, confidants and advisors, housesitters, and providers of income (Ebersole & Hess, 1981). As older adults become frail, disabled, or chronically ill, adult children may assume responsibility for the care of their aging parents. This role-reversal (as noted in Chapter 5) is often complicated and challenging for all involved.

Friendships is another important role of older adults (Lowenthal & Haven, 1968). While having extensive friendships is not necessary, the person who has a number of friendships is less vulnerable to loss of friends through death. Loss of one's partner in old age may severely disrupt life. One may lose a friend, homemaker, financial supporter, and caretaker depending on the nature of the relationship. Other role changes may accompany the loss of a partner. The surviving partner may have to take over many things previously done by the spouse.

Many older persons volunteer, serving in diverse capacities. Volunteerism provides an avenue for older adults to use their talents to benefit the community with needed services to substitute for work (Payne & Whittington, 1976).

Habits

Elderly persons often posses habits developed over a long period in a stable environment. Changes in underlying capacity and changes in environment can challenge these habits. At the same time, changing circumstances, such as widowhood or retirement, often impose demands for acquiring new habits. Moreover, as capacities decline, habits become increasingly important to sustain functional performance and quality of life.

Mind-Brain-Body Performance Subsystem

Age-related changes in the musculoskeletal, neurological, and cardiorespiratory constituents typically occur in the older adult and diminish capacity. However, substantial losses of ability are not inevitable and may be forestalled if the elderly person remains active. Consequently, age-related changes are unique to each person. Moreover, the impact of such decrements may be mitigated by adapting one's habits and environment.

CONCLUSION

As we have seen, the course of occupational development is complex and characterized by constant transformation. Some common features can be identified in the life course of most persons, but it is above all an individual journey. Indeed, one of the most remarkable characteristics of any individual journey through life are the singular incidents, the crises, the personal transformations, the setbacks, and other features which deviate from any neat or normative portrayal of development. In this chapter, I have sought to identify some of the major transformations and patterns which characterize the course of occupational development. In attempting to portray what may be typical or ordinary in the developmental course, I necessarily ignored individual differences. However, the reader should realize that it is these very differences which constitute the individual dynamics through which a particular human system undergoes the lifelong transformation we refer to as development. Moreover, these unique events, struggles, and transformations give each life its special direction, pace, and meaning. The socializing effects of the culture within which a person exists tends to give the course of development its average or characteristic pathways. The unique features which make any one life different from any other life holds the key to understanding that life. When therapists seek to understand a person's occupational development, reference to normative disruptions of the developmental course are insufficient. Rather, one must seek to grasp the particular developmental course that has brought each person to the present.

References

Alissi, A. S. (1975). Concepts of adolescence. In H. D. Thornberg (Ed.), *Contemporary adolescence: Readings* (2nd ed.). Monterey, CA: Brooks/Cole.

Allport, G. (1961). *Pattern and growth in personality*. New York: Holt, Rinehart & Winston.

Antonovsky, A., & Sagy, S. (1990). Confronting developmental tasks in the retirement transition. *Gerontologist, 30,* 362–368.

Atchley, R. C. (1972). *Social forces in later life: An introduction to social gerontology*. Belmont, CA: Wadsworth.

Bailey, D. M. (1971). Vocational theories and work habits related to childhood development. *American Journal of Occupational Therapy, 25,* 298–302.

Barker, R. G., & Wright, H. F. (1971). *Midwest and its children*. Hamden, CT: Archon.

Baruch, G., Barnett, R., & Rivers, C. (1980, December 7). A new start for women at midlife. *New York Times Sunday Magazine,* pp. 196–200.

Bernard, J. (1982). Between two worlds: The housewife. In P. L. Stewart & M. G. Cantor (Eds.), *Varieties of work*. Beverly Hills, CA: Sage Publications.

Bischof, L. J. (1976). *Adult psychology* (2nd ed.). New York: Harper & Row.

Bradley, R. H., & Webb, R. (1976). Age-related differences in locus of control orientation in three behavioral domains. *Human Development, 19,* 49–55.

Brim, O. G., Jr. (1968). Adult socialization. In J. A. Clausen (Ed.), *Socialization and society*. Boston: Little, Brown & Co.

Brown, N. S. (1971). Three-year-olds' play. In G. Engstrom (Ed.), *Play: The child strives toward self-realization.*

Proceedings of the National Association for the Education of Young Children Conference, Washington, DC.

Bruner, J. (1969). On voluntary action and its hierarchical structure. In A. Koestler & J. R. Smithies (Eds.), *Beyond reductionism*. Boston: Beacon Press.

Bruner, J. (1973). Organization of early skilled action. *Child Development, 44,* 1–11.

Burke, J. P. (1977). A clinical perspective on motivation: Pawn versus origin. *American Journal of Occupational Therapy, 31,* 254–258.

Clark, M., & Anderson, B. G. (1967). *Culture and aging: An anthropological study of older Americans*. Springfield, IL: Charles C Thomas.

Csikszentmihalyi, M., & Rochberg-Halton, E. (1981). *The meaning of things*. Cambridge, MA: Cambridge University Press.

Douvan, E., & Adelson, J. (1975). Adolescent friendships. In J. J. Conger (Ed.), *Contemporary issues in adolescent development*. New York: Harper & Row.

Duke, M. P., Shaheen, J., & Nowicki, S. (1974). The determination of locus of control in a geriatric population and a subsequent test of the social learning model for interpersonal distance. *Journal of Psychology, 86,* 277–285.

Ebersole, P., & Hess, P. (1981). *Toward healthy aging: Human needs and nursing response*. St. Louis: CV Mosby.

Elkind, D. (1981). *The hurried child*. Reading, MA: Addison-Wesley.

Elliot, M. S., & Barris, R. (1987). Occupational role performance and life satisfaction in elderly persons. *Occupational Therapy Journal of Research, 7,* 215–224.

Farrell, M. P., & Rosenberg, S. D. (1981). *Men at midlife*. Boston: Auburn House.

Frost, J. L., & Klein, B. L. (1979). *Children's play and playgrounds*. Boston: Allyn and Bacon.

Ginzberg, E. (1971). Toward a theory of occupational choice. In H. J. Peters & J. C. Hansen (Eds.), *Vocational guidance and career development* (2nd ed.). New York: Macmillan.

Goodman, E. (1984, April 3). Agreeable teenagers. *The Washington Post,* p. A-13.

Goodman, P. (1960). *Growing up absurd: Problems of youth in the organized system*. New York: Random House.

Gould, R. L. (1972). The phases of adult life: a study in developmental psychology. *American Journal of Psychology, 129,* 33–43.

Hamburg, B. A. (1974). Early adolescence: a specific and stressful stage of the life cycle. In G. V. Coelho, B. A. Hamburg, & J. E. Adams (Eds.), *Coping and adaptation*. New York: Basic Books.

Handel, A. (1987). Personal theories about the life-span development of one's self in autobiographical self-presentations of adults. *Human Development, 30,* 83–98.

Hendry, L. B. (1983). *Growing up and going out: Adolescents and leisure*. Aberdeen: Aberdeen University Press.

Hurt, J. M. (1980). A play skills inventory: a competency monitoring tool for the 10-year-old. *American Journal of Occupational Therapy, 34,* 651–656.

Johnsson, H. (1994). *Retirement from an occupational perspective: A review of theories and some empirical findings concerning the meaningfulness of work and leisure*. Unpublished manuscript, Halsohoskolan I Stockholm.

Josslyn, I. (1952). *The adolescent and his world*. New York: Family Service Association of America.

Karp, D. A. (1988). A decade of reminders: Changing age consciousness between fifty and sixty years old. *Gerontologist, 28*, 727–738.

Keniston, K. (1974). A "new" stage of life. In H. Kraemer (Ed.), *Youth and culture: A human development approach.* Monterey, CA: Brooks/Cole.

Kimmel, D. C. (1980). *Adulthood and aging* (2nd ed.). New York: John Wiley & Sons.

Konopka, G. (1976). *Young girls: A portrait of adolescence.* Englewood Cliffs, NJ: Prentice-Hall.

Kusterer, K. C. (1978). *Know-how on the job: The important working knowledge of "unskilled" workers.* Boulder, CO: Westview Press.

Kuypers, J. A. (1972). Internal-external locus of control, ego functioning, and personality characteristics in old age. *Gerontologist, 12*, 168–173.

Lambert, G. B., Rothschild, B. F., Atland, R., & Green, L. B. (1978). *Adolescence: Transition from childhood to maturity* (2nd ed.). Monterey, CA: Brooks/Cole.

Levinson, D. J. (1978). *The seasons of a man's life.* New York: Ballantine.

Lieberman, L. (1983). Second careers in arts and craft fairs. *Gerontologist, 23*, 266–272.

Lindquist, J. E., Mack, W., & Parham, L. D. (1982). A synthesis of occupational behavior and sensory integration concepts in theory and practice, part 1. Theoretical foundations. *American Journal of Occupational Therapy, 36*, 365–374.

Lowenthal, M. F., & Haven, C. (1968). Interaction and adaptation: intimacy as a critical variable. *American Sociological Review, 33*, 20–30.

Lowenthal, M. F., Thurnher, M., & Chiriboga, D. (1975). *Four stages of life.* San Francisco: Jossey-Bass.

Matsutsuyu, J. (1971). Occupational behavior: a perspective on work and play. *American Journal of Occupational Therapy, 25*, 291–294.

Mauer, P. (1971). Antecedents of work behavior. *American Journal of Occupational Therapy, 25*, 295–297.

McAvoy, L. L. (1979). The leisure preferences, problems, and needs of the elderly. *Jouranl of Leisure Resourcs, 11*, 40–47.

McGuire, F. (1980). The incongruence between actual and desired leisure involvement in advanced adulthood. *Active Adaptive Aging, 1*, 77–89.

McGuire, F. (1983). Constraints on leisure involvement in the later years. *Active Adaptive Aging, 3*, 17–24.

Mead, G. H. (1934). *Mind, self, and society.* Chicago: University of Chicago Press.

Mitchell, J. J. (1975). *The adolescent predicament.* Toronto: Holt, Rinehart & Winston.

Moor, C. H. (1976). *From school to work—effective counselling and guidance.* Beverly Hills, CA: Sage Publications.

Morgan, E. (1982). Toward a reformulation of the Eriksonian model of female identity development. *Adolescence, 27*, 199–211.

Muuss, R. E. (1975). *Theories of adolescence.* New York: Random House.

Nicholls, J. G. (1984). Achievement motivation: Conceptions of ability, subjective experience, task choice, and performance. *Psychological Review, 3*, 328–346.

Oakland, J. (1969). Measurement of personality correlates of academic achievement in high school students. *Journal of Counseling and Psychology, 16*, 452–457.

Payne, B., & Whittington, F. (1976). Older women: an examination of popular stereotypes and research evidence. *Social Problems, 2*(1), 488–504.

Perun, P. J., & Del Vento, B. D. (1981). Towards a model of female occupational behavior: A human development approach. *Psychology of Woman Quarterly, 6*, 234–252.

Piaget, J., & Inhelder, B. (1969). *The psychology of the child.* New York: Basic Books.

Reilly, M. (1974). *Play as exploratory learning.* Beverly Hills, CA: Sage Publications.

Robinson, A. L. (1977). Play, the arena for acquisition of rules for competent behavior. *American Journal of Occupational Therapy, 31*, 248–253.

Rokeach, M. (1973). *The nature of human values.* New York: Free Press.

Ryff, C. D., & Baltes, P. B. (1976). Value transition and adult development in women. The instrumentality-terminality sequence hypothesis. *Developmental Psychology, 12*, 567–568.

Santrock, J. W. (1981). *Adolescence: An introduction.* Dubuque, IA: Brown.

Schlossberg, N. K., Troll, L. E., & Leibowitz, Z. (1978). *Perspectives on counseling adults: Issues and skills.* Monterey, CA: Brooks/Cole.

Schonfield, D. (1973). Future commitments and successful aging. The random sample. *Journal of Gerontology, 28*, 189–196.

Scott, E. O., & Zoernick, D. A. (1977). Exploring leisure needs of the aged. *Leisurability, 4*, 25–31.

Shanas, E., & Streib, G. F. (1963). *Social structure and the family: Generational relations.* Englewood Cliffs, NJ: Prentice-Hall.

Sieg, A. (1975). Why adolescence occurs. In H. D. Thornberg (Ed.), *Contemporary Adolescence: Readings* (2nd ed.). Monterey, CA: Brooks/Cole.

Shannon, P. D. (1974). Occupational choice: decision-making play. In M. Reilly (Ed.), *Play as Exploratory Learning.* Beverly Hills, CA: Sage Publications.

Sheehy, G. (1978). *Passages: Predictable crises of adult life.* New York: Bantam.

Spence, D. L. (1968). The role of futurity in aging adaptation. *Gerontologist, 8*, 180–183.

Staats, S. (1974). Internal versus external locus of control in three age groups. *International Journal of Aging and Human Development, 5*, 7–10.

Stein, S. L., & Weston, L. C. (1982). College women's attitudes toward woman and identity achievement. *Adolescence, 27*, 895–899.

Stebbins, R. (1979). Amateurs: On the margin between work and leisure. Beverly Hills, CA: Sage Publications.

Stevenson, J. S. (1977). Issues and crises during middlescence. New York: Appleton-Century-Crofts.

Super, D. E. (1971). A theory of vocational development. In H. J Peters & J. C. Hansen (Eds.), Vocational guidance and career development (2nd ed.). New York: Macmillan.

Sutton-Smith, B. (1971). The playful modes of knowing. In G. Engstrom (Ed.), Play: The child strives toward self-realization. Proceedings of the National Association for the Education of Young Children Conference, Washington, DC.

Sutton-Smith, B. (1980). A "sportive" theory of play. In H. B. Schwartzman (Ed.), Play and culture. West Point, NY: Leisure Press.

Takata, N. (1974). Play as a prescription. In M. Reilly (Ed.), Play as exploratory learning. Beverly Hills, CA: Sage Publications.

Thornberg, H. D. (1975). Behavior and values: consistency and inconsistency. In H. D. Thornberg (Ed.), Contemporary adolescence: Readings (2nd ed.). Monterey, CA: Brooks/Cole.

Troll, L. E. (1975). *Early and middle adulthood*. Monterey, CA: Brooks/Cole.

Vaillant, G. E. (1977). *Adaptation to life*. Boston: Little, Brown & Co.

von Bertalanffy, L. (1966). General system theory and psychiatry. In S. Arieti (Ed.), *American handbook of psychiatry*. New York: Basic Books.

Vroom, V. (1964). *Work and motivation*. New York: John Wiley & Sons.

Winch, R. F., & Gordon, M. T. (1974). *Familial structure and function as influence*. Lexington, MA: Heath.

Wolk, S., & Kurtz, J. (1975). Positive adjustment and involvement during aging and expectancy for internal control. *Journal of Consulting and Clinical Psychology, 43*, 173–178.

10/ Occupational Dysfunction

Gary Kielhofner

INTRODUCTION

The underlying purpose of this chapter is to identify the kinds of difficulties and challenges which persons face when impairment affects their occupational choices, patterns, and performance. Most persons will experience some form of impairment in the course of their lives which forces them to cope, alter life patterns, make new decisions, and in some cases, completely retell their life story. In this chapter I will draw upon literature[a] concerning persons with a wide range of physical, psychological, and developmental disabilities to achieve a broad description of the kinds of challenges faced by persons when they experience occupational dysfunction. In order to portray the variety of problems that persons may encounter in their occupational lives, I have organized the chapter according to the three subsystems and environment. This approach dissects the human experience of occupational dysfunction and allows us to explore it in a systematic way.

---

[a]Much of the literature concerning persons with disabilities reflects the trait orientation discussed in Chapter 4. For example, studies often seek to identify the presence or extent of a particular trait (e.g., feelings of inefficacy) in a sample of persons with a particular diagnosis or disability or to correlate that trait with identified dysfunctional behavior. This is a useful body of empirical evidence concerning many of the concepts identified in this model. However, it is important to recall that these traits are extracted from individual lives wherein the full extent of their impact on function or dysfunction can be known. The constellation of factors that contribute to a particular individual's dysfunctional state remains to be discovered from careful examination of that person's total life and circumstances.

Nonetheless, the reader should remember that occupational dysfunction ordinarily involves many or all aspects of the human being and the surrounding environment. To understand occupational dysfunction in any person, consideration of all the subsystems and the environment together is necessary.

NATURE OF OCCUPATIONAL DYSFUNCTION

We recognize occupational dysfunction when an individual has difficulty performing, organizing, or choosing occupations. We also recognize it when the pattern of occupational behavior exhibited by a person fails to provide a basic quality of life to the individual and/or meet reasonable expectations of the environment. As this definition implies, it is not a precipitating disease or trauma but rather difficulty in the realm of occupation that constitutes occupational dysfunction. Occupational dysfunction is multifaceted; single sources of causation are the rare exception rather than the rule. As I already alluded to, occupational dysfunction is manifest in a cluster of factors that may include impairments of the mind-brain-body performance subsystem, disturbances of habit patterns and roles, challenges to volition, and difficulties in the person's relationship to the environment. These factors influence each other and all contribute to conditions in which the human system assembles dysfunctional occupational behavior.

Occupational dysfunction is not merely a state. Rather, it is an ongoing process in which unfolding behavior and experience both reflect and contribute to the difficulties an individual is experiencing. Within this dynamic process dysfunction is maintained, worsens, or may be ameliorated.

To understand occupational dysfunction one cannot rely on generalizations in the same way it may be possible to specify the symptoms, etiology, and consequences of a disease. For example, while the level of lesion of a spinal cord injury will predict subsequent sensory loss and paralysis, there is no similar systematic relationship between the degree of physical impairment and the degree of adjustment or maladjustment individuals exhibit, nor do all persons react to spinal cord injury in stages of denial, depression, bargaining, and acceptance as once argued (Rosenthal, 1989; Trieschmann, 1989). Rather, reaction and adjustment to such disability is a highly individual matter (Paap, 1972; Trieschmann, 1989).

Consequently, understanding the occupational dysfunction of someone with a disability requires appreciation of that person's life situation. The necessity for an individualized view of occupational dysfunction does not mean that we cannot use a systematic or common way of viewing different persons. Rather, it is helpful to have a theoretical perspective which provides a way of examining the occupational life of a person as well as cues to the types of challenges and problems which might be expected. This chapter provides such a systematic way to think about occupational dysfunction, pointing out a range of factors that may be present in any individual's occupational dysfunction.

SOURCES AND CONSEQUENCES OF OCCUPATIONAL DYSFUNCTION

Occupational dysfunction that comes to the attention of occupational therapists commonly includes impairments of the underlying mind-brain-body performance subsystem. These impairments may have their origins in a whole range of events such as genetic aberrations, biological trauma, disease, and the aging process. They may also reflect the impact of stressful or impoverished environments, learned ways of performing that are sources of trouble, or the sequelae of emotionally traumatic experiences.

While occupational dysfunctions typically include restrictions of occupational perfor-

mance skills related to some impairments in the mind-brain-body performance subsystem, their manifestation is seldom restricted to in this subsystem. Habituation, volition, and environmental factors also contribute to the occupational dysfunction. Moreover, since humans are dynamic systems, the importance of any of these factors as control parameters, maintaining or exacerbating a dysfunctional process, may shift over time.

Occupational dysfunction represents the interface of the three subsystems and the environment over time. Consequently, occupational dysfunction is nested in a complex of factors all of which reflect and contribute to sustaining the performance, patterns of behavior, identities, choices, and so on that reflect a life in trouble. The interrelationship of these factors can be illustrated by the case of children with congenital disabilities. Such children develop with a complex of biological, psychological, and sociocultural factors which tend to differ from those of children without disabilities (Molnar, 1989). For example, two of the important developmental changes of childhood that are fraught with implications of personal autonomy and social approval are achieving bladder control and walking; however, a child with spina bifida may be unable to do either. The implications of these performance restrictions on social identity, relationships with peers, family life, sense of efficacy and the impact, in turn, of these factors on choices and opportunities for learning of new skills, highlights the complex interplay of multiple factors in the unfolding nature of occupational dysfunction.

In similar fashion, traumatically acquired physical impairments have consequences which resonate throughout the human system and the environment. For example, Trieschmann (1989) describes the following adjustment challenge for the person with spinal cord injury:

The persons who acquire a spinal cord injury are often in the midst of mapping out a career or course of action that will characterize their adult lives, when they suddenly find themselves paralyzed, with no sensation in their limbs and no control over bladder and bowel. Life as they had known it will be interrupted by months of hospitalization and an often lengthy period during which new techniques must be mastered for survival and independent function. The changes in life-style will be significant. Spinal-injured persons must learn how to deal with a world designed for and dominated by able-bodied persons who are not very accepting of those with disabilities. They must learn new types of recreation and leisure activities and, in many cases, a new vocation. However, following an educational or vocational training program they must learn to face potential employers who do not want to hire them, not because of lack of qualifications for the job but because of the disability. They must learn that many of their previous friends drift away, and thus they must seek new opportunities to meet new people and to make new friends. Yet strangers tend to avoid any interaction with them; consequently, new techniques must be learned to put others at ease and to make them forget the presence of the wheelchair. Disabled persons must learn a sense of humor in order to cope with the daily frustrations and hard work that living with a disability entails. And they must learn to maintain their sense of dignity and self-worth when faced with a social welfare system that penalizes their efforts to become independent and self-sufficient. (p. 118)

What is implied in Triecshmann's description is emphasized by DeLoach and Greer (1981) who note that the most stressful aspect of an acquired disability is making the *transition* from being able bodied to living as a person with a disability. Indeed, they highlight one of the most important aspects of an acquired disability, that it requires one to remake oneself and one's life, or as Paap (1972) argues, to "reconstruct" reality.

Another large group of persons experience occupational dysfunction in concert with a psychiatric disturbance. Persons experiencing mental illness are as diverse as the talented person with borderline personality disorder who is unable to sustain a productive lifestyle and periodically engages in self-destructive behavior, the person who functioned well until the onset of a major depression that robbed him or her of all motivation, the adolescent who has been labelled a juvenile delinquent due to behavioral problems, and the person with chronic schizophrenia who is barely able to manage self-care. In the case of mental illness, occupational dysfunction is sometimes a

precipitating factor and is always closely interwoven with the disease process. For example, depression may in part result from imbalances of lifestyle and limitations of activity. Moreover, depression is recognized when the person's enjoyment of activity and activity pattern are suppressed.

The particular challenges that any individual with a disability faces depends on a host of factors that include the particularities of the impairments experienced, the point in development at which the disability occurs (e.g., congenital versus old age onset), the kind of life to which the impairment comes, the social and physical environment of the person with the disability. It must also be recognized that disability often implies long-term challenges to sustaining occupational function. As Rosenthal (1989) notes "the process of adjustment is continual and may be lifelong" (p. 44).

VOLITION

The role of volition in occupational dysfunction may vary widely depending on the nature of a person's disability and on the person's lifestyle. Volitional dispositions, self-knowledge, and life stories may lead to activities and occupational choices that are the sources of dysfunction. Acquired impairments may threaten and alter previously positive volition and can lead to a downward spiral into helplessness and demoralization. Whatever its contribution to occupational dysfunction, volition is also likely to be a strong influence on any process of adjusting to or overcoming the challenges of a disability. The importance of being able to make one's own choices (the function of volition) is underscored by the independent living movement: "To us, independence does not mean doing things physically alone. It means being able to make independent decisions." (Heumann, quoted in Frieden & Cole, 1985, p. 738). In the following sections I will examine factors related to personal causation, values, and interests that may restrict or disrupt volitional choices.

Personal Causation

When persons experience a level of impaired capacity it may affect both knowledge of capacity and sense of efficacy. The implications for personal causation depend on the nature and extent of incapacitation, its impact on one's lifestyle, as well as where in the life course it arises (Vash, 1981).

Knowledge of Capacity

Physical impairments, whether congenital or acquired in the life course, confront individuals with experiences that challenge or contradict a view of themselves as competent (Molnar, 1989; Wright, 1960). Pain, fatigue, limitations of sensations, cognition, and/or movement often mean that persons with disabilities achieve less than they desire and/or less than others; knowledge of this can permeate awareness of their own capacities (Werner-Beland, 1980). Consider, for example, the experience shared by two persons with cerebral palsy:

> Both of us were painfully aware of what it was like to be trapped inside a body that followed few directions of its mind and ignored the simple commands of speech and movement that nearly everyone takes for granted. We knew what it was like to be unable to express even one thousandth of the thoughts whirling inside our minds; what it was like to be unable to walk, or even feed ourselves . . . (Sienkiewicz-Mercer & Kaplan, 1989, p. 64)

While mental illness is not always characterized by a pronounced impairment of performance, there can often be a temporary or permanent suppression of capacity, especially when there is cognitive impairment or when symptoms interfere with competent performance. Anxiety, depression, and other symptoms of psychiatric illness can also reduce or interfere with performance. For example, Deegan (1991) describes her own experience with schizophrenia:

> At this time even the simplest of tasks were overwhelming. I remember being asked to come into the kitchen to help knead some bread dough. I got up, went into the kitchen, and looked at the dough for what seemed an eternity. Then I walked back to my chair and wept. The task seemed overwhelming to me. (p. 49)

As the example illustrates, incapacitation may not only be reflected in, but may also

partly originate in, an individual's sense of personal causation.

When one experiences a disability, awareness of capacity is a matter of great personal consequence and concern. Indeed, issues of capacity appear to hold a heightened place in considerations of self for both practical and emotional reasons. On the practical side, much of the typical competence for daily life that is ordinarily taken for granted presents major challenges or impossibilities when one has a disability. For example, Diane, a woman with quadrilateral congenital amputation, describes some of her abilities and limitations:

> I have a stool which enables me to get from the floor back up to my chair . . . I can get in and out of any bed—from w/c [wheelchair] to bed and reverse—from bed to floor (not falling out! HA) but not the reverse.
>
> I balance a glass between my face and arm . . . No one needs to place it there. I can pick up a glass, cup, or can, and drink it myself.
>
> I DO and CAN brush my teeth. I place the brush in my mouth and move it with both arms—for the uppers—with my right arm and tongue for everywhere else. No I can not floss.
>
> Doors. I can OPEN any door as long as I can get to the doorknob, which I turn with my arm and chin. I can not close a door behind me . . . (Frank, 1984, p. 641)

In the following passage Murphy (1987) shares his considerations of performing the task of lecturing which he had done automatically and effortlessly before the onset of his paralysis:

> I was much less concerned with what I would say than with how I would say it. My chest muscles had atrophied to such a degree that my ribcage was splayed. Talking for long periods tired me, and my voice had lost timbre and resonance, no longer projecting as well as it did. I was uncertain whether I could make it through a seventy-five-minute lecture, and I was apprehensive about the reaction of the students to a professor in a wheelchair. Would I be able to continue teaching? (p. 80)

A woman with chronic pain explains:

> Well, I can [vacuum] for a little while, I can't dust, because of the flicking of the wrists. It will flare it up again. Hanging the washing on the

line. The arms ache. I might get about four things on the line, then it starts to ache. Washing up I can start. I can't do the saucepans, because of the scrubbing. Cooking—oh, I can do a bit of cooking, but I can't lift heavy saucepans. I have dropped them. I have burnt myself. (Ewan, Lowy, & Reid, 1991, p. 178)

The knowledge that one is less capable than others, than one once was, or than one wishes to be can be a source of considerable psychic pain and social embarrassment. For this reason some persons with disabilities will go out of their way to avoid situations that provide occasions for failure (Cromwell, 1963; Moss, 1958). For example, emotionally disturbed adolescents indicate feelings of incompetence (Smyntek, 1983) and often prefer solitary tasks whose results are less easily judged by others (American Psychiatric Association, 1980). Mentally retarded adults are often plagued with doubts about their competence and go to great lengths to disguise their limitations (Edgerton, 1967; Kielhofner, 1983). In the following episode Doris, a mentally retarded woman, illustrates how one can be haunted by concerns about one's basic competence:

> I heard Doris saying to Paula, "I wouldn't be here [a community-based residential facility] if I wasn't okay. They discharged me from the state hospital and I wouldn't be on the outside if I wasn't okay." Then she asked rhetorically, "Isn't that right?" She talked on a while in that vein mentioning her [decade old] discharge papers in her wallet as 'proof' that she was okay. (Kielhofner, 1980, p. 172)

When shame or fear of failure dominates a person's knowledge of capacity there is disincentive to take risks, to learn new skills, or to make the best use of what one has. So long as the view of one's capacity is dominated with comparisons to previous states or others, the person may be locked into a view of self as incompetent (Wright, 1960). When this occurs, the knowledge of capacity can literally exacerbate any existing limitation of capacity.

Accuracy of Knowledge of Capacity

One's awareness of capacity expresses an understanding and belief about one's abilities that comes from experience and is influenced by cognitive and emotional factors. An issue that often arises in association with disability is whether or not one's knowledge of capacity is accurate—whether it actually reflects one's abilities and limitations. The issue of accuracy in knowledge of capacity is a complex one.

Cognitive limitations impairing comprehension of limitations, psychological pain that makes the knowledge of impairments unbearable and invites denial, fear of future pain or injury, or religious convictions that spiritual forces will lift or ameliorate the condition are examples of factors that may lead persons to over- or underestimate their capacities and limitations (Trieschmann, 1989; Tham, 1994). For example, Krefting (1989) relates that one head-injured young man "who had several cognitive deficits and gross communication problems, told me that his greatest problem was walking; if he could only walk, everything would be better" (p. 74). The consequence of his view was that his therapy program "was rendered totally ineffective because he was unable to recognize his limitations and saw no need to compensate for his deficits" (p. 74).

In contrast, when persons exaggerate their limitations they may unnecessarily limit their actions. Also, because of secondary gains related to being incapacitated (e.g., freedom from unsatisfying work conditions) persons may be motivated to overestimate their limitations. In other cases, persons who overestimate their capacities may make activity and occupational choices that can lead to injury, exacerbation of symptoms, and failure in performance.

Knowledge of capacity concerns not only what one is able to do in the present, but also in the future. Persons with a range of disabilities may not know in the early stages of a dysfunctional state, or during recovery, what their capacities will be. Persons who experience exacerbations and remissions or who have a progressive disease whose actual course cannot be known, find it impossible to know what abilities they will have in the future.

Many existing views emphasize that realistic acceptance of one's limitations is central to adjustment to disability. These views oversimplify how knowledge of capacity influences adjustment to loss of capacity. This adjustment is a highly individual process of discovering how an impairment may curtail or complicate the things one must and wants to do. This discovery may be ongoing as one's impairment and life changes. Moreover, knowledge of capacity is an expression of will (i.e., self-control and effort), as well as abilities, in the context of one's life story. Thus, the view of self as capable or incapable is not only a matter of accurate accounting, but also a reflection of one's hope and aspirations. The relative value of all these factors determine what one's view of capacity really means for adjusting to a disability. For example, some spinal cord-injured individuals may claim they will walk again, but such views are an "assertion of will and strength" (Trieschmann, 1989) which mainly reflect the substantial resources which a person will bring to coping with the disability. Given that it is often difficult, if not impossible, to know exactly what one's limits are nor to grasp the full implications of a disability, a person may need to couch any optimistic view in terms of recovery or return to a previous state. Later, when the implications of the disability are better understood and when an individual has new information with which to imagine a positive future with limitations of capacity, hope may find its expression in terms more consistent with actual impairments.

In the end, knowledge of capacity must be understood as a complex and unfolding process, not a static understanding. As the person with a disability progresses with his or her life, the implications of limitations may become more apparent. At the same time these limitations must be apprehended in the context of a life story in which it is important for a person to have hope and vision for a positive future.

Sense of Efficacy

The ability to control self (e.g., to move one's own body, to control feelings and thoughts) and to achieve desired outcomes in life may be directly challenged by disability. Children who grow up with a disability learn that they cannot do all that others do and are prone to develop feelings of inadequacy (Molnar, 1989). Such children may exhibit these

underlying feelings by insecure behavior, compensatory clowning, or aggressiveness. These children can become unnecessarily dependent and passive since they do not see their own actions as the most effective route for achieving their desires (Wasserman, 1986). Another possible liability for the child's feeling efficacious is parental overprotection. This is a difficult issue for any parent and particularly so for the parents of a child with a disability: they may know their child's vulnerabilities and have a desire to protect him or her from failure or risk. Reflecting on his own experience as a child with epilepsy Tony Greig, an English cricket player, notes:

> Maybe I was a foolhardy, a stubborn martyr. But I was lucky. I came to no harm by carrying on just the way I had always done. I never had an attack while on a bike, I never passed out while swimming, and gradually my family realized that they would take half my life away if they insisted on chaining me with safety regulations. So they let me do things my way, possibly reluctantly, possibly fearfully—but, thankfully, without disastrous consequences. (quoted in Scambler & Hopkins, 1988, p. 164)

Of course, the wisdom of allowing any degree of risk is much more easily appreciated in retrospect.

The fact that disease and trauma are visited upon one with little or no hope of escaping its consequences engenders feelings of being controlled by factors outside one's own efficacy (Trieschmann, 1989; Burish & Bradley, 1983). The loss of function accompanied by necessary dependence on medical personnel and on family or friends can exacerbate such feelings. The patient role itself may contribute to a decreased sense of personal causation (Goffman, 1961). As persons are hospitalized and lose responsibility for their daily occupations, they may come to doubt whether they can manage their own lives. Persons confronted with the sudden and overwhelming experience of a disease and subsequent treatment may feel suddenly and violently out of control:

> The patient feels he has lost power, direction, and goals—behaviors that characterize the mature adult in his interactions with others. Rather than feeling that he is in the center of activity, he

feels pushed to the periphery. He becomes an outsider dependent upon the ministrations of others. These feelings of isolated dependency and depression persist throughout the acute stages of illness and into the period of convalescence and rehabilitation. (Delaney-Naumoff, 1980, p. 87)

Concerns and fears about future success and failure also arise since the course and consequences of many conditions are uncertain or variable. Or, if the interruption of function is acute and drastic it may be difficult or impossible for individuals to imagine any possibility for success in the future.

The person with chronic progressive disease must achieve a fine balance between necessary hope for the future and unrealistic expectations. There is often little tangible information from experience or medical knowledge that can assure the individual of what the future may hold. Thus, it is important for the person to develop a belief in ability to cope with functional losses and suffering, to problem solve, and to negotiate with others over management of necessary life tasks (Burish & Bradley, 1983).

Realization that one cannot control factors in life is a reality for many persons with disability that can reach into the recesses of the most simple and intimate aspects of daily life. In this regard, Hull (1990) gives a poignant description of how something as basic as perception cannot be entirely controlled when one is blind:

While the world which greets me in this way is active, I am passive. I cannot stop these stimulations flooding me. I just sit here. The creatures emitting the noise have to engage in some activity. They have to scrape, bang, hit, club, strike surface upon surface, impact, make their vocal cords vibrate. They must take the initiative in announcing their presence to me. For my part, I have no power to explore them. I cannot penetrate them or discover them without their active cooperation. (p. 83)

Such constant reminders of one's inability to control self or the external world can result in feelings of powerlessness which sap energy, motivation, and hope. Supreme effort may be necessary to fight against the sense of power-lessness and maintain a focus on what one can control in the face of significant impairment (Murphy, 1987; Miller & Oertel, 1983).

A concomitant of many forms of mental illness is a feeling of inefficacy or helplessness (Test & Stein, 1978). Persons with mental illness often display a lowered confidence in their abilities to control life outcomes, a readiness to expect failure, and a generalized sense of being ineffective (Boskind-Lodahl, 1976; Coehlo, Silber, & Hamburg, 1971; Freedman, Donahoe, Rosenthal, & Schlundt, 1978; Hauser, 1976; Lovejoy, 1982; Manaster, 1977; Rosenberg, 1965; Strickland, 1978; Wylie, 1979; Youkilis & Bootzin, 1979). There is some evidence that the extent of psychosocial disturbance is associated with the degree of feeling ineffective (Cash & Stack, 1973; Cromwell, Rosenthal, Shakow, & Zahn, 1961; Duke & Mullens, 1973; Harrow & Ferrante, 1969; Smith, Pryer, & Distefano, 1971). Some forms of mental illness (e.g., borderline disorder) are characterized by a pervasive or periodic sense of helplessness, dependency, pessimism, and defeat (American Psychiatric Association, 1980; Gunderson & Singer, 1975; Kernberg, 1975; Meissner, 1982). Thus, it appears that feelings of inefficacy may be part of the basic dynamics of at least some forms of mental illness.

Feelings of depression may occur in persons with a wide range of disabilities. Such feelings are typically associated with the belief that one lacks control to successfully master the environment (Abramowitz, 1969; Becker & Lesiak, 1977; Dweck, 1975; Dweck & Reppucci, 1973; Lefcourt, 1976; Leggett & Archer, 1979). This feeling of depression is aptly described in the following statements of two women experiencing functional limitations imposed by repetitive strain injury:

"Quite a few times I thought I just wanted to die, that I have nothing to live for. You see, I've always been able to cope and do everything I wanted to do."

"I got to the stage where you felt that you weren't worth anything, you were good for nothing. You couldn't do anything. What's the good of me? I can't do anything." (Ewan, Lowy, & Reid, 1991, p. 184)

An extreme sense of inefficacy may extinguish any internal desire for accomplishment (Fast, 1975). Feelings of inefficacy can be behaviorally manifest as passivity or difficulty identifying goals.

Such extreme feelings of inefficacy are typified by a former client of mine. Larry had cerebral palsy and mental retardation. He lived with three other men in a single room in a residential facility. Larry was chronically bored, listless, and overtly depressed. He felt that his life was going nowhere and often reported feeling like he was "going crazy." Larry felt that his life was completely out of control. He had an extreme dislike of his living situation but saw no way of changing it. He complained about his lack of privacy and the long-standing problem of having his few resources stolen by his roommates. He lacked money to finance activities he wanted to do. He hesitated to go into the community because he feared the whispers, glances, and uncomfortable giggles that inevitably occurred. So he withdrew into passiveness and inactivity, feeling increasingly anxious and depressed, but also unable to do anything to change his situation, which he viewed as hopeless. Larry represented the extreme in feelings of inefficacy. Most importantly these feelings, reinforced by everyday experience, imprisoned Larry in a life which he could barely tolerate.

While my discussion so far has emphasized the problems of persons who feel too little control in their lives, feelings of control should not be thought of as a simple continuum in which more is better and less is worse. Persons who have very strong convictions that they can influence life outcomes are not necessarily more adaptive. For example, persons may accept too much responsibility for outcomes in their lives leading them to be overly rigid and inflexible in a constant quest for control and/or tending toward too much of a self-critical attitude (Phillips, 1980).

On the other hand, persons may need to realistically recognize that they do not have control over a variety of circumstances. For example, persons with mental retardation sometimes exhibit a very strong tendency toward feeling that others, and not they, control their lives (Gruen, Ottinger, & Ollendick,

1974; Shipe, 1971). Such a view reflects these individuals' awareness of their limitations, it can motivate an adaptive strategy of finding others more powerful to recruit as allies and benefactors.

For persons with disabilities, the challenge of maintaining appropriate feelings of efficacy is complex and difficult. By definition, most persons with significant impairments will require more external assistance than average persons. They must, in part, depend on others or on something outside themselves to accomplish what most persons do alone. It is difficult not to be constantly reminded of this reality and to have it overtake one's total view of self-efficacy. In addition, many persons must accept that they cannot control their disability and its underlying causes. Persons may have to come to grips with the fact their disability is progressive (and perhaps part of a terminal disease).

Ruth Sienkiewicz-Mercer, who has cerebral palsy, describes her own struggle with feelings of efficacy:

Despite my unavoidable dependency on others for physical assistance, I am a very independent person in thought and spirit. I have always striven to be as self-reliant as possible. For this reason, I had hoped to master feeding myself, at least partially. But disheartened as I was by my failures at this and at standing, there was one other area in which I retained high hopes . . . something that was infinitely more important to me than anything else—talking. (Sienkiewicz-Mercer & Kaplan, 1989, p.12)

While she had to go on to deal with not being able to speak, she found her voice in the autobiography, *I Raise My Eyes To Say Yes*.

The search for efficacy by persons with severe disability involves knowing disappointment, realizing what one cannot control, and finding and emphasizing what one is able to influence. As Diane, a woman who has quadrilateral congenital amputation, puts it:

I'm dependent on Jim basically, but most women are dependent on their husbands. Even in a convalescent home, I was still independent. I didn't need a lot of help from the nurses. But I am dependent on the government, financially, for what I can get and can't get. So there's a fine line between the two. (Frank, 1984, p. 644)

Summary

Personal causation is always a complicated picture of the self as actor in the world. When one experiences a disability the picture can become harder to construct and accept. It is extremely difficult to know what one's ongoing capacities will be in the face of progressive or changing diseases. Moreover, knowing one's loss or lack of capacity can be very painful to bear. Inaccurate appraisals or expectations of one's ability may nurture hope. On the other hand, when one feels that one lacks efficacy, one is more likely to be depressed and to focus on avoiding failure. By doing so one may unwittingly make choices that eliminate opportunities to develop new skills. Hence, feelings of inefficacy can lie at the core of a cycle of dysfunction in which persons already impaired are disadvantaged further by avoiding the very circumstances in which they might find their way toward a sense of efficacy. Instead, they may remain locked into a cycle of feeling and acting ineffective. Knowledge, feeling, and expectation can interweave in complex ways when one is coming to grips with a loss or absence of capacity.

Values

Values commit us to a way of life and impart commonsense meaning to the lives we lead. We are experientially, emotionally, and cognitively located in a coherent world view that gives significance to our occupations and cements our commitment to a way of life of which they are a part. Not surprisingly then, the interface of disability and value is complex and multifaceted. Some disability may have its origins, in part, in a failure of values. Values may conflict with what one is able to do and may conspire with the limitations imposed by disability to lead one toward self-devaluation. Experiencing a disability may challenge the view of the world in which our values are embedded. Finally, values may define how we experience a disability when it comes into our lives.

Origins of Disability in Values

Values are attached to our view of the future, a future toward which we are heading and to which we are willing to commit ourselves. However, persons with mental illness sometimes experience the future as distant, hopeless, or menacing (Gorman & Wessman, 1977). Adolescents identified as mentally ill sometimes appear to have little sense of themselves in the future and lack sense of the values toward which they are willing to strive (Braley & Freed, 1971; Brandt & Johnson, 1955; Cook, 1979; Offer, Ostrov, & Howard, 1981). Without a sense of value toward which one is striving, persons may question the worth of life and or find themselves alienated and without a sense of purpose (Frankl, 1978; Korner, 1970; Menninger, 1962; Mitchell, 1975; Schiamberg, 1973). A life devoid of value is the prelude to some forms of mental illness (Frankl, 1978; Strickland, 1978).

Values may be dysfunctional when they commit one to impossible ideals or to a rigid set of moral standards (Fein, 1990). Such values can result in chronic disappointment with life and/or an ongoing sense of failure when one is unable to live up to them. An example of such a problem with values is Mike, a patient I met nearly a decade ago, a man in his late 20s who was in the midst of his fourth psychiatric hospitalization. Throughout his adolescence and young adulthood Mike accepted his parents' vision that he would follow in the footsteps of his father, a successful surgeon. Upon entering a prestigious private college, Mike found the coursework overwhelming, failed his classes, became withdrawn and inactive, and finally required hospitalization for depression. Following this episode he "took a break from academics" and worked in a blue-collar position which he enjoyed. However, plagued with the idea that he was not living up to his own and his parents' ideal, he returned to college only to experience the same pattern of failure, depression, and hospitalization. Twice more he repeated the cycle of working, feeling inadequate, returning to college (each time to less prestigious and less demanding colleges) failing and needing rehospitalization. Only after these repeated failures was he able to admit that becoming a doctor was not consistent with his abilities or his interests.

Like Mike, individuals may strive after a rigid set of values in the belief that their lives will not be fulfilled or that they will not have worth unless they somehow realize those values. In such instances, values do not serve as guides for making appropriate occupational choices toward a meaningful life. Rather, they haunt and drive individuals toward choices that make life difficult to bear.

Values may also be problematic for persons exposed to subcultures which emphasize world views in conflict with that of mainstream culture. For example, it has been proposed that mentally retarded individuals may hold views and values about time that differ from mainstream society due to their unique life experiences and circumstances (Heshusius, 1981; Kavanagh, 1982; Kielhofner, 1979; Roos & Albers, 1965). As a result, they do not see the sense of striving toward goals, making appointments, and other time-related practices which characterize competence in mainstream culture. Similarly, juvenile delinquents may behave as they do because they have been socialized into a pattern of subterranean values (i.e., a premium on excitement and risk, disdain for work, and idealization of machismo) (Cavan & Cavan, 1968; Hudak, Andre, & Allen, 1980; Serok & Blum, 1979). Values which differ from mainstream culture are not inherently problematic. However, when they lead individuals to engage in behaviors which violates others' rights, which are self-destructive, or which break the law, they can be a source of occupational dysfunction.

Conflicts Between Values and Capacity

Persons with disabilities often find that their very condition is in conflict with mainstream values. As Murphy (1987) notes:

> The disabled, individually and as a group, contravene all the values of youth, virility, activity, and physical beauty that Americans cherish, however little most individuals may realize them. Most handicapped people, myself included, sense that others resent them for this reason: We are subverters of an American Ideal . . . And to the extent that we depart from the ideal, we become ugly and repulsive to the able-bodied. (p. 116–117)

In similar fashion, DeLoach, Wilkins, and Walker (1983) note that the American work ethic has "tended to discredit anyone who does not or cannot work" (p. 14). Indeed, persons with acquired disabilities may find themselves in the position of being devalued by the very values which they themselves have held all their lives.

Inasmuch as disability imposes a discontinuity between what one can do and what one values or believes one should do, it can result in a lowered self-esteem or in painful alienation from values (Zane & Lowenthal, 1960). This may be especially true for persons whose previous occupations included substantial physical ability. Physical impairment can impose a wide chasm between a previously valued self and a vastly altered self lacking the capacities that were so valued. Thus, loss of capacity can mean either rejecting old values or devaluing a self unable to live up to old values (Rabinowitz & Mitsos, 1964).

The future as one imagined it may be partially or totally invalidated by disability. Without a sense of who or what one is becoming, one may be unable to find reasons for struggling with the extra taxing problems imposed by disability (Litman, 1972; Rogers & Figone, 1978, 1979).

Disability can radically alter one's circumstances. It can challenge the whole view of life in which one's values are embedded. Consider, for example, persons who have made sense of their hard work as a means to a valued promotion and career development. After diagnosis of some progressive disease, they are no longer able to view their work in the same way since prospects of promotion are now irrelevant. The whole work ethic and the ideal of the progressive work career that they had taken for granted as a fact of life would be no longer tenable as a world view or a working plan for how to live their lives.

Values and Choice

Because it often makes doing many of the things one used to do impossible, a disability forces one to make occupational choices that affect one's lifestyle. Such choices require that persons examine what is most important to them. For example, Roberts (1989) recalls of his own experience:

> One of my therapists insisted that I learn to feed myself. Meals took hours, and I was always exhausted. After, I realized then that I could either use my time to feed myself or have an attendant feed me, allowing me to spend the time saved to go to school. I went to school. (p. 234)

Another example is Melanie, a patient I recall who had arthritis. She was the spouse of a successful businessman, routinely entertained her husband's business associates in their home, and highly valued her ability as a gourmet cook and expert hostess. However, she found that her routine of shopping for produce, preparing a complex meal, dressing, and decorating the home for guests was no longer feasible: her pain was so great by the time guests arrived that she could not enjoy the evening. Though she valued all components of the routine, she had to make difficult choices as to which aspects could be dropped or modified. She chose to have meals catered so that she would have the energy and relative freedom from pain to be a good hostess.

As both these examples illustrate, persons with disabilities are often forced to give up things they value. It becomes important not to hang on to values that cannot be realized. For example, persons with physical or emotional disabilities who experience exacerbations, whose illness is progressive, or who must depend on some forms of assistance for everyday function, can find oppressive values which stress "competition, individual achievement, independence, and self-sufficiency" (Deegan, 1991, p. 52). Indeed, because the disability experience may radically alter one's existence, it can become a source of rethinking one's values and one's fundamental view of life. Wright (1960) argues that, in order to adjust to disability, persons may need to enlarge the scope of their values to incorporate behaviors for which they are still capable. In addition, persons may need to learn new values which judge their performance given their capacities and reject old values that compare one's performance to that of others without disabilities. Such value changes make possible the occupa-

tional choices which persons need to make in order to go on with life.

Values as Definers of Disability

Values are an essential part of a person's view of life. When an individual experiences a disability, it is an event that occurs within a cultural view and way of life which that person inhabits. Moreover, the values that are a part of that world view will influence how persons experience and react to the disability. An example of how cultural values can define the experience of disability is that "people from cultures placing high valuation on physical or sexual prowess are more devastated by . . . disability than those whose traditions stress, say, scholarly pursuits" (Vash, 1981, p. 15). Values also influence the person's view of what should be done in the face of a disability. As Trieschmann (1989) notes:

> A man who belongs to a certain culture in which women are expected to take care of "incapacitated" individuals . . . may not see the necessity of learning . . . [self-care] activities because they are "woman's work." (p. 132)

Such situations can produce genuine dilemmas for therapists since the patient's or client's view of the world and dominant values can conflict directly with what the therapist believes is important or with the stated goals of a program.

Summary

Though circumstances may vary, values are always intertwined with the experience of disability. Values may simultaneously define and contribute to dysfunction in occupational life. They may lead one to make poor occupational choices; they may conflict with one's capacities and extol an impossible ideal. On the other hand, values may be a resource for coming to grips with a disability. After all, it is through values that we decide upon what is worth doing, what one should strive toward, and what kind of life is worth living. Since impairments typically invalidate some aspect of the taken-for-granted cultural responses to these questions, adjusting to disability almost invariably means embarking on an individual quest for new ways of viewing and valuing one's life.

Interests

While it is sometimes commonly overlooked, one of the most pervasive effects of disability on occupation is its influence on the experience of satisfaction and pleasure in life. The daily pleasures, comforts, and enjoyments that enliven our existence and help maintain our energy and mood become all the more important in the face of suffering that regularly accompanies any form of disability. At the same time, interests can be threatened or altered by disability.

Attraction to Occupations

Attraction is closely tied to positive experiences which emanate from exercise of capacity, sensory pleasure, and appeal to one's aesthetic sense. Children with disabilities may be at risk to fail to develop normal investment and satisfaction in occupational performance. When disability limits the range of experiences children have, they may simply not be exposed to normal opportunities to develop interests. Further, difficulties with performance and fear of being recognized as incompetent may lead a child to avoid opportunities to feel satisfaction and to develop a sense of attraction to occupations.

Physical impairments and attendant fatigue, pain, and preoccupation with failure may reduce or eliminate the feeling of pleasure in occupations. Adaptations may negatively affect the ambience and spirit of activities, making it difficult for a person to experience the same sense of satisfaction as before. Many persons with acquired disabilities describe that it is no longer worth engaging in old pastimes because they are simply no longer enjoyable, because they are not worth the additional effort required, or because necessary adaptations alter the quality of the performance that made it attractive in the first place.

Further, persons may simply be prevented by limitations of capacity from participating in activities they enjoy (Rogers & Figone, 1978; Trieschmann, 1989; Vash, 1981). For example,

persons may have to give up activities involving excessive physical stress or requiring lost sensory, perceptual or cognitive abilities. When one acquires a disability, the future may seem a bland and undesirable existence without the enjoyment and satisfaction that existed in the past.

Some psychiatric illnesses involve a loss of attraction to activities. For example, depressed persons frequently indicate few current interests, even when their past interests may have been substantial (Neville, 1987). Many depressed persons speak about losing their enthusiasm for former interests and describe that they no longer enjoy doing things that were previously fun. Supporting such individual reports, research reveals that increases in depressed mood and decreases in enjoyment in activities go hand in hand (Hammen & Glas, 1975; Lewinsohn, 1975; Lewinsohn & Graf, 1973; MacPhilany & Lewinsohn, 1974; Neville, 1987; Turner, Ward, & Turner, 1979).

While some persons with mental illness experience a short-term inability to find interest in activities, others have a history of never having been able to identify and enact interests. A failure to develop real interest and investment in the world may be part of the complex of factors that contribute to dysfunction. For example, research suggests that persons with psychiatric problems chronically express and engage in few interests (Grob & Singer, 1974; Spivak, Siegel, Sklaver, Deuschle, & Garrett, 1982). Typical of many psychiatric patients' experience is Jill, a 30-year-old single woman who has nearly completed a degree in philosophy with a straight A average, but has been hospitalized with severe suicidal ideation during each of several attempts to complete her last semester. Jill cooks and makes jewelry on an expert level but derives almost no pleasure from these activities, seeing them mainly as exercises for reducing anxiety.

Other research has found that persons with alcoholism are less likely to pursue their stated interests (Scaffa, 1982). In cases of substance abuse, it appears to be the case that the pleasure of interest is replaced by the pleasure induced by substances, or that persons feel they cannot enjoy themselves without the assistance of drugs or alcohol. In either case, the direct attraction to, and pleasure in, occupations is eroded.

In discussing how persons with spinal cord injury may experience changes in interests, Trieschmann (1989) notes:

> Reduced access to satisfying activity can certainly lower mood, which tends to lower a person's interest in activity, which further lowers mood. Thus, a vicious circle evolves. (p. 242)

Her argument is supported by the finding that when persons increase their activities, their mood improves as well (Turner, Ward, & Turner, 1979). Thus, it appears that the reduction in interest and attraction associated with many forms of disability may reflect a complex process in which decreased feelings of attraction, decreases in activity, and depressed mood interrelate in a downward spiral.

Consequently, loss of attraction to occupations may signal more than forfeiture of some previous interests. Rather, interests represent a great deal of one's investment and enthusiasm for life, and a dwindling of interest may signal a much more serious waning of a positive orientation toward life in general. Energy to put forth the effort that daily life requires emanates in part, from our interests. When attraction to occupations wanes or is disturbed, both activity choices that lead us to seek out and experience quality of life and occupational choices that involve commitment to one's lifestyle, can be compromised.

Problems Related to Preference

Persons are differentially attracted to occupations and their preferences for types of activities over others are deeply embedded in their innate differences and experiences within their culture. What a person is interested in is a powerful influence on what he or she will feel like doing. Interest pervades our choices.

Persons may develop preferences which lead to problematic activity choices. For example, there is evidence to suggest that some adolescents with psychosocial difficulties may be attracted to socially unacceptable interests (Lambert, Rothschild, Atland, & Green, 1978; Werthman, 1976) leading them to make activity and occupational choices that get them

into trouble. As another example, adults with mental retardation tend to have mainly solitary and sedentary interests (Cheseldine & Jeffree, 1981; Coyne, 1980; Katz & Yekutiel, 1974; Matthews, 1980; Mitic & Stevenson, 1981) that may reflect restricted experience, opportunities, and resources (Cheseldine & Jeffree, 1981; Coyne, 1980; Matthews, 1980; Katz & Yekutiel, 1974). These interests lead to activity choices that restrict the range and quality of occupational behavior.

One particularly fascinating finding comes from a prospective study of over 3000 aircraft workers where persons who stated that they "hardly ever" enjoyed their job tasks were two and a half times more likely to report a back injury than subjects who "almost always" enjoyed their job tasks (Bigos et al., 1991). The implication of such a study is that there may be among those persons who have work injury and disability a disproportionate number of people who do not find their work interesting. Many persons with disabilities lack access to satisfying jobs. While there is some reason to suspect that many workers today may feel disaffected from their work (Kielhofner, 1993), this may be particularly true when one has a disability. For example, Alice, who has a psychiatric disability, notes:

> I hate my job. I just hate it. It takes the mind of a seven-year-old to work there. It's boring. My supervisor is like a slave driver. I tried so many Civil Service jobs you wouldn't believe it. Sometimes two to three job interviews a week. But no one would hire me. No one. They never did tell me why. I bet I'll be stuck at Goodwill forever... (Estroff, 1981, p. 136)

Since work is a fact of life for so many adults, the degree of interest persons find in their work is no small issue.

When one acquires a disability one may simply be unable to do what one previously most enjoyed. For example, certain interest patterns such as enjoyment of physically demanding and exciting activities, make one more likely to have a disabling accident (Vash, 1981). When persons with such interests incur disability they lose the capacities that they most enjoyed exercising. Moreover, individuals may be less disposed to enjoy the exercise of remaining interpersonal and intellectual capacities. Thus, one of the challenges presented by disability is often to find new preferences for activities or new avenues for channeling one's preferences. One of my earliest patient encounters was a young man who had great promise as a swimmer and a diver. He had won regional and national championships and was an Olympic hopeful. He broke his neck in a diving accident and was rendered a high-level quadriplegic. Fortunately, he discovered that he was also a talented writer and speaker and was able to channel his interest in sports toward the field of sports journalism. For a range of reasons, others do not so easily redirect their interests. Another patient I knew at the same time was a young woman who was an accomplished dancer in a nationally famous dance troupe. Following her spinal cord injury, she became despondent over her loss of ability and her changed body image. She slowly slipped into chronic substance abuse.

The onset of disability does not change the fact that we all must have some things in our lives that we enjoy, that absorb our attention, and invite use of our capacities. Sacks (1985) provides a poignant example of the importance of interests in the case of a man without short-term memory:

> He would become keenly and briefly involved in games, but soon they ceased to offer any challenge: he solved all the puzzles, and could solve them easily; and he was far better and sharper than anyone else at games. And as he found this out, he grew fretful and restless again, and wandered the corridors, uneasy and bored and with a sense of indignity—games and puzzles were for children, a diversion. Clearly, passionately, he wanted something to do: he wanted to do, to be, to feel . . . (p. 35)

Though not always as pronounced, many persons face the same struggle to locate interests which can truly energize and fulfill them. Instead, many remain unfulfilled and unsatisfied. Jack, who is psychiatrically disabled, represents the kind of "limbo" some people with disability inhabit when they are not able to establish nor be guided by interests:

> I don't have any drive. There's nothing I really feel like working for. I guess I wouldn't mind

being a song writer. But I never wrote anything worthwhile. No, I'd like to be an architect. I'd like to design bizarre houses. I'll never do it, because I'd lose interest. I'd like to do something with my life, but what I don't know. (Estroff, 1981, p. 142)

When persons have not developed interests sufficiently, when their interests lead them toward problematic behaviors, or when they can no longer pursue their interests, they are challenged to build or rebuild their interests. Without interest life can become bleak and unattractive. How interests can infuse life with meaning and energy is aptly summarized in a story told by Christi Brown in his autobiography, *My Left Foot*. Brown, who was severely disabled with cerebral palsy, explains that as a ten-year-old boy he had become depressed and despondent over his differentness from others. He explains:

> I was now ten and a half and beginning to sink deeper and deeper into myself . . . Then, one Christmas, one of us—I think it was Paddy—got a box of paints from Santa Claus. That same year I got a box of toy soldiers, but the moment I saw Paddy's paints with all the wonderful colors and the long, slender, fuzzy-haired brush I fell in love with them at once. I felt I must have them to keep as my own. I was fascinated by the little solid blocks of paint—blue, red, yellow, green, and white. Later in the day I sat and watched Paddy as he tried to make some impression with the paints on a piece of white cardboard torn from an old shoe box, but he only made a mess and in a queer way I felt annoyed with him—and a bit jealous . . . Pushing out my box of lead soldiers towards him with my foot, I asked him, in grunts to "swop" them for his paints . . . I put them away 'til all the excitement of Christmas was past. Then one quiet afternoon when there was nobody in the kitchen but mother and myself, I crawled over to the press, opened the door with my foot and took the little black box of paints out and laid it on the floor in front of me.
>
> "What are you up to?" said mother, coming over to where I squatted with my back against the wall, "Surely you're not trying to paint!"
>
> I nodded very solemnly. I picked up the brush between my toes, wetted it in my mouth, then rubbed it on one of the paint squares—the bright blue one which I liked best. I next rubbed the brush against my other foot—and saw a blue spot on it when I took it away.

"It works!" I managed to exclaim, and I could feel my face hot with excitement. "I'll get you water," said mother, going into the pantry and coming back with a cupful which she put on the floor beside me.

I had no paper. Mother got me some by tearing a page out of Peter's sum-copy. I dipped the brush into the water and rubbed on some vivid red paint then I steadied my foot and, while mother looked on intently, painted on the open page before me—the outline of a cross . . . After the first few weeks of uncertainty and awkwardness, I settled down contentedly with my new pastime. I painted every day upstairs in the back bedroom, completely by myself.

I was changing. I didn't know it then, but I had found a way to be happy again and to forget some of the things that had made me unhappy. Above all I learned to forget myself . . . Slowly I begin to lose my early depression. I had a feeling of pure joy while I painted, a feeling I had never experienced before which seemed almost to lift me above myself. (Brown, 1990, p. 54–57)

Summary: Volitional Aspects of Occupational Dysfunction

The impact of chronic disease on personal causation, interests, and values can lead to a breakdown of morale in the individual. When the future seems bleak with goals uncertain or obliterated, pleasure in activity diminished, and meaning and purpose in life eroded, with little or no possibility of influencing the course of one's life, it is difficult or impossible for the individual to make adaptive choices to engage in occupation. Maintaining a satisfying and productive life through positive choices is a major task for all of us, and perhaps even more so when we are challenged by a disability. The strength of past success, a belief in ability to cope with problems, intense attraction to and satisfaction from performance, and strong personal values are strengths upon which persons need to draw in order to adapt to disability.

HABITUATION

Having a disability can affect habituation in a number of ways. The presence of a disability places certain restrictions and demands on the kinds of habits and roles one may establish. The onset of disability can invalidate previous habits or roles, requiring individuals to rebuild their occupational lifestyles. Moreover, one's habits and roles can themselves be a source of disability. Whatever the nature of a disability, the overriding reality is that it is a constant companion in the routines of life. Habituation is the process whereby individuals come to practical terms with a disability and organize a life which allows them to routinely function to their own and others' satisfaction.

Roles

Roles place us in relationship to the external world of people. Faced with a disability, one can find one is barred from, has failed in, or lacks opportunities to learn or enter the occupational roles which make up life in a given culture. In addition, having a disability can not only bar one from ordinary roles, but also assign one to marginal roles. In the final analysis, overcoming a disability requires that persons "place" or "replace" themselves in the social world by occupying legitimate roles.

Role Performance Difficulties Associated with Disability

Role dysfunction may be both a consequence and cause of psychosocial dysfunction. Problems with role performance due to substance abuse, alcoholism, and other psychosocial factors are the impetus for some persons' entry into the mental health care system (Black, 1976; Mechanic, 1980). Role failure may also occur when one has not internalized appropriate role scripts and, therefore, does not meet the expectations of the social group. Role scripts are based, in part, on imagining what others are seeing, thinking, and feeling (Taylor, 1982), a process which is difficult for those with cognitive limitations (Greenspan, 1979). Persons, by virtue of having a disability, may have fewer experiences in which to acquire role scripts (Smith, 1972; Versluys, 1983). For example, retarded persons are often denied access to opportunities to learn scripts of normal adult roles (Braginski & Braginski, 1971; Dexter, 1956, 1960; Guskin, 1963; Kielhofner, 1983; Wolfensberger, 1975). In such cases, limitations of capacity are magnified by the lack of experiences which would help to organize their capacities for use in roles.

Some individuals have difficulty finding and entering roles. For example, adolescents with psychosocial disorders are frequently less involved in academic, leisure, and work roles than are their peers (Holzman & Grinker, 1974; Masterson & Washburne, 1966; Offer, Ostrov, & Howard, 1981). This lack of involvement may reflect the inability to successfully make occupational choices and it may also reflect limited opportunities or roles in the environment. Adolescent girls, in particular, seem more apt to stay home in unproductive roles if they are unemployed and no longer in school (Donovan & Oddy, 1982).

Limitations of physical capacity may disrupt or terminate role performance by robbing the individual of necessary skills for performing occupational forms belonging to a role (Werner-Beland, 1980). Depending on the performance demands of a particular role, it may be impossible for an individual with progressive disability to maintain that role. If a person is to retain a role, major modifications in the expectations for the role may be required. In other cases, persons may have to find new ways to enact roles. A person may desire to continue being a worker, but be unable to engage in the old line of work, necessitating a new occupational choice. Complicating the process of achieving a worker role is that the presence of a disability often makes it harder to find employment (Erikson, 1973; Trieschmann, 1989).

Even when a disability does not remove a person from a role, it may create problems of role performance such as being unable to discharge the role in ways consistent with one's own or others' expectations for the role. For example, persons whose impairments are not visible to others may be viewed by friends, family, or coworkers as malingering (Schiffer, Rudick, & Herndon, 1983). The result can be conflicts between others' expectations and what one can actually do in the role, further adding to role stress. In other cases the conflict may be between one's own view of the role and how one is able to perform. For example, John, who has multiple sclerosis, notes of his family roles: "I feel left out of discipline over the children because I am static in an armchair and cannot even phone the school. I had lost the ability to be a real father and husband" (Robinson, 1988, p. 60). Hull (1990) similarly describes how being blind has robbed him of the ability to supervise and to participate in play with his children, eroding and constricting what kind of father he can be.

Disability may force changes in the responsibilities one assumes within roles. For example, the cord-injured person who previously was a head of a family may become the most physically dependent member of the family. Such shifts in the identity and function of ongoing roles can be sources of conflict and self-devaluation. For example, men who were accustomed to the status of being the wage earner in a family may feel a loss of worth when their wives replace them as the sole or major source of income.

Role strain may occur when a person cannot meet the multiple obligations or aspirations represented in several roles (Goode, 1960; Beutell & Greenhaus, 1983; Coser, 1974; Gerson, 1976; Gray; 1972). Role strain may arise because persons have made occupational choices to enter roles which make conflicting demands for how one should behave. Impairments may mean that persons must exert more time and energy toward maintaining such major life roles as work or homemaking, requiring them to relinquish other roles.

Consequences of Role Loss and Rolelessness

Research suggests that involvement in too few roles is even more likely to be detrimental to psychosocial well-being than having too many role demands (Marks, 1977; Seiber, 1974; Spreitzer, Snyder, & Larson, 1979). Without sufficient roles one lacks identity, purpose, and structure in everyday life.

The loss of the worker role and chronic work role problems are especially implicated in psychosocial dysfunction. Many consequences of unemployment have been suggested such as suicide, depression, stress-related physical health problems, child abuse, and increased substance abuse (Borrero, 1980; Briar, 1980). A concomitant of unemployment is the disorganization of daily routine. Unemployment means the loss of not only money and status, but also one's major form of daily activity. Work structures time. One gets up to go to work, spends significant portions of one's time in work, plans weekends and vacations around work, and develops long-term career timetables. Without work, many people find themselves unable to sleep or eat, and feeling aimless and restless (Borrero, 1980).

Women are particularly vulnerable to depression from role loss, especially in middle age (Freden, 1982). As children grow up and leave home, and as parents die, both the mother and daughter roles are suspended. Because many older women currently do not work, they lack other roles to substitute for this loss. The interaction of cultural values complicates the meaning of this loss, since Western society has traditionally valued the roles of wife and mother for women. Although these cultural standards are changing, the implication is that it is critical to occupy more than one meaningful role, so that if one role is lost, there are other roles from which to derive satisfaction (Freden, 1982). A loss of identity and self-esteem may occur as persons take on roles they believe to be less important or as they lose roles (Thomas, 1966; Werner-Beland, 1980). For example, Krefting (1989) notes:

> Most head-injured people remember parts of their old selves and recognize that the old self is gone. But they have nothing upon which to build a new self-identity. This is largely a result of lack of opportunity to fill legitimate roles in society. If an individual's personhood is not acknowledged by others, it is difficult for him or her to develop a sense of self-identity. (p. 76)

What Krefting notes is echoed throughout accounts that persons with disabilities have given of themselves. There is a substantial cost to personal identity when persons no longer are recognized as the fathers, mothers, spouses, students, workers, caretakers, or friends that they used to be or want to be.

Sick, Invalid, and Impaired Roles

A number of writers have argued that disability may not only remove or bar one from occupational roles, but also relegate one to sick and deviant roles (Bogdan & Taylor, 1989; Parsons, 1953; Werner-Beland, 1980). When a person is ill, the normal social expectations for the worker role are typically suspended. Instead, one enters the sick role and is expected to conform to the administrations and advice of medical personnel in order to get well. The sick role can be a source of problems for a person with a long-term illness or disability. For example, the sick role implies passivity and compliance (Parsons, 1953) which can be counterproductive to individuals assuming responsibility for their lives and re-entering occupational roles. A case in point is Bill, a patient I met when he was recovering from cancer. Bill was diagnosed with sarcoma, which required him to leave his job as a mechanic in order to undergo a regimen of surgery and chemotherapy with slow recovery over a period of three years. During the years of his battle with cancer Bill became accustomed to others shaping the fate and course of his life. The sick role dominated his life. His identity as a cancer patient overshadowed other aspects of his identity. His interactions with professionals, families, and friends all centered on his patienthood and his battle with a potentially fatal disease. His daily routine was dominated by the patient role even to the point of total isolation in a protected environment, necessitated by the chemotherapy that had compromised his immune system. At the end of three years, Bill, who had received a prosthetic mandible (the site of his sarcoma), was left with an able body, but found it overwhelming to consider re-entry into the work role. He described himself as stuck. He tended to look to others to provide direction and initiative, as he had become unaccustomed to making his own occupational and even activity choices.

When persons sustain such behavior beyond the course of illness the role evolves into an invalid or disabled role (Werner-Beland, 1980). Often the reactions of strangers, family, and friends can serve to reinforce this invalid or disabled role. For example, others may unnecessarily lower their expectations of the person with a disability. They may become overly protective or helpful, or consider the person to be disabled beyond his or her actual limitations. Zola illustrates in the following passage how the experience of becoming a wheelchair user transformed his social interactions:

> As soon as I sat in the wheelchair I was no longer seen as a person who could fend for himself. Although Metz has known me well for nine months, and had never before done anything physical for me without asking, now he took over without permission. Suddenly, in his eyes, I was no longer able to carry things, reach for objects, or even push myself around. Though I was perfectly capable of doing all these things, I was being wheeled around, and things were being brought to me—all without my asking. Most frightening was my own compliance, my alienation from myself and from the process. (Zola, 1982, p. 52)

As he suggests, the identity of being disabled can, of itself, trigger new expectations and behaviors. This dramatic transformation validated the sensibleness of Zola's earlier attempts to avoid being cast into the role of a disabled person:

> I had separated myself early from the physically handicapped by refusing to attend a special residential school. Later, I had simply never socialized with anyone who had a chronic disease or physical handicap. I too had been seeking to gain a different identity through my associations. (Zola, 1982, p. 75)

For children with disabilities the presence of an impaired role may restrict opportunities to explore, learn, and occupy other roles. Persons with disabilities from early in life (e.g., persons with congenital physical dysfunction or mental retardation) may also lack the experiences of normal role transitions. Such persons may be chronically frustrated as they are unable to attain a series of roles seen as highly desirable (Kielhofner, 1979, 1981).

Habits

When persons' routines fail them, their habits are sources of occupational dysfunction. Moreover, disability can place a special burden on one's everyday habits. Whole routines of living and ways of performing can be eliminated or devastated by loss of capacity.

Habits are also rich resources for overcoming the limits imposed by disabilities. Since habits regulate the routine interface between persons and their environment they can be the most natural of "prostheses," allowing one to continue to traverse the terrain of everyday life.

Dysfunctional Habit Maps

Habits themselves can be dysfunctional when they constrain effective occupational performance. Habit disorganization may manifest itself as habit patterns that are too rigid and hence do not allow for changes in routine; as habits that lack enough consistency; and as habits that do not meet the needs of the environment or the individual (Kielhofner, Barris, & Watts, 1982). For example, consistently arriving late for work is a habit that does not meet either social requirements or the needs of a person who wants to maintain a job.

The habits of individuals with psychosocial dysfunction may include difficulty organizing oneself for work, dressing to meet the demands of different social situations, and maintaining a routine of life that is satisfying. In some cases, the breakdown of habits may be precipitated by affective or cognitive disturbances. In other cases dysfunctional habits may contribute to psychosocial disorder. In either case, habits serve to sustain an overall state of dysfunction. Individuals with dysfunctional habits may find that their routines are dissatisfying, contradict their own values, and prevent them from living up to their own or others' goals.

Consider, for example, the breakdown of habits that may occur in association with depression. Time passes slowly for the depressed person (Melges, 1982), even normal routines may seem inordinately long. What had been automatic routines may now require constant effort to maintain since one feels lethargic and unmotivated (American Psychiatric Association, 1980). Eventually, the weight of depression may lead one to disregard routines rather than expend the energy. As these habits erode they begin to affect roles. For example, one neglects grooming and goes to work or school disheveled. Peers and coworkers are uncomfortable and avoid association leading one to feel further isolated and withdrawn. Sleeping habits are disrupted, and one is unable to rise on time for work or concentrate at work. One goes home exhausted and leaves behind old leisure and home care habits opting instead to stare at television. One feels worse. Life is out of control. Nothing is getting done. In such a scenario as this, habits and moods go hand in hand. They wear each other down and co-contribute to the downward spiral of occupational dysfunction.

Now consider a very different set of circumstances in which habits are challenged by disability. As the child with a disability develops, he or she may experience restrictions that affect habit patterns. Expanded time for self-care, mobility, periods of therapy time, and so on may leave less time for free play and for social interaction. A child with a disability may experience a different press from the physical environment which may result in a less flexible habit pattern. Indeed such a child may become dependent on a very rigid habit structure to feel in control.

Disruption of Habits

Habits build upon and organize one's capacities for performance in one's environment. When persons' capacities are diminished or eliminated, previously established habits can become ineffective. In some cases, entire routines of living may become so invalidated that one may be forced to develop anew habits for everyday life. For example, getting bathed and dressed in the morning after a disability is not only a matter of having lost performance capacities, but also of the loss of viable everyday routines. Describing his experience of trying to complete his morning routine from the new viewpoint of a wheelchair, Zola captures some of the subtle, but consequential invalidation of routine procedures which can take place:

Washing up was a mess. Though the sink was low enough, I nevertheless managed to soak myself thoroughly. In retrospect, I should not have worn anything. Ordinarily when washing my face, chest, and arms, I would lean over the sink, and any excess water from my splashing would drip into it. My body angle in a wheelchair was different. I could not extend over the sink very far without tipping. Thus, much of the water dripped down my neck onto me. Splashing with water was out, and the use of a damp washcloth, what I once called a "sponge bath," was in. (Zola, 1982, p. 64)

Of course, a disability can affect one's habits in other ways as well. New habits related to the need to accommodate to or manage the disability are often required (e.g., bowel and bladder care, joint protection, energy conservation needs, requirements for rest). Habits can be disturbed not only by the loss of skills, but also by the inactivity imposed by disability and hospitalization. When habits are not practiced they degenerate. Moreover, the learning of new habits may also be impeded if opportunities for practicing them are not provided during rehabilitation (Shillam, Beeman, & Loshin, 1983).

Remissions and exacerbations or progressive decreases in physical functioning make organization of habits extremely difficult. Because their physical abilities are so variable and unpredictable, some disabled persons must be extremely flexible in their habit patterns. Moreover, persons with conditions in which impairment may vary unpredictably must be ready to capitalize on "good times." For example, a gentleman with Parkinson's disease notes:

I cram in to the periods when I'm flexible all the things I would have liked to have done the rest of the day. It doesn't always work that way though. One day I may be nine-tenths of the day free, although that's very rare, and another much less. There's nothing I can do about it. (Pinder, 1988, p. 79)

The onset of severe disability can radically alter the spatial and temporal dimensions of routine performance. For example, the cord-injured person must learn to organize behavior around the constraints of where he or she can freely go in a wheelchair and how long it will take (Paap, 1972). With the onset of a disability the entire relationship of persons with their environments may change in dramatic ways, resulting in the need for new habits. In this regard Hull (1990) notes:

On the whole, my experience has been that, if I have a bad habit, it causes me some inconvenience or inefficiency in my movement, and is naturally corrected in the effort to move freely. In other words, blindness itself imposes an iron law upon the user of the white cane. Lampposts, curbs, and stairways are the best teachers. (p. 15)

Habits of the person with a disability must often accommodate a more limited number of daily activities than in the premorbid habit structure. Temporal constraints may require decisions about what activities not to perform. Temporal constraints are further imposed by the necessity of new self-care habits. Finally, persons with a severe physical disability may have to maintain unusually flexible habits since they depend on others and are more influenced by external contingencies (e.g., bad weather, crowded public places, problems of accessibility).

As a consequence of all these factors that affect habit structure, the task of organizing daily life may become daunting. Accommodations and trade-offs must take place. Some activities may need to be eliminated from one's routine. Finally, one may have to delegate some tasks to family members or an attendant in order to have time for other more valued activities. As Williams (1984) notes:

If the disabled individual is to move toward "mere" impairment, eventually alternative ways of accomplishing the tasks of everyday life will be committed to memory and habit, engrained in relationships with a new world which is once again "had." (p. 110)

Thus, when one acquires a disability, one must alter much of the manner of accomplishing the daily things that were at once taken for granted and barely noticed. Suddenly, they become hurdles to be overcome. They demand attention and they consume new energy.

The path to new habits involves leaving behind a familiar world which has been invalidated by disability. As Merleau-Ponty (1962) notes:

I am conscious of the world through the medium of my body. It is precisely when my customary world arouses in me habitual intentions that I can no longer, if I have lost a limb, be effectively drawn into it: the utilizable objects, precisely in so far as they present themselves as utilizable, appeal to a hand I no longer have. (p. 82)

Establishing new habits is to move from the known to the unknown. Only by re-encountering the world within one's altered condition can a new experience of one's relationship to the world emerge and once again become familiar and taken for granted.

This transformation of habits following the acquisition of a physical impairment is described by DeLoach and Greer (1981) in the following way:

After the initial shock of the realization of a less-than-desirable physical state which will probably not go away, a person begins to learn new ways of doing what she did before—and ways of accomplishing, as well, some brand-new things. These new, different ways are, at first, awkward, stress-producing, and frustrating. But daily chores must be done, and some of them one enjoys doing, despite the hassle; thus, little by little, a persons gets accustomed to a new modus operandi. What at first was awkward, painful, or embarrassing becomes just a regular part of living, incorporated into one's routine. After such habituation, the person begins to concentrate more on participation in life now rather than on what used to be or what might have been. (p. 251)

MIND-BRAIN-BODY PERFORMANCE SUBSYSTEM

Disabilities typically involve disturbances to the neurological, musculoskeletal, and symbolic constituents of the mind-brain-body performance subsystem. The particular disturbances to this subsystem vary with the nature of precipitating stress, trauma, or disease. However, a common denominator is that the entire subsystem is affected as the results of impairment to one constituent resonate throughout the subsystem. Whether the primary impairment is to the central nervous system, musculoskeletal system, or in the symbolic capacities of the mind, the other constituents belong to a dynamic subsystem whose overall process is altered by the impairment. For example, in the case of children who have disabilities it is difficult, if not inaccurate, to refer to a disability as located in any one part of the mind-brain-body performance subsystem. The child's primary nervous system impairment will show its effects in the musculoskeletal constituent; the child may have fewer opportunities for play with objects and people, which may constrict the development of the symbolic constituent. Consequently, understanding the nature of impairment to the mind-brain-body performance subsystem requires that we recognize this subsystem as an integrated whole and impairments as disturbances to the organization of the whole. As noted in Chapter 6, other models of practice in occupational therapy provide a range of explanations of the disturbances to the mind-brain-body performance subsystem (e.g., the biomechanical, perceptual-cognitive, and sensory integration models).

An additional way in which we can begin to understand how impairment affects this subsystem is to consider descriptions by persons with disabilities of their experiences of having an impaired mind-brain-body performance subsystem. Consider, for example, Murphy's (1987) description of his progressive loss of muscle innervation and the changes it brought about in his body:

My right hand has followed the left by about a year or two, but it is now too weak to grip things tightly. It, too, has developed a tendency for the fingers first to curl in to form claws, then to close against the palm, but it is easier to prevent this in the right hand because it is used more. (p. 187)

This change is part of a myriad of musculoskeletal changes which result in Murphy's mind being housed in a radically altered body. The changing body dominates much of conscious, mental processes both because it demands this attention for practical reasons of continuing to function and because the once familiar and taken-for-granted body has now become changed into a source of suffering and limitations. In the end, Murphy concludes that he is a prisoner in his body.

In contrasting his experience (with blindness) to that of a friend paralyzed below the neck, Hull (1990) articulates two altered mind-brain-body experiences:

Clive's situation is the opposite to my own. I, as a blind person, tend to be enclosed within my body, to be conscious primarily of it, and to be cut off from the world. He, on the other hand, is cut off from his body. He has perfect senses, and knows just what he wants his body to do in the world, but his body will not do it. My body will do perfectly well what I want it to do in the world, but it has no world within which to do it. (p. 156)

Changes in the experience of the mind-brain-body associated with disability can also precipitate the emergence of new experiences or the modification of old ones to maintain skills. Benner (1989) gives an example of the person with an amputation who rubs the stump or activates memories of the limb in order to elicit the bodily memory of the limb (sometimes referred to as "phantom limb") in order to animate a prosthesis. Similarly, she notes how blind persons ultimately learn to perceive the pressure on the hand from the cane as the physical object being probed in the environment. The different ways in which persons with disabilities experience their bodies is underscored by Brown (1990), who had no effective use of his hands; he was repulsed by having his feet covered: "When mother put shoes or stockings on my feet I felt as any normal person might feel if his hands were tied behind his back" (p. 21).

In his autobiography, Zasetsky offers poignant insights into the experiences of an altered mind following traumatic brain injury:

At first these were the only facts I had. I tried to remember whatever I could with that battered memory of mine and write it as a true story, just as a writer would. But when I started, I realized I'd never be able to do that since I didn't have enough of a vocabulary or mind left to write well. I'd get a faint idea of how to describe the beginning of the attack I was in but couldn't remember the words I needed to do it. I'd try to dig these up from my mind but I'd spend ages hunting for the right words. I had to remember and turn up words that were are at least fairly similar or close enough to what I wanted to say. But after I'd put together these second choices, I still wasn't able to start writing until I figured out how to compose a sentence. I'd go over each sentence again and again in my mind until it seemed like a sentence I'd heard or read in an ordinary book (quoted in Luria, 1972, p. 78–79).

His struggle for words, memory, and sentences illustrates the kind of mental disorganization likely shared by some persons with brain trauma.

Persons with psychiatric illness must often contend with the extremely painful emotions and symptoms which provide impediments to being able to function. Estroff (1981) provides the example of Rod who notes:

> When I'm on the job, it gets to the point where I just can't work. Everything goes wrong. I start my dreaming, my horrible dreaming. I don't like it, and I want help being set free from it. If I am ever to hold a job I have to be set free from thoughts of spacemen, gods, superheroes, and demons. (p. 143)

Medications, which may eliminate or reduce some interfering symptoms that plague persons with disabilities, may create other problems such as impairing concentration (Estroff, 1981). Many persons on psychiatric medication complain of both mental and physical changes which are unpleasant and make them feel like they are not themselves. For example, Sacks (1985) provides the following story about a man with Tourette's syndrome:

> He had diagnosed himself as having Tourette's after reading the article on 'Tics' in the *Washington Post*. When I confirmed the diagnosis, and spoke of using Haldol, he was excited but cautious. I made a test of Haldol by injection and he proved extraordinarily sensitive to it, becoming virtually tic-free for a period of two hours after I had administered no more than one-eighth of a milligram. After this auspicious trial, I started him on Haldol, prescribing a dose of a quarter of a milligram three times a day.
> He came back, the following week, with a black eye and a broken nose and said: 'So much for your fucking Haldol.' Even this minute dose, he said, had thrown him off balance, interfered with his speed, his timing, his preternaturally quick reflexes. Like many Touretters, he was attracted to spinning things, and to revolving doors in particular, which he would dodge in and out of like lightning; he had lost his knack on the Haldol, had mistimed his movements, and had been bashed on the nose. (p. 92–93)

Similar stories can be heard from patients medicated for manic symptoms who miss part of the euphoric (albeit often dysfunctional) experience of mania.

Whatever the nature of the impairment, having a disability means having a particular mind-brain-body experience of that disability. This experience may be a source of suffering, it may mean that one experiences the world in radically different ways than persons without disabilities do. Finally, it creates special circumstances for the performance of everyday occupational forms.

OCCUPATIONAL PERFORMANCE

Occupational performance involves the interface of the mind-brain-body performance subsystem with the environment. The resulting performance skills are influenced by impairments in the constituents of the subsystem. As noted in Chapter 6, one cannot assume a direct correlation between specific impairments and the actual skill persons will demonstrate. Nonetheless, it is fair to say that performance skills are often affected by impairments of the mind-brain-body performance subsystem and that decrements in the performance skills may accompany impairments to this subsystem.

Limitations of capacity that constrain how one assembles one type of skill may affect another skill. For example, Zola explains the challenge of walking as a post-polio paraplegic:

> Socialized into the role of the courteous American male, I was at one time particularly piqued that it meant my female friend, not I, must walk on the outside. My moment-to-moment concerns are even more mundane. I must be extraordinarily watchful about where I place both my cane and my leg. If not, my cane tip will slide on a water or oil slick, or I will stub my toe on an uneven piece of sidewalk, and I will lose my balance and fall. In short, I should walk as if looking for pennies. But I resist impositions which impede social interaction. If I am constantly looking down to where my foot or cane must be placed, then I cannot look directly at the person with whom I am conversing. And so I run the risk and pay the price, which means I trip, stumble, and fall all too often. (Zola, 1982, p. 208)

As the example illustrates, modifications to how he executes the motor skill of walking create problems for the communication and interaction skill of gazing. No doubt such complex interactions between skills create constant challenges in addition to those posed by direct problems in executing a skill.

On the other hand, impairment often requires that persons emphasize remaining skills and use them to replace missing skills. For example, one may need to use communication and interaction skills to compensate for motor skill losses. In the following passage, Murphy (1987) eloquently describes how he had to use process skills to compensate for his losses of motor skills:

> Whereas I could once act on whim and fancy, I now had to exercise planning and foresight. This was true of even the simplest actions. In transferring from wheelchair to toilet, bed, or armchair, I had to park in a carefully chosen position and set the brakes, lest the wheelchair fly out from under me. I next would plot my strategy for getting up, choosing my supports with care, calculating the number of steps it would take to reach my target. (p. 76)

In contrast, Brown, whose ability to orally communicate (e.g., articulate) was severely impaired, relied on less impaired motor skills as a means to communicate: "Whenever I got into difficulties and [my family] couldn't make out what I was saying, I'd point to the floor and print the words out on it with my left foot" (Brown, 1990, p. 20).

As the examples illustrate, motor, process, and communication and interaction skills represent a flexible set of operations upon which a person with disability can call to achieve any particular occupational form. Success in performance depends not so much on every skill being intact as it does on effective and integrated use of available skills for performance.

ENVIRONMENT

Environments, both physical and social, may critically contribute to occupational dysfunction. Viewed from the sociopolitical perspective embodied in the disability or independent living movement, the environment is seen as providing a number of physical, attitudinal, legal, and political barriers to function. As stated by Hahn (1985), disability also represents failure of the social environment to respond to the needs and aspirations of disabled persons, not just the inability of a disabled individual to respond to society's demands. This section considers generally how physical and social environments can affect persons with disabilities. Obviously, the specific environmental impact depends on the nature of one's disability and on the kind of interface which evolves between one and one's environments.

Physical Environment

On the face of it, the physical environment would appear to have the greatest impact on persons with physical impairments. However, as we will see, the physical environment can also affect those whose disability is psychosocial in nature.

Spaces

Physical settings pose many problems for persons with physical disabilities. Natural and architectural barriers may interfere with the performance of work, play, and daily living tasks. As Rockwell-Dylla (1992) documented, the onset of a physical disability can transform one's house from a castle to a prison: one finds oneself tethered to the physical home space and effectively separated from the external world. Even within one's house one may encounter barriers as Murphy (1987) observed:

> In common with all old houses, our floors sag in places, creating little hills and valleys so small that they are undetectable to the normal person. But when you are using weakened arms to push a wheel chair across them, you get to know every one of them. I could have made a topographic map of our floors. Every month the hills grew higher, the valleys deeper, until one day I got stuck in one, the left arm too weak to get me out, leaving me able only to go around in circles. (p. 190)

The problems encountered in one's living space can be replicated in all built spaces that persons with physical impairments encounter. As laws and social consciousness change, many such barriers are being eliminated. Physical spaces, nevertheless, will always pose some impediments and challenges to persons with severe impairments.

Natural spaces similarly can provide a variety of problems for the person with a disability. For example, Hull (1990) notes that snow is a particular problem for a person who is blind, not because of the slippery surfaces but because snow blunts the sounds and makes use of the cane difficult, robbing one piece of necessary information to navigate. As this example illustrates, the particular kind of problem represented by the physical environment may be different depending on whether one's impairment is emotional, sensory, motor, or cognitive in nature.

Objects

Man-made objects in the environment are naturally geared via their size, shape, weight, complexity, and functions for able-bodied, sighted, hearing, and cognitively intact individuals. Disabilities often make it impossible or risky to handle or interact with the objects of everyday life. Zola (1982) offers the following litany of problems posed by objects for persons like himself with motor impairments:

> Chairs without arms to push myself up from; unpadded seats which all too quickly produce sores; showers and toilets without handrails to maintain my balance; surfaces too slippery to walk on; staircases without banisters to help me hoist myself; buildings without ramps, making ascent exhausting if not dangerous; every curbstone a precipice; car, plane, and theater seats too cramped for my braced leg; and trousers too narrow for my leg brace to pass through. With such trivia is my life plagued. (p. 208)

Many physically disabled persons must also learn to use new objects which extend or substitute for motor function, replace lost senses, provide protection, or manage disease processes. Wheelchairs, braces, adaptive equipment, bottles of medication, the disability check, ramps into one's home, catheterization supplies, grab bars, and a plethora of other specialized objects fill the lives of persons with disabilities. Whether such objects are welcome resources or necessary nuisances they also carry deep symbolic messages. We saw earlier how simply being in a wheelchair can change social identity and social interactions. Since objects can symbolize dependency or disability, some persons will not use otherwise functionally helpful objects. For example, I recall vividly young men in a spinal cord unit who adamantly refused to wear splints during their Friday night poker games. For all their functional virtues, the splints simply spoiled the ambience of poker and the bravado of poker players. Consequently, the splints stayed on the bedside tables when a poker game was underway.

Bates, Spencer, Young, and Hopkins-Rintala (1993) provide an insightful chronology of how one spinal cord-injured man, Russel, struggled over the meaning of a wheelchair in his life. When first learning sitting tolerance in a wheelchair he could not yet propel, he notes:

> I hate that time then because I can't do nothing. They might as well stick me in a damn closet. Can't move, can't do nothing . . . all you can do is sit there and think how helpless you are. (p. 1016)

Later the chair came to be a symbol of his lack of ability and a reminder that his goal of being able to walk again might not be viable. Over time, he vacillates between wanting to take a blow torch to the chair and finding it necessary as a means of some mobility. Even after discharge from rehabilitation his feelings about the chair are ambivalent.

As Bates, Spencer, Young, and Hopkins-Rintala (1993) argue, there is "the potential for intense emotional responses to the introduction of wheelchairs and other devices into patients' lives. Such responses may well up, subside, and well up again repeatedly" (p. 1020). The authors also point out that these feelings influence not only what the object means to the individual, but also how that individual will learn about and use the object in therapy and whether it will be integrated into an acceptable life.

Objects are not merely things to which we direct our attention and action. In many ways, they arouse, direct, and invite our feelings, thoughts, and actions. Persons with a wide range of disabilities may end up in settings such as residential facilities which are frequently devoid of many ordinary objects. Several years ago, in a study of persons with mental retardation living in board and care homes, I was struck by how barren the rooms and apartments looked. Personal belongings (other than clothes), decorations, comfortable furniture, minor appliances, and the many other things that members of our culture take for granted as part of the ecology of our living spaces were absent. Such object-deprived contexts contribute to apathy and indifference toward one's surroundings, to feelings of helplessness and worthlessness (Gray, 1972; Magill & Vargo, 1977). Indeed, one study (Simmons & Barris, 1984) found that in the home, everyday objects that provided opportunities for activity choices were more important than specialized or adapted objects in stimulating functional behavior.

The arrangement of objects in a space can also constrain or influence task performance. For example, how furniture is arranged in a room or how food is served in an institution can encourage or discourage social interaction (Holahan, 1979; Melin & Gotestam, 1981). Too often, objects can be organized in institutional settings for purposes of organizational efficiency but with the consequence of negatively affecting the occupational behavior of inhabitants.

Whether it be the everyday objects in a home, specialized objects to enhance function, or the arrangement of objects in institutional settings, the world of objects can present special challenges and constraints to persons with disabilities. Objects can readily influence how persons choose activities and how they routinely behave.

Social Environment

The social environment is the source of attitudes and behaviors that influence how individuals view their own disabilities. The social environment also determines what roles are available, and what occupational forms will present opportunities or challenges for the person with a disability.

Social Groups

Most social groups have a deep ambivalence toward persons with disabilities. Even in societies whose laws, health care, and welfare systems are organized so as to support the persons with disabilities, the attitudes of individuals and the practices of groups often betray discomfort if not outright disgust for the person with a disability. Personal accounts of individuals with disabilities are replete with their stories of constantly having to bear the negative reactions and attitudes of others, of having to bear the painful challenges and struggles of their disabilities while maintaining a public face of cheerfulness in order to be accepted, and of experiencing outright discrimination and rejection. Society frequently imposes all manner of impediment on persons with disabilities.

The presence or onset of a physical disability means that one's social environment is forever different—different than it is for others without a disability and/or different from what it had been before one had a disability. As Murphy (1987) argues:

> Disablement is at one and the same time a condition of the body and an aspect of social identity—a process set in motion by somatic causes but given definition and meaning by society. It is preeminently a social state. And so it was that as my upper body functions became atrophied under the pressure of the growing spinal cord tumor, my social orbit shifted, my horizons shrank, my conduct of life became altered, and my sense of self underwent further deep transformation. The onset of quadriplegia, I discovered, had placed me in a new social dimension. (p. 195)

Disabilities that have their origins or manifestation in the emotional or intellectual realms equally separate persons apart from the rest of society. For example, Western cultures place a high value on intelligence so that an implied deficit in this area is tantamount to the most serious kind of personal flaw—something that strikes at the very worth of the individual (Dexter, 1956, 1960; Edgerton, 1967). In similar fashion, Western society places a high premium on physical beauty and prowess, so that the persons with a physical deformity and/or impairment, by their very nature, contradict cultural values.

The social environment also constitutes the standards against which a person's behavior can be recognized as inappropriate or unhealthy (Mechanic, 1980; Sedgwick, 1973). Social definitions of what behavior is unacceptable constitute, in part, the criteria by which persons are identified as being mentally ill.

Persons who acquire a disability may find themselves temporarily or permanently removed from the groups in which they previously enacted their roles (Sarbin, 1954). Further, those social groups in which the individual engages in occupational behavior may be fundamentally changed for that person. For example, coworkers may attribute an injured worker's accident to carelessness and thereby fear working alongside him or her. Or, coworkers may resent accommodations made for an emotionally disabled colleague or harbor fear of uncertainty about being around someone with a psychiatric impairment. Moreover, the person with a disability may experience a socially shrinking world as old friends and acquaintances are uneasy or unwilling to continue relationships or when the activities which were the basis of association are no longer possible for the person with a disability (Hull, 1990; Murphy, Scheer, Murphy, & Mack, 1988; Oliver, Zarb, Silver, Moore, & Salisbury, 1988; Vash, 1981). Much of the individual's success in maintaining or rebuilding personal abilities, habits, and roles will depend on others' willingness and ability to shift responsibilities and roles and to accommodate necessary adaptations.

Of all the social groups, the family is ordinarily the most affected by and the most influential on a member with a disability. Disability is intimately shared by those close to the person with an impairment. For example, parents share in the suffering and grief that may be a part of a child's disability (Kornblum & Anderson, 1982). Moreover, the family is also affected in a logistical way by a family member's disability. Household routines, family member responsibilities, organization of the physical home, and restraints on family spontaneity, travel, and other factors may all be a part of the reality of having a disabled member in the family. Families may be extremely taxed by the work of caring for a disabled family member. Activities such as social contact and leisure may suffer (Breslau, 1983). For example, Murphy (1987) speaks about the effect of his disability on his wife and their relationship:

> Despite brief respites, [my wife] is tied down by me, her actions are severely limited by me, and my needs are never absent from her mind . . . My very ability to survive from day to day, to satisfy both major and minor needs, is in her hands. In a very real sense, we are both held in thrall by my condition. (p. 199)

A great deal of stress may be placed on family members who must accommodate the limitations of the person with a disability (Trombly, 1983). Prolonged hospitalization may cause role strain within the patient's family. Moreover, persons with disabilities frequently have fewer nonkindred relationships, depending significantly on the family for emotional, financial, and other forms of support. Consequently, the family can be a vital influence on the successful integration or reintegration of the individual with a disability into occupational roles. Positive family adjustment is influenced by the flexibility of role partners, the strength of relationships within the family (Weissman & Kutner, 1967), the economic needs of the family (Simmons, 1965), and the shared values related to occupational roles (Versluys, 1980).

Bogdan and Taylor (1989) studied individuals who did not stigmatize, stereotype, and reject close associates with disabilities. They found that families who positively influenced their members with disabilities engaged in the following kinds of behaviors:

> . . . members coordinate getting up, taking showers, getting breakfast, accompanying each other on important occasions, preparing for holidays, going on vacation, having birthday parties, and so on. The inclusion of a severely disabled person in a family's or primary group's routines and rituals, in its private times and public displays, acknowledges to the member that he or she is one of them. The person fills a particular social place. (p. 146)

Consequently, the family is both affected by and affects the impact of a disability. Persons with disabilities often end up spending significant portions of their lives in specialized social groups. These groups may include substitutes for home such as halfway houses, residential facilities, and state hospitals. They may be short-term treatment settings such as hospitals, community mental health centers, and rehabilitation facilities or long-term social and work settings such as senior centers and sheltered workshops. The explicit purpose of such settings is to provide services which support or enhance the performance and quality of life of persons with disabilities. However, a variety of factors, from constrained resources to organizational incentives and demands, can result in less than optimal conditions for achieving their ends. Social policies that are not adequately planned or funded can contribute to such circumstances. For example, deinstitutionalization resulted in persons being suddenly dropped from state hospitals into the community with few acceptable living alternatives and scant community support structures (Jones, 1983; Scull, 1977; Taube, Thompson, Rosenstein, Rosen, & Goldman, 1983).

Many of the social groups associated with services to persons with psychosocial dysfunction may contribute to the very problems they seek to alleviate, partly because they represent a discontinuity with "normal" environments and partly because of physical and psychosocial properties inherent in these settings (Emerson, Rochford, & Shaw, 1983; Scull, 1977; Test & Stein, 1978). For example, psychiatric hospitals may encourage psychiatric patients to assume passive, marginal roles, exacerbating problems with social competence (Srivastava, 1974).

Persons who are long-term inhabitants of specialized settings may develop maladaptive habits that reflect limited opportunities or unusual subcultures of total institutions in which they live (Edgerton, 1967; Kielhofner, 1983). For example, Goode (1983) documents how a man with Down's syndrome was able to grasp the meaning of privacy; however, he did not include practices related to privacy of self and others in his daily routines because the residential facility in which he lived was not one where privacy was attainable. His overtly inappropriate public behaviors were more like that of a foreigner unaccustomed to the customs of a new setting than someone who simply was not capable of grasping and internalizing such guides to behavior. Another resident of this same facility routinely walked down the street on the edge of the curb instead of the sidewalk. While the behavior made him seem odd, it was a means of finding dropped change in the ivy around parking meters, no small windfall for a man whose income was severely limited. Other behaviors, such as gorging food during meals and hoarding belongings on one's person, were similarly encouraged by scarce food and frequent stealing in the setting (Kielhofner, 1981).

In the same way the institutional schedule can affect the habits of residents. As Suto and Frank (1994), in their ethnography of persons with schizophrenia in a residential setting, observed:

> The residents experience a type of enforced leisure resulting from a combination of factors: predominantly passive free time activities, a lack of involvement in traditional social roles, and many hours of free time. Residents spend several hours of their daily unstructured time watching television, resting on chairs or on beds, chatting with co-residents, and taking walks. (p. 14)

The combination of being severed from ordinary social groups and being placed in groups where the normal opportunities for roles and activities are severely restricted can have a profound effect on the everyday occupational life of a person with a disability.

Occupational Forms

The world of things to do—that is, of occupational forms, can be dramatically altered for the person with a disability. Performance limitations can make some forms impossible. Disease processes and/or altered physical states can make other unusual occupational forms necessary. Social prejudice may make some occupational forms inaccessible. These and other circumstances influence occupational function and dysfunction in the person with a disability.

Benignly motivated overprotection by parents and significant others may deprive persons with disabilities of opportunities to make and learn from mistakes. This denies the individual's responsibility for, and thus access to, various occupational forms.

Persons with disabilities may also find that they must give up or relinquish to others occupational forms that have become impossible to do. The temporal and social nature of occupational forms may be radically altered. More time may be required. Previously private occupational forms may need to be performed when others are available to assist. Necessary adaptive equipment may mean that occupational forms take on a qualitatively different character.

The kinds of occupational forms to which persons with disabilities are given access also communicate messages about their worth and capacity. For example:

> When assigned a consensually demeaning task, as may occur when elderly persons live with offspring, or in nursing homes, the elderly individual erroneously infers self-incompetence. If a task of sealing envelopes is viewed as unimportant, elderly persons could conclude that they are incapable of doing anything more important. If the elderly person who is living with a son, daughter-in-law, and family is included in household activities only by being asked to make his or her own bed but is capable of much more, the elderly individual feels self-incompetence and helplessness. (Miller & Oertel, 1983, p. 110)

For a variety of reasons, it seems that persons with disabilities too often find that their access to occupational forms is restricted to those which are under-challenging. In this regard, Zola makes an observation about the occupational forms available to the physically disabled in a village designed for such persons:

> The jobs here were too simple, too fragmented, too mindless, too meaningless. Granted that my fellow residents might have limited physical capacity but why such busy work, why industrial products that were marketable only with a subsidy? Could the workers possibly feel they were doing something worthwhile? Of course, many jobs in the outside world were as repetitive and meaningless but at least those workers may have had a rationalization of the job's being a means

to an end. To what end were these tasks oriented? Why was work created from the point of view of the limitations of the workers rather than their potentialities? Again and again I had been told that the residents all had good minds. Why weren't they encouraged to use them? Work is not always exclusively physical. Why in this of all places, was that myth perpetuated? (Zola, 1982, p. 71)

The questions Zola raises have been raised by both observers and disabled persons themselves over and over again. Yet it seems that access to occupational forms which are meaningful and which reflect respect for the persons with a disability remains, all too frequently, a problem.

Summary

This section gave a brief overview of some of the ways in which the physical and social environment comes into relationship with persons who have a disability. It should be clear that the environment has the potential to either mitigate or exacerbate the emotional, functional, and behavioral consequences of impairments. Indeed, where impairments are immutable, the only possibility for enhancing the function of the individual lies in environmental accommodation. This section began with an observation from the disability movement which assigns a significant responsibility to the environment for maintaining, worsening, or reducing disability. When one considers how spaces, objects, social groups, and occupational forms interface with the persons who have disabilities, it becomes amply apparent why such a perspective has been taken. For the person with a disability, the world of occupational forms, taken for granted by nondisabled persons in the course of normal life, is radically different. Because persons with disabilities live in a world of different occupational forms, their behavior is inevitability channeled differently.

CONCLUSION

Because the challenges of disability are often many and extreme, because lifestyle is a matter of individual choice, because society sometimes provides conflicting sets of values about what constitutes a good life, the largest challenge is often to determine whether, and in what ways, a person's occupational life may be said to be dysfunctional. Consequently, it is worth considering these issues at the close of this chapter.

When an individual's life demonstrates such loss, disruption of direction, lack of meaning, or purpose that the person is unable to place himself or herself in a personal narrative which has possibilities and hope, or when the personal story identifies a life in trouble, then it may be said that the persons is experiencing an occupational dysfunction. Moreover, society has a right to expect that its members do their best to care for themselves and make reasonable contributions to the collective. When persons do not use their capacities in a reasonable way to respond to these reasonable expectations of the social collective, we also recognize occupational dysfunction. Finally, we can recognize occupational dysfunction by asking what a pattern of occupational behavior is doing to the human system in question. When a person's occupational life promises to negatively affect the integrity of the human system, then occupational dysfunction exists. For example, when a person has become so inactive and passive that physiological well-being is threatened, when a person is making decisions that repeatedly result in failure and eroding personal causation, we recognize an occupational dysfunction.

Such factors may evidence the existence of an occupational dysfunction but the larger challenge is to understand the dynamics by which such a dysfunctional state is being maintained. For this, it is critical to understand which components of the human system and of the environment are most significantly contributing to the occupational dysfunction. Rarely are there simple answers. Ordinarily, multiple factors are involved. In the final analysis, the answer can only be approached by careful examination of, and consultation with, the individual in question.

References

Abramowitz, S. I. (1969). Locus of control and self-reported depression among college students. *Psychological Report, 25*, 149–150.

American Psychiatric Association. (1980). *Diagnostic and statistical manual of mental disorders.* (3rd ed.). Washington, DC: Author.

Bates, P. S., Spencer, J. C., Young, M. E., & Hopkins-Rintala, D. H. (1993). Assistive technology and the newly disabled adult: Adaptation to wheelchair use. *American Journal of Occupational Therapy, 47*, 1014–1021.

Becker, E. W., & Lesiak, W. J. (1977). Feelings of hostility and personal control as related to depression. *Journal of Clinical Psychology, 33*, 654–657.

Benner, P. E. (1989). *Primacy of caring.* Menlo Park, CA: Addison-Wesley.

Beutell, N. J., & Greenhaus, J. H. (1983). Integration of home and nonhome roles: Women's conflict and coping behavior. *Journal of Applied Psychology, 68*, 43–48.

Bigos, S. J., Battie, M. C., Spengler, M. D., Fisher, L. D., Fordyce, W. E., Hansson, T. H., Nachemson, A. L., & Wortley, M. D. (1991). A prospective study of work perceptions and psychosocial factors affecting the report of back injury. *Spine, 16*, 1–6.

Black, M. (1976). The occupational career. *American Journal of Occupational Therapy, 30*, 225–228.

Bogdan, R., & Taylor, S. J. (1989). The social construction of humanness: Relationships with severely disabled people. *Social Problems, 36*, 135–148.

Borrero, I. M. (1980). Psychological and emotional impact of unemployment. *Journal of Sociology and Social Welfare, 7*, 916–934.

Boskind-Lodahl, M. (1976). Cinderella's stepsisters: A feminist perspective on anorexia nervosa and bulimia. *Signs: Journal of Women in Culture & Society, 2*, 342–356.

Braginski, D. D., & Braginski, B. M. (1971). *Hansels and Gretels: Studies of children in institutions for the mentally retarded.* New York: Holt, Rinehart & Winston.

Briar, K. H. (1980). Helping the unemployed client. *Journal of Sociology and Social Welfare, 7*, 895–906.

Braley, L. S., & Freed, N. (1971). Modes of temporal orientation and psychopathology. *Journal of Consulting and Clinical Psychology, 36*, 33–39.

Brandt, R., & Johnson, D. (1955). Time orientation in delinquents. *Journal of Abnormal and Social Psychology, 51*, 343–345.

Breslau, N. (1983) Family care: Effects on siblings and mothers. In G. H. Thompson, I. L. Rubin, & R. M. Belenker (Eds.), *Comprehensive management of cerebral palsy.* New York: Grune & Stratton.

Brown, C. (1990). *My left foot.* London: Minerva.

Burish, T. G., & Bradley, L. A. (1983). *Coping with chronic disease: Research and applications.* New York: Academic Press.

Cash, T., & Stack, J. (1973). Locus of control among schizophrenics and other hospitalized psychiatric patients. *Genetic Psychology Monographs, 87*, 105–122.

Cavan, R. S., & Cavan, J. T. (1968). *Delinquency and crime: Cultural cross-perspectives.* Philadelphia: JB Lippincott.

Cheseldine, S., & Jeffree, D. (1981). Mentally handicapped adolescents: Their use of leisure time. *Journal of Mental Health Deficiency Research, 25*, 49–59.

Coehlo, G., Silber, E., & Hamburg, D. (1971). Use of the student-TAT to assess coping behaviors in hospitalized, normal, and exceptionally competent college freshman. *Journal of Personality and Social Psychology, 18*, 305–310.

Cook, L. (1979). The adolescent with a learning disability: A developmental perspective. *Adolescence, 14*, 697–707.

Coser, L. (1974). *Greedy institutions*. New York: Free Press.

Coyne, P. (1980). Developing social skills in the developmentally disabled adolescent and young adult: A recreation and social/sexual approach. *Journal of Leisure, 7,* 70–76.

Cromwell, R. L. (1963). A social learning approach to mental retardation. In N. R. Ellis (Ed.), *Handbook of mental deficiency*. New York: McGraw-Hill.

Cromwell, R., Rosenthal, D., Shakow, D., & Zahn, T. (1961). Reaction time, locus of control, choice behavior, and descriptions of parental behavior in schizophrenic and normal subjects. *Journal of Personality, 29,* 363–380.

Deegan, P. (1991). Recovery: The lived experience of rehabilitation. In R. P. Marinelli & A. E. Dell Orto (Eds.), *The psychological and social impact of disability* (3rd ed.). New York: Springer-Verlag.

Delaney-Naumoff, M. (1980). Loss of heart. In J. A. Werner-Beland (Ed.), *Grief responses to long-term illness and disability*. Reston, VA: Reston Publishing Co.

DeLoach, C. P., & Greer, B. G. (1981). *Adjustment to severe physical disability: A metamorphosis*. New York: McGraw-Hill.

DeLoach, C. P., Wilkins, R. D., & Walker, G. W. (1983). *Independent living: Philosophy, process, and services*. Baltimore: University Park Press.

Dexter, L. A. (1956). Towards a sociology of mentally defective. *American Journal of Mental Deficiency, 61,* 10–16.

Dexter, L. A. (1960). Research on problems of mental subnormality. *American Journal of Mental Deficiency, 64,* 835–838.

Donovan, A., & Oddy, M. (1982). Psychological aspects of unemployment: An investigation into the emotional and social adjustment of school leavers. *Journal of Adolescence, 5,* 15–30.

Duke, M., & Mullens, M. (1973). Preferred interpersonal distance as a function of locus of control orientation in chronic schizophrenics, nonschizophrenic patients, and normals. *Journal of Consulting and Clinical Psychology, 41,* 230–234.

Dweck, C. S. (1975). The role of expectations and attributions in the alleviations of learned helplessness. *Journal of Personality and Social Psychology, 31,* 674–685.

Dweck, C. S., & Reppucci, N. D. (1973). Learned helplessness and reinforcement responsibility in children. *Journal of Personality and Social Psychology, 25,* 109–116.

Edgerton, R. B. (1967). *The cloak of competence: Stigma in the lives of the mentally retarded*. Berkeley, CA: University of California Press.

Emerson, R. M., Rochford, E. B., & Shaw, L. L. (1983). The micropolitics of trouble in a psychiatric board and care facility. *Urban Life, 12,* 349–366.

Erikson, K. T. (1973). Notes on the sociology of deviance. In H. S. Becker (Ed.), *The other side: Perspectives on deviance*. New York: Free Press.

Estroff, S. E. (1981). *Making it crazy*. Berkeley, CA: University of California Press.

Ewan, C., Lowy, E., & Reid, J. (1991). 'Falling out of culture': the effects of repetition strain injury on sufferers' roles and identity. *Sociology of Health and Illness, 13,* 168–192.

Fast, I. (1975). Aspects of work style and work difficulty in borderline personalities. *International Journal of Psycho-analysis, 56,* 397–403.

Fein, M. L. (1990). *Role change: A resocialization perspective*. New York: Praeger.

Frank, G. (1984). Life history model of adaptation to disability: The case of a 'congenital amputee.' *Social Science and Medicine, 19,* 639–645.

Frankl, V. E. (1978). *The unheard cry for meaning*. New York: Touchstone Books.

Freden, L. (1982). *Psychosocial aspects of depression*. New York: John Wiley & Sons.

Freedman, B., Donahoe, C., Rosenthal, L., & Schlundt, D. (1978). A social-behavioral analysis of skill deficits in delinquent and nondelinquent adolescent boys. *Journal of Consulting and Clinical Psychology, 46,* 1448–1462.

Frieden, L., & Cole, J. A. (1985). Independence: The ultimate goal of rehabilitation for spinal cord-injured persons. *American Journal of Occupational Therapy, 39,* 734–739.

Gerson, E. M. (1976). On "quality of life." *American Sociological Review, 41,* 793–806.

Goffman, E. (1961). *Asylums*. New York: Doubleday.

Goode, D. A. (1983). Who is Bobby? Ideology and method in the discovery of a Down's syndrome person's competence. In G. Kielhofner (Ed.), *Health through occupation: Theory and practice in occupational therapy*. Philadelphia: FA Davis.

Goode, W. J. (1960). A theory of role strain. *American Sociological Review, 25,* 483–496.

Gorman, B., & Wessman, A. (1977). *The personal experience of time*. New York: Plenum.

Gray, M. (1972). Effects of hospitalization on work-play behavior. *American Journal of Occupational Therapy, 26,* 180–185.

Greenspan, S. (1979). Social intelligence in the retarded. In N. R. Ellis (Ed.), *Handbook of mental deficiency, psychological theory, and research* (2nd ed.). Hillsdale, NJ: Erlbaum.

Grob, M., & Singer, J. (1974). *Adolescent patients in transition: Impact and outcome of psychiatric hospitalization*. New York: Behavioral Publications.

Gruen, G. E., Ottinger, D. R., & Ollendick, T. H. (1974). Probability learning in retarded children with differing histories of success and failure in school. *American Journal of Mental Deficiency, 79,* 417–423.

Gunderson, J. G., & Singer, M. T. (1975). Defining borderline patients: An overview. *American Journal of Psychiatry, 132,* 1–10.

Guskin, S. L. (1963). Social psychologies of mental deficiency. In N. R. Ellis (Ed.), *Handbook of mental deficiency*. New York: McGraw-Hill.

Hahn, H. (1985). Toward a politics of disability: definitions, disciplines and policies. *Social Science Journal, 22,* 87–105.

Hammen, C. C., & Glas, D. R., Jr. (1975). Depression, activity, and evaluation of reinforcement. *Journal of Abnormal and Social Psychology, 84,* 718–721.

Harrow, M., & Ferrante, A. (1969). Locus of control in psychiatric patients. *Journal of Consulting and Clinical Psychology, 33,* 582–589.

Hauser, S. (1976). The content and structure of adolescent self-concepts. *Archives of General Psychiatry, 33,* 27–32.

Heshusius, L. (1981). *Meaning in life as experienced by persons labeled retarded in a group home: A participant observation study*. Springfield, IL: Charles C Thomas.

Holahan, C. J. (1979). Environmental psychology in psychiatric hospital settings. In D. Canter & S. Canter (Eds.), *Designing for therapeutic environments: A review of research*. New York: John Wiley & Sons.

Holzman, P., & Grinker, R. (1974). Schizophrenia in adolescence. *Journal of Youth and Adolescence, 3,* 267–279.

Hudak, M. A., Andre, J., & Allen, R. D. (1980). Delinquency and social values. *Youth and Society, 11*, 358–368.

Hull, J. M (1990). *Touching the rock: An experience of blindness*. New York: Vintage Books.

Jones, R. E. (1983). Street people and psychiatry: An introduction. *Hospital Community Psychiatry, 34*, 807–811.

Katz, S., & Yekutiel, E. (1974). Leisure time problems of mentally retarded graduates of training programs. *Mental Retardation, 12*, 54–57.

Kavanagh, M. R. (1982). *Person-environment interaction: The model of human occupation applied to mentally retarded adults*. Unpublished research project, Virginia Commonwealth University, Richmond.

Kernberg, O. (1975). *Borderline conditions and pathological narcissism*. New York: Jason Aronson.

Kielhofner, G. (1979). The temporal dimension in the lives of retarded adults. *American Journal of Occupational Therapy, 33*, 161–168.

Kielhofner, G. (1980). *Evaluating deinstitutionalization: An ethnographic study of social policy*. Unpublished doctoral dissertation, University of California at Los Angeles.

Kielhofner, G. (1981). An ethnographic study of deinstitutionalized adults: Their community settings and daily life experiences. *Occupational Therapy Journal of Research, 1*, 125–141.

Kielhofner, G. (1983). "Teaching" retarded adults: Paradoxical effects of a pedagogical enterprise. *Urban Life, 12*, 307–326.

Kielhofner, G. (1993). Functional assessment: Toward a dialectical view of person-environment relations. *American Journal of Occupational Therapy, 47*, 248–251.

Kielhofner, G., Barris, R., & Watts, J. (1982). Habits and habit dysfunction: A clinical perspective for psychosocial occupational therapy. *Occupational Therapy Mental Health, 2*, 1–22.

Kornblum, H., & Anderson, B. (1982) Acceptance: reassessed—a point of view. *Child Psychiatry and Human Development, 12*, 171–178.

Korner, I. (1970). Hope as a method of coping. *Journal of Consulting and Clinical Psychology, 34*, 134–139.

Krefting, L. (1989). Reintegration into the community after head injury: The results of an ethnographic study. *Occupational Therapy Journal of Research, 9*, 67–83.

Lambert, B. G., Rothschild, B. F., Atland, R., & Green, L. B. (1978). *Adolescence: Transition from childhood to maturity* (2nd ed.). Monterey, CA: Brooks/Cole.

Lefcourt, H. M. (1976). *Locus of control: Current trends in theory and research*. Hillsdale, NJ: Erlbaum.

Leggett, J., & Archer, R. P. (1979). Locus of control and depression among psychiatric patients. *Psychology Report, 45*, 835–838.

Lewinsohn, P. M. (1975). Engagement in pleasant activities and depression level. *Journal of Abnormal and Social Psychology, 84*, 729–731.

Lewinsohn, P. M., & Graf, M. (1973). Pleasant activities and depression. *Journal of Consulting and Clinical Psychology, 41*, 261–268.

Lovejoy, M. (1982). Expectations and the recovery process. *Schizophrenia Bulletin, 8*, 605–609.

Litman, T. J. (1972). Physical rehabilitation: A social-psychological approach. In E. G. Jaco (Ed.), *Patients, physicians and illness: A sourcebook in behavioral science and health* (2nd ed.). New York: Free Press.

Luria, A. R. (1972). *The history of a brain wound: The man with a shattered world*. (L. Solotaroff, Trans.). New York: Basic Books.

MacPhilany, D. J., & Lewinsohn, P. M. (1974). Depression as a function of desired and obtained pleasure. *Journal of Abnormal and Social Psychology, 83*, 651–657.

Magill, J., & Vargo, J. (1977). Helplessness, hope, and the occupational therapist. *Canadian Journal of Occupational Therapy, 44*, 65–69.

Manaster, G. (1977). *Adolescent development and the life tasks*. Boston: Allyn and Bacon.

Marks, S. R. (1977). Multiple roles and role strain: Some notes on human energy, time, and commitment. *American Sociological Review, 42*, 921–936.

Masterson, J., & Washburne, A. (1966). The psychiatric adolescent: Psychiatric illness or adolescent turmoil? *American Journal of Psychiatry, 122*, 1240–1280.

Matthews, P. R. (1980). Why the mentally retarded do not participate in certain types of recreational activities. *Therapeutic Recreation Journal, 14*, 44–50.

Merleau-Ponty, M. (1962). *Phenomenology of perception*. (Collins & Smith, Trans.). New York: Humanities Press.

Mechanic, D. (1980). *Mental Health and Social Policy* (2nd ed.). Englewood Cliffs, NJ: Prentice-Hall.

Meissner, W. W. (1982). Notes on the potential differentiation of borderline conditions. *Psychoanalytic Review, 70*, 179–209.

Melges, F. T. (1982). *Time and Inner Future: A temporal approach to psychiatric disorders*. New York: John Wiley & Sons.

Melin, L., & Gotestam, G. (1981). The effects of rearranging ward routines on communication and eating behaviors of psychogeriatric patients. *Journal of Applied Behavioral Analysis, 14*, 47–51.

Menninger, K. (1962). Hope. In S. Doniger (Ed.), *The nature of man in theological and psychological perspective*. New York: Harper Brothers.

Mitchell, J. J. (1975). *The adolescent predicament*. Toronto: Holt, Winston.

Mitic, T. D., & Stevenson, C. L. (1981). Mentally retarded people as a resource to the recreationist in planning for integrated community recreation. *Journal of Leisure Research, 8*, 30–34.

Miller, J. F., & Oertel, C. B. (1983). Powerlessness in the elderly: Preventing hopelessness. In J. F. Miller (Ed.), *Coping with chronic illness: Overcoming powerlessness*. Philadelphia: FA Davis.

Molnar, G. E. (1989). The influence of psychosocial factors on personality development and emotional health in children with Cerebral Palsy and Spina Bifida. In B. W. Heller, L. M. Flohr, & L. S. Zegans (Eds.), *Psychosocial interventions with physically disabled persons*. New Brunswick, NJ: Rutgers University Press.

Moss, J. W. (1958). *Failure-avoiding and stress-striving behavior in mentally retarded and normal children*. Ann Arbor, MI: University Microfilms.

Murphy, R. F. (1987). *The body silent*. New York: WW Norton.

Murphy, R. F., Scheer, J., Murphy, Y., & Mack, R. (1988). Physical disability and social liminality: A study in the rituals of adversity. *Social Science and Medicine., 26*, 235–242.

Neville, A. M. (1987). *The relationship of locus of control, future time perspective and interest to productivity among individuals with varying degrees of depression*. Unpublished doctoral dissertation, New York University.

Offer, D., Ostrov, E., & Howard, K. (1981). *The adolescent: A psychological self-report*. New York: Basic Books.

Oliver, M., Zarb, G., Silver, J., Moore, M., & Salisbury, V. (1988). *Walking into darkness: The experience of spinal cord injury*. London: MacMillan Press.

Paap, W. R. (1972). The social reconstruction of reality: The rehabilitation of paraplegics and quadraplegics. *Dissertation Abstracts International, 33,* 45-A. (University Microfilms No. 72-19, 234).

Parsons, T. (1953). Illness and the role of the physician: A sociological perspective. In C. Kluckhohn, H. Murray, & O. Schneider (Eds.), *Personality in nature, society, and culture* (2nd ed.). New York: Alfred A. Knopf.

Phillips, W. M. (1980). Purpose in life, depression, and locus of control. *Journal of Clinical Psychology, 36,* 661–667.

Pinder, R. (1988). Striking balances: Living with Parkinson's disease. In R. Anderson & M. Bury (Eds.), *Living with chronic illness: The experience of patients and their families.* London: Unwin Hyman.

Rabinowitz, H. S., & Mitsos, S. B. (1964). Rehabilitation as planned social change: A conceptual framework. *Journal of Health and Social Behavior, 5,* 2–13.

Roberts, E. V. (1989). A history of the independent living movement: A founder's perspective. In B. W. Heller, L. M. Flohr, & L. S. Zegans (Eds.), *Psychosocial interventions with physically disabled persons.* New Brunswick, NJ: Rutgers University Press.

Robinson, I. (1988). Reconstructing lives: Negotiating the meaning of multiple sclerosis. In R. Anderson & M. Bury (Eds.), *Living with chronic illness: The experience of patients and their families.* London: Unwin Hyman.

Rockwell-Dylla, L. A. (1992). *Older adults meaning of environment: Hospital and home.* Unpublished master's thesis, University of Illinois at Chicago.

Rogers, J. C., & Figone, J. J. (1978). The avocational pursuits of rehabilitants with traumatic quadriplegia. *American Journal of Occupational Therapy, 32,* 571–576.

Rogers, J. C., & Figone, J. J. (1979). Psychosocial parameters interacting the person with quadriplegia. *American Journal of Occupational Therapy, 33,* 432–439.

Roos, P., & Albers, R. (1965). Performance of retardates and normals on a measure of temporal orientation. *American Journal of Mental Deficiency, 69* 835–838.

Rosenberg, M. (1965). *Society and the adolescent self-image.* Princeton, NJ: Princeton University Press.

Rosenthal, M. (1989). Psychosocial evaluation of physically disabled persons. In B. W. Heller, L. M. Flohr, & L. S. Zegans (Eds.), *Psychosocial interventions with physically disabled persons.* New Brunswick, NJ: Rutgers University Press.

Sacks, O. (1985). *The man who mistook his wife for a hat.* New York: Summit Books.

Sarbin, T. R. (1954). Role theory. In G. Lindzey & E. Aronson (Eds.), *The hand-book of social psychology* (Vol. 1). Reading, MA: Addison-Wesley.

Scaffa, M. (1982). *Temporal adaptation and alcoholism.* Unpublished master's thesis, Virginia Commonwealth University, Richmond.

Scambler, G., & Hopkins, A. (1988). In R. Anderson & M. Bury (Eds.), *Living with chronic illness: The experience of patients and their families.* London: Unwin Hyman.

Schiamberg, L. B. (1973). *Adolescent alienation.* Columbus, OH: Merrill.

Schiffer, R. B., Rudick, R. A., & Herndon, R. M. (1983). Psychologic aspects of multiple sclerosis. *New York State Journal of Medicine, 3,* 312–316.

Scull, A. T. (1977). *Decarceration: Community treatment and the deviant—A radical view.* Englewood Cliffs, NJ: Prentice-Hall.

Sedgwick, P. (1973). Illness, mental and otherwise. *Hastings Center Studies, 1,* 19–40.

Seiber, S. D. (1974). Toward a theory of role accumulation. *American Sociological Review, 39,* 567–578.

Serok, S., & Blum, A. (1979). A treatment vehicle for delinquent youths. *Crime Delinquency, 25,* 358–362.

Sienkiewicz-Mercer, R., & Kaplan, S. B. (1989). *I raise my eyes to say yes.* New York: Avon Books.

Shillam, L. L., Beeman, C., & Loshin, P. (1983). Effect of occupational therapy intervention on bathing independence of disabled persons. *American Journal of Occupational Therapy, 37,* 744–748.

Shipe, D. (1971). Impulsivity and locus of control as predictor of achievement and adjustment in mildly retarded and borderline youth. *American Journal of Mental Deficiency, 76,* 12–22.

Simmons, J. E., & Barris, R. (1984). *The relationship between the home environment and the occupational behavior in the post-CVA patient.* Unpublished manuscript.

Simmons, O. (1965). *Work and mental illness.* New York: John Wiley & Sons.

Smith, C. A. (1972). Body image changes after myocardial infarction. *Nursing Clinics of North America, 7,* 663–668.

Smith, C., Pryer, M., & Distefano, M. (1971). Internal-external control and severity of emotional impairment among psychiatric patients. *Journal of Clinical Psychology, 27,* 449–450.

Smyntek, L. E. (1983). *A comparison of occupationally functional and dysfunctional adolescents.* Unpublished master's project, Virginia Commonwealth University, Richmond.

Spivak, G., Siegel, J., Sklaver, D., Deuschle, L., & Garrett, L. (1982). The long-term patient in the community: Life-style patterns and treatment implications. *Hospital Community Psychiatry, 33,* 291–295.

Spreitzer, E., Snyder, E. E., & Larson, D. L. (1979). Multiple roles and psychological well-being. *Social Focus, 12,* 141–148.

Srivastava, R. K. (1974). Undermining theory in the context of mental health care environments. In D. H. Carson (Ed.), *Man-Environment interactions: Evaluations and applications, Part II.* Stroudsberg, PA: Dowden, Hutchinson & Ross.

Strickland, B. (1978). Internal-External expectancies and health-related behaviors. *Journal of Consulting and Clinical Psychology, 46,* 1192–1211.

Suto, M., & Frank, G. (1994). Future time perspective and daily occupations of persons with chronic schizophrenia in a board and care home. *American Journal of Occupational Therapy, 48,* 7–18.

Taube, C. A., Thompson, J. W., Rosenstein, M. J., Rosen, B. M., & Goldman, H. H. (1983). The "chronic" mental hospital patient. *Hospital Community Psychiatry, 34,* 611–615.

Taylor, A. R. (1982). Social competence and interpersonal relations between retarded and nonretarded children. In N. R. Ellis (Ed.), *International Review of Research in Mental Retardation* (Vol. 11). New York: Academic Press.

Test, M. A., & Stein, L. I. (1978). Community treatment of the chronic patient: A research overview. *Schizophrenia Bulletin, 4,* 350–364.

Tham, K. (1994, April). Volitions in persons with unilateral neglect. Paper presented at the World Federation of Occupational Therapists, London, England.

Thomas, E. J. (1966). Problems of disability from the perspective of role theory. *Journal of Health and Human Behavior, 7*, 2–14.

Trieschmann, R. B. (1989). Psychosocial adjustment to spinal cord injury. In B. W. Heller, L. M. Flohr, & L. S. Zegans (Eds.), *Psychosocial interventions with physically disabled persons*. New Brunswick, NJ: Rutgers University Press.

Trombly, C. A. (1983). *Occupational therapy for physical dysfunction* (2nd ed.). Baltimore: Williams & Wilkins.

Turner, R. W., Ward, M. F., & Turner, D. J. (1979). Behavioral treatment for depression: An evaluation of therapeutic components. *Journal of Clinical Psychology, 35*, 166–175.

Vash, C. L. (1981). *The psychology of disability*. New York: Springer-Verlag.

Versluys, H. P. (1980). The remediation of role disorders through focused group work. *American Journal of Occupational Therapy, 34*, 609–614.

Versluys, H. P. (1983). Psychosocial adjustment to physical disability. In C. A. Trombly (Ed.), *Occupational therapy for physical dysfunction* (2nd ed.). Baltimore: Williams & Wilkins.

Wasserman, G. A. (1986). Affective expression in normal and physically handicapped infants. Situational and developmental effects. *Journal of the American Academy of Child and Adolescent Psychiatry, 25*, 393–399.

Weissman, R., & Kutner, B. (1967). Role disorders in extended hospitalization. *Hospital Administration, 12*, 52–55.

Werner-Beland, J. A. (Ed.) (1980). *Grief responses to long-term illness and disability*. Reston, VA: Reston Publishing Co.

Werthman, C. (1976). The function of sociological definitions in the development of the gang boy's career. In R. Giallombardo (Ed.), *Juvenile delinquency: A book of readings* (3rd ed.). New York: John Wiley & Sons.

Williams, R. S. (1984). Ability, disability and rehabilitation: a phenomenological description. *Journal of Medicine and Philosophy, 9*, 93–112.

Wolfensberger, W. (1975). *The origin and nature of our institutional models*. Syracuse, NY: Human Policy Press.

Wright, B. A. (1960). *Physical disability: A psychological approach*. New York: Harper & Row.

Wylie, R. (1979). *The self-concept: Theory and research* (2nd ed.). Lincoln, NE: University of Nebraska Press.

Youkilis, H., & Bootzin, R. (1979). The relationship between adjustment and perceived locus of control in female psychiatric in-patients. *Journal of Genetic Psychology, 135*, 297–299.

Zane, M. D., & Lowenthal, M. (1960). Motivaiton in rehabilitation of the physically handicapped. *Archive of Physical Medicine and Rehabilitation, 41*, 400–407.

Zola, I. K. (1982). *Missing pieces: A chronicle of living with a disability*. Philadelphia: Temple University Press.

11/ Gathering and Reasoning with Data During Intervention

Gary Kielhofner and Trudy Mallinson

INTRODUCTION

In this chapter we will discuss the process by which a therapist, using the model of human occupation as a theoretical framework, gathers data and uses them to reason about patients and their life circumstances. This data gathering and reasoning process enables therapists to plan and carry out a beneficial course of therapy.

We refer to this process as gathering and reasoning with data to emphasize two points. First, we wish to underscore that the process of gathering and reasoning with data is an interactive, analytical process; that is, a therapist moves back and forth between obtaining data and thinking about data in order to come to an understanding of complex factors involved in a particular client's circumstances. Moreover, gathering and reasoning with data is a *theoretically informed* process that occurs within a framework provided by the model(s) of practice a therapist is using.

Data should be collected not simply as a prelude to drawing conclusions, but as a part of a process of active, analytic questioning. Therapists should seek out data for the specific purpose of answering questions they have generated in order to understand a client from a theoretical perspective. For example, therapists using the model of human occupation will initiate the following possible queries: Is this person's habit pattern contributing to his substance abuse? How has the onset of chronic pain affected this person's enjoyment of previous interests? Is this person's sense of efficacy interfering with her ability to make an important occupational choice with which she is faced? Does this child hesitate to move because of the anxiety of being out of control? It is precisely because therapists generate such questions that they need to gather data. Therapists then use the data to make theoretically-informed judgements about the answers to such questions.

Our second point is that therapists use data to make moral judgements. When therapists decide what *should be done in therapy*, they are engaging in a form of moral reasoning (Mattingly & Fleming, 1993). That reasoning asks: What is currently not in the best interest of this person and those in his or her environment? What future state of affairs would be better than the present state?

Therapy is always a process of trying to enable a patient or client to move from a current dynamic state to some future state which is deemed better. Arriving at the judgement about what future state would be better is a deeply complex process. It requires the occupational therapist to have enough data to understand the dynamics of a person's dysfunction, to grasp essential features of a person's life and often of others who are part of that life. Finally, it requires the therapist to take a stance about the data's significance to form a vision of how the person's life ought to unfold. No small amount of responsibility is attached to this requisite moral judgement.

GATHERING AND REASONING WITH DATA IN THE CONTEXT OF THERAPY

The process of gathering and reasoning with data goes on throughout the entire course of intervention; it is not finished until the client has left therapy. Moreover, the process extends beyond the end of therapy when therapists retrospectively reflect upon how intervention affected a person's life.

In a very real sense, therapists learn as they gather and reason with data. Learning takes place in the course of a relationship with any patient as the therapist becomes more knowledgeable about that patient and his or her circumstances. Learning also takes place over the career of the therapist as experiences with clients augment one's store of therapeutic wisdom.

Gathering and reasoning with data is ordinarily most intensive at the early stage of therapy and is essential for therapists to: (1) construct a nascent understanding of the patient and (2) to envision the outcomes toward which therapy is aimed. Ongoing data gathering in the course of therapy serves three important processes: (1) revising and sharpening understanding of the patient, (2) reconsidering the good that should emerge from therapy, and (3) determining how therapy is working with an eye toward refining the therapeutic method for this person and for subsequent clients.

The extent of data gathering will vary with time available. However brief the therapeutic encounter, it will be more beneficial to the patient when the therapist has the kind of data which allow a determination of what is in the best interest of this unique person. Changes in health care delivery, with emphasis on shorter periods of intervention, should not mean that therapists abandon the means, or the goal, of knowing their patients. Rather, these changes should challenge therapists to sharpen their abilities to gather and reason with data. In discussing this process, we have tried to be mindful of the constraints that therapists face in everyday practice. In this and the next chapter, we will outline a flexible approach to using formal and informal data-gathering methods which can be integrated into the therapeutic process. Readers should recognize that implementing the model of human occupation in gathering and reasoning with data is not predicated on the use of any particular instrument. Rather, therapists should engage in a thoughtful process, using concepts from the model to guide information gathering. The strategies used to get the information should be those that work best in the situation.

In sum, gathering and reasoning with data is the process which serves to guide the course of therapy. It is necessary to create an understanding of the patient, to imagine desirable outcomes, to plan a course of therapy to achieve those outcomes, and to watchfully monitor whether the course of therapy is fitting with the client's situation and achieving the desired direction of change. The process of therapy, whether short or long, should be directed and redirected on the basis of data which are gathered and with which the therapist reasons.

NATURE OF DATA

The data which occupational therapists use in reasoning about therapy pertain to patients or clients, their social worlds and physical environments, and the dynamic process of the patient or client engaging in occupational behavior (including that which occurs in therapy). Most of the data that are used in occupational therapy are generated in four ways: (1) therapists observe, informally or through some formal, structured instrument, what the patient does, (2) the client reports data to therapists through verbal or written means, (3) therapists obtain information from others who make up the client's social groups (e.g, family members, coworkers, supervisors, teachers), and (4) therapists observe the physical and social environments in which the client lives and performs.

Data may take on many forms. The kind of data gathered depends on the kind of method used to collect and record the data. For example, informal observation yields behavioral data that are typically described in oral reports or written reports. However, the same observed behavior might be captured on a structured rating scale.

Self-report forms typically elicit data in the form of simple indications of what one does, likes, values, and so on. These descriptive data take the form of patterns and profiles. Interview methods which ask patients or others to relate how they see, understand, or feel about things that have happened in their lives can yield data in the form of life stories. Whether it takes the form of numbers, descriptions, profiles, or stories, data always constitute information with which therapists reason. Consequently, data should be collected with the reasoning process in mind.

GENERATING THEORETICAL QUESTIONS TO GUIDE DATA COLLECTION

We have emphasized that the process of gathering and reasoning with data should be theoretically informed. Coles (1989) notes that theory comes from the Greek, Θεαωραι, which means "to behold." When theory is used well, it is in the eye of the beholder—meaning that to use theory is to adopt a particular viewpoint. In the process of gathering data, theory should provide a systematic way of looking for information.

We already noted that theory influences data gathering by suggesting the questions that therapists seek to answer through the data they collect. The model of human occupation provides a theoretical viewpoint for generating such questions. The particular nature of the questions a therapist seeks to answer depends on a number of factors emanating from the patient and the therapeutic situation. For example, these factors may include the age of the client, the patient's disability, the educational, rehabilitative, or preventative mission of therapy, the anticipated duration of therapy, and the hospital, home, school, work or other setting in which therapy will be implemented.

While the questions that guide the data gathering and reasoning process must be tailored to such contingencies, it is possible to identify the kinds of questions which can be derived from the model. We have identified a number of these questions in three areas: (1) the human system's organization, (2) environmental influences, and (3) systems dynamics. The questions we identify should be taken only as examples. They do not exhaust, by any

means, the generative possibilities of the theoretical constructs. Therapists should use these questions as a starting point for developing more specific and tailored questions. Moreover, the best questions emerge from within the therapeutic context. When a therapist is beholding a client from a theoretical perspective, questions should naturally arise. As more is known about the client, newer and more refined questions should emerge.

Questions Concerning the Internal Organization of the System

When persons experience difficulties with occupational functioning, therapists should ask whether and how the internal organization of the volition, habituation, and mind-brain-body performance subsystems may be contributing. Importantly, the subsystems may also reflect important strengths to support the person's struggle to adapt. By gathering data on the status of the subsystems, the therapist gains important information about both assets and liabilities that the person brings to everyday occupational performance.

Personal Causation

In the area of personal causation, therapists should seek to know about the persons' knowledge of their own capacities and about their sense of efficacy. The goal of questioning about knowledge of capacity should be, first, to comprehend how persons organize their common-sense understanding of current and potential abilities. The following questions can be considered:

- What abilities are emphasized in this person's view of self?
- In what ways does this person's view of capacity consider physical, intellectual, or social abilities or limitations?
- Does this person tend to evaluate capacities by comparison to others, or in terms of some other standard?
- What areas of performance evoke this person's strongest reactions to being able or unable?
- What specific abilities or impairments stand out in this person's view of self? For

example, what capacities are most prized and what limitations create the most negative emotional response?

For persons with longstanding or lifelong impairments, therapists might consider additional questions such as:

- What areas of limitation does this person recognize?
- What abilities has this person been able to identify despite impairments?
- Is this person's view of capacity saturated with concern over inability or does it emphasize things that can be achieved?
- How does this person deal with areas of incapacity? For example, does this person go ahead and perform at the level at which he or she is capable? Or, does this person avoid such areas of performance altogether?
- In what ways does this person use intact capacities to compensate or substitute for areas of inability?
- How does this person approach situations that challenge ability? For example, does he or she tend to focus on the gap between capacity and challenge? Or, does the person look for ways to meet the challenge?

For individuals with more recently acquired impairments, other questions may be useful:

- How has the limitation this person is experiencing changed his or her sense of capacity?
- What is the overall impact of any changed view of self?
- Does this person's impairment affect only a few or many areas of perceived self-competence?
- Has this person experienced a significant loss of capacity in his or her own view? Does this person grasp the actual losses of capacity (if they are clearly known)?
- Does this person believe that he or she has capacities for achieving the things that most matter and that others in his or her life deserve or expect? Does this person have worries about having capacities equal to what is demanded or desired in social groups to which he or she belongs?

- Is the person's knowledge of capacity commensurate with actual performance?
- Does this person have an unrealistic (under- or overestimated) view of capacity? Does he or she overemphasize or fail to recognize deficits?
- What are the consequences of any disparity between actual and perceived capacity for this person?

Many persons do not have fixed impairments. Some may improve; others have conditions involving exacerbations and remissions. Still others have progressive disorders. For such persons therapists may want to ask:

- How is this person's knowledge of capacity influenced by the fluctuating nature of his or her disability or illness?
- In what ways is this person struggling with uncertainty about what he or she will be able to do because of unknown outcomes?
- How do declining physical or mental capacities figure in this person's knowledge of things he or she can and cannot do?

Since knowledge of capacity sometimes must be inferred from observation, occupational therapists may ask the following of clients' actions:

- Does this person take reasonable risks, try things within capacity, know when to avoid problems or danger, or otherwise demonstrate a sense of capacity that is accurate? If not, what are the consequences for this person?
- Does this person appear to seek out opportunities for occupational performance within his or her capacity? When does this person challenge or constrain him or herself?
- Does this person recognize whether he or she has demonstrated the capacity for a task? What is done with such information?

Finally, therapists can consider how knowledge of capacity may affect other factors through questions like this:

- What is the emotional impact of this person's knowledge of his or her abilities? Is there motivation to change, demoralization, or anxiety?

- What role might misestimation of capacity be playing in this person's view of self and his or her activity choices?
- How does this person experience the performance of daily occupations? When is he or she frustrated or encouraged by performance?
- What particular experience of limitation of capacity does this person have and what is its emotional impact?
- What it is like for this person to have difficulty performing?

The concept of sense of efficacy leads therapists to consider an individual's beliefs and feelings about controlling self and outcomes in life. Beginning with the idea of self-control, therapists may ask:

- Does this person appear to feel in control of her or his own thoughts, feelings, and actions? In what ways does he or she demonstrate this?
- In what ways does this person experience the inability to control self? For example, does he or she complain of being unable to discipline self, of being unmotivated, stuck, or trapped?
- Does this person report extreme emotions, compulsive thoughts, or even hallucinatory experiences that rob him or her of control?
- Does this person show self-control through determination in the face of challenges, tolerance for frustrating situations, and so on?

Beyond controlling self, the sense of efficacy is concerned with one's ability to effect desired outcomes. In regard to this, therapists may consider:

- What things appear, to this person, to be in the scope of personal control? What things seem beyond control?
- Is this person more likely to attribute control of desired outcomes to self or to other people or factors outside himself or herself?
- Is this person's sense of control realistic?

- What possibilities for being out of control does this person fear most?
- In which situations does this person most want to be in control?

Observation of individuals' behavior and reactions to situations can provide a great deal of information about their feelings of efficacy. Observation can be guided by such questions as:

- What kinds of situations cause this person to be anxious or worry that he or she might not be able to cope?
- In what situations does this person appear to feel confident?
- When does this person appear able or unable to manage her or his own feelings and thoughts?
- What strategies does this person use to increase feelings of control or to avoid situations of failure or maximize possibilities of success?
- Does this person accept too little or too much responsibility for outcomes in life? What are the consequences of this approach to control for this person?

The experience of disease and disability (and its uncertain outcomes) can give persons a powerful sense of being unable to control their lives, which affects their morale and activity choices. Therapists should consider:

- How does this person's sense of being controlled by such factors as pain, incapacity, emotions, etc., influence her or his willingness to engage in daily activities and make occupational choices?
- What situations have led this person to feel overwhelmed by loss of control? What areas of control can this person still identify?
- How might an unpredictable future influence this person's sense that he or she can set and work towards goals?

Occupational therapists should also consider the consequences of the persons' sense of efficacy for their view of life and volitional choices. For example, the following questions raise these issues:

- Has this person's sense of control changed his or her involvement in tasks?
- How does this person's sense of being controlled by illness or incapacity affect her or his willingness to engage in occupations (activity choices, occupational choices)?
- In what ways has disability challenged this person's belief that he or she can achieve a worthwhile life or can engage in important occupations?

Persons often reveal the most about their sense of efficacy by the kind of life story they tell or in the way they relate incidents. By using certain images (e.g., having life "ruined" versus "having a cross to bear") they may tell a great deal about their sense of being able to achieve what they want in life. Other imagery, such as the metaphors they employ, can also reveal a great deal about their sense of efficacy. Therefore, the following questions are important to consider:

- What kinds of stories or incidents does this person relate about her or his life? What do these stories portray about this person's sense of efficacy? For example, does this person self-characterize as a "failure," "fighter," "survivor," or "victim"? Does this person relate being "stuck," "slowed down," or "trapped"? What kind of future does this person anticipate or imply in his or her stories? Is the future hopeful and positive, unknown and threatening, or hopeless and negative?

Values

Values are concerned with what persons hold as significant and important in their lives and to what ends and behaviors they are committed. Since values are part of a coherent world view, occupational therapists should begin with questions that help identify the way an individual assigns significance to life:

- What is the organizing theme in this person's sense of values? Is it deep religious conviction? Is it a set of cultural or subcultural values (e.g., the strong work values of a Vietnamese immigrant or the

streetwise values of a gang member or drug dealer?)
- What is the depth of conviction about these values and what emotional strength do they have for this person?
- Is this person clear as to what his or her values are? Is he or she in a period of disillusionment or disintegration of values?
- What do the stories this person tells about his or her life reveal about what he or she most wants from life?
- What values figure in this person's choices and reactions to circumstances in these stories? What moral do his or her stories appear to have and what does this reveal about what matters to this person?

Values often play a strong role in how persons make sense of their disabilities. To determine how values are affecting a person's situation, the following questions can be considered:

- How do this person's values match or conflict with his or her abilities? Do any conflicts lead to devaluation of self and in what ways is this so?
- How do this person's values influence the way he or she experiences disability and believes he or she should deal with it? What meaning does this person assign to the disability?
- How do family and cultural values shape this person's view of what it means to be a person with a disability? Do those values support or restrict options for this person?

Disability can also serve to invalidate values; therapists may ask such questions as:

- In what ways do the consequences of this person's disability challenge his or her own values and aspirations?
- In what ways has disability led this person to struggle to redefine his or her own values?
- Is this person having to make difficult choices about giving up valued activities or routines?

Sometimes values are themselves a source of problem for individuals in this regard. Therapists should consider such questions as:

• Does this person ascribe to values that are not really his or her own? Does this person hold values that lead to choices not in his or her own best interest?

• In what way is this person acting from a deviant set of values that conflict with those in occupational behavior settings?

• In what ways do this person's values place him or her in a negative future trajectory or limit choices for the future?

Interests

Interests have to do both with the experience of pleasure in occupations (attraction) and with the specific preferences that characterize each person. Some questions that help identify these dispositions in an individual are:

• Around what activities and to what degree does this person report experiences of pleasure in occupations?

• What are the aspects of activities that this person has enjoyed most (e.g., physical challenge, intellectual stimulation, social contact, aesthetic experience)?

• Does this person have many interests done infrequently? Or, does he or she have a few very focused and intense interests?

• Has a change in this person's life (e.g., new job) significantly changed the pleasure or satisfaction this person experiences?

• Does this person have any very passionate interests that are a special source of motivation, hope or joy?

• When this person tells stories about good times, what were the events, settings, activities, and other elements that were so enjoyable?

• Does this person look forward to upcoming events? Does he or she plan for and positively anticipate involvement in occupations?

Similar information can be gathered through observations which consider:

• Does this person get involved or excited in occupations? What physical or vocal signs show that this person is having a good time?

• What activities appear to sustain this person's attention and draw out the most positive affect?

• In what activities does this person show investment and satisfaction?

• Will this person show preference by seeking out certain opportunities for activity? What are they?

To determine whether interests might be a source of problems for persons, therapists can ask such questions as:

• Is this person's pattern of interests too narrow, solitary, or passive?

• Does this person lack experiences to develop attraction to, and preference for, occupations that lead to difficulties in making activity choices?

• Does this person seem oblivious to opportunities for pleasure in action?

To identify factors which may interfere with interest, therapists may ask:

• In what ways is physical or psychic pain interfering with the attraction to occupations or the feeling of pleasure and satisfaction in performance? Is this person too anxious, fatigued, distracted, depressed, or otherwise indisposed to enjoy activity?

• In what ways has loss of capacity taken away possibilities for participation in interests? Has this person been forced to give up a whole area of interest or some particularly strong interests?

• How do adaptations which allow this person to perform an activity change his or her experience of pleasure in the activity?

• Did this person lose skills he or she most enjoyed using?

The impact of interests on other aspects of an individual's life can be considered:

• In what ways have loss of interest, or inability to engage in interests, influenced the mood of this person?

• What does any loss of attraction or ability to pursue interests mean for this person's routine and activity choices?

• How extensive is any loss of satisfaction and pleasure in this person's life? Is there a significant drop in quality of life?

• Does the lack of attraction or loss of ability to pursue interests isolate this person from classmates, previous friends, etc?

Habits

Habits organize behavior to fit one's ecologies. They are manifest in one's style, use of time, and ways of doing occupational forms. Consideration of habits can begin with the following questions:

• Has this person had well-established habits? What kind of routine characterized this person when he or she was most adaptive? How does it differ from the present routine?
• What is this person's characteristic style of performance? How does this style fit with the social groups and occupational forms in this person's occupational behavior settings? Does this style support or interfere with effective performance?
• Is this person's routine effective for the occupational behavior settings in which he or she performs?
• What quality of life is provided by the habitual routine of this person?
• Do certain habits create problems in performance and how so?

Habits can be affected in a number of ways by disability; related questions are:

• In what ways has the disability disrupted or changed this person's daily routine?
• How have deficits in performance skills altered this person's ability to carry out occupations in habitual ways? Has he or she been able to acquire new habits? How do new habits affect overall lifestyle?
• What old habits need to be relinquished or modified as a result of the disability?
• What new habits will be required for this person to manage her or his disability?
• How do the vagaries of this person's illness stymie establishing new habit patterns or periodically interfere with the performance of old ones?
• How do barriers in the environment place constraints on the habit patterns this person can develop?

Roles

Roles provide a sense of identity, organize one's time and locate one in social groups. For competent role performance, persons must have internalized appropriate role scripts. Therapists can begin to ask about roles with consideration of these issues:

• What are the roles with which this person has identified and currently identifies? What is the overall pattern of role involvement of this person? Is the person over- or under-involved in roles? How important are each of these roles to the person?
• Has this person internalized functional role scripts for each of his or her roles? That is, can he or she organize his or her behavior to meet the expectations of the social groups to which each role belongs? In what situations can this person take on roles, knowing how to behave and anticipating and understanding what others expect, think, and feel?
• How might limited access to opportunities be influencing this person's ability to enact various roles? What succession of roles has this person experienced and how does this influence his or her present role identity?

Therapists should also consider how disability affects roles:

• In what ways might the lack or loss of necessary skills be affecting this person's ability to enact roles? What are the consequences for this person?
• What are the implications of role alteration or loss on this person's sense of identity, use of time, and involvement in social groups?
• How might a reduction in the task responsibility affect this person's sense of making a valued contribution to a group?
• Does this person experience conflict between others' expectations of role requirements and what he or she can actually do?
• Is there a conflict between this person's view of what successful enactment of a role entails and what he or she can actually do?
• How might fluctuating or unpredictable periods of dysfunction affect this person's

willingness and ability to assume role responsibilities?

- When do role requirements become too demanding or make conflicting demands on this person?

Changes in roles brought on or required by disability can significantly alter many aspects of a person's life. The following are some questions concerning the impact of role changes on loss:

- Will changes in performance require this person to find new groups in which to assume meaningful roles? What are the implications for this person's sense of identity?
- What challenges or opportunities are available for this person to replace lost roles?
- How does the loss or alteration of a significant role (such as the worker role) affect this person's enactment and satisfaction in other roles (such as parent or friend)?
- How has role loss influenced the economic, social, and other resources in this person's life?
- What impact does loss or alteration of roles have on this person's daily routine?

Disability can dramatically change the social role to which others assign an individual. In this regard therapists can consider:

- What impact does the reactions of friends and family have to validate or devalue the significance this person ascribes to new or altered roles? Is this person assigned by others to a disabled role and, if so, how does this affect her or his identity?
- How do values of the prevailing culture influence this person's adjustment to role loss?
- How might features of an extended sick role experience prove problematic in the resumption of this person's occupational roles?
- Why might this person feel that negotiating changes in role responsibilities might result in subsequent feelings of conflict and self-devaluation?

Mind-Brain-Body Performance Subsystem

Impairment of the mind-brain-body performance subsystem is common in persons with occupational dysfunction. Since many of the questions which might be asked about the subsystem emanate from other models of practice (e.g., biomechanical, sensory integrative), we will not discuss them here. However, as noted in Chapter 6, therapists should be aware of, and select, appropriate models when they wish to examine the symbolic, neurological, and musculoskeletal constituents of this subsystem.

One set of questions which can be raised about the mind-brain-body performance subsystem from the way we have conceptualized it in this text are concerned with the experience of performing with an altered or impaired subsystem. For example:

- How does this person describe the experience of being inside a body or mind they cannot entirely control?
- What particular body and/or mind experiences interfere with this person's performance and how do they do so?
- What kinds of changes in the mind and/or body has this person experienced? How does he or she describe them?
- How does this person feel about being in a body that will always be different from others and from the way he or she once was?
- What emotional or cognitive experiences are troubling for this person and how do they interfere with performance?
- What are the consequences of changed sensory, motor, or other capacities for this person's experience of performing activities?
- How do experiences of pain or fatigue influence this person's performance of occupational forms?
- How do alternative approaches to completing activities affect this person's experience and views of the meaning of occupations?

Such questions are aimed at gaining insight into the phenomenology of disability. That is, they provide insights to what a person with a disability experiences as he or she uses an impaired mind-brain-body to perform and to experience the world.

Questions Concerning the Environment

The second area of concern is the influence of the environment. Within this arena questions must be raised about how a person's environments may be affording or pressing for occupational behavior. Consequently, therapists consider the impact of spaces, objects, occupational forms, and social groups within the person's occupational behavior settings. The following are some questions related to the environment's influence:

- What performance and experience do space and objects in this person's occupational behavior settings afford and press for?
- Does this person encounter physical barriers to performance? Are previously used objects creating difficulty for the person now? Do the available objects discourage performance?
- Does the environment provide appropriate occupational forms in which this person can engage?
- Are some occupational forms too challenging or impossible for this person? Do the occupational forms sufficiently challenge this person and provide a sense of worth?
- Do the expectations of others in social groups support or inhibit this person's performance?
- How do the social groups of which this person is a member support the assumption of meaningful roles?
- What are the reactions of others in occupational behavior settings to this person's disability?
- How do the routines of occupational behavior settings support or challenge this person's occupational behavior?

Questions Concerning Systems Dynamics

This next and final area of concern is the dynamic process in which the person is lo-

cated. The first type of questions in this area will have to do with the skill which persons demonstrate when engaging in occupations in their environments. Chapter 8 provided a detailed set of definitions of motor, process, and communication/interaction skills. Each of those definitions (summarized at the end of that chapter) provides a concrete basis for asking the appropriate conceptual questions about skill in performance. Therefore, we have not listed or specified these questions here.

The second type of questions in this area have to do with the character or nature of the overall pattern of occupational behavior. Chapter 2 emphasized that the organization of the human system is influenced by an ongoing process—that is, by the occupational behavior in which the person engages. It is important that therapists focus not only on the various structures or organizational features of the person and of the environment, but also on the processes that characterize the person's interaction with the environment. This latter area also incudes the therapeutic process, since therapy represents organized attempts to forestall loss of abilities, maintain function, or achieve change through influencing persons' occupational behavior in the therapeutic session and beyond. The following are some generic questions to guide the therapist in this kind of inquiry:

- What is the quality of occupational behavior that characterizes this person now? Is he or she engaged in normal role behavior and maintaining habitual routines? Is this person involved in a variety of environments? Or, has the dynamic process of maintaining and changing organization become threatened by a cessation or reduction of occupation? That is, are skills and habits eroding due to disuse?
- What kind of experiences is this person having and how are they affecting his or her interests, personal causation, and values?
- Are there parts of this person's ongoing behavior and experience that support maintenance of the system or positive change? How can these behaviors be supported or enhanced?

As noted in Chapter 2, any factor in the person or the environment can become a control parameter for initiating and sustaining a particular kind of behavior. Thus, therapists should ask:

- Are parts of the system acting as control parameters sustaining incompetent performance? For example, is any of the following serving as a control parameter: fear of failure, lack of good habits, deficits in skills, or some object in the environment?

Generating One's Own Theoretical Questions

This discussion has illustrated some ways in which a therapist can translate the theory into conceptual questions to guide data collection. However, as we have noted, a therapist must both tailor these questions and generate additional questions to fit the emerging circumstances of gathering data on each particular patient. When translating concepts into theoretical questions, the therapist is seeking the relevance of the theory for *this* person's life.

A given question can result in a wide range of answers. For example, in response to questions one has about interests, a therapist may find one of the following:

- a passionate interest is sustaining a person's motivation to continue an occupation in the face of severe performance limitations, or
- an individual who has lost interest in previously pleasurable activities because of the interference of physical limitations and pain, and is depressed as a consequence.

Each of these different pieces of information suggest new questions:

- How can the first person be supported to continue involvement in the passionate interest?
- What was enjoyable about the lost interests for the person and what are opportunities to alter or replace these interests?

As the example illustrates, therapists must be prepared to generate new questions as the data collection process unfolds.

ANALYTIC REASONING WITH THEORY AND DATA

Therapists should use theory as a context for exploring and deciding what to make of, and where to go next, from the data one has gathered. For example, consider an occupational therapist gathering data from a client in work rehabilitation following an injury. An important consideration becomes understanding the place of the worker role in the person's habituation. Let us say the therapist learns that the client has a history of solid employment, identifies strongly with the work role, has a well-defined role script for the kind of work he or she has done for a long time, and envisions himself as moving beyond his current impairment to return to the work role.

At this point, the therapist may feel satisfied that the work role component of habituation is well-ordered and represents a strength for the patient. In such a case, the therapist can move on to other questions such as exploring the nature of the occupational forms the person performs on the job, asking if any gaps exist between the person's present and long-term limitations and what is required on the job. Next, the therapist may ask what changes in the skills or habits of the individual may be necessary to support the role and what modifications are possible in the workplace.

The therapist is able to move to each new question because previous data are made sense of in the context of the theory. That a client identifies strongly with the worker role and has a good role script (i.e., a thorough working knowledge of what the work entails), is what the theory specifies as a strength for occupational performance. The therapist knows that what this part of the system will contribute to the assembly of work behavior is positive; however, the therapist also knows from the theory that another part of the system may be serving as a control parameter preventing competent work performance. Using the theory the therapist will use other concepts to raise further questions. For example, the concept of skills provides a way of observing and thinking about how this person performs with his or her new impairment. If the data indicate that the person has permanent limitations in motor skills, they lead to new questions concerning whether process skills can be substituted for the permanently impaired motor skills. In addition, the concept of habits would lead the therapist to ask about how the person's work routine can be altered to accommodate limitations in motor skills. The therapist may also ask how the objects used, and the occupational forms performed on the job, affect performance.

As the therapist reasons with data, moving from one set of emerging data to the next, he or she is able to do so with a cognitive framework provided by the theory. The theory both provides a collection of concepts which can remind the therapist of what to consider and serves as a framework for integrating what is known about one aspect of a client with what is known about another aspect.

Reasoning with data is to create an explanation of the patient's circumstances. This explanation emerges in a dialectic between the data the therapist is gathering and the theory which the therapist is using to make sense of the data. What should result is a *particular theory of the circumstances of the individual patient in order to begin or continue therapy*. The therapist's reasoning serves to bridge the general concepts of the theory with the concrete particulars of the client. The former attempts to explain persons in general and the latter to explain a person in particular.

The theoretical constructs offered by the model are abstract categories for a class of phenomena, the individual expressions of which are as many as the individuals to which we apply the concept. For example, no one's experience of value is exactly the same. One person may have a value system tightly organized around a set of fundamental religious beliefs. In such a person's value system certain themes concerning morality, personal obligations, and ideals for conduct may predominate. In the case of another individual values may be approached in a very different way with different issues emphasized. In either case, the important thing to discover in data collection is how the particular individual's way of experiencing and expressing value influences his or her occupational life.

It should also be remembered that the definitions given for various concepts in the first chapters of this book are meant to orient therapists to what is meant by a particular construct. The language of the definition or the discussions in this text should not be taken for the sum total of what can be an expression or instance of a construct in practice. This is not an invitation for therapists to improvise what the concepts are intended to mean. However, therapists should take the definitions and theoretical discussions as a point of departure, providing a way of beholding patients or clients. With time, and with using a concept to view one's patients or clients, the concept should become both richer and clearer. In applying the theory, therapists should seek a course between ambiguous thinking that invites misunderstanding and strict orthodoxy which hampers application of the general theory to particular individuals.

In the same way, these theoretical arguments represent possible circumstances that may influence function or dysfunction. Systems concepts point out how important it is to gain an understanding of the dynamics that represent a given person's situation at a given point in time. For example, one theoretical argument of this model is that volition influences the activity choices of individuals. It further points out that volition may be a source of strength, sustaining a level of occupational functioning because of the person's value commitments, satisfaction, and/or sense of being able to achieve desired outcomes. Conversely, volition may be impaired, leading to poor activity choices or preventing persons from making choices. In such cases, loss of important life goals, inability to experience pleasure in action, and a sense of helplessness may all contribute to the problem. The therapist collects data in order to figure out what particular set of conditions represent *this* patient's occupational dysfunction.

The therapist who collects and reasons with data in therapy becomes, for those purposes, an investigator and theorist; that is, the therapist, like the researcher, collects data to answer questions derived from theory. Moreover, the therapist interprets the data in light of the theoretical framework and creates new theory in light of the data. This act of creating a local theory of a given person's situation is the core of theory use in clinical practice. It represents the most critical reasoning process performed by a therapist. Ultimately, it is the reason that general theories such as the model of human occupation exist. That is, the model of human occupation serves its purpose when it is a basis upon which therapists create their own theory-based explanations of their clients.

MORAL REASONING

We noted earlier that therapists make moral decisions that have to do with how a patient's life should unfold, what should be the outcome of therapy, and the good toward which therapy is aimed. These moral decisions are not easily made.

For moral reasoning, therapists must approach data in two ways. First, therapists use data to come to know *about* a client. That is, the therapist gathers and examines data from the point of view of someone looking in on the person's circumstances. Thus, for example, therapists gather and use data to draw conclusions about the level of skill of which a person is capable and about the impact that habits have on a person's ability to compensate for impairment. Such data are gathered and used to generate an understanding of the person's occupational functioning.

In addition, therapists must collect and use data to help them understand *how clients see themselves and their worlds*. These data, which represent the subjective viewpoint of clients, contain information about what they envision as the good in life or, said another way, what meaning they attribute to their lives.

As we saw in Chapter 4, persons experience meaning in their lives through volitional narratives which organize their knowledge of self and circumstances (i.e., personal causation, interests, and values) into a coherent schema. These narratives relate past, present, and potential life events into wholes that illustrate what one most desires or holds as important in life (Geertz, 1986; Gergen & Gergen, 1988; Mattingly, 1991; Mattingly & Fleming, 1993;

Schafer, 1981; Spence, 1982; Taylor, 1989). Discovering the life perspective of the patient as told in the volitional narrative should be done whenever possible since it represents the patient's view of the good worth pursuing in life.

The moral judgement which a therapist makes about what should be done in therapy represents an attempt to reconcile data which inform the therapist about the patient and that which allow the therapist to see the world through the perspective of the patient. Because the nature of this moral reasoning is imbedded in the specific situation it is impossible to specify ahead of time how therapists should interweave their evaluations and consequent action plans with the patient's life narrative. The process of moral reasoning is best illustrated then by example.

Thelma

We will take as our example Thelma[a] who is in her mid-thirties and a patient in a psychiatric day hospital program; she carries a diagnosis of bipolar disorder. Data *about* Thelma can be summarized as follows:

She was much more functional in the past. An honors student in high school, she was also a student council member and active in athletics. She entered junior college, majoring in Spanish and aspired to be an interpreter for the United Nations. She worked part-time in an office for two years to support herself in college. However, following the onset of her illness 25 years ago, she dropped out of school. Since that time she worked for varying lengths of time (never more than two years) in several jobs; she has not worked for 11 years. Thelma is amicable and verbal; while her work skills have undoubtedly suffered from disuse, she appears to have the basic capacities for work. Her habit patterns reflect a

[a]Thelma was previously discussed by one of the present authors and other colleagues in two articles: Helfrich, C., & Kielhofner, G. (1993). Volitional narratives and the meaning of therapy. *American Journal of Occupational Therapy, 48*, 319–326; Helfrich, C., Kielhofner, G., & Mattingly. C. (1993). Volition as narrative: Understanding motivation in chronic illness. *American Journal of Occupational Therapy, 48*, 311–317.

largely passive and inactive lifestyle that contributes, along with overeating, to her present obesity. Now, her roles are limited to a sporadic family role and her periodic role as a psychiatric patient. She has a variety of interests that include crafts and cooking and she still expresses some interest in working. She expresses a desire to have a more active lifestyle and possibly return to work, but both of these prospects appear to create a great deal of anxiety for her.

This understanding of Thelma represents the kind of explanation that is often generated about a patient. The understanding of the patient becomes much fuller if we peer inside the patient to see the world as she does through her volitional narrative. In Thelma's volitional narrative she is tragically transformed from an attractive, bright, ambitious, athletic, young woman into an unemployed, overweight, and undesirable woman. Rejected by others who see her as a "nut head, fruitcake" and who "don't take you serious or anything," she lives in public housing where it is not safe to be outside her apartment. From Thelma's own point of view, bipolar disorder has meant that her "hopes and dreams went down the tubes!" Within this story of a life gone down the tubes, she ponders her prospects for work as follows:

> I can't think of what I would excel with. I don't know. I type pretty good. I could do stuff like that. That wouldn't be so good just typing all day long for somebody like term papers and stuff, assignments here and something small or something. That would sort of dwindle down to nothing.

Similarly, she considers whether it would make sense to return to school:

> I wouldn't mind going back to school if I knew it would help me, but I don't know. Sitting in the classroom all those weeks and months and not get anything out of it, it would be a very sour experience. And if I ever got a job I got to pay full fee for my apartment. I don't want to be making the wrong move and then I'll be stuck with nothing, you know. I don't want to open up any doors I couldn't close.

Indeed, it seems to Thelma that attempting to make her life better could instead make it worse:

> It's hard getting a job out there. You see, you may get one and then you may get sick again, or have a relapse. You're out in the cold again trying to get back on disability. You might not even get as much as you have now. I've got to weigh the situation very kindly before I go out there and bite the dust again.

Clearly, Thelma's volition is dominated by a narrative in which any attempt to make life much better carries the risk of a further downward slide, making life even worse.

In providing therapy for Thelma, the therapist is faced with the question: What should be the goal of therapy? Or more broadly: How can Thelma's life be improved? The answer does not come easily and must involve consideration of both data about Thelma and the way that Thelma sees her life. The therapist knows that Thelma's life is not satisfactory to her nor does it meet societal expectations for a productive and independent adult. Given her early history and remaining skills, there appears to be a strong rationale for Thelma improving her life by becoming more active and possibly returning to work.

However, such objectives would make little sense from the perspective of Thelma's volitional narrative. Therefore, should therapy aim at returning her to work and possibly risk making her life even worse than now? Should Thelma get out of her apartment more, even though it may expose her to violent crime? These are moral questions with which the therapist and Thelma should struggle in therapy. The answers require more data about Thelma's actual options for living and working. They may depend on a more detailed determination of Thelma's skills and potential for employment. Indeed, the answers can only emerge out of ongoing data collection and reasoning by the therapist who must collaborate with Thelma in the formation of a vision of where her life might go and how therapy can help it get there.

The moral questions of therapy most often emerge when a therapist must weigh alternatives, deal with dilemmas, and arbitrate between conflicting interests. Such considerations may weigh, for example, (1) the need of a physically disabled child for frequent therapy against family needs for a normal life pattern;

(2) the need of a worker for job modification against the concerns of coworkers whose jobs will change or become more complicated as a result; (3) the dilemma of a person with quadriplegia over whether to expend the energy necessary to be independent in self-care or to save energy for other occupations by having an attendant. Such dilemmas permeate the necessary moral reasoning in therapy. The answers are never easy, but they are more forthcoming when therapists ask the right questions and have the appropriate data with which to reason.

References

Coles, R. (1989). *The call of stories: Teaching and the moral imagination*. Boston: Houghton Mifflin.

Geertz, C. (1986). Making experiences, authoring selves. In V. Turner & E. Bruner (Ed.), *The anthropology of experience* (pp. 373–380). Urbana, IL: University of Illinois Press.

Gergen, K. J., & Gergen, M. M. (1988). Narrative and the self as relationship. In L. Berkowitz (Ed.), *Advances in experimental social psychology* (pp. 17–56). San Diego: Academic Press.

Mattingly, C. (1991). The narrative nature of clinical reasoning. *American Journal of Occupational Therapy, 45,* 998–1005.

Mattingly, C., & Fleming, M. (1993). *Clinical reasoning: Forms of inquiry in a therapeutic practice*. Philadelphia: FA Davis.

Schafer, R. (1981). Narration in the psychoanalytic dialogue. In W. J. T. Mitchell (Ed.), *On narrative* (pp. 25–49). Chicago, IL: University of Chicago Press.

Spence, D. P. (1982). *Narrative truth & historical truth: Meaning and interpretation in psychoanalysis*. New York: WW Norton.

Taylor, C. (1989). *Sources of the self: The making of the modern identity*. Cambridge, MA: Harvard University Press.

12/ Methods of Data Gathering

Gary Kielhofner, Trudy Mallinson, and Carmen Gloria de las Heras

METHODS OF DATA GATHERING

Therapists gather data through both structured and situated means. Structured means of data gathering (typically referred to as assessments, evaluations, or instruments) employ protocols which must be followed for the method to work according to its design. Situated methods are devised by the therapist in the course of therapy to obtain data. We refer to them as situated methods since they arise out of therapists' efforts to get data in ways that match a specific situation. As we will see, both methods have their place in the course of intervention. Structured methods use tested means for gathering information, guard against bias, and provide data which are readily interpretable. Situated methods capitalize on therapists' more intimate knowledge of patients and upon unique opportunities that arise for getting useful information in informal, spontaneous, and creative ways. Gathering data is optimal when therapists select and use both methods systematically and thoughtfully.

STRUCTURED METHODS OF DATA GATHERING

Structured data-gathering procedures: (a) have a specified protocol for use, (b) have been systematically developed with research to determine that the assessment is dependable, and (c) have some formal basis for interpreting the data obtained.

Protocol

Through experience, field testing, and research, investigators develop and determine optimal methods for gathering particular data. Once these methods have been determined they become part of the formal protocol of a data-gathering method. Protocols may consist of such things as a standard context in which observation is done, a set of questions to ask in an interview, or a specific scale used in making ratings. Depending on the nature of the assessment these protocols may be very strict or they may allow some adaptation to circumstances. Following the protocol allows one to know that a proven method of getting data is being used; that is, since one is replicating a procedure which has been developed through research, the data should be dependable.

Evidence of Dependability

When we say a data-gathering method is dependable, we mean two things. First, a dependable data-gathering method is reliable; it will give the same information within reasonable variations of administration (e.g., in different circumstances, on different clients, when different therapists use it). Second, a dependable data-gathering method is valid in that it really measures what it is intended to measure.

The science of developing standardized data-gathering methods employs a variety of statistical approaches to examine the properties of the method in actual use. Ordinarily series of studies are conducted to appraise whether a particular data-gathering procedure consistently provides the kind of information one intends. In the course of these studies refinements in the data-gathering method are made to approximate the ideal of dependability.

Structured methods of data collection, including those presented in this chapter, vary widely in how thoroughly they have been studied. Moreover, all methods—no matter how thoroughly researched—have some limitations. Therapists should have an awareness of the known properties of the structured methods they use. This knowledge allows the therapist to know how much confidence should be placed in the data collected. The confidence one places in a method should be commensurate with what is known about the data collection method from both research and practical experience.

Means of Interpretation

Structured methods provide data in the form of categorization, designation of degree, or determination of amount. By categorizing, a method may determine, for example, whether a person belongs to one group or another or whether a person does or doesn't have a given problem. Designation of degree determines whether a person has more or less of some characteristic. Determination of amount refers to how much of a characteristic someone has. Structured methods may also guide the user to generate descriptive information. Importantly, structured methods incorporate a means of interpreting or determining the meaning of the data obtained from the method.

Some data-gathering methods used in occupational therapy provide a single score or series of scores to be interpreted by the therapist. Scores obtained through such assessments may be interpreted in terms of their deviation from some norm or average. For example, therapists can compare scores that persons receive on tests of ability or developmental level to determine whether persons have less ability than average or whether they are delayed in development. Some authors have pointed out that such approaches have limited functional significance, may be culturally biased, and fail to recognize that individual differences can be adaptive (Fisher, 1993; Spencer, Krefting, & Mattingly, 1993).

An alternative means of interpreting data is by reference to some criteria. Assessments that use criteria have the advantage that the functional significance of a score can be specified (Fisher, 1993). For example, in the context of work hardening, a therapist may use the crite-

ria of what a worker has to do on the job in order to interpret a score. If a worker must be able to lift 100 pounds to do her or his job, then the functional significance of the ability to lift 80 pounds can be more readily interpreted than by comparing it to what persons are, on average, able to lift.

Still other assessments are interpreted according to the patterns they reveal. Data-gathering methods which rely on the pattern of scores for interpretation require the therapist to interpret each person's pattern individually. For example, therapists interpret the Interest Checklist and Role-Checklist (which are discussed later in this chapter) by identifying such patterns as having only solitary interests or having several currently interrupted roles. The patterns themselves may be evidence of a problem or they may be useful in determining the nature of a person's dysfunction.

Benefits of Structured Data Collection Methods

Writers have correctly encouraged occupational therapists to make use of standardized or formal assessments (Bonder, 1993; Fisher & Short-DeGraff, 1993; Watts, Brollier, Bauer, & Schmidt, 1989). Some reasons behind such exhortations are: (a) When therapists use structured assessments they benefit from the systematic effort which has gone into creating a methods of data gathering. (b) Consumers and other professionals have some assurance that the procedure is worth the therapist's time and effort and yields useful information. (c) Such methods are less likely to yield data which is misleading or personally biased. Consequently, when appropriate structured data collection methods are available and feasible, therapists are well advised to use them. Coordinating the use of structured methods with situated methods into a comprehensive plan of data gathering will be discussed later in this chapter.

STRUCTURED DATA COLLECTION METHODS USED WITH THE MODEL

The three most common structured data collection methods developed for, and used in association with, the model of human occupation are observational measures, self-report questionnaires and checklists, and structured interviews. In the following three sections we will briefly describe those assessments and their use. In the appendix to this chapter, more detailed descriptions of each of these data collection methods are found along with information about the procedure's reliability and validity, intended use, required skills or training, availability, and references in the literature. The materials in the appendix will provide the reader with the necessary information to decide whether a particular assessment would be appropriate for a particular kind of use. It will also give the therapist all the necessary information about how to obtain the instrument in order to learn to use it properly.

Observational Measures

The methods discussed in this section gather data from observation of a patient's or client's behavior. Performance is rated by the observing therapist and the ratings are used to produce a measure of some observed capacity or characteristic.

Observational Measures of Skills

The Assessment of Motor and Process Skills (AMPS) (Fisher, 1994) and the Assessment of Communication and Interaction Skills (ACIS) (Salamy, Simon, & Kielhofner, 1993) have been developed to measure skill. The AMPS employs observation of patients performing occupational forms. The ACIS uses observations of persons involved in social groups. Both the AMPS and the ACIS are based on the skills noted in Chapter 8. Each of the motor, process, or communication/interaction skills appear as items on the rating scales used by the AMPS and ACIS.[a]

---

[a] The same is true of the social interaction scale, which is an alternative approach to measuring communication/interaction skills as discussed in Chapter 8. Since the scale is not yet available in English—it was originally developed and studied in Sweden—it is not discussed here. In the future the scale is likely to be available as an independent scale or alternately as a hybrid scale incorporating ideas from the social interaction scale and the ACIS.

The AMPS and ACIS represent a unique approach to the problem of assessing a patient's ability to function in everyday life. As discussed in Chapter 8, many assessments observe performance and attempt to make inferences about underlying capacity (e.g., strength, range of motion, perception, cognition). These include tests specifically designed only to test underlying impairments (e.g., tests of perception, strength, and mental status). They also include tests designed to measure underlying performance based on observation of a more global task. While such instruments can be helpful in determining impairments in the mind-brain-body performance subsystem that may contribute to performance difficulties, they are limited as explanations or predictors of actual performance as they still must be based on performance. Conversely, assessments such as typical activities of daily living checklists and other similar tests provide information about what a person can or cannot do, but they do not tell the therapist why a patient cannot perform an occupational form.

The AMPS and ACIS have been designed with an eye toward overcoming some of these limitations of traditional strategies of data collection. They provide detailed information about the actual performance difficulties a person experiences in a given occupational form. The AMPS consists of two scales that separately measure process and motor skills. The two scales are administered simultaneously, and this allows for direct evaluation of the interactive nature of motor and process skills (e.g., use of process skills to compensate for limitations in motor skills). A more detailed description of the AMPS can be found in the appendix at the end of this chapter and in the case of Diane in Chapter 14.

The use of the ACIS to evaluate communication/interaction skills can be illustrated through the case of Gilbert, a student in a special education classroom. Gilbert had Down's syndrome and was considered moderately retarded. He was enrolled in a class which included other students with intellectual deficits. Like a number of other students in the class, Gilbert exhibited aggressive behavior and was deemed a troublemaker by the teacher and aide who ran the classroom. The occupational therapist was asked to evaluate Gilbert's social skills and make recommendations concerning managing his aggression.

The occupational therapist observed Gilbert in the classroom, during recess, and during lunchtime. The ratings and comments on the ACIS score sheet (illustrated in Figure 12.1) were made from the composite of these observations.

As the ratings and comments demonstrate, Gilbert had competent language skills. In contrast, he had problems with physicality. When he was excited or angry he tended to use physical forms of expression which made others uncomfortable or upset. He also had problems engaging with others, respecting social norms and in asserting himself. Based on the assessment, the therapist could recommend two strategies. The first was to provide training and feedback to Gilbert about his physical use of self in communication and interaction. The therapist recommended and devised examples

Figure 12.1.   Gilbert: Scores* and comments on the Assessment of Communication and Interaction Skills.

*4 = COMPETENT 3 = QUESTIONABLE 2 = INEFFECTIVE 1 = DEFICIT					
PHYSICALITY					
Gestures	1	2	3	④	
Gazes	1	②	3	4	Avoids eye contact in many interactions. When angry, he stares.
Approximates	①	2	3	4	Often invades others' space; is overly affectionate or aggressive.
Postures	1	②	3	4	Sometimes looms threateningly over others.
Contacts	①	2	3	4	Hits others to get attention. Hits others when angry.
LANGUAGE					
Articulates	1	2	3	④	
Speaks	1	2	3	④	
Focuses	1	2	3	④	
Emanates	1	2	③	4	Sometimes gets over excited and raises voice and speed of speech.
Modulates	1	2	3	④	
RELATIONS					
Engages	1	②	3	4	Is ineffective at initiating conversation often uses poor strategies to engage others (e.g., hugging, hitting)
Relates	1	2	③	4	Can be genuinely nice to be with, but has problems when upset.
Respects	①	2	3	4	Takes other people's food; forces his way in line.
Collaborates	1	②	3	4	Can work with others in a structured game or task, but needs support and supervision.
INFORMATION EXCHANGE					
Asks	1	2	3	④	
Expresses	1	2	③	4	Mainly communicates when he is upset.
Shares	1	2	3	④	
Asserts	①	2	3	4	Is aggressive instead of assertive.

of role-playing situations to practice appropriate skills. The therapist also recommended the use of videotape to help Gilbert become more aware of how he behaved and how this behavior affected others, as well as to allow him to see the difference in his own behavior when he used more skillful ways of interacting. The second recommendation was to provide Gilbert with specific training in how to initiate interactions with others and how to assert himself without becoming aggressive, since these were two major problem areas for him. Once again, role-playing and use of videotape was also recommended to allow Gilbert to see his own behavior. As this case illustrates, the ACIS is useful for providing a profile of strengths and weaknesses in communication and interaction skills and, in so doing, in enabling the therapist to target specific skills for intervention.

Volitional Questionnaire

Another measure which is based on observation of behavior is the Volitional Questionnaire (de las Heras, 1993b). This observational rating scale was developed as a means of obtaining information about volition from persons who could not effectively report on their own volition (e.g., persons with substantial cognitive limitations). Prior to development of the Volitional Questionnaire, there was no structured volitional assessment available to occupational therapists for use with persons who were unable to complete the checklists or respond to the interviews ordinarily used to gather data on volition.

Working in a state hospital with a population of patients who had mental retardation and/or mental illness, de las Heras (1993a) began the development of this method of gathering data on volition from observation of patient participation in occupations. Occupational therapists administer this scale by observing and rating patients while they engage in work, leisure, or daily living tasks. The ratings are summed to produce a score indicating the amount of volitional spontaneity (versus passivity or need for support and encouragement) the individual demonstrates. This instrument is intended for examining the effect of different environments on volitional spontaneity and for tracking volition over time. For example, the instrument's original author used it to monitor the impact of motivational programs on improving volition. Additionally, the instrument can be used to provide insights into individuals' reactions to different occupational forms and circumstances (e.g., when they become involved versus passive). Finally, the individual items on the scale (shown in Figure 12.2) highlight areas of volitional strengths and weaknesses.

In addition to the ratings obtained on the scale, the instrument provides a structured means of describing a person's volition; the scale and the descriptive data together provide detailed information on volition.

To examine the use of the volitional questionnaire in the context of intervention, let us consider Alexander, a 30-year-old man who has lived in state institutions since he was ten years old. Currently hospitalized due to his inability to cope with frustration and a tendency to become extremely physically aggressive, he has not been allowed to leave the ward for reasons of safety. Recently, staff have been work-

I. Intrinsic Motivation	II. Personal Causation
Demonstrates interest in the environment	Shows initiative
III. Values/Interests	Tries new things
	Indicates pride
Demonstrates preferences for activity	Shows satisfaction when complimented
Shows enjoyment in particular activity	Is willing to try to fix own mistakes
Stays within an activity	Is willing to try to solve problems
Is lively/energetic in particular activities	Attempts to support others
Indicates/pursues simple goals	
Shows that an activity is special to her/him	

Figure 12.2. Items on the Volitional Questionnaire.

ing with Alexander to enable him to attend work outside the ward. Alexander has begun to attend a work program where he is learning how to work on computers and do other clerical tasks. Alexander also is interested in painting and has begun to go to the art studio in the hospital. He still must be kept on the ward frequently for not complying with rules. On such occasions, he becomes even more upset and is sometimes physically aggressive. Staff are concerned that such behavior may occur when he is off the ward.

The therapist determined that Alexander was not likely to provide a great deal of verbal information on his own volition. He does not verbalize self-reflective information and would likely have difficulty talking about or responding to questionnaires that asked about his volition. Consequently, it was decided that the best method to learn about his volition was through observation. The Volitional Questionnaire was used in order to observe Alexander's personal causation, interests, and values and determine what would be the most appropriate way to help him control himself in the work center, art studio, and during activities of daily living on the ward. His ratings on the Volitional Questionnaire for these three settings are found in Figure 12.3. The following is a description of Alexander's behavior as the therapist observed it in the work center. By comparing the following description with the ratings and comments from this observation shown in Figure 12.3 the reader can see how the Volitional Questionnaire is used to structure and summarize observations of volition.

The Work Center consists of a computer room and a clerical functions room. It is a very busy place that handles numerous contracts that require word processing, designing and making fliers and invitations, collating, copying, and mailing. Up to six people work in the center at any one time with one or two vocational counselors available to provide training and assistance.

Alexander arrived at 9:15 a.m. and apologized to the supervisor, explaining that he was 15 minutes late because he didn't change his clothes on time. He repeatedly asked not to be docked in payment, but the supervisor explained that he could not be paid for time he missed. Alexander accepted the explanation and went into the computer room to work. Looking around, he commented that things were busy, and there was a lot to do. The supervisor asked him to choose between collating, copying, and mailing since all the computers were in use at the time. Alexander protested that he always started work on the computer and persisted in requesting to use the computer. Then, he approached another worker at a computer, asking him to leave. The supervisor offered him the other alternatives again, which he didn't accept. He insisted that his favorite activity was the computer and that he wouldn't do anything else, whereupon the supervisor asked him to leave the room and calm down. Despite resting for ten minutes, Alexander still insisted on using the computer, again apologizing for being late. However, after some discussion, he agreed to work on another task—copying. He had to make 100 copies of a flier and 50 of a memo. After he made the first copy of the flier he realized that he needed to reduce the size or use a bigger paper. He asked the supervisor for assistance, but when the supervisor began to demonstrate the task, Alexander stopped him, saying that he couldn't do it, that it was too hard for him, and that he had never done it before. The supervisor tried to convince him to try it, but he resisted. Then the supervisor made the necessary adjustments on the machine and Alexander completed the job successfully. Smiling, he showed the copies to the supervisor indicating he didn't make any mistakes. Carefully placing the copies in separate boxes, he put a sign on each box. Asking the supervisor for more work, he requested the occupied computer again, but finally accepted working on collating a document of twenty pages. Though he had only collated five pages together previously, he smiled and began to do the job. In the middle of the work, he realized he had mixed up two pages of the document, increasing his pace as he continued. After reviewing the document twice, he switched the pages to the right order. He continued working and telling the supervisor that he really liked it because it was the same all the time and volunteering

Figure 12.3. Alexander: Ratings on the Volitional Questionnaire worksheet.*

Area to Evaluate	Environment	Rating	Rationale
Intrinsic Motivation			
Demonstrates Interest/ Curiosity in the Environment	WORK	4	Spontaneously looked around and commented about the amount of work to do
	ART STUDIO	4	Asked for people to come. Recognized other people's work, said hello, spontaneously.
	ADL	2	Generally passive in participating in most of the ADL, but he is actively participating in community meeting.
Personal Causation			
Shows Initiative	WORK	4	He initiated all tasks assigned. He initiated spontaneously.
	ART STUDIO	4	Initiated all tasks spontaneously
	ADL	2	Generally passive even after reminding. Only takes initiative in tasks he is interested in. He initiates work only when there is strict prompting from therapist.
Tries New Things	WORK	2	Shows hesitation to try new work, needs significant support.
	ART STUDIO	3	Spontaneous in trying new colors and different colors of paper, but he needed extra support and encouragement from therapist to be involved in cleaning the crayon box.
	ADL	1	Totally passive and overreacts to changes in that environment (change time in lunch, move rooms).
Indicates Pride (verbally or non-verbally)	WORK	4	He shows products and good results to others.
	ART STUDIO	4	Shows products to others in group. Makes positive comments of his painting spontaneously.
	ADL	4	When successful in writing minutes, he shows to others spontaneously.
Shows Satisfaction When Complimented	WORK	4	Thanks and smiles spontaneously when complimented.
	ART STUDIO	4	Spontaneously thanks and smiles. Confirms verbally others feedback.
	ADL	4	Thanks and smiles when receives feedback spontaneously.

continued

Figure 12.3.   Personal Causation—*continued*

Area to Evaluate	Environment	Rating	Rationale
Is Willing to Try to Fix Own Mistakes	WORK	4	*(Pages on collating & computer button) he tries to solve mistakes spontaneously.*
	ART STUDIO	N/A	*No opportunity to assess*
	ADL	1	*He was quite passive on this indicator, does not recognize responsibilities for lateness/ overreacts, although therapists remind him.*
Is Willing to Try to Solve Problems	WORK	2	*When problems presented, he shows hesitation in trying to solve them and needs a substantial amount of support from supervisor.*
	ART STUDIO	4	*He spontaneously tries to solve problems emerged from the tasks though the strategies he adopts are not always appropriate.*
	ADL	1	*Needs a lot of prompting from therapist to deal with inconveniences, (opening door, late for work, example).*
Attempts to Support Others	WORK	N/A	*No opportunity to assess*
	ART STUDIO	4	*Spontaneously gives positive comments on others at the beginning of the session.*
	ADL	N/A	*No opportunity to assess*
Values/Interest			
States/Demonstrates Preferences for Activity	WORK	4	*Clearly prefers computer work. From three alternatives he spontaneously chose copying.*
	ART STUDIO	4	*Demonstrates preferences for drawing with bright crayon colors.*
	ADL	4	*Spontaneous preferences for taking minutes in meeting and going off the ward.*
Shows Enjoyment in Particular Activities	WORK	4	*Spontaneously asks for more work. Smiles, spontaneously says he will do things again.*
	ART STUDIO	4	*Pace of production, immediate initiation of tasks, plans to return*
	ADL	2	*Does not demonstrate enjoyment of any ADL, but shows enjoyment when in community meeting, e.g., shows note to therapist.*
Stays With an Activity	WORK	4	*He completes all work even if it was new to him.*
	ART STUDIO	4	*He stayed spontaneously in activities of choice, i.e., community meeting.*
	ADL	2	*Has great difficulty in finishing self-care activity.*

continued

Figure 12.3. Values/Interest—*continued*

Area to Evaluate	Environment	Rating	Rationale
Is Lively/Energetic in Particular Activities	WORK	4	*Spontaneously increases pace and creativity in particular tasks.*
	ART STUDIO	4	*He also shows creativity and fast rate of production, changes shapes and colors of papers.*
	ADL	2	*He is especially energetic in community meeting.*
Indicates/Pursues Simple Goals	WORK	4	*Makes decisions spontaneously on flier, activities to do, activities to choose. Makes decision on keeping the products safe.*
	ART STUDIO	4	*Changes styles of drawing, creativity, goal directed behavior during whole session.*
	ADL	4	*Makes decisions on what to do. Clear demonstration of when he needs to go to work.*
Shows that an Activity Is Special or Significant to Her/Him	WORK	4	*Stores products safely, constant interest in computer, functioning well and spontaneously with recognition.*
	ART STUDIO	4	*Enjoys company of OT, drawing with crayons. Keeps his materials in box. Takes care of materials spontaneously.*
	ADL	4	*When asked to go to work, when taking notes in meetings, values his belongings and structure.*

*Readers should note that Figure 12.3 is *not* an example of the Volitional Questionnaire score sheet. Refer to the Appendix for more details.

that he would do it again if he couldn't work on the computer. He was congratulated for his success and for considering other alternatives when the computers were not available. Smiling, he acknowledged this.

Half an hour before the session was over a computer became available, and he immediately asked if he could do some work on the computer. He had to design a recruitment flier for the art studio. While there were some directions, the flier needed composition and design of logos and letters. Smiling, Alexander asked the supervisor if he could improvise on that flier. He chose new logos and changed some of the organization of the letters. He then began to compose it on the computer. After trying one key for a while to call up a logo, he realized he was pressing the wrong key, and corrected his mistake. After finishing the flier, he made a copy that he proudly

showed to his supervisor and showed the other workers his work.

Figure 12.3 also includes the ratings and comments obtained from the art studio and activities of daily living observations. As the ratings and comments show, Alexander showed similar volitional strengths in each of the occupational forms, but had more problems in self-care tasks. From these and other observations, the therapist completed the final brief summary report (see Figure 12.4) which is part of the Volitional Questionnaire. For instance, she was able to conclude that Alexander's enjoyment and sense of efficacy in activities often depended on the amount of social support available in a given environment. She was therefore able to make appropriate treatment recommendations.

As the ratings and summary report show, a great deal of information about a person's volition can be gleaned from this assessment. Both the ratings, which show areas of strength and weakness, and the written report structured by the volitional questionnaire are useful in gaining a detailed understanding of a person's personal causation, values, and interests.

Self-Report Checklists and Questionnaires

The self-report instruments discussed in this section have been designed so that they can be self-administered, paper and pencil inventories. In practice, therapists can use these methods of data collection in different ways to accommodate limitations of both the patient and the treatment environment. For example, they are sometimes administered verbally; they may be completed from reports of family members when the patient is incapable of reporting. Sometimes they are completed in group discussion sessions.

The self-report instruments we will discuss here are the Role-Checklist, the Interest Checklist, the Occupational Questionnaire, the Activity Record, and the Self Assessment of Occupational Functioning. With the exception of the Interest Checklist which existed prior to the introduction of the model, these data collection methods were first developed as part of efforts to research and apply the model in practice.

Role-Checklist

The Role-Checklist (Oakley, Kielhofner, & Barris, 1985) was developed as a means of identifying clients' role-identification as well as determining the value a person attached to roles. Using the taxonomy of 10 roles presented in Chapter 5 (see Table 5.1), the checklist asks the respondents to indicate for each role: (a) whether they have held the role in the past, (b) whether they are currently in the role, (c) whether they expect to be in the role in the future, and (d) how much they value the role. Brief lay-oriented definitions of each role are given on the checklist. Since the model is concerned with how roles structure occupational behavior, the definitions employ the criteria of at least weekly involvement in each role. Thus, for example, being a family member is defined

not merely as a relationship but as *doing something* with a family member at least once a week.

The instrument can be filled out in a few minutes. It may be filled out independently or with therapist assistance. Occupational therapists find it very useful to discuss the pattern of responses with the client in order to obtain more detailed information on the person's role-pattern and its meaning for function. Some therapists have clients fill it out along with several other persons in a group where discussion can be used to search for the meaning of each person's responses. In this context, the checklist can facilitate planning future role-behavior.

The Role-Checklist is interpreted by examining the pattern of responses; a summary sheet aids in the visual examination and interpretation of the response pattern. We will illustrate the interpretive process through two contrasting examples. Figure 12.5 shows the Role-Checklist Summary Sheet for Ray, a 36-year-old man hospitalized during an acute episode of mental illness.

Ray's pattern of role-identification and value shows a tendency to overload himself with roles, which leads to the inability to maintain any roles (his current circumstance). Ray's occupational therapist was able to use this information to share with him her observation about this tendency, as reflected in his expectations for future roles and assignment of high value to almost every role. She helped Ray to prioritize which roles were most important and to identify which roles he wanted to reinstitute first.

In contrast, Velma, a 71-year-old woman who has hemiplegia as the result of a recent stroke, indicated on the Role-Checklist that, of her past roles as a worker, home-maintainer, friend, and family member, she most wanted to maintain in the future her home-maintainer and family member roles since these are the ones she most valued (Figure 12.6). Velma's clear identification of her roles is interpreted as a habituation strength and a resource for her rehabilitation. This information served as a basis for treatment planning which emphasized those skills necessary for maintaining her valued roles.

Motivation: *Alexander is highly motivated for leisure and work. He is curious and spontaneously explores alternatives offered or conditions in the environment. His motivation for self care activities is lower than for work or leisure.*

Personal Causation: *Alexander demonstrates better personal causation in valued environments such as work or leisure. He is able to recognize personal accomplishments and responds well to praise. He is able to confront new situations, problems or mistakes only if constant social support and clear expectations are provided. He loses control when no support is given or when situations are confusing. He tends to get frustrated even with minimal changes to his environment. He also loses control under hectic conditions or in rigid environments and when not involved in valued activities.*

Values: *Alexander strongly values work, structure, art, his own belongings, staff, company and attention. He does not value self care activities, being on his ward, and being under control of the staff.*

Interests: *Alexander demonstrates strong interest in working on computers, writing, drawing with crayons and watching and talking about Science Fiction movies. His pattern of interests is mostly isolated and intellectual.*

Final Conclusion: *Alexander functions better when participating in valued occupations with clear limits and expectations and when consistent social support is given. He can become very spontaneous, creative and helpful to others when these conditions are provided. His personal causation is negatively influenced by the rigidity of his ward environment where he gets the most attention if he loses control. There is a significant difference in his ability to cope with undesirable outcomes when he is in supportive environment that provides*
(Including *opportunities for processing the difficulties, allows him time to calm down*
Nursing *and gives help to confront changes. His low level of enjoyment in self-care*
Questionnaire) *activities is questionable in the sense that it may be related to how he feels in his ward.*

Figure 12.4. Alexander: Summary Report of the Volitional Questionnaire.

Occupational therapists find that sharing interpretations of the Role-Checklist with clients is helpful. Clients tend to find the checklist revealing since the responses provide a concrete pattern to which persons can often relate. For example, one depressed patient, having filled out the form, noted his several past roles. He reflected that he had been feeling very incompetent, but on having seen how many roles he was able to fill in the past, he felt better about his abilities and more hopeful for the future. Sharing interpretations can also be a way of understanding better what clients meant when filling out the form and it can begin a process through which patient and therapist come to a common understanding of the patient's occupational role-pattern.

Interest Checklist

The Interest Checklist was originally developed by Matsutsuyu (1969). Later, when the checklist was being routinely used in associa-

tion with the model, it was modified by Scaffa (1981) and by Kielhofner & Neville (1983). The original Neuropsychiatric Institute (NPI) Interest Checklist (Matsutsuyu, 1969) has 68 interests toward which the respondent indicates "strong," "casual," or "no" interest.

The current modified version of the Interest Checklist also includes opportunity for the respondent to indicate how interests have changed and to indicate whether the activity is one in which a person participates or wishes to participate in the future. The additional responses in the modified version gather data about interest changes associated with occupational dysfunction, about how interests influence activity choices and about desires to participate in interests in the future, which could have implications for therapy. Both the original version of the checklist and the modified form are in use.

The Interest Checklist is a leisure interest inventory. While it can be used to gather information relevant to a person's overall occupa-

ROLE	Role Identification			Value Designation		
	PAST	PRESENT	FUTURE	NOT AT ALL	SOME-WHAT	VERY
Student	✓		✓			✓
Worker	✓		✓			✓
Volunteer	✓				✓	
Care Giver					✓	
Home Maintainer	✓		✓			✓
Friend	✓		✓			✓
Family Member	✓		✓			✓
Religious Participant	✓		✓			✓
Hobbyist/Amateur	✓		✓			✓
Participant in Organizations						✓
Other:						

Figure 12.5.   Ray: Role Checklist summary sheet.

ROLE	Role Identification			Value Designation		
	PAST	PRESENT	FUTURE	NOT AT ALL	SOME-WHAT	VERY
Student						
Worker	✓					✓
Volunteer						
Care Giver						
Home Maintainer	✓		✓			✓
Friend	✓					✓
Family Member	✓		✓			✓
Religious Participant						
Hobbyist/Amateur						
Participant in Organizations						
Other:						

Figure 12.6.   Velma: Role Checklist summary sheet.

tional interests, its main focus is on obtaining information about avocational interests that influence activity choices. This checklist is interpreted by examining the pattern of interests. Originally, it was thought that the check-list would be useful in determining clusters of interests (i.e., whether a person's interests were manual versus intellectual or cultural). Research failed to establish the validity of such clusters of interests (Rogers, Weinstein, &

Figone, 1978) and practical use suggests that the main value of the checklist is in what it reveals about each individual's unique pattern of interests. For example, Erik, a young man with a diagnosis of schizophrenia, indicated the following strong interests on the checklist: radio, walking, listening to popular music, movies, listening to classical music, attending lectures, and reading. All of these interests he pursued alone, despite the fact that he complained of being lonely. The only strong interests that involved interaction with others were holiday activities, which his family organized, and bowling, which was an activity organized by the day hospital he attended. What the pattern illustrated was that, given his own interest pattern, Erik would make activity choices that kept him isolated from others. Erik's interest checklist and the clarification his occupational therapist received when discussing it with him provided necessary information to develop a conclusion that his interest pattern led to dissatisfying activity choices. This discussion also helped to develop treatment objectives that helped Erik find ways to pursue some of his current interests with others and of developing new, more socially-oriented interests.

The checklist reflects middle-class, mainstream American interests at the time of its development in 1969. Therefore, some of the interests on the list may not be relevant (or even known) to some populations and cultures. More importantly, other interests currently popular may not be reflected in the checklist. For this reason, therapists have modified the items on the checklist. While this makes practical sense, one limitation of checklists in such modified forms is that they have not been examined in research. However, given that the assessment is interpreted by examining the pattern of interest, the value of having a culturally and lifestyle-relevant assessment would appear to outweigh using a standard form with limited relevance.

Occupational Questionnaire and the NIH Activity Record

Activity configurations in which clients report their actual or typical activities over a period of time (e.g., a day) have traditionally been used by occupational therapists to examine how persons use their time as well as the activities that fill that time. The NIH Activity Record (Furst, Gerber, Smith, Fisher, & Shulman, 1987) and the Occupational Questionnaire (Smith, Kielhofner, & Watts, 1986) are similar in this regard; each of these self-report forms ask the client to indicate what activity he or she engages in over the course of a weekday and weekend day.

The Occupational Questionnaire, upon which the Activity Record is based, is the simpler form. As illustrated in Figure 12.7, it asks persons to report, for each half-hour period in which they are awake, what activity they are performing. Then each activity is rated by the respondent in the following ways: (a) whether he or she considers the activity to be work, leisure, a daily living task, or rest, (b) how much he or she enjoys the activity, (c) how important the activity is, and (d) how well he or she does the activity. The latter three questions give insight into the volitional characteristics of the activity pattern; that is, they reveal the personal causation, interest, and value experienced in the activity. The questionnaire also provides data about: (a) habits (i.e., the typical use of time) and (b) balance of work, play, daily living tasks, rest, and sleep in daily life.

The Activity Record, developed for use with persons who have physical disabilities, asks additional questions pertaining to pain, fatigue, difficulty of performance, and whether one rests during the activity. Consequently, in addition to the information provided by the Occupational Questionnaire, the Activity Record provides detailed information about how a disability influences performance of everyday activities.

Both forms are organized to be used as self-reports, but can be administered as semi-structured interviews.

The forms may be used to report on an actual period of time, being filled out as diaries periodically throughout the day or at the end of a day. Alternatively, they may be used to report on what is a "typical day." Each of these methods have their advantages (e.g., diaries tend to be more accurate but may reflect an unusual day). Actual use depends on the purpose and circumstances of therapy.

Typical Activities	Question 1 I consider this activity to be: 1 – work 2 – daily living work 3 – recreation 4 – rest	Question 2 I think that I do this: 1 – Very well 2 – Well 3 – About average 4 – Poorly 5 – Very poorly	Question 3 For me this activity is: 1 – Extremely important 2 – Important 3 – Take it or leave it 4 – Rather not do it 5 – Total waste of time	Question 4 How much do you enjoy this activity: 1 – Like it very much 2 – Like it 3 – Neither like it nor dislike it 4 – Dislike it 5 – Strongly dislike it
For the half hour beginning at:				
5:00 am	1 2 3 4	1 2 3 4 5	1 2 3 4 5	1 2 3 4 5
5:30	1 2 3 4	1 2 3 4 5	1 2 3 4 5	1 2 3 4 5
6:00	1 2 3 4	1 2 3 4 5	1 2 3 4 5	1 2 3 4 5

Figure 12.7.   Format of the Occupational Questionnaire.

These instruments potentially give the occupational therapist important information about (1) particularly troublesome times or activities in the daily schedule, (2) disorganization in the person's use of time, (3) lack of balance in time use, (4) problems such as a lack of feeling competent, a lack of interest or value in daily activities.

The instruments can be used to produce scores which represent the amount of value, interest, personal causation, pain, fatigue, etc. experienced in a day. When this is the case, the therapist can calculate average levels. In addition to the possibility of getting numbers from the instruments, the results of the instruments can be graphically portrayed to (by) the person. For example, the time spent in work, play, rest, etc. can yield a "pie of life" in which slices of the pie represent the percentage of the day devoted to each of these life spaces. Doing the pie of life can be used as an individual or group exercise. Similar pies of life can be made with percentages of time spent doing things not valued, valued somewhat, and so on. Used in this way, these instruments are also useful for collaborating with individuals to discover their strengths and weaknesses and to set therapeutic goals.

Self Assessment of Occupational Functioning

The Self Assessment of Occupational Functioning (SAOF) (Baron & Curtin, 1990) and its corresponding children's version (Curtin & Baron, 1990) are designed to assist collaborative treatment planning between the occupational therapist and the client. While this instrument provides valuable data to the therapist concerning client's perceptions of their areas of strength and weakness, its purpose and design is broader than simply collecting data. It is designed as a process in which a client reports self-perceptions followed by discussion with the therapist to achieve consensus on problems and strengths. Finally, it results in mutually agreed upon goals for intervention.

The SAOF consists of a series of self-statements that correspond with the components of the model of human occupation. Figure 12.8 shows the items related to personal causation.

As indicated in Figure 12.8, the patient rates each statement as either an area of strength, adequacy, or needing improvement. The result is a profile of strengths and weaknesses from the patient's point of view. The respondent also identifies, from among the weaknesses, personal priorities for change. The form is designed so that the entire process of self-assessment and goal prioritization is represented visually. This affords both patient and occupational therapist a quick overview of the patient's view of his or her own level of function.

The version shown in Figure 12.8 is used with adults and some adolescents age 14 and older. As noted, there is also a children's SAOF designed for younger respondents. The children's version may be more appropriate for some adolescents, depending on their level of development. The children's version (ordinarily used with children who are at least nine years of age) is written in more age-appropriate language as illustrated by Personal Causation items shown in Figure 12.9.

The occupational therapist may read the statements and record the patient's responses, or the patient may complete the form independently depending upon the clinical situation and on the patient's individual needs. After the patient completes the form, the instrument then becomes the vehicle for a discussion of treatment planning. Next, a collaborative treatment plan is then written in the patient's words.

Therapists find that an additional benefit of this assessment is what it tells patients about occupational therapy. The form, by identifying and framing strengths and weaknesses in a unique way, conveys a message about what will be the concerns addressed in occupational therapy. Since the aim of the SAOF is to increase collaboration between the therapist and patient, it can often result in patients becoming more committed to therapy. The case of Kim presented in Chapter 14 provides an illustration of the use of the SAOF in the process of planning intervention.

Interviews

Whether through formal or informal conversations, interviews with patients are the method whereby therapists gather a large portion of the data by which they come to know their clients. Four interviews have been developed for use with the model of human occupation. Each has a distinct format and purpose. The Occupational Case Analysis Interview and Rating Scale is based on a case analysis approach to using the model of human occupation (Cubie & Kaplan, 1982). This assessment was originally designed for short-term psychiatric treatment settings, although it has been applied in other settings. The Assessment of Occupational Functioning was originally developed for use in long-term settings (Watts, Kielhofner, Bauer, Gregory, & Valentine, 1986); later revision of the scale resulted in a more generic version (Watts, Brollier, Bauer, & Schmidt, 1989). The Occupational Performance History Interview (Kielhofner & Henry, 1988) was developed with funding from the American Occupational Therapy Association and American Occupational Therapy Foundation and reflects the mandate for a generic instrument which can be used from adolescence through old age with a variety of populations. The Worker Role Interview (Velozo, Kielhofner, & Fisher, 1990) is the most recent in this family of interviews and was designed for use with injured workers in work-rehabilitation settings. More recently, the interview has been modified for use with psychiatric populations (Handelsman, 1994).

Together, these interviews represent a range of applications and foci. However, they all share some common features. Each interview has a designated domain of concern around which occupational therapists conduct a semi-

	Strengths	Adequate	Needs Improvement	Priority
I. Personal Causation: 1. Knowing my abilities.				
2. Expecting success from my efforts rather than failure.				
3. Believing I can make things happen at work, in school, during recreation and/or at home.				

Figure 12.8. Personal causation section of the Self Assessment of Occupational Functioning.

Area of Occupational Functioning	Strengths (Good)	Adequate (OK)	Needs Improvement (Get Better)	Most Important
1. I know what I am "good at" or can do well.				
2. I feel proud about what I can do.				
3. I expect things I do to turn out well.				
4. I think I can do or say something to make things happen.				
5. I can make up my own mind when given choices.				
6. I can stay with a hard activity.				

Figure 12.9.   Personal causation section from the children's Self Assessment of Occupational Functioning.

structured interview. The goal of some of these interviews is that the therapist using the interview will eventually become so cognizant of the necessary data to be gathered that he or she can construct questions which are more natural and emerge out of a conversation between the therapist and the client.

After the interview is conducted, the therapist must have some means of analyzing the data. Each of these interviews has a rating scale which the therapist completes after conducting the interview. The items on the scale reflect the model of human occupation concepts and allow a shorthand representation of what is learned in the interview. Additionally, each of the interview scales can be summed to achieve a total score. The practice of summing the items for a total score is more common in research than in clinical practice. More commonly, therapists use the ratings on the items as a profile of strengths and weaknesses. This will be illustrated further when we discuss particular interviews.

The qualitative data which emerges from the interview is equally important for understanding the client. The Occupational Performance History Interview includes a narrative section in which the occupational therapist writes a brief life history of the patient and relates it to one of several life history patterns. The other interviews simply provide a section for therapists to enter comments about the patient along with making the ratings. We have recently begun to develop a means of narrative analysis of interviews (Mallinson, Kielhofner, & Mattingly, 1994) and expect a more formal means of narrative analysis to emerge in the future. We will discuss this further after presenting the interviews.

Occupational Case Analysis Interview and Rating Scale

The Occupational Case Analysis Interview and Rating Scale (OCAIRS) (Kaplan & Kielhofner, 1989) is composed of a semi-structured interview, a rating scale, and a summary form. The instrument was originally designed for discharge planning with short-term psychiatric inpatients. It provides a structure for gathering, analyzing, and reporting data on the extent and nature of an individual's occupational adaptation. The interview is used to collect information on personal causation, values and goals, interests, roles, habits, skills, and other areas related to the environment and system dynamics.

This instrument is conceptually sound, clinically useful, and reasonably consistent as a measurement tool. It employs a different rating format for each of the concepts. For example, Figure 12.10 presents the rating for the concept of personal causation.

Because the rating form is so specific, the interview questions recommended for this assessment need to be followed more closely than other interviews or the therapist will have difficulty making the rating. The rating scale has the virtue of specificity, but this specificity sometimes makes it harder to rate patients whose circumstances do not neatly fit the descriptions given for the individual items.

The instrument also employs a brief, one-page summary form which is appropriate for short-term settings and effective for communicating the results of the interview. In general, occupational therapists who want an interview with more structure find this one to be helpful. In contrast, some therapists find it too constraining.

Assessment of Occupational Functioning

The Assessment of Occupational Functioning (AOF) was originally developed as a screening tool for collecting a broad range of information thought to influence a person's occupational performance (Watts, Kielhofner, Bauer, Gregory, & Valentine, 1986). Subsequent revision and investigation of the instrument resulted in it being appropriate for a range of populations and settings (Watts, Brollier, Bauer, & Schmidt, 1989). It does provide a more comprehensive evaluation than its original purpose of being a screening tool. However, the AOF does not attempt evaluation of specific daily living skills or environmental variables directly but aims to efficiently gener-ate a picture of many factors that influence a person's ability to function.

The interview employs a semi-structured interview format which allows the user to make parenthetical probes or clarifications as needed. But like the OCAIRS, the interviewer must be certain to collect the appropriate data for the ratings to be made. The interview rating scale employs a five-point rating format (5 = Very Highly to 1 = Very Little).

Figure 12.11, from the area of Personal Causation, illustrates the kind of items that are rated for this interview.

Occupational Performance History Interview

As a historical interview, the Occupational Performance History Interview (OPHI) (Kielhofner & Henry, 1988) seeks to gather information about a patient or client's past and present occupational performance. It is designed as a generic interview for use with a variety of patients or clients. The OPHI is comprised of two parts. The first part is the interview itself, consisting of a set of recommended questions that cover five content areas relevant to occupational performance. The occupational therapist uses these questions (or his or her own modified version of them) to conduct the inter-

Figure 12.10.   Personal causation rating from the Occupational Case Analysis Interview and Rating Scale.*

5.	Expresses much confidence about abilities and anticipates very successful outcomes of action. Identifies at least three skills proud of, startes at least one item is improving, and indicates that anticipates stress.
4.	Expresses pretty much confidence about abilities and anticipates pretty successful outcomes of action. Identifies one or two skills proud of, states at least one step taken to improve, and indicates that anticipates being somewhat successful.
3.	Expresses some confidence about abilities and anticipates somewhat successful outcomes of action. Identifies one or two skills, no areas or steps taken to improve, and indicates that anticipates being mostly unsuccessful or lists no areas of unsuccessful performance and is overly confident about skills.
2.	Expresses little confidence about abilities and anticipates barely successful outcomes of action. Does not identify anything to be proud of and indicates that anticipates being unsuccessful.
1.	Does not express feelings about abilities or outcomes.

* Taken from Kaplan, K., & Kielhofner, G. (1989). *The Occupational Case Analysis Interview and Rating Scale*. Thorofare, NJ: Slack, p. 10

view, making sure to cover all five content areas. Additionally, the questions for each content area are accompanied by a set of yields that are to be used to guide the therapist as to the type of information that should be collected for each content area. The yields should be used by the therapist to formulate any additional questions or probing that might be needed.

The second part consists of a standard form for reporting the results of the interview, called the OPHI Rating and Life History Narrative Form. It includes a rating scale that allows the therapist to quantify information collected during the interview. The rating scale consists of ten items—two items for each of the five content area of the interview. After completing the rating form, the therapist identifies the respondent's life history pattern. Next, the therapist composes a description of the patient's life history on the Rating and Life History Narrative Form.

As the only historical interview in this group, the OPHI is designed to gather an individual's history of work, play, and self-care performance. It can be used with psychiatric and physically disabled adolescents and adults.

The OPHI's recommended questions and ten items cover five content areas: (a) organization of daily living routines; (b) life roles; (c) interests, values, and goals; (d) perceptions of ability and responsibility; and (e) environmental influences. Each of the five content areas is represented by two items on the interview rating scale. As an example, the following two items on the scale belong to the area of perception of ability and responsibility: (a) acknowledgment of abilities and limitations and (b) assumption of responsibility. These two items correspond to the volition concept of personal causation.

Each item on the scale is rated using a five-point rating system (5 = adaptive through 1 = maladaptive). Separate ratings are made for the respondent's past and present function. To establish these ratings, the therapist must identify individually with each interviewee a demarcation point that defines what is considered present and past functioning. Such markers as the onset of disability or major change in life roles are used.

The strength of the OPHI is that it does provide a historical approach to interviewing and thereby lends itself to gathering information about the patient's life story. This aspect, as we will discuss shortly, may be one of the important new directions for interview development.

Worker Role Interview

The Worker Role Interview (WRI) is a semistructured interview originally designed to gather data from the injured worker (Velozo, Kielhofner, & Fisher, 1990). The interview is designed to have the client discuss various aspects of his or her life and job setting. The WRI is unique among interviews in that the occupational therapist makes ratings by combining

Figure 12.11.   Rating for personal causation from the Assessment of Occupational Functioning.*

Personal Causation					
1. Does this person demonstrate personal causation through an expressed belief in internal control?	5	4	3	2	1
2. Does this person demonstrate personal causation by expressing confidence that he/she has a range of skills?	5	4	3	2	1
3. Does this person demonstrate personal causation by expressing confidence in his/her skill competence at personally relevant tasks?	5	4	3	2	1
4. Does this person demonstrate personal causation by expressing hopeful anticipation for success in the future?	5	4	3	2	1

* Taken from Watts, J.H., Brollier, C., Bauer, D., & Schmidt, W. (1989). The assessment of occupational functioning: The Second Revision. *Occupational Therapy in Mental Health, 8*(4), 61–87.

information from the interview with observations made during the physical and behavioral assessment procedures of a physical and/or work capacity assessment. The intent is to identify the system and environmental variables that may influence the ability of the injured worker to return to work.

The WRI Rating Form uses a four-point rating scale that indicates the impact that each concept rated has on the likelihood of return to work. The items rated are derived from the model of human occupation; they are shown in Figure 12.12. As noted earlier the WRI has recently been adapted for use with psychiatric populations (Handelsman, 1994).

Interviews in Perspective

All the interviews share a common feature of gathering information via semi-structured interviews, using a rating scale to record the results, and providing a wealth of descriptive information. These features of the interviews can be illustrated through the following example with the Worker Role Interview.

The interview was used to explore vocational difficulties experienced by Bill. Following an extended period of treatment, Bill's cancer was considered successfully treated and his physician and occupational therapist had both encouraged him to begin efforts to return to work. Prior to the onset of cancer, Bill worked as a mechanic. Since he had no physical impairment as a result of the cancer, it was reasonable to expect that he could return to his old line of work. After several months, Bill still was unable to make any serious moves toward return to work. At this point, it was decided that Bill should be evaluated to determine the source of his difficulties in returning to work. The occupational therapist's ratings from the Worker Role Interview are summarized on WRI Summary Form (Figure 12.13).

The ratings show that Bill's volition is a strength while his habituation is clearly a source of difficulty. While this is helpful to know, the real utility of the interview data is contained in the descriptive information about Bill's life. We will highlight the critical things learned from the interview and reflected in the rating scale.

Bill was an average high school student who jumped at the chance to receive vocational training in his senior year. The training provided him knowledge and skills in the field of automotive mechanics where he immediately found a job upon graduation. Bill was a dependable worker who followed the routine of a 45-hour work week. He valued his work, was engaged to be married, and looked forward to buying a house and settling down with a family. Bill especially enjoyed work as a mechanic since it combined his manual interests with the challenge of diagnosing and fixing the problems on cars. He was confident in his skills and saw himself as a good employee. He expected to spend his work life as a mechanic.

The onset of cancer changed all that. Bill notes that the physicians told him he'd have a lot of time on his hands during which he would be receiving treatment and recovering from the cancer. Surgical removal of the cancer, followed by a long course of chemotherapy, interrupted Bill's career for three years. During this time his major life role was that of being a patient—a role in which he had to rely on the expertise and actions of health professions and comply with their procedures. During both his illness and convalescence Bill acquired, by his own admission, "a lot of bad habits." He describes a typical day in which he rises, dresses, and takes nearly the whole morning to complete a leisurely breakfast. His afternoon may be punctuated with an errand or task. Following an evening shower, he watches television until bedtime. It is a schedule in which Bill "pretty much does nothing." He is ashamed of his routine but feels held at bay by it. He recalls three years ago saying to his father, who is retired on disability, that he thought "it would be hard to sit around the house all day and do nothing." It is a surprise to Bill just how easy it has become to do the same. Now Bill literally feels "stuck." He cannot seem to get himself going; it is as though he has completely lost momentum and now needs a monumental effort to restart himself. Bill's substantial anxiety and worry about whether he can successfully get started is contributing to

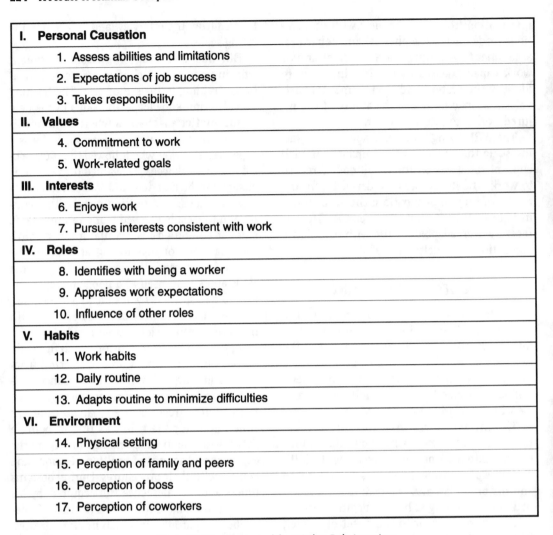

I.	**Personal Causation**
	1. Assess abilities and limitations
	2. Expectations of job success
	3. Takes responsibility
II.	**Values**
	4. Commitment to work
	5. Work-related goals
III.	**Interests**
	6. Enjoys work
	7. Pursues interests consistent with work
IV.	**Roles**
	8. Identifies with being a worker
	9. Appraises work expectations
	10. Influence of other roles
V.	**Habits**
	11. Work habits
	12. Daily routine
	13. Adapts routine to minimize difficulties
VI.	**Environment**
	14. Physical setting
	15. Perception of family and peers
	16. Perception of boss
	17. Perception of coworkers

Figure 12.12. Content of the Worker Role Interview.

his inability to make an occupational choice about returning to work, which is one concern reflected in the rating scale.

The erosion of his worker role and the extreme disorganization of his habits of routine are also reflected in the rating. Bill has become disabled, not by any physical sequela of his illness (his skills are intact), but by the loss of habituation structure to maintain his daily routines. Indeed, habituation seems to be serving as a control parameter maintaining him in a pattern of inaction and anxiety. His awareness of his capacities is good, since he knows he has the skills for a mechanical job, but his sense of efficacy is in question because he does not feel very confident that he can achieve his desired goal of returning to work.

Together the profile provided by the rating scale and the descriptive data on patient's lives, provide substantial information from which to construct an explanation of occupational dysfunction. While the scales on the interviews provide a structured means of organizing data from the interviews, there is, as yet, no comparable way to organize the life story that is told in interviews.

Future of Interviews: Narrative Analysis

Chapter 4 argued that individuals experience meaning in their lives through volitional narratives which organize their knowledge of self and circumstances (i.e., personal causation, interests, and values) into a coherent schema. These volitional narratives relate past,

Strongly Supports	Supports	Interferes	Strongly Interferes
4	3	2	1
Strongly supports client returning to job	Positive qualities outweigh negative qualities: advantage for returning to job	Negative qualities outweigh positive qualities: disadvantage for returning to job	Strongly interferes with returning to job

NA = NOT APPLICABLE

BRIEF COMMENTS WHICH SUPPORT RATINGS

PERSONAL CAUSATION

1. Assesses abilities and limitations	④	3	2	1	NA	Is aware of both strengths and weaknesses
2. Expectation of job success	4	③	2	1	NA	Is worried about ability to "get started" but has a strong will to work
3. Takes responsibility	4	③	2	1	NA	Has become passive since illness

VALUES

4. Commitment to work	④	3	2	1	NA	Strong values of work
5. Work related goals	④	3	2	1	NA	Apartment, wife, etc.

INTERESTS

6. Enjoys work	④	3	2	1	NA	Likes problem-solving of mechanics, likes physical work
7. Pursues interests	4	③	2	1	NA	Since illness less pursuit

ROLES

8. Identifies with being a worker	4	③	2	1	NA	Yes, but father is poor role model. Also has been in sick role for 3 years
9. Appraises work expectations	④	3	2	1	NA	Is aware of what it takes to work
10. Influence of other roles	4	③	2	1	NA	Family role mixed, father is disabled, mother is supportive

HABITS

11. Work habits	4	3	②	1	NA	Many work habits lost
12. Daily routines	4	3	2	①	NA	Current routine is not functional
13. Adapts routine to minimize difficulties	4	3	2	1	⊘NA⊘	

ENVIRONMENT

14. Perception of work setting	④	3	2	1	NA	Sees mechanics as a positive place to work
15. Family and peers	4	③	2	1	NA	Family generally wants him to return to work
16. Perception of boss	4	3	2	1	⊘NA⊘	
17. Perception of co-workers	4	3	2	1	⊘NA⊘	

Figure 12.13. Bill: Scores on the Worker Role Interview.

present, and potential life events within a plot that gives them meaning.

One of the challenges in future development of the interviews will be to develop better means of eliciting and analyzing narrative data. In a preliminary study, Mallinson, Kielhofner, and Mattingly (1994) explored patients' use of metaphor in their responses to the Occupational Performance History Interview. Metaphors such as being slowed down or being trapped provided substantial insight into patients' volition in particular. For example, persons using metaphors of having lost momentum (like Bill) were expressing concern over the challenge they faced, but also expressing hope concerning their ability to achieve desired outcomes in life. Patients who described themselves as trapped were expressing complete feelings of inefficacy (i.e., they could not see ways in which they could change their lives). While more work remains to be done in developing the narrative content and analysis of narrative data in interviews, it promises to be an important direction for the future development of interviews.

Selecting and Using Other Structured Methods of Data Collection

As we noted earlier there are still a limited number of structured assessments designed specifically for use with the model of human occupation. Therapists using the model as a conceptual model for practice sometimes will use other structured methods of data collection for a variety of reasons.

First of all, therapists often use the model in association with other conceptual practice models which have their own assessments. For example, other models may be used to provide a better understanding of the mind-brain-body performance subsystem. In such cases the structured methods of data collection are derived from those models.

Second, therapists may chose other assessments of occupational performance. As discussed in this chapter and Chapter 8, a unique approach to conceptualizing and gathering data on skilled performance has been developed through the model. However, therapists

may also choose other methods of gathering data on performance. They may include activities of daily living assessments, standardized developmental assessments, standardized assessments of motor performance, formal work evaluations, and so on. Such methods of data collection are chosen when the therapist needs the kind of data on performance that these provide. While such methods were not developed for use with the model of human occupation, they are compatible with it.

Third, a therapist may choose standardized assessments which gather data directly or partly related to constructs in the model of human occupation. One kind of assessment that has often been used are locus of control scales. These self-administered scales indicate a person's degree of internal or external locus of control—this data is easily related to the patient's sense of efficacy. The case of Kim in Chapter 14 illustrates the use of such a scale.

Another example is the use of structured interest inventories. Since the Interest Checklist focuses mainly on leisure interests, therapists wishing to gather data on work-related interests will ordinarily use one of a number of available standardized vocational interest assessments. Additionally other assessments developed for use with special population such as persons with cognitive and/or reading limitations are sometimes selected. These assessments ordinarily have been developed by other professionals such as vocational counselors. However, the construct of interests and its operationalization in the assessments make these data-gathering tools compatible with the model.

When selecting structured assessments to provide data relevant to the model of human occupation, the therapist should be careful to understand the degree of relevance or overlap of the construct measured to the construct in the model of human occupation about which he or she wants data. For example, therapists have sometimes used measures of self-esteem to provide data relevant to personal causation. Self-esteem measures ordinarily include items that tap a wider range of phenomena than is meant by personal causation. That is, while self-esteem scales ordinarily include items concerning one's appraisal of one's abilities, other items may pertain to one's assessment of one's physical attractiveness, social acceptance, and other factors that are not included in the concept of personal causation. For this reason, therapists should take care that any instrument they use is closely connected to the theoretical concept for which it is intended. Moreover, they should be aware of any difference in what the instrument measures and about what they want information.

It is always complicated to find methods of data collection developed outside a particular theory that will work well in association with that theory. While it is not impossible to do it, it takes thoughtful consideration in selecting, and care in using, such a method of data collection.

Structured Methods of Data Collection in Perspective

The model of human occupation is still a relatively new conceptual model. Development of structured methods of data collection began in earnest about a decade ago. The methods we have just presented are the fruits of these years of effort. It ordinarily takes a significant period of time to conceptualize, pilot, study, revise, and reinvestigate a structured method of data collection. In fact, the process never really ends. For example, the interviews discussed in this section represent studies initiated in the early 1980s and, as noted above, we are still in the process of improving these interview methods of data collection. Despite the ongoing efforts of many investigators, a limited number of structured methods of data collection specifically based on the model of human occupation are currently available. Moreover, many still require further development. As we noted above, it is possible to incorporate the use of related structured methods of data collection. However, as we also noted this practice also has its limitations.

SITUATED METHODS OF DATA GATHERING

An occupational therapist wishing to apply the model in a particular situation will not al-ways find sufficient structured methods of data collection based on the model for a comprehensive evaluation. In such cases the therapist will use situated methods of data collection. As we will see, such situated methods can be more than an alternative when structured methods are not available. Indeed, they serve a complementary role to the structured methods already discussed. Under certain circumstances they will be preferred to available structured methods.

Situated methods of data collection differ from structured methods in two respects. First, the therapist does not follow an established protocol. Second, since the methods do not have the guarantee of dependability that go with proper use of a structured method, the therapist is obligated to safeguard the process of data collection through careful planning and judgement.

For this reason, situated methods require substantial thought on the part of the occupational therapist. The best situated methods are those which are systematic and reflective. The therapist using situated methods uses them systematically when they are planned, clearly linked to theory, and done in ways that maximize the dependability of the data gathered. Methods are reflective when the occupational therapist actively determines the need for data, selects a situated method to collect data, and considers how to best analyze and report the data.

Situated data collection ordinarily takes one of two forms. The therapist observes the client or the therapist interviews the client. In either case, the occupational therapist should be guided by the kinds of conceptual questions which were identified in the previous chapter. These conceptual questions inform therapists about the kind of data they are seeking and guide therapists in developing situationally appropriate methods of collecting data.

The following are some common circumstances in which the use of situated methods are called for: (a) there is no appropriate structured method available, (b) the client is threatened by a more formal method, (c) the therapist wishes to augment data collected by structured assessments, (d) available structured methods take more time than is available in the setting, (e) the therapist questions the cultural relevance of the existing structured assessment.

Situated assessments also provide a means of gathering more comprehensive data about such environments as the family, institutional living setting, workplace, and so on.

Finally, situated methods are an important means of continuing the data collection process throughout the course of therapy. Though it is not always the case, structured methods are often used at the beginning of therapy when the most intensive data collection occurs, and again at the end when therapists wish to determine and document changes or to have data for discharge planning. However, the treatment process along with other ongoing observations of clients and continuing opportunities to talk with clients provide a constant source of situated data. If therapists use such opportunities wisely, they can gather a wealth of data in an efficient way.

One of the advantages of situated methods is that they can be adapted to the unfolding situations in therapy. The therapist can periodically obtain data relevant to conceptual questions which are still unanswered or which emerge in the course of intervention. Situated data collection can occur in a wide range of circumstances such as having a conversation with a patient while beginning an activity, observing a client's performance in the classroom, listening to a patient's comments about the workplace where he was injured, noting the affect of a client during a group session, or listening to a client's occasional stories about what happened since he was last seen.

Since situated methods often occur serendipitously, during a treatment session or an informal opportunity to observe or interact with a client, they may appear, at first, to be much less important than structured methods. However, all situated data collection is potentially very valuable. Moreover, situated data collection can often be very detailed and sophisticated.

Proper Use of Situated Methods

When using situated methods to gather data, therapists use much of the same kind of logic and safeguards that qualitative researchers use when they gather data from field observation and interviews. While it is not possible to review here all the kinds of concerns and practices that qualitative researchers have in mind when collecting and interpreting data, we will offer some guidelines for situated data gathering.

First of all, since therapists do not rely on a structured and tested method of gathering data, they must think about and undertake their own steps to assure that the data is dependable. Two important steps are evaluating the circumstances surrounding the data collection and comparing different sources of data.

Circumstances have an important influence on the kind of data one gets. For example, a patient has a particularly bad day struggling with some problem and breaks down while confiding in a therapist about all his fears for the future. From that encounter, the therapist may have much more honest and useful data than the data previously gathered in a formal interview. Here, the circumstances tell the therapist that the data can really be interpreted as the patient's greatest fears about the future. On the other hand, circumstance may make the data suspect. For example, if a patient is reporting on her performance in a group where it is clear she is trying to impress another group member, the therapist may have reasons to suspect that the report is exaggerated.

One method of helping to assure that data is accurate is to compare it with another source of data. Thus, for example, one may compare what patients say they can do with observation of performance or with what a spouse or caretaker says the person can do. Another way to ensure accuracy is to compare the same type of data collected over time. Observing performance or asking about a patient's view of the future more than once is a way of checking whether the one observation was truly representative of how the person performs or feels.

The second consideration in using situated methods is to ask whether one's interpretation of the meaning of data is valid. Once again, there are some steps drawn from qualitative research which can be helpful in assuring the validity of one's interpretations of data. First, a therapist should ask whether an interpretation corresponds logically and structurally with the general picture obtained from earlier data. If it does, then one has a stronger basis to consider the interpretation. The therapist may also ask whether the interpretation corresponds with case examples and other discussions offered by the theory upon which the data collection is based. Another important method of checking the validity of one's interpretations is to continue to collect data which will either support or refute the interpretation of the previous data's meaning. Finally, one can check interpretations of data by checking them with the patient. For example, an observation of a patient's behavior in a task situation suggests that he was anxious and the therapist interprets this data as meaning the patient's sense of efficacy in a particular task is poor, the therapist can share that inference with the patient to ask whether he or she agrees with the interpretation.

As this brief discussion should have illustrated, much of what a therapist does to assure dependability is to employ a careful attitude in which one reflects upon and checks up on data and its interpretation. If the therapist makes the effort to do this, situated methods can be a very useful source of data.

A final but important comment on the use of situated data collection methods is that these methods should be carefully linked to questions which emerge from the theory as discussed in the previous chapter. Since one does not have the structure of a formal method, the theory provides the kind of structure which guides one in seeking certain data through situated methods and in selecting which spontaneously available data is most relevant to understanding the patient.

An Illustration of Situated Data Collection

We will use the following example to illustrate how observational methods and informal interviewing were used in the case of a very young, severely involved child in order to assess volition. Mary is a three-year-old being following in a developmental clinic. She has a rare genetic disorder which has resulted in extreme delay of growth and development of cognitive, motor, and social functions.

The evaluation of Mary included an attempt to understand how her volition influenced her activity choices. These activity choices were important as they determined what opportunities she had to develop new skills. She was observed during two 30-minute therapy sessions and her mother was informally interviewed.

During these sessions the occupational therapist made the following observations of Mary. While she had no formal language Mary was effective in communicating desires and displeasures. She cried or made sounds of disapproval when things were not going as she wanted. For example, the therapist presented a toy which made music and when the music stopped Mary began crying. The therapist started the music again and Mary stopped crying immediately demonstrating her communicative intent. In contrast to her obvious sense that she could have control and achieve desires by influencing those around her, Mary appeared to have very little awareness of how to make things happen through movement. She kept her flexed arms tight against her chest. She made no attempts to reach for objects, grasp or otherwise motorically act on her environment. It was as if it did not occur to her to physically do things to the environment. These observations led to the conclusion that Mary's belief in skill and sense of efficacy was organized around her basic awareness of being able to influence others. It was corroborated by her mother that at home Mary was surrounded by many family members who readily understood much of her primitive communication and did things for her that she wanted. In contrast, she rarely made any attempts to move her body.

It was also observed during the sessions that Mary valued and responded intensely to human contact. In her own way, she connected with the therapist and was very aware of attention by others. She also displayed a number of interests through orienting and maintaining attention (e.g., music and vibratory stimulation from a vibrating pillow). Additionally, she vocalized pleasure at vestibular stimulation through a pleasant grunting sound and through laughing while being bounced on a ball.

This information about Mary's values, interests, and personal causation was used to construct a treatment plan in which the occupational therapist would challenge her to use her motor system (i.e., reaching, touching, grasping, rolling) to generate social, vestibular, musical, and tactile experiences that she enjoyed. The occupational therapist also instructed the family in how to encourage her to generate these experiences with their help instead of doing everything for her. Over the course of one month Mary began more active reaching toward novel objects. She displayed a primitive grasp and was able to pick up some objects such as her socks. She was able to use a foot operated switch to provide vibratory and auditory (music) stimulation. Careful observation of her volitional responses during therapy sessions to determine, for example, when she was too challenged by the demands presented or when she was attending to an interest, were important for the occupational therapist to guide therapy.

As the example illustrates, Mary was unable to report on her volition, but from observation and from discussion with Mary's mother, the occupational therapist was able to gather data that allowed an understanding of her volition to emerge and be used in therapy.

Situated Methods in Perspective

For a variety of reasons occupational therapists will collect data with situated methods. As discussed, such methods allow for spontaneous, situationally imbedded, but still systematic collection of data. Situated data collection requires the therapist to be guided by sound theory and to actively reason in the course of collecting data. When properly used, they can be invaluable sources of data.

ACHIEVING A BALANCED AND COMPREHENSIVE APPROACH TO DATA COLLECTION

In this chapter, we have discussed both structured and situated methods of data collection. Each of these approaches have their special strengths and contributions to the process of gathering and reasoning with data.

Structured methods of obtaining data about a patient typically provide us with details about such things as how much, how far, how often, and how different this person is at time two from time one. This is important and necessary information to gather and use in implementing and evaluating intervention. Situated methods typically provide occupational therapists with qualitative details that complement the information gathered in structured data collection.

For example, consider an elderly client, Joe, who has returned to living on his own following a moderate right cerebrovascular accident. Joe experiences some motor difficulties, tactile disturbances, and hemianopia.

Consider the following question from Chapter 11: What are the consequences of changed sensory experiences on this person's performance of activities? In this case, the Assessment of Motor and Process Skills may determine that he is ineffective in a number of activities of daily living, having consistent difficulty with manipulation, calibration, gripping, noticing/responding, and searching/locating.

During a visit to Joe's home we observe that he is embarrassed at having others watch his unskillful attempts at eating. We further learn from his wife that he no longer goes out to dinner in public places. Later, he confides that he is concerned about the difficulty he is having finding objects in his environment and, as a result, is reluctant to go to the supermarket alone.

It is equally important for the therapist to have all this information on Joe. The clinical data regarding the hemianopia, the formal AMPS data that provides details about performance skill deficits, the report of the client's embarrassment in a social setting, and the informal interview regarding difficulty in the supermarket each provide different data, all critical to the understanding of this client, which will be necessary to carry out a therapeutic course of occupational therapy.

All methods are simply means to obtaining data. What is important is that therapists can work back and forth, asking themselves the kinds of conceptual questions that grow out of knowing a theory well and taking every appropriate opportunity to use structured and situated methods to gather data for answering those questions.

References

Baron, K., & Curtin, C. (1990). *A manual for use with the Self Assessment of Occupational Functioning*. Unpublished manuscript, Department of Occupational Therapy, University of Illinois at Chicago.

Bonder, B. (1993). Issues in assessment of psychosocial components of function. *American Journal of Occupational Therapy, 47*, 211–216.

Curtin, C., & Baron, K. (1990). *A manual for use with the Children's Self Assessment of Occupational Functioning*. Unpublished manuscript, Department of Occupational Therapy, University of Illinois at Chicago.

Cubie, S., & Kaplan, K. (1982). A case analysis method for the model of human occupation. *American Journal of Occupational Therapy, 36*, 645–656.

de las Heras, C. G. (1993a). *Validity and Reliability of the Volitional Questionnaire*. Unpublished master's thesis, Tufts University, Boston, MA.

de las Heras, C. G. (1993b). *The Volitional Questionnaire*. Unpublished manual, Santiago, Chile.

Fisher, A. (1993). The assessment of IADL motor skills: An application of many-faceted rasch analysis. *American Journal of Occupational Therapy, 47*, 319–329.

Fisher, A. (1994). *The Assessment of Motor and Process Skills* (Version 8.0). Unpublished test manual, Colorado State University, Occupational Therapy Department, Fort Collins.

Fisher, A., & Short-DeGraff, M. (1993). Improving functional assessment in occupational therapy: Recommendations and philosophy for change. *American Journal of Occupational Therapy, 47*, 199–201.

Furst, G. P., Gerber, L. H., Smith, C. C., Fisher, S., & Schulman, B. (1987). A program for improving energy conservation behaviors in adults with rheumatoid arthritis. *American Journal of Occupational Therapy, 41*, 102–11.

Handelsman, D. (1994). *The construct validity of the worker role interview for the chronic mentally ill*. Unpublished master's thesis, University of Illinois at Chicago.

Kaplan, K., & Kielhofner, G. (1989). *The Occupational Case Analysis Interview and Rating Scale*. Thorofare, NJ: Slack.

Kielhofner, G., & Henry, A. (1988). Development and investigation of the Occupational Performance History Interview. *American Journal of Occupational Therapy, 42*, 489–498.

Kielhofner, G., & Neville, A. (1983). The modified interest checklist. Unpublished manuscript, University of Illinois at Chicago.

Mallinson, T., Kielhofner, G., & Mattingly, C. (1994). *"Like being stuck in fly paper:" Understanding volition through metaphor*. Manuscript submitted for publication.

Matsutsuyu, J. (1969). The Interest Check List. *American Journal of Occupational Therapy, 23*, 323–328.

Oakley, F., Kielhofner, G., & Barris, R. (1985). An occupational therapy approach to assessing psychiatric patients' adaptive functioning. *American Journal of Occupational Therapy, 39*, 147–154.

Rogers, J., Weinstein, J., & Figone, J. (1978). The Interest Check List: An empirical assessment. *American Journal of Occupational Therapy, 32*, 628–630.

Salamy, M., Simon, S., & Kielhofner, G. (1993). *The Assessment of Communication and Interaction Skills* (Research version). Department of Occupational Therapy, University of Illinois at Chicago.

Scaffa, M. (1981). *Temporal adaptations and alcoholism*. Unpublished master's thesis, Virginia Commonwealth University, Richmond.

Smith, N., Kielhofner, G., & Watts, J. (1986). The relationship between volition, activity pattern and life satisfaction in the elderly. *American Journal of Occupational Therapy, 40*, 278–283.

Spencer, J., Krefting, L., & Mattingly, C. (1993). Incorporation of ethnographic methods in occupational therapy assessment. *American Journal of Occupational Therapy, 47*, 303–309.

Velozo, C., Kielhofner, G., & Fisher, A. (1990). *A user's guide to the Worker Role Interview* (Research version). Department of Occupational Therapy, University of Illinois at Chicago.

Watts, J. H., Brollier, C., Bauer, D., & Schmidt, W. (1989). The Assessment of Occupational Functioning: The second revision. *Occupational Therapy in Mental Health, 8*(4), 61–87.

Watts, J. H., Kielhofner, G., Bauer, D., Gregory, M., & Valentine, D. (1986). The assessment of occupational functioning: A screening tool for use in long-term care. *American Journal of Occupational Therapy, 40*, 231–240.

Appendix: Structured Methods of Data Collection Used with the Model of Human Occupation

INTRODUCTION

This appendix contains further information on the twelve methods of structured data collection outlined in the earlier part of this chapter. The reader will find the discussion of each method divided into a number of sections. Each discussion begins with an overview of each method, followed by a summary of research on the dependability of the method. There is an overview of the method's application in practice, as well as information on obtaining and learning to use the method. Each section concludes with a comprehensive reference list.

Figure 12.A1 provides a brief guide to the structured methods of data gathering outlined in this appendix. It is designed to help the reader identify quickly the methods available for evaluating a particular construct, and the kinds of clients for whom that method is suitable. In the relatively short time since the model first appeared in the literature, a range of observational assessments, checklists, and interviews, covering a range of model constructs have appeared. By looking over the table, the reader will see that some constructs have been extensively covered, while others are still in early stages of development. For example, there are a range of tools available for gathering data on volition, designed for a variety of patient needs. Some constructs, such as the environment are less extensively covered and work continues in these areas.

OBTAINING INSTRUMENTS

In outlining where various structured methods of data gathering can be obtained, we have tried to keep things as simple as possible. In this regard, we have given a single contact name and address for each method. You should contact this person or entity directly. It is the reader's responsibility to inquire about costs incurred to acquire a particular assessment.

Many of the data-gathering methods are available through the Model of Human Occu-

pation Clearinghouse. The Clearinghouse is a not-for-profit service of the Center of Research, Department of Occupational Therapy, University of Illinois at Chicago. A charge is made to cover services. When the Clearinghouse is cited as the source for obtaining an instrument, you should fax or mail your name, address, and/or fax number to:

> Coordinator, Model of Human Occupation Clearinghouse
> Department of Occupational Therapy M/C 811
> University of Illinois at Chicago
> 1919 West Taylor Street
> Chicago, IL 60612
> UNITED STATES OF AMERICA
> FAX: (312) 413-0256

When contacting the Clearinghouse, state which instrument(s) you are interested in obtaining. *Do not* send money with your preliminary request. You will receive an order form detailing how to complete your request.

For example:

> To: Coordinator, Model of Human Occupation Clearinghouse
> From: John Doe
> FAX: (123) 456-7890
> 111 Green Street
> Brownsville, IL 65432
> RE: Please send information about requesting the Children's Self Assessment of Occupational Functioning.

1. ASSESSMENT OF COMMUNICATION AND INTERACTION SKILLS

The Assessment of Communication and Interaction Skills (ACIS) is a formal observational tool designed to measure an individual's performance in the area of personal communication and group interactions. The instrument aims to assist occupational therapists in determining a client's ability in discourse and social exchange in the course of daily occupations. To date, the ACIS has been developed for use pre-

	Volition			Habituation		Performance			Environment		Method of Data Gathering			Population C = children Y = adolescents A = adults E = elderly
	Personal Causation	Values	Interests	Roles	Habits	Motor	Process	Communication /Interaction	Physical	Social	Observation	Checklist	Interview	
1. Assessment of Communication & Interaction Skills								✓			✓			YAE
2. Assessment of Motor and Process Skills						✓	✓				✓			CYAE
3. Assessment of Occupational Functioning	✓	✓	✓	✓	✓	✓	✓	✓					✓	YAE
4. Interest Checklist			✓									✓		YAE
5. NIH Activity Record	✓	✓	✓		✓							✓		AE
6. Occupational Case Analysis Interview and Rating Scale	✓	✓	✓	✓	✓	✓	✓	✓	✓	✓			✓	AE
7. Occupational Performance History Interview	✓	✓	✓	✓	✓	✓	✓	✓	✓	✓			✓	AE
8. Occupational Questionnaire	✓	✓	✓	✓								✓		YAE
9. Role Checklist		✓		✓								✓		YAE
10. Self Assessment of Occupational Functioning	✓	✓	✓	✓	✓	✓	✓	✓	✓	✓		✓		CYAE
11. Volitional Questionnaire	✓	✓	✓						✓	✓	✓			YAE
12. Worker Role Interview	✓	✓	✓	✓	✓				✓	✓			✓	AE

Figure 12.A1. Structured methods of data gathering using the model of human occupation.

dominantly in group settings for clients with psychiatric illnesses; however, it would appear to have relevance for a broader population. Observations are carried out during a group activity following which the occupational therapist completes an 18-item rating form. Data can be combined with observations from other settings to give a more complete picture of the client's skills in communication and interaction.

Test Format and Administration

Administration of the ACIS consist of two steps: (1) observation of the client in a group activity and (2) rating and entering comments on the score sheet.

The ACIS consists of 18 skill items divided into six domains as presented in Chapter 8. These items were devised following extensive literature review. The items are arranged into domains by commonality among items.

To administer the ACIS, the occupational therapist observes the client in a group activity (observation periods are approximately 30–60 minutes); it may be possible to observe more than one person during a group. The rating is completed following conclusion of the group. Skills are scored on a four-point scale (4 = competent, 3 = questionable, 2 = ineffective, 1 = deficit) following the scoring criteria for each item provided in a manual. Comments that describe behaviors for a given rating may be entered on the form.

Dependability

Simon (1989) developed the first version of the ACIS and studied its interrater reliability. She found modest interrater reliability and concluded that further refinement of item definitions was needed along with a reorganization of the verbs and clarification of scoring criteria. Following reanalysis of Simon's data using Rasch methods, Salamy (1993) made revisions to the ACIS. Salamy then further tested the instrument in a clinical setting. Utilizing Rasch analysis her study supports the conclusion that the items do form a single unidimensional scale (construct validity). The ACIS reflects an instrument in the early stages of development. Further development of this in-

strument is anticipated. Meanwhile, occupational therapists may wish to use the ACIS as an informal guide for observation and to use the score sheet to give basic profiles of strengths and weaknesses in communication and interaction.

Application in Practice

Due to the early stage of development of this instrument, it is recommended that occupational therapists utilize this instrument as a guide to observation of communication and interaction skills. Although formal development of the instrument has centered on psychiatrically disabled clients, the instrument has been successfully used on a wide range of clients. Occupational therapists are advised to use the ACIS as an aid to making clinical judgements until further research on this instrument is available.

Resources

Copies of the ACIS and User's manual are available at cost through the Model of Human Occupation Clearinghouse. In addition to describing the construct of communication/interaction and reviewing research to date, the manual provides a descriptive summary of skill items, detailed rating guidelines for each of the 18 skill items, guidelines for raters, and a score sheet.

Collected Writings About the Instrument and Its Development

Salamy, M. (1993). *Construct validity of the Assessment for Communication and Interaction Skills*. Unpublished master's thesis, University of Illinois at Chicago.
Salamy, M., Simon, S., & Kielhofner, G. (1993). *The Assessment of Communication and Interaction Skills*. (Research version). Department of Occupational Therapy, University of Illinois at Chicago.
Simon, S. (1989). *The development of an assessment for communication and interaction skills*. Unpublished master's thesis, University of Illinois at Chicago.

2. ASSESSMENT OF MOTOR AND PROCESS SKILLS[a]

The Assessment of Motor and Process Skills (AMPS) (Fisher, 1994) represents a fundamen-

---

[a] This section was prepared by Anne G. Fisher and Day Bennett.

tal and substantive reconceptualization in the development of occupational therapy functional assessments. The AMPS is used to evaluate the quality or effectiveness of the actions of performance (motor and process skills) as they unfold over time when a person performs daily life tasks. The daily life tasks included in the AMPS are domestic or instrumental activities of daily living (IADL) (e.g., meal preparation, home maintenance). The 56 tasks included in the AMPS manual vary in difficulty from simple to complex, with the easiest tasks being less difficult than many self-care tasks, including dressing and toileting.

Since the occupational therapist using the AMPS rates specific motor and process skills according to how each skill contributes to successful task performance, the results provide the occupational therapist therapeutically useful details about (a) why a person is having difficulty completing a task and (b) how complex a task the person has the ability to perform. These capabilities are possible because the use of many-faceted Rasch analysis has enabled the development of hierarchies of task challenges and skill item difficulties, as well as the capacity to calibrate raters with regard to the severity of the ratings that they assign clients. Through computer scoring of the client's test results, ability measures for IADL motor skills and IADL process skills can be generated that take into account the challenge of the tasks the client performed and the severity of the ratings of the therapist who observed and scored the performance.

An important feature to the AMPS is that the occupational therapist who administers the AMPS does not evaluate impairments of the mind-brain-body performance subsystem. Instead, he or she evaluates how underlying motor and process skill capacities are manifested in the context of performance of simple meal preparation and other household tasks. Motor skills are observable actions that the person uses to move the body or the task objects during performance (e.g., lift, reach, manipulate). Process skills are actions the person uses to logically organize and adapt behavior over time in order to complete a task (e.g., search and locate, sequence, accommodate). The interpretation of the AMPS, therefore, ad-

dresses the question: does this person have adequate motor and process skills to perform IADL tasks? Another purpose of AMPS is to identify areas of deficit that should be targeted for intervention.

Test Format and Administration

The AMPS is a structured, observational evaluation. The AMPS is intended to be administered and scored within a 30- to 60-minute period. In most cases, the client completes two or three tasks that take 10–20 minutes each to perform. The administration of the AMPS involves six steps: (1) interviewing the client, with the interview culminating in the client choosing two or three AMPS tasks that he or she will perform; (2) establishing collaboratively the constraints of the tasks to be performed (setting the task contract); (3) setting up the environment; (4) reviewing the contract; (5) administering the assessment; and (6) scoring and interpreting the results.

Before administering the AMPS, the occupational therapist carefully interviews the client and/or the client's care giver to ensure that the client performs tasks he or she has experience performing and that are relevant to the client's daily life needs. From the 56 tasks in the AMPS manual, a short list of four or five tasks is identified by the occupational therapist, who then offers them to the client as possible choices. The short list is selected based upon two criteria: (1) the familiarity and relevance of the tasks to the person to be evaluated and (2) the level of challenge that the tasks will offer the client. From this list, the client chooses which two or three he or she will perform for the AMPS evaluation.

Prior to initiating each AMPS observation, the occupational therapist ensures that the client is fully oriented to the testing environment. This includes confirming that the client knows where all needed tools and materials are located. In unfamiliar or clinic environments, this is accomplished by having the client actually place all tools and materials where he or she would typically store them. Moreover, as part of the interview, the occupational therapist and the client negotiate a specific "task contract" that specifies the occupational form or the constraints of the task to be performed. Knowing the specific task the client intends to perform provides the structure needed for the occupational therapist to evaluate the effectiveness of the client's motor and process skills as they are observed during the IADL task performance.

For each task performed the client is rated on 16 motor skill items and 20 process skill items. These motor and process skill items were derived from theoretical constructs described in the literature and have been validated through research. Each motor and process skill is rated by a trained occupational therapist who uses a four-point rating scale from 4 (competent) to 1 (deficit). The skill item definitions and specific criteria for scoring are set forth in the AMPS training manual.

Because the motor and process skills are observable actions expressed in the midst of occupational behavior, they can be evaluated in terms of how they contribute to the logical progression and outcome of task performance. What is logical is determined by the constraints of the task and by the culture of the person being evaluated. Therefore, scoring criteria that the occupational therapist learns in AMPS training courses emphasize that the effectiveness of the client's performance is to be judged based on what is appropriate given the client's cultural background and the constraints of the task performed.

Upon completion of the AMPS observation, the occupational therapist scores the client's task performances and enters these item raw scores into the computer. The AMPS computer program is used to generate AMPS IADL motor and process ability measures and a variety of reports that can be used for documentation, treatment planning, and research.

Summary of Dependability

Numerous studies supporting the validity and reliability of the AMPS are listed below. The results of these validity and reliability studies support the internal consistency of the AMPS motor and process skills scales, the stability of the AMPS measures over time, and the ability of the measures to remain stable when the AMPS is scored by different raters. Evi-

dence of the validity of the AMPS scales is provided by the ability of the AMPS motor and process skills scales to differentiate levels of IADL motor and process ability among (a) persons who vary in the level of assistance needed to live in the community, (b) older and younger community-living well persons, and (c) well persons and persons with a variety of disabling conditions. The AMPS also has been shown to be valid in cross-cultural applications. These results point to the sensitivity of the AMPS motor and process scales to detect subtle, but clinically meaningful differences in IADL motor and process ability within and between individuals.

Application in Practice

The AMPS has been shown to have applicability in a wide range of clinical, community, and educational settings. Appropriate populations tested using the AMPS include children five years of age and older, adolescents, adults, and older persons with developmental, psychosocial, neurological, or musculoskeletal conditions that may affect independence in occupational performance. The person evaluated must also have a need to perform IADL tasks. Thus, the AMPS is not appropriate for use with persons who are confined to bed, require total care, or are unwilling or have no need to perform IADL tasks.

The results of the AMPS can be used to answer two questions. The first question is: Why does this person experience difficulty? The answer is derived from a profile of that person's motor and process skill raw scores, and the raw scores provide the basis for treatment planning. The second question is: What level of task challenge can this person manage? The AMPS motor and process ability measures are numbers that place the person on two continua of ability, one for IADL motor skills and one for IADL process skills. These IADL motor and process ability measures are computer generated and provide an objective basis for measuring change and the effectiveness of intervention. The Rasch measurement model used to develop and computer score the AMPS allows a therapist to predict how well the client can be expected to perform on any of the

56 instrumental IADL tasks that are calibrated into the AMPS system (e.g., making a salad, doing the laundry, making the bed) even though that individual is only observed performing two or three of these tasks. An example of how the AMPS is used in clinical practice is presented in "Diane: The Use of the Assessment of Motor and Process Skills in Treatment Planning for an Adult with Developmental Disabilities" (see Chapter 14).

Valid and reliable administration and interpretation of the AMPS requires that interested individuals (a) participate in a training workshop and (b) become calibrated as a rater. See the section on resources below for details.

Resources

In order to validly and reliably use the AMPS in clinical practice or research, the occupational therapist must attend a five-day training and calibration workshop and develop skill in the administration and interpretation of the AMPS. Workshops are regularly held in North America, Scandinavia, the United Kingdom, New Zealand, Australia, as well as in other countries around the world. Occupational therapists interested in attending an AMPS workshop should contact the AMPS Project, Occupational Therapy Building, Colorado State University, Fort Collins, CO 80523, or the local AMPS coordinator in the country where the person resides.

Selected References

Baron, K. B. (1994). Clinical interpretation of "The assessment of motor and process skills of persons with psychiatric disorders." *American Journal of Occupational Therapy, 48*, 781–782.

Bernspång, B., & Fisher, A. G. (1994a). Comparison of functional performance between persons with right or left CVA based on the Assessment of Motor and Process Skills. Manuscript submitted for publication.

Bernspång, B., & Fisher, A. G. (1994b). Validation of the Assessment of Motor and Process Skills for use in Sweden. Manuscript submitted for publication.

Dickerson, A. E., & Fisher, A. G. (1993). Age differences in functional performance. *American Journal of Occupational Therapy, 47*, 686–692.

Dickerson, A. E., & Fisher, A. G. (in press). Culture-relevant functional performance assessment of the Hispanic elderly. *Occupational Therapy Journal of Research*.

Doble, S. E., Fisk, J. D., Fisher, A. G., Ritvo, P. G., & Murray, T. J. (1994). Evaluating the functional competence of community-dwelling persons with multiple sclerosis using the Assessment of Motor and Process Skills. *Archives of Physical Medicine and Rehabilitation, 75*, 843–851.

Fisher, A. G. (1993). The assessment of IADL motor skills: An application of many-faceted Rasch analysis. *American Journal of Occupational Therapy, 47*, 319–338.

Fisher, A. G. (1994). *Assessment of Motor and Process Skills* (version 8.0). Unpublished test manual, Department of Occupational Therapy, Colorado State University, Fort Collins, CO.

Fisher, A. G. (in press). Development of a functional assessment that adjusts ability measures for task simplicity and rater leniency. In M. Wilson (Ed.), *Objective measurement: Theory into practice* (Vol 2). Norwood, NJ: Ablex.

Fisher, A. G., Bryze, K. A., Granger, C. V., Haley, S. M., Hamilton, B. B., Heinemann, A. W., Puderbaugh, J. K., Linacre, J. M., Ludlow, L. H., McCabe, M. A., & Wright, B. D. (in press). Applications of Rasch analysis to the development of functional assessments. *International Journal of Educational Research*.

Fisher, A. G., Liu, Y., Velozo, C. A., & Pan, A. W. (1992). Cross-cultural assessment of process skills. *American Journal of Occupational Therapy, 46*, 876–885.

Fisher, W. P., & Fisher, A. G. (1993). Applications of Rasch analysis to studies in occupational therapy. *Physical Medicine and Rehabilitation Clinics of North America: New Developments in Functional Assessment, 4*, 551–569.

Magalhnães, L., Fisher, A. G., Bernspång, B., & Linacre, J. M. (1994). Developing the Assessment of Motor and Process Skills as a cross-cultural evaluation of IADL. Manuscript submitted for publication.

Nygård, L., Bernspång, B., Fisher, A. G., & Winblad, B. (1994). Comparing motor and process ability of persons with suspected dementia in home and clinic settings. *American Journal of Occupational Therapy, 48*, 689–696.

Pan, A. W., & Fisher, A. G. (1994). The assessment of motor and process skills of persons with psychiatric disorders. *American Journal of Occupational Therapy, 48*, 775–780.

Park, S., Fisher, A. G., & Velozo, C. A. (1994). Using the Assessment of Motor and Process Skills to compare occupational performance between clinic and home settings. *American Journal of Occupational Therapy, 48*, 697–709.

3. THE ASSESSMENT OF OCCUPATIONAL FUNCTIONING

The Assessment of Occupational Functioning (AOF) is a semi-structured interview, designed to identify strengths and limitations in areas of occupational functioning derived from the model of human occupation (personal causation, values, roles, habits, and skills).

Test Format and Administration

The AOF includes two parts: (1) an interview schedule and (2) a rating scale. The interview consists of 24 questions. While occupational therapists should use the questions as they appear, they are also encouraged to use probes and clarifications of questions as necessary. The questions are designed to elicit information regarding a client's perception of his or her occupational functioning. The interview takes approximately 30–40 minutes to complete. The occupational therapist then scores the rating scale which includes 20 items.

Dependability

A number of studies have been conducted to establish the test-retest and interrater reliability, content and concurrent validity of this instrument. Overall, the data suggest the AOF is reliable and valid. The original AOF was studied in 1986. Later research resulted in two revisions of the AOF. The most recent version has subsequently been studied while being used with alcoholic clients (See references below).

Application in Practice

While the AOF has been predominantly researched with psychiatric clients, the authors also recommend the instrument for use in physical disability settings. The instrument assists occupational therapists to identify those areas of a client's occupational functioning that require more in-depth evaluation. Further, clinicians have reported that the AOF is useful for assisting treatment and discharge planning, particularly in acute care and outpatient settings. The AOF is particularly useful for occupational therapists in acute care settings where there is pressure to develop specific, focused assessment protocols for each client.

Resources

Copies of the second revision of the AOF can be made directly from Watts, Brollier, Bauer, and Schmidt (1989a). Readers should consult the reference list below for articles which discuss the use of the AOF in practice.

Collected Writings About the Assessment and Its Development

Baber, K. P. (1988). *Validity inferences about occupational functioning based on the assessment of occupational functioning for persons with physical disabilities.* Unpublished master's thesis, Virginia Commonwealth University, Richmond.

Brollier, C., Watts, J. H., Bauer, D., & Schmidt, W. (1989a). A content validity study of the Assessment of Occupational Functioning. *Occupational Therapy in Mental Health, 8*(4), 29–47.
Brollier, C., Watts, J. H., Bauer, D., & Schmidt, W. (1989b). A concurrent validity study of two occupational therapy evaluation instruments: The AOF and OCAIRS. *Occupational Therapy in Mental Health, 8*(4), 49–59.
Hopkins, S., & Schmidt, W. (1986). *A comparison and concurrent validity examination of two evaluation instruments used with psychiatric patients.* Unpublished master's thesis, Virginia Commonwealth University, Richmond.
Viik, M. K., Watts, J. H., Madigan, M. J., & Bauer, D. (1990). Preliminary validation of the Assessment of Occupational Functioning with an alcoholic population. *Occupational Therapy in Mental Health, 10*(2), 19–33.
Watts, J. H., Brollier, C., Bauer, D., & Schmidt, W. (1989a). The Assessment of Occupational Functioning: The second revision. *Occupational Therapy in Mental Health, 8*(4), 61–67.
Watts, J. H., Brollier, C., Bauer, D., & Schmidt, W. (1989b). A comparison of two evaluation instruments used with psychiatric patients in occupational therapy. *Occupational Therapy in Mental Health, 8*(4), 7–27.
Watts, J. H., Kielhofner, G., Bauer, D., Gregory, M., & Valentine, D. (1986). The Assessment of Occupational Functioning: A screening tool for use in long-term care. *American Journal of Occupational Therapy, 40,* 231–240.

4. INTEREST CHECKLIST

Although the Interest Checklist was developed prior to the introduction of the model of human occupation, both the instrument and the theory have strong ties to the occupational behavior tradition. The Interest Checklist has been modified and utilized extensively over the years in studies based in the model of human occupation because of this tool's utility in identifying clients' past and present interests and the degree of attraction clients express towards those interests.

Test Format and Administration

Although a number of versions of the Interest Checklist exist, the revised version appears to be the one most commonly used by occupational therapists utilizing the model of human occupation and will be the one referred to in this discussion. This version consists of 68 activities or areas of interest. The client is asked to place checks in each column in order to describe his or her level of interest (strong, some, or no interest) in each of the activities. Clients are asked to rate his or her level of interest in each activity over two time frames:

the past ten years and the past year. Further, clients are asked whether or not they actively participate in each activity now and whether or not they would like to pursue this activity at some point in the future.

It is suggested that following completion of the checklist the occupational therapist and client discuss the client's pattern of interests.

Dependability

While the Interest Checklist has been used fairly widely in studies, only limited psychometric data is available. Factor-analytic studies aimed at establishing the validity or interest patterns identified by the instrument do not support the practice of formal scoring of activities by category of interests. Other studies that compare disabled and nondisabled populations do suggest that both overall attraction to occupations and patterns of interest may be different for the two groups. Occupational therapists are encouraged to use the checklist for what it reveals about the person's patterns of interests. Often the checklist is most useful when used in conjunction with other structured and unstructured methods. For example, Scaffa (1991) used the Hourly Time Log with the Interest Checklist in a study of clients with alcoholism. She found that while clients newly in rehabilitation and those with extended periods of sobriety recorded similar numbers of strong interests, those newly in rehabilitation spent less time pursuing a narrower range of activities. Those clients with longer periods of sobriety appeared to have established routines that supported more frequent periods of participation in pleasurable activities.

Application in Practice

In clinical use it is common for occupational therapists to follow up the administration of the checklist with an informal interview. The interview is helpful in clarifying responses. This would seem to be particularly important if the occupational therapist is to appreciate the impact that disability has had on how the client is experiencing pleasure from an activity or the significance disability has had in altering a client's attraction to particular kinds of activities.

Resources

The Modified Interest Checklist is available from the National Institutes of Health.

Occupational Therapy Department
Department of Rehabilitation Medicine
National Institutes of Health
Building 10, Room 6S235
Bethesda, MD 20892

Readers should consult the reference list below, particularly Rogers (1988) for details on how the instrument can be used in practice.

References

Collected Writings About the Assessment and Its Development

Barrows, C. (1988). *Stability of self-report measures of volition in bipolar affective disorder.* Unpublished master's thesis, Boston University.

Katz, N. (1988). Interest checklist: A factor analytical study. *Occupational Therapy in Mental Health, 8*(1), 45–56.

Matsutsuyu, J. (1969). The Interest Checklist. *American Journal of Occupational Therapy, 23,* 323–328.

Rogers, J. (1988). The NPI Interest Check List. In B. Hemphill (Ed.), *Mental Health Assessment in Occupational Therapy.* Thorofare, NJ: Slack.

Rogers, J., Weinstein, J., & Figone, J. (1978). The Interest Check List: An empirical assessment. *American Journal of Occupational Therapy, 32,* 628–630.

Collected Writings in Which the Assessment Was Used

Barris, R., Kielhofner, G., Burch, R. M., Gelinas, I., Klement, M., & Schultz, B. (1986). Occupational function and dysfunction in three groups of adolescents. *Occupational Therapy Journal of Research, 6,* 301–317.

Bauer, J. (1988). *The relationship of self esteem to value goals, interests, personal causation in adolescents with severe disability and those without severe disability.* Unpublished master's thesis, University of Southern California, Los Angeles.

Ebb, E. W., Coster, W., & Duncombe, L. (1989). Comparison of normal and psychosocially dysfunctional male adolescents. *Occupational Therapy in Mental Health, 9*(2), 53–74.

Fronczek, V. (1985). *A study of the comparison of the roles, locus of control and interests of the acute hand injured patient.* Unpublished master's thesis, Virginia Commonwealth University, Richmond.

Katz, N., Giladi, N., & Peretz, C. (1988). Cross-cultural application of occupational therapy assessments: Human occupation with psychiatric inpatients and controls in Israel. *Occupational Therapy in Mental Health, 8*(1), 7–30.

Katz, N., Josman, N., & Steinmetz, N. (1988). Relationship between cognitive disability theory and the model of human occupation in the assessment of psychiatric and non-psychiatric adolescents. *Occupational Therapy in Mental Health, 8*(1), 31–44.

Kavanaugh, M. (1982). *Person-environment interaction: The model of human occupation applied to mentally retarded adults.* Unpublished master's thesis, Virginia Commonwealth University, Richmond.

Oakley, F., Kielhofner, G., & Barris, R. (1985). An occupational therapy approach to assessing psychiatric patients' adaptive functioning. *American Journal of Occupational Therapy, 39,* 147–154.

Scaffa, M. (1991). Alcoholism: An occupational behavior perspective. *Occupational Therapy in Mental Health, 11*(2/3), 99–111.

Smyntek, L., Barris, R., & Kielhofner, G. (1985). The model of human occupation applied to psychosocially functional and dysfunctional adolescents. *Occupational Therapy in Mental Health, 5*(1), 21–40.

5. THE NATIONAL INSTITUTES OF HEALTH ACTIVITY RECORD

The NIH Activity Record (ACTRE) was developed as an outcome measure for a study of patients with rheumatoid arthritis. This instrument provides a 24-hour log of a patient's activities and is an adaptation of the Occupational Questionnaire (described later in this appendix). The ACTRE aims to provide details on the impact of symptoms on task performance, individual perceptions of interest and significance of daily activities, and daily habit patterns. Specific information gathered covers frequency and/or percentage of time spent in role activity and resting, frequency of rest periods during activity, frequency and/or percentage of time with pain and fatigue and time of day or activity with which it occurs, plus volitional concerns such as interests, meaning, enjoyment, and perception of personal effectiveness.

Test Format and Administration

The ACTRE is a self-administered questionnaire and is essentially a 24-hour time log. The log is completed at three points during each of the two days which are being recorded. This helps improve the accuracy of the instrument, since recall is of a very recent past.

The person begins by recording the major activity that they were doing for each half-hour block of time. Then for each of those activities the person records the following information:

- level of energy required (3 levels)
- type of activity (8 categories, e.g., rest, self-care, treatment, recreation)
- amount of pain experienced (4 levels)
- amount of fatigue experienced (2 questions, 4 levels)
- perception of ability (2 questions, 4 levels)
- personal significance of activity (4 levels)
- amount of pleasure in activity (4 levels)
- rest taken during activity (yes/no)

The client should read the instructions and do a sample form with the occupational therapist prior to taking the ACTRE home to complete. The ACTRE should be completed for two full days, either two weekdays or one weekday and one weekend day. The authors suggest that this instrument is particularly suitable for persons whose activity is limited by pain or fatigue.

Dependability

The initial validation of the ACTRE was undertaken with a group of clients with rheumatoid arthritis. It appears that the ACTRE correlates well with other measures of pain, fatigue, and ADL performance. Additionally, although actual measures of reliability do not exist, one study does suggest that this instrument is reasonably able to consistently discriminate between different patient groups.

Application in Practice

The ACTRE has been used as an outcome measure in patients with progressive neuromuscular and neurological conditions (e.g., rheumatoid arthritis, Parkinson's disease, postpolio syndrome). The authors suggest that since it provides an individualized account of a person's daily pattern of activity it can act as a valuable aid to treatment planning. They also suggest that the ACTRE can be useful for tracking patients over the course of their illness. Since the ACTRE can detect changes over time it can be used to see if a client's activity patterns are changing as a result of therapy (e.g., if education programs are effective). The ACTRE is also useful to document results of treatment for insurance and research as it provides a means to quantify otherwise subjective data.

The ACTRE is appropriate for use with adolescents and adults. It should be completed in the problem-generating environment (i.e., home, school, work, etc.). Instructions can be read to the patient, but the ability to read each question is necessary to complete the form.

The ACTRE is a performance-based evaluation in the problem-generating environment. It is most useful as one of several evaluations when it is necessary to quantify frequency and/or percentage of waking hours.

- pain and/or fatigue (amount, intensity, time of day and associated activity).
- level and patterns of physical activity and/or rest which may be contributing to patient's functional limitations.
- changes in participation in role activities which may be contributing to patient's functional limitations.
- information on how patient feels about daily activities (meaningful, enjoyable) as in psychosocial disorders and when disability results in changed role activities.
- patients' perception about their performance (difficulty).

To assist clinicians and researchers in scoring, a computer-based method of scoring and summarizing the ACTRE using a spreadsheet is currently available from NIH (see address in resource section).

Resources

Copies of the NIH ACTRE can be obtained directly from the authors at the National Institutes of Health. This information packet contains details on how to use the instrument, instruction sheets, activity record logs, and other necessary materials. In addition, an updated method of scoring the ACTRE using a computer spreadsheet can also be obtained from Gloria Furst at NIH. Computer scoring is recommended over the existing manual scoring method that has been reported in some current literature.

Contact:

Gloria Furst, MPH, OTR
Department of Rehabilitation Medicine
Warren Grant Magnuson Clinical Center
National Institutes of Health
9000 Rockville Pike, 10/6S235
Bethesda, MD 20892

References

Collected Writings About the Assessment and Its Development
Gerber, L. & Furst, G. (1992a). Validation of the NIH activity record: A quantitative measure of life activities. *Arthritis Care Research, 5*, 81–86.
Gerber, L. & Furst, G. (1992b). Scoring methods and application of the Activity Record (ACTRE) for patients with musculoskeletal disorders. *Arthritis Care and Research, 5*, 151–156.

Collected Writings in Which the Assessment Was Used
Furst, G., Gerber, L., Smith, C., Fisher, S. & Shulman, B. (1987). A program for improving energy conservation behaviors in adults with rheumatoid arthritis. *American Journal of Occupational Therapy, 41*, 102–111.
Packer, T. L., Martins, I., Krefting, L., & Brouwer, B. (1991). Activity and post-polio fatigue. *Orthopedics, 14*(11), 1223–1226.

6. OCCUPATIONAL CASE ANALYSIS INTERVIEW AND RATING SCALE

The Occupational Case Analysis Interview and Rating Scale (OCAIRS) was developed primarily to aid discharge planning for psychiatric clients in short-term treatment settings. The instrument organizes the gathering, analysis, and reporting of information concerning an individual's occupational functioning.

Test Format and Administration

With practice the interview takes about 20–35 minutes to administer and a further 30–50 minutes to score, record, and interpret the information gathered. The procedure for administering the OCAIRS consists of three parts: interview, rating scale, summary sheet.

This is a semi-structured interview. The manual provides a number of questions aimed at gathering details on various aspects of the person's function as conceptualized in the model. The occupational therapist must be familiar with the intent of the questions so that he or she can probe for further details when required. Suggestions for probing for further information are provided in the manual.

To score the assessment, the occupational therapist rates the client's level of adaptation using a five-point ordinal scale for each of 14 components. A score of 5 indicates that this area facilitates adaptive daily living, a score of

1 indicates that this component impedes daily living or is not adaptive. The manual provides details for each item as to the kind of information and responses which would be considered adaptive at each level of the scale. Four of the items ask the occupational therapist to make global judgements of the individuals' function. These include: dynamic—how the various components interacts in this person to determine adaptation; historical—how the person has adapted over the course of his or her life; contextual—how does the environment support performance; system trajectory—overall, where do you think the person's life is headed?

On the summary form, scores are used to create a clinically useful profile of this person's occupational status. This can then be used to document on findings in the patient's chart.

Dependability

Two studies have been undertaken to establish the content validity of the OCAIRS. In both studies a panel of experts were used to validate that the content of the interview and the items rated reflected the content of the model of human occupation. After revisions following the first study, the second study supported the assumption that the OCAIRS has adequate content validity.

Two studies comparing the OCAIRS with the Assessment of Occupational Functioning indicate that this instrument has adequate concurrent validity.

Interrater reliability has been demonstrated to be acceptable. Following an initial study which resulted in some revisions, a second study was undertaken and found the OCAIRS to be generally acceptable in terms of interrater reliability.

Application in Practice

The OCAIRS was developed primarily for use in short-term psychiatric settings where pressures of time put efficient data gathering and discharge planning at a premium. It seems likely that the OCAIRS would be applicable in a variety of settings, although therapists should think carefully about the kind of data needed to be gathered with their particular clients.

Resources

All occupational therapists wishing to use this assessment should purchase a copy of the manual which explains in detail how to conduct the interview, provides scoring criteria, and blank score sheets.

To order a manual, please contact:

BOOK ORDER DEPARTMENT
SLACK Incorporated
6900 Grove Road
Thorofare, NJ 08086-9447
Phone 1-800-257-8290 or FAX (609) 853-5991
Please quote order number 30543

References

Collected Writings About the Assessment and Its Development
Brollier, C., Watts, J. H., Bauer, D., & Schmidt, W. (1989). A concurrent validity study of two occupational therapy evaluation instruments: The AOF and OCAIRS. *Occupational Therapy in Mental Health, 8*(4), 49–59.
Cubie, S., & Kaplan, K. (1982). A case analysis method for the model of human occupation. *American Journal of Occupational Therapy, 36*, 645–656.
Hopkins, S., & Schmidt, W. (1986). *A comparison and concurrent validity examination of two evaluation instruments used with psychiatric patients.* Unpublished master's thesis, Virginia Commonwealth University, Richmond.
Kaplan, K. (1984). Short-term assessment: The need and a response. *Occupational Therapy in Mental Health, 4*(3), 29–45.
Kaplan, K., & Kielhofner, G. (1989). *The Occupational Case Analysis Interview and Rating Scale.* Thorofare, NJ: Slack.

7. Occupational Performance History Interview

The Occupational Performance History Interview (OPHI) is a semi-structured interview designed to gather an individual's history of work, play, and self-care performance. The instrument can be used with both psychiatric or physically disabled adolescents and adults. The instrument has two interview forms to accommodate occupational therapists using the model of human occupation and those using an eclectic approach.

Test Format and Administration

The first part of the OPHI, the interview, consists of 39 recommended questions covering five content areas. The content areas include: (1) organization of daily living routines;

(2) life roles; (3) interests, values, and goals; (4) perceptions of ability and responsibility; and (5) environmental influences.

The interview takes approximately 45–60 minutes to complete. The interview is structured to assist the patient to relate his or her life story, with the occupational therapist and patient identifying a "turning point" which divides the interview, and the subsequent life history, into past and present.

The second part of the OPHI, the rating form, requires the interviewer to quantify the information collected during the interview. The interviewer scores 10 items (two for each of the five content areas). Each item is rated on a five-point scale, indicating the degree of adaptive occupational function the client reports.

Finally, a Life History Narrative form is used to report qualitative data from the interview and a five-item nominal scale called the Life History Pattern is used to characterize the individual's overall history.

Dependability

The first study of the OPHI with psychiatric clients found modest test-retest and interrater reliability (Kielhofner & Henry, 1988). The investigators concluded that, among other factors, the conceptual model which occupational therapists employed differentially influenced their implementation and rating of the interview and contributed to rater disagreement.

Consequently, a second study (Kielhofner, Henry, Walens, & Rogers, 1991), looked more closely at the influence of conceptual practice models on the interrater stability of the interview. Despite revisions to the interview and the participation of occupational therapists who were matched and trained in the use of conceptual models, the results did not show any significant improvement in interrater reliability.

A more recent study (Mallinson, Kielhofner, & Mattingly, 1994), rephrased the issues by more closely examining the actual content of the interview and the data it provides. This study yielded implications for the way historical interviews are conducted, including the importance of using narrative-evoking strategies and attention to how patients interpret their lives.

Application in Practice

The OPHI seeks to objectify data of the life history; i.e., the occupational therapist is to elicit from the respondent the facts of his or her life and then analyze what those facts mean in terms of adaptiveness as exhibited in a potential life pattern. This interview can be used successfully with patients with a range of diagnoses and disabilities, given that the patient has adequate skills in communication and attention. The OPHI is most significant for its ability to give the interviewer a means of understanding the way a patient perceives her or his life to be unfolding.

Resources

All occupational therapists wishing to use this assessment should purchase a copy of the manual which explains in detail how to conduct the interview, lists recommended questions, and provides scoring criteria and score sheets.

The OPHI manual may be purchased from:

The American Occupational Therapy Association, Inc.
4720 Montgomery Lane
PO Box 31220
Bethesda, MD 20824-1220
(301) 652-2682
FAX: (301) 652-7711
Please quote order number 1690

References

Collected Writings About the Assessment and Its Development

Gutkowski, L. (1992). *A generalized study of the revised occupational performance history interview*. Unpublished master's thesis, University of Illinois at Chicago.

Kielhofner, G., & Henry, A. D. (1988). Development and investigation of the Occupational Performance History Interview. *American Journal of Occupational Therapy, 42,* 489–498.

Kielhofner, G., Henry, A., & Walens, D. (1989). *A user's guide to the Occupational Performance History Interview*. Rockville, MD: American Occupational Therapy Association.

Kielhofner, G., Henry, A., Walens, D., & Rogers E. S. (1991). A generalizability study of the Occupational Performance History Interview. *Occupational Therapy Journal of Research, 11,* 292–306.

Mallinson, T., Kielhofner, G., & Mattingly, C. (1994). *"Like being stuck in flypaper": Understanding volition through metaphor.* Paper submitted for publication.

Collected Writings in Which the Assessment Was Used
Bridle, M. J., Lynch, K. B., & Quesenberry, C. M. (1990). Long term function following the central cord syndrome. *Paraplegia, 28*, 178–185.

8. THE OCCUPATIONAL QUESTIONNAIRE

The Occupational Questionnaire (OQ) is a pen and paper, self-report instrument which asks the individual to provide a description of typical use of time and utilizes Likert-type ratings of competence, importance, and enjoyment during activities.

Test Format and Administration

The OQ asks the client to complete the instrument in two parts. First, he or she completes a list of the activities he or she performs each half-hour on a typical weekday. After listing the activities, the client is asked to answer four questions for each activity. The questions ask the client to rate whether they consider the activity to be work, daily living tasks, recreation, or rest, and to consider how well he or she does the activities, how important they are to him or her, and how much he or she enjoys doing them. The occupational therapist can use the scores to calculate the quality of waking activities in terms of value, interest, and personal causation, along with the actual number of half hours spent in activity. While a variety of scores can be calculated, what matters most is what the client and therapist are able to deduce from them. The numbers obtained should provide insight into the person's pattern of occupational activity in daily life.

Dependability

This instrument was pilot tested in a study by Riopel (1982) which was interested in establishing how patterns of daily activity affected volition and life satisfaction. This preliminary evidence suggested the OQ had adequate test-retest reliability and concurrent validity. Since that time, little psychometric work has been added although the instrument has been used extensively in clinical research studies to compare the difference in patterns of time use between occupationally dysfunctional clients and their well peers.

Application in Practice

The OQ is a valuable clinical tool for establishing not only how a client spends their time but also for gaining information on how a client interprets the activity (does it seem like work or leisure) and also how confident and satisfied they are in their performance of those activities. Like all pen and paper instruments, the OQ is best supplemented with an in-depth discussion with the client about the consequences for them of their daily use of time, and the meaning and satisfaction they feel in the performance of those activities.

Resources

A brief guide to using the OQ, including use and interpretation of scores, and score sheets may be obtained from the Model of Human Occupation Clearinghouse.

References

Collected Writings About the Assessment and Its Development
Smith, N. R., Kielhofner, G., & Watts, J. (1986). The relationship between volition, activity pattern, and life satisfaction in the elderly. *American Journal of Occupational Therapy, 40*, 278–283.

Collected Writings in Which the Assessment Was Used
Barris, R., Kielhofner, G., Burch, R. M., Gelinas, I., Klement, M., & Schultz, B. (1986). Occupational function and dysfunction in three groups of adolescents. *Occupational Therapy Journal of Research, 6*, 301–317.
Ebb, E. W., Coster, W., & Duncombe, L. (1989). Comparison of normal and psychosocially dysfunctional male adolescents. *Occupational Therapy in Mental Health, 9*(2), 53–74.
Kielhofner, G., & Brinson, M. (1989). Development and evaluation of an aftercare program for young and chronic psychiatrically disabled adults. *Occupational Therapy in Mental Health, 9*(2), 1–25.
Knapp, J. (1984). *An investigation of occupational behavior, leisure values & life satisfaction of the older adult.* Unpublished master's thesis, Virginia Commonwealth University, Richmond.
Rust, K., Barris, R., & Hooper, F. (1987). Use of the model of human occupation to predict women's exercise behavior. *Occupational Therapy Journal of Research, 7*, 23–35.
Simmons, J. (1984). *The correlation of home environments' physical and social dimensions with occupational performances of post stroke victims.* Unpublished master's thesis, Virginia Commonwealth University, Richmond.
Smyntek, L., Barris, R., & Kielhofner, G. (1985). The model of human occupation applied to psychosocially functional and dysfunctional adolescents. *Occupational Therapy in Mental Health, 5*(1), 21–40.

9. ROLE CHECKLIST

The Role Checklist is a self-report checklist that can be used to obtain information about the types of roles people engage in and which organize their daily lives. This checklist provides data on an individual's perception of his or her roles over the course of their life and also the degree of value, i.e., the significance and importance that they place on those roles. The Role Checklist can be used with adolescents, adult, or geriatric populations.

Test Format and Administration

The Role Checklist asks the client to consider each of ten roles described on the form. These roles are student, worker, volunteer, care giver, home maintainer, friend, family member, religious participant, hobbyist/amateur, participant in organizations. See Chapter 5 for more discussion on these occupational roles. There is also an "other" category in which clients may enter additional roles not listed. Each role is accompanied by a brief description and a reference to the frequency with which the role is enacted. Since the intent of the checklist is to identify roles which organize an individual's daily life, reference to frequency of performance is included for each role definition.

The checklist itself is in two parts. Part One asks the client to check those roles they have performed in the past, are currently involved in, and/or plan to perform in the future. For example, if an individual volunteered in the past, does not volunteer at present, but does anticipate volunteering in the future, he or she would check the role "volunteer" in both the past and future columns. "Past" refers to any time up to preceding week. "Present" includes the week prior, up to and including the day of administration of the checklist. "Future" refers to tomorrow or any day thereafter.

In Part Two of the checklist, the client is asked to indicate how much worth or importance, i.e., how valuable, each of the 10 roles is for them. Each role is rated as to whether the person finds it "not at all valuable," "somewhat valuable," or "very valuable."

The Role Checklist takes approximately 15 minutes for a client to complete. The occupational therapist is encouraged to remain with the client in order to answer or clarify questions.

Dependability

The majority of the psychometric work on the Role Checklist was carried out during the development of the instrument (Oakley, Kielhofner, Barris, & Reichler, 1986). Content validity was established by an extensive review of the literature and a review by a panel of occupational therapists, which resulted in revisions to some aspects of the checklist. Initial measures of test-retest reliability indicated that the instrument was reasonably stable over time with adults.

Since that time, little psychometric work has been added, although the Role Checklist has been used frequently in research. Many of the studies use the checklist as a measure of changes in role performance or value that is linked to understanding clients' future orientation and life satisfaction. The checklist has been used in studies of clients with multiple personality disorder, HIV infection, psychiatric adolescents, and normal adults. It has also been used to compare well and psychiatrically disabled populations, as well as level of engagement in ADL following total hip replacement surgery.

Application in Practice

The checklist can be a valuable tool for understanding what roles an individual perceives themselves as occupying and also the significance or importance they place on those roles. This can usefully lead to understanding the degree of identification a person has with a particular role, and the interest they have in engaging in tasks necessary to enact that role. When followed up with an interview, the Role Checklist can further help the occupational therapist and client identify patterns in role selection, preference, and performance. For example, looking at the kinds of roles the person has been successful at over the course of their life, the kinds of roles they have avoided or given up, if roles focus around particular kinds of occupational forms (e.g., social relationships, service delivery). The occupational therapist might also learn that the client has many roles but gains little satisfaction from them or that they have one special role about which they are passionate and which they have sustained over a long period of time.

Resources

Discussion on the use of the Role Checklist in practice can be found in Barris, Oakley, and Kielhofner (1988).

Copies of the Role Checklist can be obtained from NIH:

Frances Oakley, MS, OTR/L
Building 10, Room 6S235
National Institutes of Health
9000 Rockville Pike
Bethesda, MD 20892

References

Collected Writings About the Assessment and Its Development

Barris, R., Oakley, F., & Kielhofner, G. (1988). The Role Checklist. In B. Hemphill (Ed.), *Mental Health Assessment in Occupational Therapy*. Thorofare, NJ: Slack.

Barrows, C. (1988). *Stability of self report measures of volition in bipolar affective disorder*. Unpublished master's thesis, Boston University.

Duellman, M. (1983). *Impact of available activity and perceived environmental congruency on the institutionalized elderly*. Unpublished master's thesis, Virginia Commonwealth University, Richmond.

Fronczek, Y. (1985). *A study of the comparison of the roles, locus of control and interests of the acute hand injured patient*. Unpublished master's thesis, Virginia Commonwealth University, Richmond.

Lerder, J., Kielhofner, G., & Watts, J. (1985). Values, personal causation and skills of delinquents of the acute hand injured patient. *Occupational Therapy in Mental Health, 5*, 59–77.

Oakley, F., Kielhofner, G., Barris, R., & Reichler, R. K. (1986). The Role Checklist: Development and empirical assessment of reliability. *Occupational Therapy Journal of Research, 6*, 157–170.

Pezzulli, T. (1988). *Test-retest reliability of the role checklist with depressed adolescents in short term psychiatric hospitals*. Unpublished master's thesis, Virginia Commonwealth University, Richmond.

Collected Writings in Which the Assessment Was Used

Barris, R., Dickie, V., & Baron, K. (1988). A comparison of psychiatric patients and normal subjects based on the model of human occupation. *Occupational Therapy Journal of Research, 8*, 3–37.

Barris, R., Kielhofner, G., Burch, R. M., Gelinas, I., Klement, M., & Schultz, B. (1986). Occupational function and dysfunction in three groups of adolescents. *Occupational Therapy Journal of Research, 6*, 301–317.

Bränholm, I., & Fugl-Meyer, A. R. (1992). Occupational role preferences and life satisfaction. *Occupational Therapy Journal of Research, 12*, 159–171.

Duellman, M. K., Barris, R., & Kielhofner, G. (1986). Organized activity and the adaptive status of nursing home residents. *American Journal of Occupational Therapy, 40*, 618–622.

Ebb, E. W., Coster, W., & Duncombe, L. (1989). Comparison of normal and psychosocially dysfunctional male adolescents. *Occupational Therapy in Mental Health, 9*(2), 53–74.

Egan, M., Warren, S. A., Hessel, P. A., & Gilewich, G. (1992). Activities of daily living after hip fracture: Pre- and post discharge. *Occupational Therapy Journal of Research, 12*, 342–356.

Elliott, M., & Barris, R. (1987). Occupational role performance and life satisfaction in elderly persons. *Occupational Therapy Journal of Research, 7*, 215–224.

Oakley, F., Kielhofner, G., & Barris, R. (1985). An occupational therapy approach to assessing psychiatric patients' adaptive functioning. *American Journal of Occupational Therapy, 39*, 147–154.

Pizzi, M. A. (1990). The model of human occupation and adults with HIV infection and AIDS. *American Journal of Occupational Therapy, 44*, 257–264.

Rust, K., Barris, R., & Hooper, F. (1987). Use of the model of human occupation to predict women's exercise behavior. *Occupational Therapy Journal of Research, 7*, 23–35.

Sepiol, J. M., & Froehlich, J. (1990). Use of the role checklist with the patient with multiple personality disorder. *American Journal of Occupational Therapy, 44*, 1008–1012.

Smyntek, L., Barris, R., & Kielhofner, G. (1985). The model of human occupation applied to psychosocially functional and dysfunctional adolescents. *Occupational Therapy in Mental Health, 5*(1), 21–40.

10. Self Assessment of Occupational Functioning

The Self Assessment of Occupational Functioning (SAOF) and its corresponding children's version were developed out of a belief that collaborative treatment planning between patient and occupational therapist is a prerequisite to effective occupational therapy intervention. This view is consistent with the recent trend of viewing patients as consumers, with rights to information regarding their treatment.

Test Format and Administration

The SAOF is a checklist that consists of a series of statements; these statements correspond with the components of the model of human occupation. The patient rates each statement as a strength, adequate, or an area needing improvement. Priorities are then identified from among the latter, and listed. The form is designed so that the entire process of self-assessment and goal prioritization is represented visually; this affords both patient and occupational therapist a quick overview of the patient's level of function. The instrument then becomes the vehicle for a discussion of treatment planning. A collaborative treatment plan is then written in the patient's words.

The clinician must determine the method of administration: either the occupational therapist reads the statements and records the patient's responses, or the patient completes the form independently. This decision depends on the clinical situation and on the patient's individual needs. Both a long and short version of the SAOF have been created to fit the needs of the patient.

Dependability

Two content validity studies have been completed on the adult/adolescent version of the SAOF. These indicate that the SAOF is theoretically sound. Occupational therapists can be reasonably sure that the statements represent the concepts of the model of human occupation.

A survey was also completed to examine the usability of this instrument in clinical practice. As a result the instrument was revised in order to improve its "user friendliness."

Application in Practice

This instrument in suitable for use with a wide range of clients with varying degrees of occupational dysfunction. Clients with impaired written and verbal comprehension and expression may find this approach challenging in its original form. Adaptations such as reading items to the client and simplifying language should be implemented where indicated. Clinical judgement should be exercised when using this instrument with clients whose illness or disability impairs their ability to make accurate assessments of their abilities. Adolescents with learning disabilities or attention deficit disorder may find they are able to

complete the children's version more easily than the adult version.

Resources

The SAOF and the Children's SAOF are available from the Model of Human Occupation Clearinghouse. The manual includes background information and a full discussion of the collaborative treatment planning process, as well as detailed instruction on the administration of the SAOF and CSAOF. Client instructions and rating forms (short and long versions) are also included.

Collected Writings About the Assessment and Its Development

Baron, K. (1991). *The Self Assessment of Occupational Functioning: An efficacy study*. Unpublished master's thesis, University of Illinois at Chicago.

Baron, K. B., & Curtin, C. (1990). *A manual for use with the Self Assessment of Occupational Functioning*. Department of Occupational Therapy, University of Illinois at Chicago.

11. VOLITIONAL QUESTIONNAIRE

Traditionally, it has been difficult to assess volition in clients who have communication and cognitive limitations due to the complex language requirements of most assessments of volition. The Volitional Questionnaire is an attempt to recognize that while such clients have difficulty formulating goals or expressing their interests and values verbally, they are often able to communicate them through actions. The client is observed in a number of occupational behavior settings so that a picture of the person's volition and the environmental supports required to support the expression can be identified.

Test Format and Administration

The Volitional Questionnaire is of most benefit when the client is observed over multiple sessions in a variety of occupational behavior settings. The author recommends that a person be observed in self-care, work, and leisure environments for a combined total of five sessions. The person's performance in each session is rated.

Before beginning the evaluation, it is important to make adaptations to the setting if needed. Once the person arrives, he or she is invited to go in and explore the different alternatives for activity. Following this, he or she is invited to choose an activity. After the person has participated in the activity for some time, the occupational therapist starts to introduce novelty into the activity situation and to offer different levels of demands in order to evaluate personal causation indicators. When the activity is complete, the occupational therapist talks with the person about his or her feelings of competence, satisfaction, and personal goals related to the type of activities and environment. Following the session the occupational therapist completes the rating form.

The Volitional Questionnaire consists of 14 indicators in three areas: (1) intrinsic motivation; (2) personal causation; and (3) values/interests (see Figure 12.2).

The person is rated in terms of the degree of spontaneity with which they demonstrate behavior reflective of the indicators. The ratings are on a four-point scale: 4 = Spontaneous—the person engages in and responds to their environment with minimal support, structure, or stimulation; 3 = Involved—the person engages in the environment with moderate support; 2 = Hesitant—the person requires substantial support and structure to engage in the environment; 1 = Passive—the person can engage in the environment only with a maximal amount of support or structure. The manual outlines specific examples of these ratings for each indicator.

The occupational therapist concludes by writing a brief narrative which details the person's interests and values, the amount and kind of support required for a person to accomplish a behavior, the influence of this person's values, interests, and personal causation on the person's motivation to engage in activities, and the influence of different environments on this person's volition.

Dependability

The first study to examine the reliability and validity of the Volitional Questionnaire was completed by de las Heras (1993a, 1993b). Content validity was established through a review of the literature and by a panel of experts who were familiar with this model. Preliminary evidence of construct validity was similarly established using a panel of experts. Analysis suggested that members generally concluded items reflected the model constructs they were intended to reflect. Measures of reliability for the instrument showed reasonable stability and interrater reliability was adequate. Differences in client performances between occupational behavior settings supported the belief that volition is influenced by the environment and highlights the importance of evaluation in all three settings.

A second series of two studies to examine the validity of this instrument was recently completed (Chern, 1994). This study utilized the Rasch measurement model to establish that the items of the Volitional Questionnaire do indeed reflect a single construct of volition. This study also found that the instrument was not as effective in separating out persons of different abilities. As a result, the scale was revised to reflect spontaneity of behaviors rather than frequency. Following the recommendations of de las Heras, item descriptions were clarified. A second study found that with these revisions the instrument was more discriminating (i.e., it was able to separate out more effectively persons of varying levels of volitional ability). This instrument was originally developed for use with clients with chronic psychiatric disabilities and cognitive impairments. This second study indicates that some items may be too easy for clients with less involved difficulties. Further studies on a wider range of clients will be needed to establish if such a ceiling effect exists and if scale revision is necessary.

Application in Practice

The Volitional Questionnaire was designed to assess, through observation, volition in those clients for whom traditional interview and pen and paper approaches were not appropriate. This is a frequently neglected and misunderstood group of individuals. One of the real advantages of this instrument is that rather than focusing on the multitude of deficits these people have, it is geared to ask and answer such questions as "When, and under what conditions, does this person demonstrate useful and appropriate volition?" and "What kinds of supports or environments facilitate spontaneous expressions of volition in this person?" Since the instrument also requires the occupational therapist to write a detailed narrative of the person's behavior that reflects volition, he or she must be particularly observant of and sensitive to both the person and the environment. At present the instrument is more particularly suited to individuals with marked deficits in occupational behavior. Further work will need to be done to extend its use among other groups of clients.

Resources

The Volitional Questionnaire and User's Manual can be obtained from the Model of Human Occupation Clearinghouse. The manual includes background on the use of the instrument, detailed descriptions of each indicator, scoring guidelines, discussion on implementation and interpretation, as well as two case simulations. Rating forms, narrative form, and case analysis forms are also included.

References

Collected Writings About the Assessment and Its Development
Chern, J. S. (1994). *The validity and reliability of Volitional Questionnaire—A rasch analysis.* Unpublished master's thesis, University of Illinois at Chicago.
de las Heras, C. G. (1993a). *The Volitional Questionnaire.* Unpublished manual. Santiago, Chile.
de las Heras, C. G. (1993b). *The Volitional Questionnaire.* Unpublished master's thesis, Tufts University, Boston, MA.

12. WORKER ROLE INTERVIEW

The Worker Role Interview (WRI), is a semi-structured interview designed to be used as the psychosocial/environmental component of the initial rehabilitation assessment process for the injured worker. The interview is designed to have the client discuss various aspects of his or her life and job setting that have been associated with past work experiences. The WRI combines information from an interview with observations made during the physical and behavioral assessment procedure of a physical and/or work capacity assessment. The intent is to identify the psychosocial and environmental variables that may influence the ability of the injured worker to return to work.

Test Format and Administration

Administration of the WRI consists of five steps: (1) interview preparation; (2) conducting the semi-structured interview, which is completed at the beginning of initial assessment of the injured worker; (3) the usual physical/work capacity assessment procedures used in the rehabilitation setting; (4) scoring the WRI Rating Form following initial evaluation; and (5) rescoring the WRI Rating Form at discharge from the treatment program.

The WRI has six content areas with subcontent areas (see Figure 12.12). These subcontent areas were devised from an extensive review of the literature of factors that seem to impact on return to work.

The semi-structured interview includes 28 recommended questions covering the areas outlined below. The interview can be administered in approximately 30–60 minutes. The occupational therapist rates each of the subcontent areas on a scale of 1 to 4 depending on how strongly the interview findings appear to support this client returning to his or her previous employment or work in general, whichever is more appropriate for this client. The occupational therapist is encouraged to write brief comments to support each rating (see Figure 12.12).

Dependability

The WRI is still in initial stages of test development although a number of early studies support the internal validity of the instrument (Velozo, 1992), test-retest reliability (Biernacki, 1994), interrater reliability, and construct validity (Gern, 1993). The instrument appears to effectively evaluate the range of abilities with which work hardening clients present, with no apparent "ceiling" or "floor" effects.

To date, the test has been predominantly validated on clients with physical disabilities (e.g., low back pain, hand injuries); however, one study developed and examined a version for clients with psychiatric illness (Handlesman, 1994).

Application in Practice

The WRI was originally designed for use with work hardening clients, although it is proving robust with a wide range of client groups. This instrument is designed to be used alongside other assessments of work-related skills. It is generally suggested that it be used as part of an initial assessment protocol and can be useful for indicating areas of occupational functioning that require more detailed evaluation. Studies have also showed that the WRI may be useful in facilitating discharge planning.

Resources

Copies of the WRI user's manual and a videotape detailing interview administration can be obtained from the Model of Human Occupation Clearinghouse. The manual includes background to the instrument, administration procedures, recommended questions, scoring instructions, and rating scale for each subcontent area. Rating forms are also included.

Collected Writings About the Assessment and Its Development

Biernacki, S. (1993). Reliability of the Worker Role Interview. *American Journal of Occupational Therapy, 47,* 797–803.

Gern, A. (1993). *Validity of the Worker Role Interview*. Unpublished master's thesis, University of Illinois at Chicago.

Handlesman, D. (1994). *The construct validity of the Worker Role Interview for the chronic mentally ill*. Unpublished master's thesis, University of Illinois at Chicago.

Lin, F. L. (1994). *The Worker Role Interview: Construct validity across diagnoses*. Unpublished master's thesis, University of Illinois at Chicago.

Velozo, C., Kielhofner, G., & Fisher, G. (1990). *A user's guide to the Worker Role Interview*. (Research version). Department of Occupational Therapy, University of Illinois at Chicago.

13/ Change Making: Principles of Therapeutic Intervention

Gary Kielhofner

INTRODUCTION

Life is change. Whether the catalyst be biological development, novel experiences, the aging process, necessary adjustment to trauma or disease, or alterations in one's environment, change is part and parcel of human life. Even those periods of life that appear relatively stable are marked by a series of ongoing smaller changes.

Occupational therapists encounter patients and clients whose lives are in particular need of change. Whether it be enabling a child to develop and adapt despite a lifelong disability, helping a person to adjust to an acquired physical impairment, enabling a person with limited cognitive capacity to make a life transition (e.g., from school to work), or supporting someone with psychiatric disability to achieve a more adaptive lifestyle—therapy always involves some kind of change.

When viewed in totality, adjustment to any kind of disability, even one characterized by permanent and inalterable limitations of capacity, requires change. Acquired impairments are themselves changes which demand the human system and often the environment to adjust. Compensation for permanent impairments inevitably involves alteration of life routines, goals, or other factors affected by altered capacity. Moreover, even when limitations of capacity are stable, developmental, environmental, and other factors may change requiring the human system to adjust accordingly. Thus, it is necessary to think of therapy as always involving changes in lives.

Therapeutically supported change becomes necessary when persons' ways of living are challenged, compromised, or threatened by internal and/or external conditions and when such individuals need assistance to make necessary or desired changes in their lives. I use the phrase *therapeutically-assisted (or supported) change* to emphasize that patients or clients, through their own efforts, accomplish the most essential aspects of change. Therapy is not the *cause* of change. Rather, therapy provides various forms of assistance to change. When therapy is successful, it enables persons to make choices for, perform, and engage in patterns of occupational behavior that continue their lives in a positive direction.

This chapter will present a number of principles related to therapeutically-assisted change that are derived from the concepts and themes of the model of human occupation. Before presenting and discussing these principles, however, a few caveats are in order. First, the principles I will present here should not be considered exhaustive. Indeed, therapists employing the model in practice should discover additional ways in which the theory provides general insights into achieving therapeutically-assisted change. Second, these principles are derived from a theoretical conceptualization which has some empirical support, but they are not empirically demonstrated facts. Their worthwhileness and accuracy as explanations of the change process will need further verification. Third, the principles offered here are generalizations. Therapists will need to recognize them in the particular circumstances of therapy with each individual client or patient. In the end, therapists should select strategies of intervention based on an understanding of a given patient's or client's problem. The principles stated here propose broad themes about how change may take place in highly complex human systems. However, "There is no longer any universally valid law from which the overall behavior of the system can be deduced. *Each system is a separate case*" (Prigogine & Stengers, 1984). Good therapy never substitutes generalized principles or strategies for detailed knowledge of the individual's situation. Rather, knowledge of each patient should infuse any general principles with local meaning.

Indeed, in this regard, the occupational therapy process is very different from that of medicine. The medical diagnostician seeks to gaze beyond the idiosyncratic features of a person's life and symptoms to uncover the nature of the disease process or trauma. It is identification of the underlying pathology and general knowledge of its etiology and prognosis that directs medical intervention. The details of an individual's life and experiences add little useful information for most medical procedures.

In contrast, the occupational therapist requires a local knowledge of the individual to know what the occupational implications of any disease or trauma might be. Occupational therapists readily learn that similar impairments can produce vastly different consequences in the lives of clients. This point can be illustrated by considering two patients with a diagnosis of hemiparesis secondary to a cerebrovascular accident. The diagnosis tells us each individual will have a motor impairment on one side of the body which affects ambulation and upper extremity strength and coordination. What is not known from this information is the specific occupational behavior that is interrupted by this disability. Suppose the patient is a retired individual living in a rural setting with a supportive extended family. He occupies himself with entertaining grandchildren, doing small chores around the farm, fishing in the nearby pond, and spending long hours playing checkers and talking with other elderly neighbors on his front porch. The implications of his hemiparesis might be quite

different from that of a 55-year-old, single, female dance instructor living in a high-rise apartment in mid-Manhattan, whose major recreation is travel. While the status of the two persons may be similar in respect to some basic functional abilities, each faces a very different set of needs in order to go on with their respective lives.

In the same way that we can only know through careful, local examination what impact an impairment of capacity has for an individual, specific details about the individual are also necessary for therapists to know in order to anticipate and understand the change process. For example, the model of human occupation suggests that improvement in a person's sense of efficacy requires positive experiences of undertaking and completing occupational forms that are valuable and interesting. Which occupational forms should best serve as media in therapy depends on what a particular client enjoys and finds important. However, while some patients positively respond to modification of old interests so that they can be pursued, others find diminished performance in highly valued occupations too painful and must instead explore new occupations. Moreover, how many positive experiences it will take to shift a person's perception concerning efficacy cannot be specified ahead of time. It is simply impossible to anticipate what scenario will unfold. Therapy then, often means experimenting to find out a client's reaction to a particular occupation. Importantly, patients often discover, along with the therapist, what their reactions will be only once they engage in various occupations. With each successive therapeutic encounter the therapist gains important information about how the specific individual is changing. That emerging information is essential for anticipating what might come next and what strategy might help the patient go the next distance.

Consequently, the principles I will outline are neither recipes for change nor detailed instructions for how to implement the model of human occupation in intervention. They are intended to be used as a way of thinking about change as one plans and evaluates the implementation of therapy. These principles should suggest useful ways to envision and to interpret the events of therapy. Occupational therapists who use this theory in practice should find that the instructions for how to intervene emerge when general principles are considered in light of the particular circumstances of therapy. A therapist's theoretically guided appreciation of the patient's situation, and of the unfolding events of therapy, provide insights for what to try next. If a priori instructions could be substituted for this therapeutic reasoning we would have little need of theory[a].

The following discussions are ordered into the categories of general, performance, habituation, and volition principles. I have not included a separate category of environmental principles since environmental issues are integrated throughout each of the principles. Indeed, the view which should emerge through these principles of intervention is that occupational therapy is, first and foremost, an environmental therapy. That is, by both altering and utilizing a variety of conditions in the environment, therapy becomes a milieu which assists persons to activate their own development, recovery, or adjustment.

Therefore, these principles of therapeutic intervention should not be viewed in isolation. Rather, all the principles shared in this chapter should be considered as a whole. Together, they should provide a perspective on therapeutically-assisted change and provide a framework for appreciating, planning, and implementing therapy.

GENERAL THERAPEUTIC PRINCIPLES

Principle: Therapy is an event that comes into a life in progress and must be understood and undertaken in that context.

The role of occupational therapy is to enter into a life that has a history and/or future extending beyond the therapeutic process. Ther-

---

[a]Therapists, like other complex systems, encounter the instructions for how to behave in the dynamics of unfolding situations. From our theoretical viewpoint we would hardly expect therapists to know ahead of time all that they could or should do in therapy. Rather, they should have a well-developed appreciative capacity, which is what theory aims for.

apy is a unique and bounded event, the goal of which is to contribute positively to the course of an individual's life. Consequently, therapy should always proceed with appreciation of the life the individual has lived and might live in the future (Helfrich & Kielhofner, 1994).

What therapy can be for any person depends on the person and where he or she is going. In daily life, persons solve, more or less successfully, fundamental occupational issues that confront everyone: How shall one fill one's time? How does one find satisfaction in life? What constitutes a worthy or good life? How does one accomplish what one desires?

Human systems are organized so as to address these fundamental issues of occupational life. The particular organization of each human system is achieved over time. Persons encounter a particular cultural world and come to experience, interpret, anticipate, and choose their activities and occupations. This volitional process of choosing leads to recurrent performance in specific environments which serves to establish certain roles and habits and evoke and sustain skilled performance. This organization represents a dynamic whole, brought into a specific organization by the course of acting out one's personal history.

Whether a disability comes as a condition in the beginning of life, as a traumatic event in the prime of life, as an insidious and progressive encroachment on life, as recurring interference with life, or as a waning near the end of life, its specific impact depends on the life it has entered into and of which it is now a part. Impairments of capacity, such as blindness, paralysis, or cognitive deterioration, bring on occupational dysfunction not only because they reduce capacities, but also because they interrupt and disrupt that unfolding dynamic order. Their most far-reaching impact is on the life course. Impairments interfere with the way of living that both reflects and sustains the organization of the human system.

In other instances, it is the ongoing dynamic order which is itself the source of occupational dysfunction. The following are examples: a way of life overburdened with achievement and stressed with insatiable internal and external demands; a way of life without satisfying occupation and anesthetized through substance abuse; a restrained life of inaction and understimulation in an institutional setting; or the life paralyzed by fear, anxiety, and eroded capacities, which make getting started or going on too large a burden to be borne.

Therapy has the ominous challenge of enabling a human system to achieve a new dynamic order. To do so it must be a bridge between what has come before and what is to come. Therapy comes into and becomes an event in this dynamic unfolding and dysfunctional life course; it becomes, if successful, a means by which the life course is redirected and achieves a new dynamic unfolding order. Even when a client's goal is to reinstitute, as much as possible, a previous way of life, a new dynamic order will be required to approximate life as it was before the onset of impairment. To be useful to a patient or client, therapy must enter into the particular life stream affected by disability and become part of charting a new course or maintaining an old course in new ways.

Principle: The focus for change should be the action or process underlying the human system.

As presented in earlier chapters, the human system (i.e., the bounded organization of biological and symbolic components, conceptualized in this text as comprised of three subsystems) is maintained and shaped by the unfolding personal history of action. Occupational dysfunction is primarily a disorder of this active process. The primary focus of occupational therapy must be on enabling an adaptive process that replaces a maladaptive one and minimizes the impact of any impairments on the history of action. Consequently, therapeutically-assisted change must begin with an alteration in ongoing action.

How therapy focuses on the process of action as opposed to the human system's structures can be illustrated through an example. In the case of a child with cerebral palsy, therapy can target the child's identified problems such as impairments of motor control, lack of a mobility, and limited communication/interaction skills. If, instead, the therapist focuses

on the dynamic occupational process, consideration is also given to how the child fills time, what kind of actions and occupations make up the child's typical action, how the physical and social environments support or constrain this occupational behavior, and where the system of action is taking the child. The therapist then selects interventions to support an adaptive dynamic system of action. The following case illustrates such an approach.

Julie is four years old and lives with her mother, father, and six-year-old brother in a small town. She has severe cerebral palsy resulting from anoxia at birth. She experiences fluctuations in tone, i.e., she is very "floppy" much of the time but also has a marked extensor thrust. She has limited head control and at times disconjugate eye movements. She cannot talk and has other oral-motor problems. It is likely that she has some cognitive limitations. However, Julie can make her preferences clear and she is generally cheerful and interested in things going on around her. For example, Julie is passionate about computer games and single-switch toys.

Despite her communication impairments, Julie very much wants to interact with other children. Her mother has observed that Julie is becoming more irritable, particularly when her brother goes out to play in the street with other children. Since Julie spends most of the day in an adapted chair or buggy (which are difficult to get out of the house), she cannot readily go out and join the other children. Instead, she watches the other children playing in the street from the front windows of the house. It is clear that this pattern of passive watching is increasing Julie's frustration and sense of isolation.

The major goal of therapy, then, became helping Julie to begin to play with neighborhood children. To reach this goal Julie needed a means of mobility. Upon the therapist's recommendation, a ramp was installed at the front door of the home to make access in and out easier. Julie was quite fearful of being in a powered chair, since she had difficulty controlling her body and the chair often moved faster or in directions other than what she had planned. However, sitting in the buggy did not allow her to be in a position in which she could play. The therapist tried out a number of different seats and wheelchairs with Julie, finally settling on one with small wheels which needed to be pushed by another child or attendant, and from which she could safely play in the street. Soon she was routinely part of the group of children and learning how to communicate with them in simple ways.

While working on getting a chair for Julie that she could use without fear, it was certainly necessary to work on improving her head control, finding seating positions that enabled her to hold her head up without invoking an extensor thrust, improving her concentration, and increasing her tolerance to frustration. However, this was not the primary focus of therapy. Rather, the focus was enabling Julie to do what other four-year-old children do and that she wished to do—namely, play with friends.

Bolstered by a growing success in joining and interacting with friends at play, Julie was more ready to try out in occupational therapy a variety of self-powered go-carts until she found one with which she was comfortable. When Julie went to school a year later, she was using her own motorized chair.

By enabling and supporting the underlying action the therapist capitalized upon and supported the natural processes that maximized Julie's motor capacities, mobility, and communication/interaction skills. But the therapy focused only secondarily on these problems. As with Julie, it is the system of action which carries the client forward toward any improved state, which should always be the focus.

The importance of focusing on process becomes even more apparent in situations where it is this system of action itself which has become the source of occupational dysfunction. An illustrative case is John, who is middle-aged and lives in a comfortable suburb with his wife and four sons. John was recently hospitalized for depression, complaining of insomnia, increased heart rate, decreased appetite accompanied by a 20-pound weight loss, anxiety, suicidal ideation, and a lack of energy. John first began experiencing these symptoms two years ago; they have been intermittent and varying, but have become most intense in recent weeks.

As the therapist began to gather data about John, the following picture emerged about his life history. John is a nurse who has worked his way up through the ranks over the years. A few years ago, he attended night school while working full-time as a nurse in order to obtain a Master of Business Administration degree. Two years ago he accepted an administrative post in a company that owns and operates a chain of nursing homes. This new position removed him from clinical management and placed him in a new context where his managerial decisions had less and less to do with the quality of care and more and more with the profit of the company. Additionally, there was significant pressure on John to work long hours and to hold the bottom line within the company. John's new position paid significantly more than he previously earned, enabling him to move his family to a larger home in a more affluent suburb.

John is a dedicated family man who always enjoyed spending time with his wife and sons. Before the move John lived in a tightly-knit ethnic neighborhood where he was involved in a number of community and church-related activities. He has always been an avid fisherman and bowler. When John took his new position he found that the increased work hours and longer commute left him less and less opportunity to shoot a few hoops with his sons. He frequently missed the evening meal, which had been a family ritual for years. He couldn't recall having gone fishing in the last year and his bowling ball had been undisturbed in the hall closet. Additionally, as John began to experience his current symptoms, he found he had to spend even larger amounts of time to get the same amount of work done. This, in turn, increased his long hours and a growing sense that he was pressured by forces which he could not control. Another important source of stress for John was that he found himself increasingly forced to make decisions (e.g., reducing staff to resident ratios in the nursing home) which went against his longstanding and deeply held views of good care. John had begun to feel like he had gotten on an out-of-control roller coaster ride from which he could not escape.

The therapist was able to identify that much of the source of John's dysfunction was the occupational lifestyle he was pursuing. In fact,

John's values, interests, prior sense of personal causation, roles, habits, and skills were all ordered so as to support the way of life he desired. Now the threat to them was the roller coaster lifestyle in which he felt trapped and the press of his current work environment for occupational behavior inconsistent with his strongly preferred way of life. Thus, the focus of intervention was to enable and support John in making changes to the system of action which had carried him to such a dysfunctional state.

As the two previous examples illustrate, therapeutically-assisted change always focuses on the alteration of the current system of action which is contributing to, maintaining, failing to overcome, or compensate for impairments. The change process begins when a person is helped to assemble new choices and/or new behaviors. For John, whom we just discussed, the first action was to recommence leisure activities with his family. The long-term decision he faced was whether he could alter his work style in the current job or whether he needed to make a new occupational choice.

Choosing and engaging in new behavior (repeated and elaborated over time) leads to experiences which elicit a new organization in the human system. Consequently, the crux of all therapy is to get the patient to *do something anew* which starts the process of self-driven change. The onset of action begins the process of change. It may, as Price (1994, p. 187–188) notes, "break the inward gaze" at the "withering self" and instead force one to "move outward." It may begin the process of overcoming inertia or being stuck. It may re-evoke the sense of physically moving in the world. It may place one back into association with others. It may return one to a familiar and satisfying territory of being useful. It may confront paralyzing anxiety and fear. It may rekindle a sense of pleasure in completing something. However small, whatever its nature and its intended impact, all change begins with one action followed by another.

Principle: Change does not mean simply more or less; it means a different organization.

The human system is an organized whole in which change must always be more than a linear alteration of isolated components. In an organized system it is impossible for isolated change to take place. An alteration in one part shifts the configuration of the whole network of parts. This is true both for changes associated with disability and for therapeutically-assisted change. As discussed in Chapter 2, acquired limitations of capacity can serve as new control parameters in the human systems dynamics, shifting the system into a state of occupational dysfunction. That is, they alter overall system dynamics so that the occupational behavior assembled initiates or worsens a dynamic state of dysfunction. For example, a loss of capacity may be accompanied by a sense of despair about one's ability to effect desired outcomes in the environment. Together the decrement in ability and the changed sense of personal causation represent new conditions that may lead a person to abandon previous activity choices. Hence, the person does not engage in and experience satisfaction and success in old occupations. Nor does the person engage in actions that might help restore or reorganize ability. Suppressed activity choices and consequent lack of positive experiences may, at best, keep the person locked in a dysfunctional pattern of incompetence and poor sense of efficacy. At worst, they may contribute to a downward trend of negative thought and feeling, inactivity, role loss, and habit and skill deterioration. Dysfunction is located in the circumstances of the whole.

Traditional ideas of therapeutically-assisted change have emphasized linear and unidimensional changes. For example, the idea of grading activities implies that change involves an incremental process in which a person simply acquires more ability, more confidence, and so on. Only when viewing parts of the human system in isolation is it possible to conceive of change as occurring in this linear fashion. When the person is considered as a whole system, we recognize that change is much more than a process of incremental improvement. Consider, for example, a patient attending a work hardening program who experiences an increase in work-related capacities. Such change in capacity is likely accompanied by change in her or his knowledge of capacity. Further, this change in capacity may alter or create differences in activity or occupational choices. Further, a change in work skill confidence and choices may lead the person to reenter the work environment where a new set of circumstances will emerge and transform the human system even further. In this way we see, as discussed in Chapter 2, that change involves reverberating effects throughout the system.

In sum, change in the human system always involves reorganization; i.e., change in the overall order of the human system. Consequently, change will require that the therapist recognize the overall pattern of dysfunction which is maintained by the client's system of action. Then the therapist must consider how the client can be enabled to alter the system of action to facilitate movement toward a new organization. While the new organization may resemble a previous functional order, it will also be different in important ways. Changes in personal causation, interests, values, roles, and habits may all be required. Moreover, the environment may need to be modified in a number of ways. All this change cannot be completely preplanned in its details; rather, the therapist must carefully monitor how the system of action is unfolding and what new organization is being achieved. As this occurs, useful therapeutic strategies can be devised to support the unfolding reorganization.

The following case example illustrates how therapeutically-assisted change involves reorganization over time. Harold is 42 years old, married, and has one child. Several months ago he began work as a corrections officer for a federal prison. He was engaged in on-the-job training, preparing to take a series of physical and mental exams which would certify him for the job. At the same time, he rented and farmed several acres of land. During the spring wheat harvest he accidentally caught his right, dominant hand in a combine mechanism, resulting in a crush amputation of his thumb, index, middle, and ring fingers at the metacarpophalangeal level. Following surgery and a continuing course of therapy in a hand clinic, he has been able to develop a marginally functional grasp using his thenar eminence and the remaining fifth digit which is restricted in active flexion and extension.

Harold has reorganized his occupational functioning to offset the impact of the impairment on his life course. From the beginning of his rehabilitation, Harold identified that he wished to continue his training and pursue his goal of permanent employment as a corrections officer. Because his ability to physically respond to prisoners in an emergency is affected, he has secured a placement as the officer in charge of a main gate so that direct contact with prisoners was minimized. This position, however, required that he do additional paperwork related to prisoners' coming and going. Harold has a prosthesis which allows him to write with his dominant hand, but he feels that wearing it inside the prison might disadvantage him against a potential assailant. Thus, he chose instead to change hand dominance, learning to write with his left hand. His writing is legible but slow. Because prison reports must be error free and completed quickly, he could not afford to lose further time by having to redo reports. Therefore, he developed a new habit of composing the report in his head before writing it down.

Harold made other adaptations to a number of routines necessary for his job and for preparation to take certification exams. For example, he requires more time to take notes from books in preparation for exams. This means that he must devote more time to studying. Consequently, he has decided not to attempt to farm, giving up this second work role, at least temporarily.

Because of his impairment, he had to learn to be more assertive in negotiating role responsibilities. For example, he requested and secured permission to take written exams under altered conditions so as not to be penalized by his slow writing. To pass the performance component of the corrections certification exam he had to deliver a number of accurate shots to a target with both a shotgun and a .38 caliber revolver, accurately firing two rounds of ammunition during a timed test. He had to acquire a new way of completing this occupational form of firing, unloading, reloading, and firing the guns with the dual challenges of changed handedness and an impaired right hand. He readily managed to develop a process for reloading the shotgun without trouble, but getting small bullets in and out of the 6-shot revolver was more of a challenge. The test requires delivering ten accurate shots out of 12. After experimenting with different solutions, he developed the following routine. He fired one round of six shots. Then, to save time, he loaded and fired only four additional bullets. By delivering ten well-placed shots within the time period, he passed the exam.

In a whole range of situations, Harold encountered problems with the injured hand. He consistently substituted process skills (e.g., adapting, accommodating) for impaired motor skills such as handling and gripping. Moreover, he modified his habits of performance so as to compensate for the lost function and still be able to carry out some important occupations. For example, Harold chose to retain his hobby of cutting firewood. He managed to do this by changing the chain saw he uses. He sold his large saw and purchased a smaller one which he could handle safely. Moreover, he learned to rely on good planning to avoid unsafe situations in which he might lose control of the saw. Harold also had to develop new communication and interaction skills related to his stigmatized upper extremity. Children reacted most strongly to it, some expressing fear. Harold really liked children and figured out that he could assuage children's fears by offering them soda and candy with his partly amputated hand.

The changes which Harold made in objects, occupational forms, skills, habits, and roles have allowed him to retain a sense of efficacy and pursue his values and interests despite clear changes in his capacity. Most importantly, he was able to continue his volitional narrative; he successfully completed the entire certification process, passed probation, and secured a permanent job as a corrections officer. This continuation of his life was made possible through an underlying substantial reorganization.

Principle: Changes can and should occur in many aspects of the human system simultaneously.

The model of human occupation points out that occupational dysfunction ordinarily involves many different contributing and affected factors. For example, a child with a physical incapacitation not only has impaired motor skills, but these impairments may also negatively affect her or his sense of efficacy, development of interests, entry into the player and student roles, and development of habits of self-care.

All of these and other related problems faced by persons with occupational dysfunction can and should be addressed in therapy. It is tempting to oversimplify the therapeutic process and only address some of the problems or to address them sequentially. However, the most effective therapeutic route is to attempt to address simultaneously as many parts of the human system as possible. For example, the child who develops an increased sense of efficacy will naturally seek out new opportunities for motor learning, creating a synergy between the development of increased motor skill and strengthened personal causation. Therapy should always be aimed at capturing and capitalizing upon such synergies.

There is increasing evidence that such synergies will be at the core of the most effective kind of occupational therapy intervention. For example, Trombly (1994) recently pointed out that motor relearning following brain injury is likely to be more effective in real occupational forms (i.e., reaching into a closet or drawer to obtain clothing for dressing) than in simulated movement tasks such as stacking cones. Real life occupational forms afford and press for movement differently from simulated tasks and potentially invite more effective motor learning. The use of occupational forms which address a person's concerns about being able to pursue an interest or sustain an occupational role have the dual advantage of being more appropriate for motor relearning and for continuing one's volitional life story.

It further stands to reason that synergies between gaining new hopefulness in returning to one's way of life will have further advantages for enhancing skill development. The human system is, by nature's design, an integrated system in which the various components are meant to work together, augmenting and complementing each other. Good therapy builds upon the system's natural tendency to achieve its ends by assembling its various components in accomplishing occupational behavior.

Carefully planned occupational forms can be chosen in therapy to provide persons simultaneous opportunity to develop skill, enact a role, pursue an interest, and strengthen the sense of efficacy. In the context of an increasingly resource-limited and accountability-oriented health care system, therapists may feel pressured by time constraints to avoid considering the potential, multiple impacts of therapy. However, when viewed in light of the implied goal of reformed health care, which is to reach the best outcomes with the most restrained use of resources, a therapeutic process which is able to address multiple factors and elicit synergies of change in the human system makes sense.

Principle: Change is often disorderly.

Dynamical systems theory emphasizes that chaotic states are often necessary for transitions from one state of order to another. It should be expected, then, that therapeutically-assisted change involves periods of stability and instability, dramatic transformation, and uneven progression. We noted in Chapter 2, for example, that linear change in one element of a system will not necessarily be accompanied by linear change in other elements or behaviors of the system. For example, increasing strength may not result in changes in skill (e.g., reaching, lifting) until a critical threshold is reached. Thus, it is possible to observe incremental improvement in strength without a commensurate change in skill. On the other hand, a small change in strength that crosses a critical threshold can result in a significant change in skill.

This nonlinearity in change can be manifest in all aspects of the human system. Consider, for example, an adolescent patient with whom I worked in a psychiatric setting. During several successive occupational therapy sessions, Jim engaged in woodworking projects. Despite increasing skill and success in each subsequent session, Jim persisted in downgrading his own capacities. Moreover, he needed encouragement and support to get started and to continue during each therapy session. Unsure of each new step, he required reassurance and guidance. After each session Jim was quick to attribute positive outcomes to my assistance and difficulties to his own lack of skill. Over several sessions he seemed to become even more agitated and upset over minor failures, despite the fact that his overall performance was visibly increasing. At the end of one therapy session he disavowed interest in the woodworking and pronounced it "a stupid waste of time."

A couple of days later Jim arrived at therapy to announce that he had been working on a plan to make a piece of furniture and requested additional time in the woodshop to undertake this project. Needless to say, I was surprised and a bit puzzled. However, Jim's behavior is comprehensible if we consider the following. He entered therapy with a particular, stable volitional pattern: a sense that he could not succeed accompanied by a defensive conviction that being able to perform didn't matter to him. It became clear in therapy that Jim did see working with the kind of equipment that was in the woodshop (e.g., table and band saws, electric drill press) as symbolizing a world of technology and competence—a world he dared not imagine entering despite his attraction to it. By avoiding it, he could avoid the pain of failure and by bringing him into it, I raised the stakes for him. Jim's protestations of disinterest were defensive maneuvers against the possibility of painful failure. Until his skill and sense of efficacy reached a critical level, he was unable to reinvent his view of the situation. Only when he reached a critical threshold of confidence could he dare to imagine success and allow his interest and value to energize him toward an occupational choice for a personal project. Importantly, this choice proved to shift him into a new mode of action.

Jim was soon proudly showing other patients and therapists the progress of his work and insisting that I let him do the project on his own. By the time he was discharged, he had negotiated access to a neighbor's workshop and had several woodworking projects planned to help furnish the semi-apartment in which he lived in the basement of his parent's home.

Every therapist can recall such incidents in which therapy appears to be failing or halting, only to be followed by surprising shifts in choices, behavior, and investment. These occur when some critical factor in the person or environment shifts the dynamics of the system into a new order.

The disorderliness of change in therapy also comes from the fact that new states of organization are fragile and easily fall apart. Persons may seem to have made important gains only to revert to less functional behaviors. Maladaptive patterns once overcome are repeated. Deegan (1991, p. 52), speaking of her own recovery from psychiatric illness and that of an acquaintance with physical disability, aptly points out the small and halting steps that often characterize the reorganization of life:

> It is important to understand that for most of us, recovery is not a sudden conversion experience. Hope does not come to us as a sudden bolt of lightning that jolts us into a whole new way of being. Hope is the turning point that must quickly be followed by the willingness to act. The paralyzed man and I began in little ways with small triumphs and simple acts of courage: he shaved, he attempted to read a book, and he talked with a counselor: I rode in the car, I shopped on Wednesdays and I talked to a friend for a few minutes. He applied for benefits, he got a van and learned to drive; I took responsibility for my medications, took a part-time job, and had my own money. He went to college so he could work professionally with other disabled people; I went to school to become a psychologist so I could work with disabled people. One day at a time, with multiple setbacks, we rebuilt our lives.

Often the role of the therapy is to provide a place to regroup after a setback and to provide encouragement to go on despite failures. Whether it be the nonlinearity of change or the fragility of new states of organization, therapeutic change is often marked by the unexpected, by unevenness in change, and by occasional reverses in behavior. The role of therapy is to provide a source of steady support and direction that serves as scaffolding or bracing to help hold together new order

which is being realized as a human system changes.

Principle: Therapy should involve experimentation to find best solutions.

I have already noted that one cannot enter into therapy with detailed plans for what will occur. The disorderly way in which change sometimes unfolds means that best laid plans must frequently be put aside. It is helpful to recall that each successive change in the human system results in a new dynamic order. Once that new order emerges, new strategies and directions may be called for.

Moreover, when a human system is in a state of disorder following the onset of impairment or as the result of some transition, the correct solution for accomplishing the next step may not be apparent. Hull, a professor who lost his sight, provides a telling account of his own experimentation over a four-year period with how to conduct lectures without the possibility of reading notes:

> I experimented in making a summary on microcassette which I would use as a prompt. The problem was that, if I happened not to need the reminder until later in the lecture, I would have to run the cassette through all the material until arriving at the point, and this would take a few seconds. Locating the exact point was very difficult, and it was an embarrassing disclosure to an audience that one had lost the way.
>
> Sometimes I would record a brief summary of what I proposed to say, divided into sections. I would actually play this short summary to my audience, and would simply talk around it. This was only a partial success. Sometimes my listeners found it difficult to hear what was coming out of the tape recorder and I would have to repeat it, which was time-wasting. It was also inflexible, in that it committed me to an invariable sequence and to a great deal of laborious preparation, and these factors impaired my informal style and my capacity to respond to the needs of the moment.
>
> I tried dictating to myself by making a recording of the whole speech, or a summary, and using an earplug. For a while I actually tried to listen and speak at the same time, but after one or two disastrous experiences I gave this up. I tried using braille headings. This not only involved laborious preparation, but my braille was

just not good enough. I could not scan quickly enough to get myself out of the difficulty which arose when I forgot what to say next.

In the end, I developed the habit of making a précis on cassette and of listening and re-listening to this right up to the moment when I had to deliver the lecture. I would take the tape recorder to the lecture, since it gave me a sense of security, although I seldom needed to refer to it. (Hull, 1990, p. 122–123)

By encouraging patients to vary their strategies and by varying the conditions in which patients try out successful strategies, good solutions to problems can be discovered. A recurring impediment to change is holding on to old strategies which are suboptimal for solving a problem or facing a challenge.

An important corollary to this principle is that a solution which is good for one client may not be useful to another. One patient will find a given piece of adaptive equipment a particularly good solution to a functional problem. Another will find it stigmatizing and prefer to avoid the problem altogether or accept a less efficient method of accomplishing the task without the equipment. If therapists pay careful attention to the range of ways in which clients manage solutions to similar problems, they will have a variety of suggestions to provide future patients. Offering suggestions and opportunities for trying out alternatives are some of the most useful assistance occupational therapists can provide to the change process.

Principle: The only tool which therapists have at their disposal is to change the relevant environment to support or precipitate a change in the human system.

Occupational therapy does not directly alter the human system. While physicians have at their disposal drugs, surgery, and other methods that produce direct changes in the human system, occupational therapists, as noted earlier, seek to assist change through influencing the active process underlying the human system's organization.

Consequently, the therapist's only tool for affecting the system's process is to produce some change in the person's relevant environment. This is accomplished in one of the following ways:

1. The therapist may purposefully alter the physical setting to shift the network of conditions, thus eliciting new assembly of behavior. Examples of this process are when a ramp is built to replace inaccessible front steps to a home or when a kitchen is modified to accommodate a wheelchair-using homemaker.
2. The therapist may provide a person with a new object. For example, the entire use of assistive technology is based on this strategy of environmentally enhancing change. For example, providing a computer-based, augmentive communication device for a child with a severe motor disability or providing an elderly person with limited range of motion a pair of reachers are both examples of using objects in the environment to evoke changes in function.
3. The therapist may provide, monitor, or seek to change social groups which are a context of a person's occupational performance. In this category are included such strategies as: therapist's consultation to families, the use of therapeutic groups, making recommendations to the workplace for accommodating a person with a psychosocial disability. The use of leadership skills in groups and providing social expectations and support to patients are examples of how therapists modify social conditions through the use of self.
4. The therapist may provide (or help a client select) occupational forms to undertake. Alternately, the therapist may suggest modifications of an occupational form that afford the patient opportunities for performance.

Therapy often involves the simultaneous use of more than one of these environmental strategies. In the end, the success of therapy depends on the therapist's ability to know how to manage the environment so as to provide conditions which will afford and press for the desired behaviors on the part of a patient or client.

PERFORMANCE AND SKILL CHANGES

Principle: Changes in skill (as opposed to underlying capacity) should be the primary target of therapy.

Occupational therapy literature and practice often emphasizes that occupational performance is built upon various underlying capacities. For example, therapists have been traditionally trained to consider the impact that biomechanical, cognitive, neurodevelopmental, and other underlying capacities have on performance. Moreover, therapists are encouraged to know and use strategies in intervention that remediate limitations of such underlying capacities. Thus, for example, increasing strength, perceptual abilities, and cognitive orientation are frequently goals of therapy.

There is nothing problematic about envisioning such increases in capacity as resulting from therapy, but it is more efficient and effective to focus the attention of therapy at a different level of concern, the level of skilled performance. There two important reasons for this. First of all, as noted in Chapter 7, correlations between underlying capacity and actual skilled performance are far less than perfect. This means that one may achieve changes in underlying capacity without enabling a person to attain changes in the more important functional skill. Readers should recognize this as an example of nonlinearity, as discussed earlier. Secondly, whatever changes will be achieved in underlying capacity are best achieved in the context of focusing on improving skills. As alluded to earlier, when persons are engaged in actual or real life occupational forms, the total dynamic evokes the skills necessary for executing those occupational forms. Hence, natural movement, problem solving and communication occur when person engage in occupational forms. Moreover, by exercising skill one engages underlying capacity. Consequently, when change in capacity is desired, that change is best achieved through skill-based performance in occupations.

Principle: Change in performance can involve learning to call upon different configurations of skills.

Motor, process, and communication and interaction skills may be enacted in different combinations to achieve a desired functional outcome. When one or more skills are impaired, other skills can be used in their place to achieve an acceptable level of performance in an occupational form. For example, a person whose limited range of motion in the upper extremity affects the motor skills of reaching and bending may be able to use process skills (e.g., adjusting the environment, accommodating how actions are done, organizing materials alternatively in space) or communication and interaction skills (i.e., asserting oneself to request assistance) to achieve the same functional outcome. Consequently, learning to perform adaptively sometimes means learning to substitute remaining skills for those which are limited or unavailable.

Principle: Occupational forms have a powerful influence on changes in skill.

Occupational forms, by virtue of being culturally coherent units of action with socially understood meanings, purposes, and procedures, provide rich informational contexts which can help reorganize skills following disruption of function. Appreciating the importance of occupational forms is helped if we consider for a moment how skill in occupational performance is assembled. As noted in Chapters 2 and 6, the various components of the human system and the environment must collaborate in the assembly of behavior. Each of these components brings something to the performance. When the human system has been compromised by incapacitation, what the environment brings becomes even more important.

Occupational forms represent structured, information-rich, and meaningful contexts for eliciting maximal performance. Both Mathiowetz (1994) and Trombly (1994) recently underscored this point with reference to the impact of occupational forms on organizing motor behaviors of persons with central nervous system-related motor dysfunction. They concluded that when persons engaged in true occupational forms from daily life, the motor behavior is more organized than when moving in simulated activities or in response to requests to move.

This same principle holds for all forms of skill. Since skill is assembled in the context of the environment and in the dynamics of unfolding performance of an occupational form, these contextual factors serve as important parts of the network of conditions that elicit and sustain skill. When these contexts are impoverished or absent, the potential for exercising and learning skill are reduced.

HABITUATION CHANGE

Principle: Habits and roles are naturally resistant to change since their basic function is to preserve patterns of behavior; sustained practice is necessary to cement change in habituation.

Habits and roles are organized so as to resist change. They preserve patterns of behavior operating semi-autonomously and asserting themselves. Each of us can readily recall how resistant even minor habits of action are to change. For example, who has not repeatedly gone to the closet, the drawer, or cabinet to retrieve objects which are no longer there, having been relocated recently during a reorganization of one's household or office. Habits and roles not only assert old ways of doing things, but by evoking the assembly of habituated behavior they sustain themselves through practice.

Habit maps and role scripts represent well-worn solutions to particular problems. Whether the problem be how to fill time, how to get dressed in the morning, how to study for an exam, how to complete a series of typical work tasks, or how to deal with coworkers, habits and roles represent established solutions. They are used over and over again as solutions for the problems because they have become paths of least resistance. However ineffective or problematic habits or roles may be,

they typically represent that which is most natural and comfortable to do.

At the same time, new habits and roles are fragile organizations. Without a history of repeated assembly, new behavioral forms lack the stability of old forms of behavior. Thus old tendencies can readily outweigh new strategies until the latter are strengthened by repetition.

Consequently, a change in habits or roles requires sustained practice of the new strategies. If a new habit or role is not performed repeatedly, it will not be established and it will not successfully replace old patterns which will instead reassert themselves. When the goal of therapeutically-assisted change is to establish new habits or roles, the therapist must look for multiple opportunities for the client to practice the new behavior. This often requires practice outside the therapeutic context which of itself is too infrequent or too short for establishing new patterns of habituation.

Principle: Habituation organizes behavior for specific ecologies; new habits must often be learned in new ecologies.

Habituation organizes behavior to fit some set of circumstances in a particular environment. For example, habits of time use are sustained because conditions in the environment afford opportunity for and press for those habits. Therefore, to change habits and roles, one must often change the environment. This means that therapeutically-assisted change in habituation will often require the therapist to intervene in the environment (e.g., consulting with staff in a nursing home who encourage a particular maladaptive habit pattern or cast a resident in a particular dysfunctional role). It may also require that the therapist search for alternatives to the client's current occupational behavior settings.

A second consideration emanates from the observation that roles and habits are particularly sensitive to the environments in which they are practiced. Indeed, habits and roles organize humans so as to be a good fit to particular ecologies. For this reason habits learned in environments that differ significantly from the environment where the person will perform will likely be ill-suited to support competent occupational behavior. Therapeutically-assisted change in habits and roles must, therefore, take place in the natural environment where the behavior will be routinely enacted or in environments which carefully replicate the physical and social conditions of the true occupational behavior setting.

For example, Callahan (1990) points out how his own rehabilitation following spinal cord injury involved practicing personal hygiene, bathing, and eating skills in a highly adapted environment within a regulated schedule. Upon discharge he found himself in an apartment with a bathroom too small for him to use and in a kitchen that required him to eat off a cutting board pulled out of the cabinet. He had to reorganize his daily habits to fit this apartment. Unfortunately, most of the routines he learned in rehabilitation proved of limited or no use to him.

Principle: The loss of roles and habits requires swift replacement.

As we saw in Chapter 5, habit and roles are the source of security, familiarity, and identity for individuals. The whole fabric of the familiar world and the known self is dependent on the recurrent patterns of behavior and experiences sustained by habits and roles.

When habituation is disrupted (as in the case of a sudden loss of capacity that invalidates roles and habits), the individual may suffer tremendous disorientation and discomfort. For example, those robbed of the worker role find themselves without an identity which has been a source of self-esteem and which located them as legitimate members of the social world. Robbed of the familiar routine of a 40-hour work week, these persons are suddenly faced with large portions of uncommitted time.

Loss of such roles and habits can seem as though the scaffolding which held up much of everyday life has suddenly collapsed. This loss can occasion a strong emotional reaction followed by disorganization of a person's way of life (Fein, 1990). Consider, for example, the role loss and habit changes that result from the death of a spouse. Persons who lose the identity of being a spouse are immediately assigned a new and unfamiliar identity of being a widower or widow. Unfortunately, this new role does not so much replace the old role as it signals an alteration from a previous identity. Old role scripts may now fail the individual; the widow whose relationships to friends were on a couple-to-couple basis may be very unsure as to how to continue those relationships. At the same time, the widow may be faced with the requirement to develop new habits (e.g., mowing the lawn, paying bills). These new roles or role challenges may evoke strong reactions of anxiety. Thus, a person making the transition from a spouse role to these new roles may experience a wide range of negative emotions which must be supported in therapy. Nonetheless, the surest means of restabilizing both the emotional and behavioral disruption which comes with role loss is to assist the person's resocialization into a new role or roles to replace any roles which are being left behind (Fein, 1990). For example, research suggests that the grieving process for persons who have lost spouses concerns the loss of roles as well as the loss of a loved one. Persons who find ways to replace lost roles and routines are less susceptible to depression (Fein, 1990).

Helping persons establish new roles and habits in a timely way is often complicated by the fact that a person may be extremely distraught over the recent losses and become anxious when faced with the new role and habit demands. However, it appears that a prolonged period without finding roles and habits to replace old ones only invites further degeneration.

Principle: Acquiring a new role script and related habits is a process of socialization and negotiation.

Taking on a new role involves learning a new role script to guide effective assembly of role-related behavior. The role script is learned through a process of socialization in which persons learn what is expected of them in a role and of figuring out what behaviors will satisfy others' expectations. It is also a process in which persons negotiate with others in the environment for how the role will be filled.

Role script change involves multiple and sustained transactions, the new role being acquired in fragments over time and in many and varied encounters with others in the social group of which the role is a part. Therapeutically-assisted change must provide opportunities for these multiple social encounters and for a clear sharing of information concerning what others expect of the person in the new or altered role. Additionally, the person undergoing change in roles scripts may need assistance in identifying and negotiating specific role expectations.

Changes in role scripts do not ordinarily occur in the confines of a hospital or rehabilitation center; rather, they occur in the home, the workplace, the classroom, or other occupational behavior setting where individuals enact their life roles. In such settings, the occupational therapist often serves as a coach, assisting persons to sort out what their new role scripts and related habits will be. The therapist also acts as an arbitrator and advocate, helping the negotiation process between persons with disabilities and the social groups in which they enact their roles and habits.

A case in point is the role that occupational therapists play in assisting persons with disabilities to request and receive reasonable accommodations in the workplace, which are guaranteed under the Americans with Disabilities Act. Requests for reasonable accommodations are often requests for modification in the ordinary expectations for persons in a role or for alternative ways of enacting role scripts. An example of this is Laverne, who works in an advertising firm. Her job is to interact with customers concerning their various accounts and projects. Laverne had always felt somewhat marginal in her role in the firm since most other employees were directly involved in producing the advertisements for the clients. She sometimes felt that she lacked the technical and creative skill that others had and she sought to overcompensate for what she considered to be her own inadequacies on the job. This resulted in Laverne feeling a high level of stress in her worker role and in her spending more and more extra hours at work. However, stress and fatigue made her less effective and efficient at work, thus increasing both her levels of felt stress and her perception that her work was inadequate. She, in turn, tried to compensate by putting forth more time and effort on the job, but this only exacerbated the problem. Eventually, Laverne became depressed and needed intervention. In occupational therapy, she was able to identify how she had interpreted others' expectations of her and created role scripts for herself that were impossible to sustain. By identifying to her employer that she had a stress-related disability, she was able to ask for reasonable accommodations on her job that included reallocating the more stressful parts of her job to others. She could then readily take over and accept more responsibility for work functions for which she felt she had unique skills. She also modified a number of her habits of time use and altered habitual ways of carrying out job tasks. The result was that Laverne felt more effective and comfortable in her job and internalized a more realistic work role script and work habits while becoming a more valuable worker.

VOLITIONAL CHANGE

Principle: Volitional anticipation, experience, interpretation, and choice are at the core of what is referred to as meaning in therapy.

It is a long-standing adage that, to be effective, occupational therapy must be meaningful to the patient. However, there is limited discussion in the literature of the field concerning how patients actually experience meaning in therapy. One useful way of approaching the problem of therapeutic meaning is to conceptualize it as involving the volitional processes of anticipation, experience, interpretation, and choice discussed in Chapter 4.

Each person is differently disposed to experience the occupational forms used in therapy. That is, the patient brings to each occupation a tendency to enjoy or not enjoy the actions involved, an idea of its worth and relevance, and expectations concerning how well he or she could do what is required to complete the occupation. These volitional tendencies, combined with what actually happens in the successive moments of a therapeutic session, generate the experience which a client has while performing an occupational form in therapy.

The quality of experience in the course of therapy can serve to energize or paralyze motivation, to draw in or alienate a client, and to raise fears or engender hope. Thus, the nature of moment-by-moment experience cannot be underestimated. Therapists can maximize the clients' experience in the therapeutic process by (a) carefully selecting occupational forms which have highest potential to be relevant to a patient's volition, and (b) seeking ongoing data about what the patient is experiencing in order to make appropriate modifications that maximize experience. Therapists should take care to observe, when possible, how the patient appears to be acting and reacting in therapy, looking for cues as to the patient's enjoyment, anxiety, boredom, investment, outrage, shame, excitement, and so forth. Similarly, therapists can "check in" with clients during and after each therapeutic process to appreciate what each experienced.

It would appear that the importance of the patient's experience in therapy is obvious, but the reports of many person with disabilities suggest this experience is not always carefully considered. I offer two examples:

> When I was able to sit up in the chair long enough, I began two hours . . . of occupational therapy daily . . . I remember having my hands harnessed for long periods of time to a rolling-pin-like apparatus that sanded a piece of wood. A bright future as a finish sander stretched before me if I played my cards right. (Callahan, 1990, p. 74)

> I was also doing well in occupational therapy, although I thought some of the exercises ridiculous. Nonetheless, visitors to our house still scrape their feet on the doormat that I made in O.T. Yolanda is the only person who knows its origins, a sign of the care I have taken to keep secret the indignities visited upon me in my disability. (Murphy, 1990, p. 54–55)

It is an indictment of the failure to carefully consider patient's experience, that a number of former patients complain of the irrelevance and indignity of the things they were asked to do in occupational therapy.

Interpretation occurs as a client reflects upon an experience or series of experiences in terms of the significance for the volitional self. That is, it is when persons reflect on what experience has told them about how enjoyable certain actions are, about the worth of engaging in certain occupations, and about their own competence. For example, interpretation is the process whereby an individual may reflect that an old interest is no longer enjoyable under the new conditions imposed by disability, that an activity that seemed to be too difficult was actually within reach, that there is new value to be found in activities that previously were not considered important. The interpretive process is also important for how persons will remember their experiences and for what they will expect to experience and are likely to choose in the future. Interpretation places experience in a particular perspective. Interpretation occurs in such reflections as: "I was extremely anxious during this group activity, but I hung in there, did okay and actually enjoyed myself near the end . . . maybe I'll do that again."

Occupational therapists can abet and influence interpretation by informally and formally reflecting with clients on their course of therapy. For example, the therapist may offer new ways of viewing experience to a patient who has a tendency to interpret his or her own behavior in light of negative views of self and life.

The process of choice involves translating expectations into decisions to engage in specific activities (activity choices) and it involves making commitments to acquire new roles or habits or to take on personal projects (occupational choices). Activity choices are pivotal since they are spontaneous processes by which an individual is brought into action. Occupational choices are essential since they are the processes of commitment by which persons sustain themselves in a course of action over time. Therapists can enhance a patient's experience with making choices by both providing opportunities for and supporting choices.

The application of this principle in practice is aptly illustrated in the following example of Charlie, a man who experienced a cerebrovascular accident (CVA) with residual left hemiparesis and hemianopia four months before his planned retirement from running the family business. Charlie had recently purchased a new boat and fishing equipment: he intended to pursue an interest for which he had little time during his years as a worker. He was engaged in what was routine for stroke patients in the setting: he was placed on a skateboard to range the affected upper extremity and offered a deltoid assist. However, Charlie's occupational therapist observed that he was extremely unmotivated. She found that he would not range his arm unless constantly cajoled; he tended to be sullen and tearful. Charlie complained about the skateboard and the deltoid aid and indicated that he hated therapy. When the therapist further explored the source of Charlie's dissatisfaction with therapy she learned that his real concerns centered on the uncertain future of his business, and on his expectation that his plans for retirement leisure were shattered.

Armed with this information about Charlie's experience and interpretation of the events of therapy, the occupational therapist set about to use occupational forms that would allow Charlie to address the real life choices with which he was faced. She began by working with Charlie to allay his first concern by developing a business and logistic plan to maintain the business and later transfer the responsibility to someone else. Next, the occupational therapist asked his wife to bring in Charlie's new fishing rod. She attached graded sized fish (weights) to the leader line so Charlie could practice casting and reeling, first using the affected extremity as an assist and later using it to cast the rod. Through such activities as using a leather strop to sharpen his fishing knife blade, Charlie also redeveloped his grasping skill. Later, he developed sufficient coordination to tie his own lures and leader lines. Both Charlie's outlook and his motor skills improved dramatically. By paying attention to Charlie's experiences and interpretation of therapy and by addressing the occupational choices with which he was faced in life, his occupational therapist was able to make therapy meaningful.

Principle: Volitional change means finding a direction for one's personal narratives.

When persons experience disability, they also experience a threat to the integrity of their ongoing life stories. Whether due to a deterioration of the life story from within, or to an impairment imposed from without, a core problem for the persons experiencing occupational dysfunction is to figure out where life will go next. As noted in Chapter 4, a coherent sense of where life has been and is headed is achieved through the experience of narrating one's own life story.

Telling and living a story which makes sense of one's life requires finding an appropriate plot and supporting metaphors to infuse the events of a life with coherence, wholeness, and direction (Helfrich, Kielhofner, & Mattingly, 1994; Mallinson, Kielhofner, & Mattingly, 1994). The person with a disability often faces great challenges to finding a meaningful life plot. Indeed, because of the physical and emotional barriers faced by persons with disabilities, the plot of the life story may need to be even more powerful and explicit.

For example, when faced with his own saga of life-threatening disease and disability, the novelist, poet, and lyricist Reynolds Price, clearly outlined how he set about to narrate his experience:

> Now at last I must enter what was plainly a war, with life-or-death stakes, and assume the fight in the only way I knew to fight—in the arts of picture-making and story-telling that I'd worked at since childhood. I'd be myself to the outer limit of all I could be, resourceful as any hunted man in the bone-dry desert, licking dew from cactus thorns. So, even that early, I'd cast myself as the hero of an epic struggle, and I saw both the ludicrous melodrama of that role and the urgent need for it. (Price, 1994, p. 31)

A decade after the battle has begun, Price emerges clearly victorious:

> I know that this new life is better for me, and for most of my friends and students as well. . . . As I survived the black frustration of so many new forms of powerlessness, I partly learned to sit

and attend, to watch and taste whatever and whomever seemed likely or needy, far more closely than I had in five decades. The pool of human evidence that lies beneath my writing and teaching, if nothing more, has grown in the wake of that big change . . . in the ten years since the tumor was found, I've completed thirteen books—I'd published a first twelve in the previous twenty-two years . . . I sense strongly that the illness itself either unleashed a creature within me that had been restrained or let him run at his own hungry will; or it planted a whole new creature in place of the old . . . I'm left today, as I write this page, with an odd conclusion that's risky to state. But since it's not only thoroughly true but may well prove of use to another, I'll state it boldly—I've led a mainly happy life. I write six days a week, long days that often run 'til bedtime; and the books are different from what came before in more ways than age. I sleep long nights with few hard dreams, and now I've outlived both my parents. Even my handwriting looks very little like the script of the man I was in June of '84. Cranky as it is, it's taller, more legible, with more air and stride. It comes down the arm of a grateful man (Price, 1994, p. 189–193).

While most persons do not possess the eloquence of Reynolds Price, each must find a story plot which is compelling enough to empower him or her to move forward with the necessary courage and fortitude that it takes to deal with the suffering, disappointment, and challenge that are a part of living with disability.

Learning to live with a disability is a matter of finding, at minimum, an acceptable and, at best, fulfilling and joyful life. It has little or nothing to do with living a life which is normal or dictated by one particular set of values. For example, Deegan (1991) notes that:

Too often we project traditional "American" values on disabled people, for example, rugged individualism, competition, personal achievement, and self-sufficiency . . . For some psychiatrically disabled people, especially those who relapse frequently, these traditional values of competition, individual achievement, independence, and self-sufficiency are oppressive. (p. 52)

Each person with a disability must discover and enact ways of thinking, feeling, and acting that lead to a viable lifestyle in the face of limitations of capacity and challenges from the environment. As Vash (1981) notes:

Acceptance of disability evolves gradually, for most people, over a span of years filled with instructive experience. It comes seldom, if ever, as a *coup de foudre* followed by getting on with life. Instead, the process of living teaches, little by little, that disablement needn't be viewed as an insurmountable tragedy . . . As the struggles to survive, work, live, and play show evidence of some success, individuals find awareness of disablement slipping longer and oftener into the background of consciousness. Eventually, for some, it may come to be seen as a positive contributor to life in its totality—a catalyst to psychological growth. Since these changes take time, trial, error, and correction to unfold, forward movement does not always look like progress. (p. 124)

What form a person's attitude toward disability takes is, of course, a highly personal matter. Each person must construct his or her own story of what it means to be a person with a disability. All therapists have encountered persons who truly believe that their lives have been destroyed by disability and who go on to live lives much more constrained and unhappy than might have been otherwise. Moreover, among those who make a positive adaptation to their disabilities, there are many differences. Consider for example Robert Murphy's (1990) reflection on his experience of having a spinal cord tumor which resulted in progressive paralysis:

I gradually learned to live day by day, to block from my consciousness any thoughts about the final outcome of the illness, to repress from awareness any vision of the unthinkable. I have maintained this perspective for the past ten years. In the many stages of my progressive debility, I have guarded against meditation about what would come next. And as I have confronted every affront to my body, whether inflicted by nature or medicine, I have lived for the moment. Lest this be misunderstood as an attempt to escape the truth, I did (and still do) know what could happen to me, but I knew also that there wasn't a damned thing I could do about it. It's the worst kind of human foolishness to worry over things that are inevitable. It's like fretting over death; you can spoil your life that way. (p. 25)

John Callahan is a cartoonist and recovering alcoholic who is quadriplegic from a car accident. In his autobiographical book, *Don't worry, he won't get far on foot,* he reflects:

> ... I'm more surprised than anyone that I have adapted to this way of life. Sometimes I still wake in panic in the night when I discover I cannot move my legs, just as I did sixteen years ago on that night in L.A. And I panic again at the thought of having to spend the rest of my life in this condition. I wonder if I will survive it. It's true I've had to be a scrapper. I've had to work exceedingly hard to survive; before all else, it takes me three hours just to get ready in the morning.
>
> But deep inside I know I'm always right where I'm supposed to be at the time. I don't want self-pity. I don't allow it. I want to grow. My life certainly has a black side but in other ways it's almost charmed. I always knew it would be. It's really satisfying in quite a wonderful way. (Callahan, 1990, p. 217)

While Robert Murphy and John Callahan reflect differently on their lives, they both agree that adjustment to disability is ongoing, done in each moment of living and requires that one look forward, not back. Vash (1981) notes in this regard:

> I have been disabled since I was sixteen, yet hardly a week goes by, nearly thirty years later, that I don't make some discovery or improvement that in one way or another makes my disability less handicapping. Since I hope that happy process never stops, I have to say that I hope I am never fully "rehabilitated." My physical abilities are still increasing. When, with age, they begin to decrease I fully expect to continue or accelerate in the psychological and spiritual discoveries that make my disability not only less handicapping, but a matter of trivia compared with the nonphysical realms of discovery and improvement I am experiencing. (p. 2, 3)

If there is any quality which seems to represent an adaptive life story in the face of disability it is a quality which Vash (1981, p. 132) speaks about. That is, that disability fades into the background (still present) while going on with life comes into the foreground. Stories that are saturated with disability leave little room for anything else. It appears that those persons who are able to find satisfying or at least acceptable stories for themselves are those who have found a place in their story for the disability, but whose stories are primarily about themselves, not about the disability.

Occupational therapy can play a very important role in assisting persons to construct and live their volitional stories. As DeLoach and Greer (1981) note early in the process of living with a disability:

> Both the miracles we hope for and the miseries we fear are failures of the imagination, which tends to use the imagery supplied by daydreams and nightmares to fill what is at first a vacuum, virtually devoid of any experience, with relevant facts. (p. 251)

In occupational therapy the experiences of encountering the everyday world can be generated. The occupational therapy process should facilitate movement back and forth between the telling and living of a life story. Through therapy, the client can test the reality of his or her imagination and in therapy the courage to imagine can be fashioned.

CONCLUSION

In this chapter I have outlined a number of principles for therapeutic intervention. As should be obvious by now, these are general principles. They can only instruct therapists by way of suggesting a means for looking at, and thinking about, therapy. It still remains, and should remain, for each therapist to decide with regard to each client or patient where and how a principle may be relevant. The everyday events of therapy should serve to bring alive and give deeper meaning to the principles herein. To the degree that therapists can "own" these principles as operational ways of therapeutic reasoning, they will have served their purpose.

These principles form a whole. They will be much less useful if taken as isolated notions about practice. Instead, therapists are encouraged to think about the overall view of therapy which emerges when the principles are considered together. Each event in therapy is potentially an instance of almost every principle in this chapter. Consequently, therapy should be comprehended from a viewpoint that transcends any individual principles and reflects the attitude behind them all.

Finally, these principles are only points of departure. They should serve as examples of how therapists can go about seeking more general wisdom about the therapeutic process. Experience in practice should teach therapists additional principles which can be drawn from the model of human occupation. These principles are also only a beginning in attempting to articulate how therapy based on this model can best be carried out to have optimal effects. There remains much to be done in empirically validating and exemplifying them.

ACKNOWLEDGMENT

I am indebted to Fran Oakley, Theresa Plummer, Renee Moore, and Trudy Mallinson who provided a number of the case materials and anecdotes shared in this chapter.

References

Callahan, J. (1990). *Don't worry, he won't get far on foot.* New York: Vintage Books.

Deegan, P. E. (1991). Recovery: The lived experience of rehabilitation. In R.P. Marinelli & A.E. Dell Orto (Eds.), *The psychological and social impact of disability* (3rd ed.). New York: Springer-Verlag.

DeLoach, C., & Greer, B. G. (1981). *Adjustment to severe physical disability: A metamorphosis.* New York: McGraw-Hill.

Fein, M. L. (1990). *Role change: A resocialization perspective.* New York: Praeger.

Helfrich, C., & Kielhofner, G. (1994). Volitional narratives and the meaning of therapy. *American Journal of Occupational Therapy, 48,* 319–326.

Helfrich, C., Kielhofner, G., & Mattingly. C. (1994). Volition as narrative: Understanding motivation in chronic illness. *American Journal of Occupational Therapy, 48,* 311–317.

Hull, J. M. (1990). *Touching the rock: An experience of blindness.* New York: Vintage Books.

Mallinson, T., Kielhofner, G., & Mattingly, C. (1994). *"Like being stuck in fly paper:" Understanding volition through metaphor.* Manuscript submitted for publication.

Mathiowetz, V. (July, 1994). *Informational support and functional motor performance.* Paper presented at the American Occupational Therapy Foundation Research Colloquium, American Occupational Therapy Association National Conference, Boston.

Murphy, R. F. (1990). *The body silent.* New York: WW Norton.

Prigogine, S. C., & Stengers, I. (1984). *Order out of chaos.* New York: Bantam Books.

Price, R. (1994). *A whole new life.* New York: Atheneum.

Trombly, C. A. (July, 1994). *Occupation: The effects of goal-directedness.* Paper presented at the American Occupational Therapy Foundation Research Colloquium, American Occupational Therapy Association National Conference, Boston.

Vash, C. L. (1981). *The psychology of disability.* New York: Springer.

14/ Application of the Model in Practice: Case Illustrations

Gary Kielhofner and Trudy Mallinson

INTRODUCTION

This chapter contains eleven cases that illustrate application of the model of human occupation. The cases were chosen to illustrate a range of issues. For example, some cases exemplify a thorough approach to data gathering using formal methods, while using others emphasize informal methods of data gathering. Moreover, each case may highlight one or another aspect of the process of therapeutically-assisted change. For example, one case may have a stronger emphasis on volition while another stresses performance skills.

The cases are presented as realistic examples of how therapists apply the model. We can imagine a variety of ways in which therapy for each of the persons described herein might have been done differently or improved upon. However, we selected cases that represent the realities of practice. Such realities do not always allow as much time as desired for data gathering and intervention. Under such conditions, a therapist may elect to emphasize methods of data gathering and intervention that have the best chance of doing the most good. By presenting the kinds of cases we have provided here, we hope to give examples of theory use which can be imitated in the real world.

Each of the cases can stand alone as a partial example of applying concepts from the model of human occupation. Because of the length of the chapter and the number of different cases, readers are advised not to attempt to read this chapter all at once. Indeed, each case can be treated as a separate "mini-chapter." We

have organized the cases into one large chapter to stress the importance of viewing them collectively as illustrations of a range of approaches to applying the model. No single case employs every idea or concept from the model. Indeed, good use of the model of human occupation involves recognizing which concepts are most useful in formulating an understanding of a particular patient or client and deciding a course of intervention. Consequently, while we do not recommend attempting to digest this chapter in a single reading, we do strongly advise readers to consider the collection of cases as a whole. Having read the cases, one should have a better appreciation of a range of ways in which the model can be applied. We hope that therapists can take helpful instructions from each of the cases and, with the lessons taught by all the cases together, have a fuller appreciation of the model's application in practice.

In many of the cases presented here, the therapists used a combination of conceptual models of practice along with other supporting knowledge. Indeed, what most often characterizes best practice is the judicious use of more than a single conceptual model of practice (Kielhofner, 1992). However, in presenting the cases here, we have emphasized aspects of each case which highlight the contribution of the model of human occupation to gathering and reasoning with data, and to the intervention process. We will make brief reference to how therapists employed other models of practice, but not with the same level of detail we have tried to provide in presenting the application of the model of human occupation. This emphasis reflects the goal and purpose of this book, which is to present the concepts and applications of the model of human occupation. The emphasis of the cases should not be read as a statement of the relative contribution of different theoretical ideas to the total therapy that each individual received. We wish to underscore that it was often the combination of more than a single model of practice which characterized good therapy.

The cases in this chapter have been partly fictionalized for two reasons. First, we have sought to preserve the identity of the persons involved. Second, we have written the cases to best reflect current versions of data collection methods and current concepts. While not all details of the cases are literal, we have sought to preserve the nature of the therapist's gathering and reasoning with data, the actual course of intervention, and the outcomes of the case.

Finally, a word about authorship. We have selected, organized and prepared the final presentation of the cases in this chapter. In some cases, persons shared the case materials with us and we created the case presentation. In other cases, we were given a fully written case presentation which we edited. In order to give due credit, we have listed beside each case any person(s) who provided the case materials or initially wrote up the case.

Alex: Rebuilding Life Following Spinal Cord Injury
by Jayne Shepherd

Persons with spinal cord injury face sudden and life-shattering changes in their abilities and in their way of life. A number of physiological challenges (such as losing bowel and bladder control and being infection- and decubiti-prone) require special dietary and hygienic practices. The major loss of sensory and motor capacities also requires adjustment in how almost all basic functions of life are performed. The biomechanical model (Kielhofner, 1992) provides a major framework for understanding and addressing the movement problems faced by a person with spinal cord injury. Moreover, occupational therapists draw upon a large store of specific knowledge for enabling persons with spinal cord injury to learn to manage their special health needs and challenges.

Persons with spinal cord injury also face major challenges in continuing their occupational lives. For example, they may lose or have dramatically altered a number of life roles. They must completely reorganize their habit patterns. They must relearn motor skills as well as learn to substitute process and communication and interaction skills for lost motor skills. Moreover, their social and physical environments often must undergo tremendous change. It is these and other related aspects of the necessary adjustment to spinal cord injury which the model of human occupation can be helpful in addressing.

We will illustrate how the model can be used to guide treatment in such situations by presenting Alex, who is 30 years old. Alex sustained a complete C7 spinal cord lesion when he dove into unexpectedly shallow water in a local creek. After four weeks of acute care, he was transferred to a rehabilitation unit in a halo vest. At the time, his condition was complicated by sacral pressure sores, a urinary tract infection, and orthostatic hypotension. Our discussion of his occupational therapy program begins in the rehabilitation unit.

Initial Data Gathering and Reasoning

Since Alex was still experiencing high fevers and unstable blood pressure, his occupational therapist began the process of gathering data at bedside. Since Alex's major life role was as a worker supporting a family, the therapist chose to conduct the Worker Role Interview (WRI) to assess Alex's work history and future. The interview was administered very informally over two sessions since Alex's endurance and attention was limited by continuing medical problems. Alex tended to give brief, unelaborated responses but the therapist was able to put together a reasonable picture of his unfolding history as a worker and complete the WRI ratings as illustrated in Figure 14.1. Alex completed the Interest Checklist and the Role Checklist. Figure 14.2 summarizes his responses on the Role Checklist. He discussed his responses with the occupational therapist to get a picture of his other life roles and his interests outside of work. Since Alex lacked the motor skills to complete the assessments as paper and pencil forms, and since the therapist wanted to use them as a basis from which to learn more about Alex's volition and habituation, these tools were administered as semi-structured interviews.

Figure 14.1. Alex's ratings* on the worker role interview (WRI).

PERSONAL CAUSATION					
1. Assesses abilities and limitations	4	③	2	1	NA
2. Expectation of job success	4	3	②	1	NA
3. Takes responsibility	4	③	2	1	NA
VALUES					
4. Commitment to work	④	3	2	1	NA
5. Work related goals	4	③	2	1	NA
INTERESTS					
6. Enjoys work	4	3	②	1	NA
7. Pursues interests	④	3	2	1	NA
ROLES					
8. Identifies with being a worker	④	3	2	1	NA
9. Appraises work expectations	4	③	2	1	NA
10. Influence of other roles	4	③	2	1	NA
HABITS					
11. Work habits	4	3	②	1	NA
12. Daily routines	4	3	②	1	NA
13. Adapts routine to minimize difficulties	4	3	②	1	NA
ENVIRONMENT					
14. Perception of work setting	4	3	2	1	⊘NA
15. Family and peers	4	3	②	1	NA
16. Perception of boss	4	3	2	1	⊘NA
17. Perception of coworkers	4	3	2	1	⊘NA

* 4 = Strongly Supports; 3 = Supports; 2 = Interferes; 1 = Strongly Interferes.

Since Alex was not very verbal, the detailed structure and partial redundancy of these three data-gathering methods helped elicit a more comprehensive understanding of Alex. What the occupational therapist learned from these assessments is summarized below.

Alex dropped out of school after tenth grade "to start earning money." He first went to work on a maintenance crew for the city and later was hired by a road construction firm. During this time, Alex became heavily involved in drug abuse; the problem grew until he was unable to work and realized he needed help. He accepted hospitalization and was treated in an inpatient substance abuse unit. Alex's experience in drug rehabilitation introduced him to a new way of thinking about himself and relating to others. He began to identify with others' struggles to overcome substance abuse problems. Following his rehabilitation for substance abuse, he entered a federally funded work-training program where he worked as a counselor with persons who were handicapped. Alex tremendously enjoyed this kind of work. In what was a departure from his life story thus far, Alex began to seriously think about becoming a rehabilitation counselor. Unfortunately, due to a cut in federal funding for the program, Alex's on the job training as a counselor was terminated. Realizing that his status as a high school dropout disadvantaged him and discouraged by the loss of opportunity for training, he reluctantly returned to a physical labor job. Alex

Role	Past	Present	Future	Not At All Valuable	Somewhat Valuable	Very Valuable
Student	X		X		X	
Worker	X		X			X
Volunteer			X		X	
Care giver	X		X			X
Home Maintainer	X		X			X
Friend	X	X	X			X
Family Member	X	X	X			X
Religious Participant	X		X			X
Hobbyist/ Amateur	X		X			X
Participant in Organization				X		
Other:						

Figure 14.2. Alex's responses on the role checklist.

worked as a plumber's apprentice for six months. However, disinterested in this line of work, he quickly became disillusioned with his coworkers and with the tediousness of the job, so he quit. Left with narrowing options, he next found employment as a stock clerk for a large supermarket. He was working at this job at the time of his injury.

Alex still had a very strong desire to pursue a counseling career, but he was uncertain of what would be possible for him. He was acutely aware of some major challenges that loomed ahead. Though still denying the permanency of his paralysis, he realized that he faced some sort of impairment that might limit his work possibilities. He realized that his work history was sporadic and that he had had difficulty keeping a job. He also recognized that his limited education was a deterrent to a career. However, he was still able to envision some possibilities and was willing to investigate and pursue training options. In his future story, Alex portrayed himself as someone who

had struggled to overcome one kind of disability and was struggling to overcome another. By envisioning himself as counseling others who were challenged by a disability, Alex was able to integrate into a coherent whole his experiences in struggling with two very serious forms of impairment. Becoming a counselor represented survival and triumph over his adversities. He would turn his experiences into something useful for others. It was clear that the power of this story for Alex was what made him willing to commit himself to efforts to achieve such an outcome.

Alex's other major life commitments related to family and friends. Prior to his accident Alex lived with his wife, their three-year-old son, and two children from her previous marriage. At the time of the accident, they were expecting another child. Alex identified being a family member and a friend as the only roles which survived his accident. Still, he recognized that these roles were very different than they had been in the past. He was very concerned that his family role had changed from his being a provider and care giver to his child and wife, to his being cared for or dependent on others. Being a care giver and being a family member were very valuable roles to Alex and were closely related to his working role. In Alex's midwestern, working class view of the world, a man of worth worked hard and supported his family. Any other scenario just didn't fit with Alex's world view. His perspective on life also stressed physical strength and prowess. His strong leisure interests had been in sports and other physically demanding occupations. Being paralyzed was not something he could fully comprehend or imagine as part of his life. Indeed, Alex persisted in announcing that he would "walk out of the hospital." In part, this seemed a strategy to avoid an overwhelming sense of despair. Moreover, Alex has only just begun to realize what it meant to be in his vastly altered body and had yet to find out what gains in capacity would result from therapy.

One of Alex's immediate concerns was how his son would react to him in a wheelchair. He was very attached to his son, and feared his son would be frightened or reject him. Moreover, he was also worried about his own ability to care for both his son and the new baby. In many ways, the future of his being a father was very vague and uncertain for Alex at that time.

The initial evaluation yielded data which clearly illustrated that Alex faced a number of challenges in continuing his life. Prior to the spinal cord injury he had already begun to identify that he saw himself evolving into some type of counselor. This view of himself emerged as part of his recovery from substance abuse, which was a major transition for him. Indeed it appeared that his sporadic work history was related to being in jobs and training that did not fit his interests and image of himself. He appeared to have the conviction to stick with something that fit with the image of his unfolding life, but often found himself sidetracked into other worker roles in which he could not sustain the effort to be successful. His threatened sense of efficacy showed in his anxiety and uncertainty about his ability to fulfill a worker role in the future. He was also apprehensive about others' reactions to his changed physical appearance.

Alex's view of life placed a high premium on his family obligations and relationship to his children. In this area, as in other aspects of his life, he was first beginning to deal with the dramatic transformation which spinal cord injury had brought about. Much of his immediate feelings of

inefficacy related to his relationship with his child and expected baby. Alex's occupational therapist was able to see how the continuation of his life pattern and life story needed to resolve his previously unsettled occupational choice of a worker role, to continue his family role, and to incorporate the reality of his new physical limitations into alternate role scripts and supporting habit maps.

Much of Alex's challenge for the future was dependent on what capacities he had remaining and could develop. As is ordinary for persons with spinal cord injuries, comprehensive data concerning Alex's sensory and motor capabilities were gathered as guided by the biomechanical model (Kielhofner, 1992; Trombly, 1989). Briefly this evaluation yielded the following picture of Alex's capacities. Alex did not have a measurable grip in either hand and he had difficulty doing fine motor tasks (e.g., he could not dial a phone or manipulate money). He had no sensation below the C7 dermatome. Alex's endurance for activity was low; he could only do an upper extremity activity for five minutes before needing a rest or experiencing dizziness. With built-up handles and someone's assistance in setting up necessary objects, Alex could wash his face and arms, brush his teeth, and feed himself (though he didn't have the endurance for an entire meal). He couldn't dress himself or bathe his lower body. He had no bowel and bladder control. He needed assistance to transfer with a sliding board and to roll from side-to-side. Alex's sitting balance in his wheelchair was precarious and, with great effort, he could slowly propel his wheelchair about 150 feet on a flat surface before becoming fatigued.

In order to go forward with both his work and family roles, Alex was faced with the challenge of developing new repertoires of skills and habits. Thus, therapy began by emphasizing how this infrastructure could be developed. It was also expected that working on these areas would provide Alex with experience that would bring into relief the permanent nature of his disability, allowing him to construct realistic knowledge of his capacities and to grapple with how he would live out his future narrative. Also, since Alex's sense of efficacy was so threatened, some means of giving control was needed.

His occupational therapist decided to gather further data about Alex's routine in the rehabilitation unit. Alex reportedly felt that his whole day was controlled by others or by his medical conditions (e.g., if his skin was too red, if his blood pressure dropped, if he spiked a fever, or if he had a bowel accident, the whole routine changed). He depended on others for his self-care, transfers, and being wheeled to therapies, so what he did and when he did it depended on them. Even his visitors came when they wished.

Treatment Process

Alex was an inpatient coming to occupational therapy twice a day. As in most rehabilitation centers, treatment was based on a team approach. This was especially crucial since the program of therapy for developing necessary skills and self-care habits needed to be discussed and integrated with the efforts of other disciplines such as nursing and physical therapy.

The first phase of treatment for Alex included learning about his medical status and necessary self-care, as well as learning how to direct others to undertake his care (since he was still in a halo vest, he needed complete assistance for most self-care). By receiving information and being given the responsibility to direct others in his care, Alex began to realize some feeling of efficacy.

Together the occupational therapist and Alex developed a workable time schedule for daily routine care and leisure time. Alex was put in charge of his schedule and given responsibility for adhering to it. Later, when the halo vest was removed, Alex shifted from directing to performing his own care as he acquired the needed skills. These steps put Alex back in control of parts of his life and set the stage for him to progressively reclaim his life story. Additionally, it provided Alex with a new routine for which he was responsible. The latter assisted him in developing the necessary habit maps to accommodate his changed capacities.

Since Alex had a number of concerns about his role as a parent, and had lost the capacity to pursue most of his previous interests, his occupational therapist carefully selected occupational forms which appealed both to his role as a father and to his male-oriented interest pattern. For example, with therapist guidance, Alex chose to make a toy wooden truck for his new son. This occupation also provided him opportunity to address the biomechanical goals of increasing upper extremity strength and fine motor coordination. He used the bilateral sander with weights, a paint brush, hammer and nails, glue and a wax dabber while constructing his truck. He had to problem-solve how to stabilize and position himself and the wood, how to use the tools, how to sequence the construction steps, and how to maneuver his wheelchair to gather needed items.

Consequently, the occupational form of woodworking afforded him opportunities to relearn motor skills and substitute process for motor skills when necessary. Here, one can readily see in action, the principle noted in Chapter 13 that multiple areas of change can take place simultaneously.

In other occupational therapy sessions, Alex learned how to use such adapted equipment as a reacher, a long-handled sponge, a long and short transfer board, a button hook, a zipper pull, an adaptive can holder/dispenser, and wheelchair gloves to perform necessary mobility and self-care. By learning how to incorporate these new objects into old and new occupational forms, he became more skillful in their performance.

To assist Alex in thinking about his future life, his therapist spent time with him to discuss where he saw his life headed and what was important to him. These ideas were translated into short-term goals for each week and into long-term goals, which were reviewed periodically. This process was important since it gave Alex a concrete opportunity to tell his future story to his occupational therapist while receiving her help in figuring out how to begin living that story in small steps. This gave a stronger sense of reality to Alex's volitional narrative.

Ongoing Data Collection

Observation of and discussion with Alex about his progress in occupational therapy were constant sources of data for his therapist. Alex worked hard in therapy and made good progress in his self-care, transfers, mobility, and fine motor manipulation. He was gaining a sense of efficacy in his ability to control his routine and skillfully complete self-care tasks. His interest in these and leisure activities showed a generally optimistic view toward his future.

A home visit was done in anticipation of discharge as Alex was approaching his expected level of functional independence, given the nature of his spinal cord injury. Alex and his therapist visited his home together. The therapist used this home visit as an opportunity to observe the family as a social group and to examine the physical spaces and objects of the home. She was concerned to learn how this environment would afford and press Alex in his everyday occupations.

The therapist observed that Alex and his wife had difficulty controlling their son and resorted to spanking or hitting him when he misbehaved. Their frustration level was high. It was also apparent that Alex and his wife had difficulty working together as a parent team. However, Alex's son interacted with him quite naturally. He asked Alex questions. He sat on Alex's lap. He got items that Alex requested, and he kissed his father affectionately. Alex also held his second son (who was born during Alex's rehabilitation) and spontaneously played peek-a-boo with him. Alex's warm and spontaneous connection with his children contrasted with the strained interaction between Alex and his wife.

Upon discharge, Alex planned to share his two-bedroom apartment with his wife, her brother, her two children from a previous relationship, their three-year-old son, and their two-month-old second child. The entrance to the apartment was wheelchair accessible, but the bedrooms and bath were up 14 steps. Consequently, Alex planned to live in the living room, sleep on the couch, have a bedside commode, and wash in the kitchen sink. Unfortunately, there was no way to divide the small crowded living room to give Alex some privacy. While the physical space was much less than ideal, Alex did not have the financial resources for a better arrangement.

Preparation for the Return Home

The occupational therapist discussed data from the home evaluation with Alex. Together, they decided to focus during the remainder of therapy on Alex's re-entering his roles as a father and homemaker. The following are examples of the kinds of sessions that occurred in therapy. Alex first practiced how to diaper a baby, how to discipline a child, and how to react to emergency situations. Alex's two children were then brought into therapy where he was responsible for their care. These sessions occurred in a private environment and began with Alex using a doll for diapering and dressing. During the first three sessions with his own children, the therapist stayed with Alex, made suggestions, modeled appropriate disciplinary action, and provided immediate feedback to Alex. Later, Alex cared for the children himself, first in the hospital setting and then when he went home for the weekend. Alex also practiced homemaking tasks such as cooking, cleaning, and laundry. He went out in the community for grocery shopping, went to the store and used a local public transportation system for persons with handicaps.

Alex's functional abilities for being able to return home were progressing well. However, there was increasing evidence that Alex's relationship with his wife was deteriorating. Alex confided that, prior to his injury, they had had difficulty getting along and, in particular, coping with their extremely active three-year-old son. Through the course of his hospitalization, their relationship had grown increasingly stormy with frequent disagreements and periods of not talking with each other. As Alex's discharge date came closer, they appeared to move increasingly apart, and began to speak of the other as a former or lost spouse. Both were beginning to express a sense of defeat about being able to preserve their relationship.

As Alex's return to his wife and children began to look less promising, it became necessary to explore alternatives. As noted in Chapter 13, such detours in therapy are not unusual; neat, linear progress seldom characterizes the entire therapeutic course. Finding an alternative scenario for Alex's discharge was abetted by the fact that Alex's parent's and siblings were very supportive. His parents, younger brother, and a married sister participated in occupational therapy in order to be trained in Alex's care. His parents offered their house as an alternative living situation for Alex in the event that things did not work out with his wife. As it turned out, Alex did move to his parents' home.

At the time of his discharge, Alex's occupational performance in such areas as wheelchair mobility, transfers, handwriting, manipulating money and letters improved to the point that he had reached the maximal independence expected for a person with his level of spinal lesion. Alex lived in the hospital apartment for a week prior to discharge home. This environment more nearly simulated his expected conditions upon discharge and allowed a more realistic picture of Alex's capacities and needs to emerge. He was able to do almost all self-care independently. He dressed, cooked, cleaned, made his bed, did laundry, took his medicines, and kept his own schedule independently. The occupational therapist observed as the week went on that Alex increasingly resorted to talking others into assisting him in these activities. When the therapist explored this with Alex he expressed concern over whether his energy level was sufficient to be independent in all activities and he noted that he found it a source of nurturance to get some assistance. Consequently, the therapist and Alex agreed that some balance between total independence and overreliance on others was ideal. Alex and his parents and siblings came to therapy together in a subsequent session and they identified activities in which assistance could be given if both parties were agreeable at the time.

Throughout therapy, Alex grew more firm in his desire to enter the counseling field. As it became clear that Alex did not see himself returning for a lengthy education, alternatives were explored. Alex agreed that some form of shorter term vocational training to prepare him for work with persons who had handicaps would be acceptable, so this option was pursued. Following discharge, Alex went to another facility for vocational training and three months later began work for Goodwill Industries as a cashier and assisting in the supervision of workers with handicaps.

A few months after discharge, he was happily working at Goodwill Industries. He pursued interests as a sports spectator, did some woodworking, and swam regularly at a local YMCA. He was on the waiting list for an apartment designed for persons with handicaps and hoped to move to these more accessible quarters within a few months. Alex studied for and successfully passed the test for a learner's permit for driving. He completed his behind-the-wheel training at the vocational center and was successful in learning to drive with hand controls. This represented one more step in Alex's plan to eventually live on his own.

Although his marriage ended in divorce, he received joint custody of his children. He both visited his children at his ex-wife's apartment and had them over to his parents' home where he babysat them regularly. He looked forward to a time when he could have them to his apartment for more extended visits. He met new friends and renewed friendships which were extremely important to him.

Although Alex continued to maintain hope for more improvement and occasionally spoke of being able walk again, he began to develop and pursue a realistic long-term vision for himself. Overall, Alex felt confident in his capabilities and saw himself as pursuing the life he desired.

Barbara: The Transformation from Victim Back to Heroine

Barbara was a 33-year-old single mother. She was diagnosed as having multiple sclerosis three years before. As long as five years prior to when she was diagnosed she had intermittent symptoms such as weakness and pain in her back and lower extremities, blurred vision, and some slurring of her speech.

Barbara was admitted to a rehabilitation center after several months of exacerbation of the disease process. During this period of exacerbation,

Barbara had dramatically decreased endurance and ascending muscle weakness that even produced difficulty breathing and swallowing. During the worst of this period, she was unable either to walk on her own or to propel a wheelchair. Just before beginning this first rehabilitation experience, Barbara had been on bedrest while receiving corticosteroid therapy. She was clearly very depressed and hopeless; her occupational therapist was quite concerned about Barbara's motivation for rehabilitation.

Gathering and Reasoning with Data

Given Barbara's emotional and motivational state, her therapist felt it was most critical to understand from Barbara's point of view what had happened to her life. In order to get an initial picture of how the disease process had affected Barbara's life, she decided to begin with formal methods of data gathering. She interviewed Barbara using the Occupational Performance History Interview (OPHI) and she collaborated with Barbara to complete the Interest Checklist and the Role Checklist. Her plan was first to get an overall picture of Barbara's life and how the multiple sclerosis had affected it, then to go on to assess Barbara's physical functioning and to gather other data as needed.

Transformation in Barbara's Life Story

During her interview, Barbara related the following life story. During her senior year in high school she became pregnant. Upon graduation she married the father and her daughter was born soon after. She had only worked briefly as a waitress on weekends during school. Barbara did not enjoy this job; she disliked working with customers on a daily basis. She saw herself as more of a private person. For the next two years, Barbara's time was taken up with being a homemaker and mother. A second daughter was born two years after her first.

In the meantime, Barbara's relationship with her husband had badly deteriorated. Shortly, after the birth of her second daughter she divorced her husband. He was an alcoholic and occasionally abused Barbara when he was inebriated. He also had been unable to hold a steady job because of multiple absences and a temper which got him in trouble with supervisors. The financial stress and uncertainty, combined with the knowledge of her husband's self-destructive drinking problem and his abuse of her, made life practically unbearable for Barbara. As it became clear to her that her husband was not going to do anything about his drinking and abuse and had no prospects for work, she decided it would be better to be on her own with the children.

Forced by the financial realities of being a single mother without the benefit of child support (her husband deteriorated further after the divorce and had no income to contribute for child support), Barbara returned to work. This time she was able to find employment as a secretary in a construction firm. In this job, Barbara filed papers, did some typing and bookkeeping, and acted as a receptionist. With a great deal of effort she managed to balance the demands of being a single mother of two children, working full-time, and maintaining a household for nearly a decade. During this time Barbara viewed herself as a fighter and a survivor who overcame a number of hurdles to be a good mother and provider.

Barbara was forced to resign her job three years ago when her multiple sclerosis had progressed to the point that she was unable, despite extreme effort and a supportive work environment, to fulfill her job responsibilities. In the two years before her resignation, Barbara frequently missed work due to her fatigue and weakness.

In retrospect, Barbara felt that she enjoyed her job. She liked the moderate contact with other people that her job demanded and felt that she did it well. She felt a sense of accomplishment in being able to hold the dual role of single parent and breadwinner for the family. While it was hard, it was nevertheless a source of satisfaction to her that she had pulled her life together. However, Barbara had also felt guilty about not being with her children during the day. Barbara's values were organized around her view of her responsibility as a mother and her hard-won independence. Her children, and the family which she and they constituted, were of central importance. Fiercely independent, she wanted to be financially secure and therefore not reliant on anyone else.

The advent of multiple sclerosis threatened all Barbara's most basic values. She was plagued by the idea that she could neither be a good mother nor a source of income for her family. The entire life story she had constructed and lived had now come crumbling down. Her financial picture had become more and more negative as she lost her income and had to rely on Social Security. She had grown dependent on her children and her parents; she had relinquished the independence and self-reliance she had worked so hard to achieve after leaving her husband. The transformation of Barbara's lifestyle after the interference

of multiple sclerosis is illustrated on the past and present ratings, which her therapist made on the OPHI rating form (see Figure 14.3).

At this point, Barbara felt her life was in a shambles; she was unable even to take care of herself. The future loomed ahead as a great blank. Despite the great strength Barbara had shown in the past, when confronted with the life change wrought by multiple sclerosis she had no idea of where to begin in imagining a future for herself.

Consistent with her interview, Barbara identified family member as her only continuous role for the past, present, and future on the Role Checklist (see Figure 14.4). At this time, her daughters were 14 and 12 years old. She had been completely out of touch with her husband for 12 years and had depended only on the occasional support of her parents to assist in child rearing. Nonetheless, she didn't indicate on the form that she was a care giver to her children. When her therapist questioned why she didn't consider herself presently in the role of care giver to her children, she responded, "No, I'm inadequate and unable to do those responsibilities; my parents are their care givers."

Barbara identified the following roles as disrupted: worker, care giver, home maintainer, and friend. She felt that she had lost her friends; they had become uncomfortable as her disease progressed and slowly faded away. Barbara missed the lack of social contact with others outside her family.

Barbara rated the roles of care giver, home maintainer, and family member as very valuable; when the therapist pointed this out, Barbara agreed that if she could choose her future, these would be the roles she wanted to fulfill. Discussing the Role Checklist brought out that Barbara's biggest concern was being a burden to her children as they were coming to an age when they needed more independence. Her concern about being a burden was even more acute, since she very much wanted for her daughters to have a better start in life than she had had.

Together, the OPHI and the Role Checklist gave a detailed picture of how Barbara's overall life had been transformed by the steady progress of her multiple sclerosis. A previously self-reliant and determined women, she had been transformed into someone who felt victimized and helpless. This transformation was also reflected in her change from a life filled with valued roles to one filled with losses and haunted by the possibility of entry into the invalid role, being a burden rather than a mother.

		PAST	PRESENT
INDIVIDUAL			
Organization of Daily Living Routines	Maintenance of organized functional daily routines	⑤ 4 3 2 1	5 4 3 2 ①
	Achievement of a balance in work, play, and daily living tasks	⑤ 4 3 2 1	5 4 3 2 ①
Life Roles	Maintenance of involvement in life roles	⑤ 4 3 2 1	5 4 3 ② 1
	Fulfillment of expectations of life roles	⑤ 4 3 2 1	5 4 3 ② 1
Interests, Values, and Goals	Identification of interests, values, and goals	⑤ 4 3 2 1	5 ④ 3 2 1
	Enactment of interests, values and goals	⑤ 4 3 2 1	5 4 3 2 ①
Perception of Ability and Responsibility	Acknowledgment of abilities and limitations	⑤ 4 3 2 1	5 4 ③ 2 1
	Assumption of responsibility	⑤ 4 3 2 1	5 4 ③ 2 1
ENVIRONMENTAL			
Environmental Influences	Influences of the human environment	5 4 ③ 2 1	⑤ 4 3 2 1
	Influences of the nonhuman environment	5 4 ③ 2 1	5 4 ③ 2 1

Figure 14.3. Therapist's rating of Barbara's strengths and weaknesses on the occupational performance history interview.

Other Shifts in Lifestyle

Barbara identified eight strong interests on the 80-item modified Interest Checklist. These interests mostly centered around socialization or sports. Despite Barbara's regular involvement in these interests in the past, she had recently participated in only one interest, watching television. She agreed with her occupational therapist's feedback that she needed to identify, develop, and pursue new interests.

As suggested in the Interest Checklist responses, Barbara had seen a significant decline in the quality of her everyday occupational behavior. Her therapist decided to explore the issue of her lifestyle further by conducting an informal interview concerning the details of her everyday occupational behavior pattern just prior to hospitalization. Her responses gave a vivid picture of how her lifestyle had been affected by the disease process.

Barbara spent 70% of her waking day in bed watching television or talking to family members on the phone. The other major portion of her day was spent talking with or directing her children in getting household chores completed. Barbara had no set schedule for meals or self-care activities. Household chores were completed sporadically by her children or her parents. When Barbara had more energy, she would get up and spend an hour or two folding clothes or straightening the house. As a consequence, she would be exhausted for the next two or three days.

Overall, her low energy level and easy fatigability meant that Barbara was unable to sustain even a resemblance of the active lifestyle she previously had when working as a single mother. Moreover, she no longer had access to the occupational forms which she enjoyed and valued and which gave her a sense of competence. Finally, the highly organized habits which had supported her earlier function had disintegrated to a haphazard and passive daily routine.

Barbara's Functional Decrements

As indicated through the data of Barbara's life story and lifestyle, the multiple sclerosis had im-

Role	Past	Present	Future	Not At All Valuable	Somewhat Valuable	Very Valuable
Student	X					
Worker	X		X			
Volunteer				X		
Care giver	X					X
Home Maintainer	X		X			X
Friend	X		X		X	
Family Member	X	X	X			X
Religious Participant				X		
Hobbyist/ Amateur				X		
Participant in Organization					X	
Other:						

Figure 14.4. Barbara's responses on the role checklist.

posed functional limitations that severely affected Barbara's occupational functioning. Since the disease affects the ability for movement, the therapist gathered data related to the biomechanical conceptual practice model (Kielhofner, 1992; Trombly 1989). She began with manual muscle testing, a range of motion evaluation, and sensory testing. While her range of motion was normal she had proximal upper extremity and trunk weakness. Her fatigability was abetted by inefficient breathing. Barbara could not maintain her balance and fell to her left side when attempting functional activities from the wheelchair. This evaluation provided a picture of how extensive were the decrements in Barbara's motor capacities.

At admission, Barbara could not completely dress herself or bathe; she reported that she had not been in a shower for well over a year and instead took sponge baths. She was unable to transfer from her wheelchair without assistance and could only propel it about 200 feet on a level sur-face, requiring two or three rest stops to catch her breath.

Since Barbara's major life role at the time was as a homemaker, the occupational therapist continued an ongoing informal evaluation of Barbara's homemaking performance. Barbara reported that, for the past five months, she had managed to make only two or three meals for her family and had relied on her children or parents to do most homemaking tasks. She confessed that she was unsure of how to approach these tasks from a wheelchair. During an informal observation of her performance in the kitchen, Barbara was unable to maneuver her wheelchair, to effectively transport items from the cabinets, stove, or refrigerator. It took her about 15 minutes to transport a single item from the refrigerator to a counter across the room.

Course of Intervention

Barbara was an inpatient who came to occupational therapy twice a day. She came in a wheelchair or on a stretcher if she was too fatigued to sit. Her occupational therapist felt that the overall focus of her therapy would be to help her find a way out of her story of victimization and helplessness and to reinstate life roles. She realized that this would mean enabling Barbara to maximize her functional abilities within her extreme motor limits and that it would also require adjustments in her environment.

Barbara's program of occupational therapy was developed in conjunction with physical therapy and nursing; it was modified weekly according to Barbara's endurance level and increased strength. Her various therapies and self-care activities were scheduled hourly with half-hour rest periods between major activities.

The occupational therapist began by educating Barbara about multiple sclerosis: the symptoms, possible precursors to exacerbations, and how she would need to have a flexible habit pattern in the future to accommodate fluctuations in her motor skills. In relating this information to Barbara, her therapist also began to portray ways in which she could retake control over her life and reinstate important parts of her former life. She began to help Barbara give her story possible endings other than being totally helpless. Throughout the hospitalization, Barbara's children and parents were also educated about multiple sclerosis and encouraged to support Barbara to envision her life in a more positive way.

Prior to relearning any self-care or homemaking skills, Barbara was also taught work simplification techniques. Once she had the basic information, she practiced work simplification within the hospital routine and occupational therapy sessions. Barbara also learned to use objects which would compensate for her limited motor skills—e.g., a reacher, a dressing stick, and a long-handled bath sponge.

During self-care and homemaking tasks, Barbara increasingly learned how to plan her actions ahead of time to complete the task with efficiency and minimal energy expenditure. Because Barbara still had a limited energy level, her therapist gave her hypothetical problem situations. Barbara would then identify solutions and choose the most efficient and comfortable solution for her. With her therapist's assistance, Barbara also identified when it was acceptable to ask for help from her children or parents to complete tasks.

For two weeks, Barbara kept an hourly time log of her activities in the hospital and on the weekends when she went home. She also reported her level of fatigue for each hour. Prior to each weekend at home, Barbara developed a schedule with the occupational therapist and then compared the schedule with her actual activities. In doing this, Barbara learned the value of both planning ahead and of being flexible with her time according to her strength and endurance.

The occupational therapist worked with Barbara to gradually identify a future for herself. Together they explored what roles and activities were most important to her, using these as a basis to set goals. Barbara decided to set daily, weekly, and monthly goals and to identify which of these were of highest priority for her. In selecting occupational forms to use in the course of therapy, her therapist had two interrelated goals: (1) giving Barbara an opportunity to explore various occupational forms which might become new interests and (2) improving her strength, coordination, and endurance. For example, Barbara chose to learn macramé. She learned the basic knots while sitting at a table and then was able to macramé with her arms up in the air, with the macramé secured to an overhead stationary object. As her strength and endurance improved, time spent doing macramé was increased and the wheelchair seat belt and armrests were removed. Later, she sat on the edge of a plinth while doing macramé to increase her stability.

As Barbara increased her functional motor skills, her occupational therapist began to emphasize ways that her environment could be modified to accommodate her limitations. Her therapist helped her identify bathroom equipment that would enable her to be independent in self-care. The therapist fitted Barbara for an appropriate wheelchair and cushion, and she helped her learn wheelchair control and maintenance. In preparation for her return home, Barbara also planned environmental adjustments to her house to improve accessibility. Finally, she began to participate in community excursions where she was able to put together all she had learned about energy conservation, work simplification, and use of adapted equipment. For example, she shopped in a local grocery store using a wheelchair grocery cart. In the final stage of her therapy, Barbara identified that she wanted to be independent in getting around in her community and needed to be able to drive a car. So she received driving instruction and learned to drive with hand controls.

Throughout the course of therapy Barbara had to come to grips with the fact that the life she had built and would have preferred to continue living was not going to be possible in the way she had previously imagined. Her therapist recognized this and also anticipated that Barbara would need a new life story to sustain her motivaiton in the face of both further decrements in capacity and periods of exacerbation. Barbara commented that she had successfully faced adversity before when she became a single mother and that, by doing it again, she would continue to enact for her daughters a powerful example. Over time, Barbara was able to reframe her experiences in this way and increasingly saw herself as a kind of heroine struggling against a mighty adversary, multiple sclerosis. The transformation from victim back to heroine ultimately gave Barbara much of the volitional strength she needed to go on with her life.

Preparing for the Return Home

About two weeks prior to her discharge Barbara's occupational therapist accompanied her on a home visit. Barbara and the therapist were met there by Barbara's parents who participated in the review of possible home modifications. Barbara lived in a one-floor ranch home. Neither of two entrances to the home were wheelchair accessible, but a ramp and sidewalk could be constructed at the front entrance. The home was small and crowded with excess furniture. By re-arranging the furniture, all the rooms were made wheelchair accessible except the utility room and the bathroom. Since neither of these rooms could be modified for improved accessibility, Barbara and her occupational therapist identified and practiced a system of transfers onto a chair and the commode. They were able to determine that the transfers were feasible so that Barbara could use the bathroom independently.

Barbara's father and mother were impressed with the improvement therapy had brought about in Barbara's ability for transfers and in her mobility throughout the house. They added suggestions for further possible home modifications. Both of Barbara's parents were extremely supportive and acknowledged Barbara's new physical capabilities. Her father planned to make the necessary home modifications with the help of Barbara's two brothers who lived nearby. Both of Barbara's daughters were accepting of their mother's illness and did extra household chores with few complaints. Her family admitted that in the past their willingness to help Barbara may at times have made her overly dependent and agreed to cooperate with her in the future to maintain the level of independence that she wanted to have in her life.

Return to an Acceptable Life

As therapy proceeded, Barbara continued to recognize and accept her reduced capacities and other consequences of her disease. Importantly, she had begun to develop an image of how she could have a satisfying life which operationalized her values of independence. In part, this meant that she had a new definition of independence which allowed her to rely to some extent on her family while being on her own in every way that she reasonably could. Her life story and long-term goals were organized around being an independent homemaker and a care giver to her children. She came to see herself as an example to them of how to rise above adversity. Barbara no longer felt helpless. She was in "control" of her life; she felt competent and was indeed in a state of occupational functioning; and she was able to return to and achieve in her homemaker and mother roles, albeit in altered ways.

At discharge, Barbara's sitting tolerance had increased to 12 hours a day and she complained very little of back pain. Her sitting balance had improved so she could do bilateral activity for 30 minutes with no rest periods. She was independent in self-care, advanced homemaking, and wheelchair management. Barbara could propel her wheelchair up and down ramps, on flat level surfaces and over rough terrain; she balanced her wheelchair on the rear wheels to ascend a curb and was able to maneuver the chair around objects and through small hallways. Barbara completed adapted driving training, was able to drive using hand controls, and was able to put her own wheelchair in and out of her car. She identified this accomplishment as her "ticket to freedom." After discharge, Barbara was referred to a vocational counselor at the Department of Rehabilitation Services. Her stated goal of independent homemaking was recognized by the department as a vocation and it financed the recommended home modifications and the hand controls for car.

Barbara no longer required her parents' assistance on weekends and she managed the cooking and cleaning and her own self-care independently with minimal help from her children. Barbara began socializing again with some of her old friends and neighbors and joined a bimonthly bridge club. Barbara continued her new-found interest in macramé and has given many of her projects as gifts and was "even paid for a macramé pocketbook."

Though Barbara will have more exacerbations, remissions, and loss of skills over time, she has been able to identify an acceptable lifestyle for herself and she has been able to reinstate her most important roles. Barbara also remade her life story. The multiple sclerosis which had recently dominated her life and her volitional narrative, victimizing her and making her helpless eventually faded to the background. Like her experience in leaving behind an alcoholic husband and getting control of her life, the current struggle had become another episode in which her fierce determination has allowed her to prevail and create the kind of life she wants. The strength she had rallied and vision she created would be her greatest asset as the disease continued its likely course.

Carl: Finding a Life Role
by Frances Oakley

Carl is a 32-year-old single man with a diagnosis of chronic schizophrenia who was admitted for an acute psychiatric hospitalization. Carl had an eighth grade education and had always lived with his parents and older brother in a two-bedroom apartment in a low-income neighborhood. None of his family members were employed. Both of Carl's parents had a history of mental illness and Carl himself had a long history of psychiatric hospitalizations dating back to when he was 16 years old.

Carl stopped taking his medications approximately six weeks prior to his admission and, according to his parents, his behavior had gradually deteriorated. When Carl was referred to occupational therapy, he was disoriented and reported hearing voices. He often wandered into other patients' rooms, taking their plants and flowers into his own room. He was extremely withdrawn and did not respond to verbal approaches. Carl required staff assistance for personal hygiene, grooming, and eating. He was unable to share any information about himself and preferred to stay in his room in the dark.

The primary purpose of this acute setting was to stabilize Carl on medication and quickly return him to the community. Thus, given the restraints of the setting and Carl's decompensated status, his occupational therapist had to decide how to accomplish the most within a limited time and given Carl's chronic condition. Specifically, the occupational therapist considered how she could: (a) chart a new course for Carl once his acute symptomatology subsided, (b) attempt to break the revolving door syndrome, and (c) address simultaneously as many parts of the human system as possible.

The therapist knew from experience that medication would decrease Carl's psychosis; that is, his symptoms would remit. However, she also expected that upon discharge Carl would go back to watching television and in several months would likely be psychotic and back in the hospital. The therapist decided to see if Carl could identify an occupational role around which he could organize his daily life. She knew what a tremendously organizing influence roles have on the human system.

Therefore, in planning the data gathering process the occupational therapist was guided by three theoretically based questions: In his background, did Carl have interests and experience that would suggest an appropriate life role for him? How could Carl meaningfully fill his time with behaviors related to roles? How could he find identity and satisfaction in his life?

Since Carl was initially too disorganized to participate in any formal data gathering, the therapist began by talking with Carl's parents. They related that Carl had never worked and had no friends. He spent almost all his time watching television. They also noted that when his illness was in remission, he was able to attend to his self-care and to help a bit around the house. Finally, they mentioned that occasionally Carl would ride the bus to the local park where he would pick flowers and bring them home. This final bit of information stood out in the therapist's mind. While she was not yet sure exactly what to make of it, she decided to use it as the entry point for therapy.

Wooing Carl

At this point, Carl was so withdrawn that the first step was to attempt to woo him back into interacting with the environment. From the discussion with Carl's parents, the occupational therapist knew that plants and flowers seemed to be the one thing that attracted Carl. Since there were several plants in the occupational therapy room, Carl's therapist invited him to care for them. The strategy worked. Carl perked up and agreed to come into the occupational therapy room. Almost immediately he was repotting plants, planting seeds, and watering and pruning the existing plants. His therapist observed that Carl did all of these things very well despite his previously regressed state. Carl immensely enjoyed this activity with plants and stayed totally absorbed in it. The occupational forms of horticulture clearly had an organizing effect on Carl's behavior. Since

Carl was still dysfunctional in his self-care, the occupational therapist decided to use his motivation for horticulture to influence his performance in this area. She insisted that Carl come to therapy appropriately dressed and groomed. The next day he started performing personal hygiene and dressing without staff intervention. It was clear that when motivated, Carl could function at a much higher level than when he had nothing to motivate him and organize his behavior.

The occupational therapist also observed that Carl preferred to work alone, remaining on the fringes of the group. He rarely interacted with others. The therapist decided that this aspect of Carl's behavior likely reflected a lifelong pattern and was not nearly as problematical for him as was his inactivity. Therefore, she decided to accept his continued engagement in mainly solitary activity.

As Carl became more organized his occupational therapist assisted him to complete an Interest Checklist and the Role Checklist. Her rationale in selecting these assessments was as follows. First, she wanted to determine whether Carl had any other strong interests which could be capitalized upon to motivate him. Second, because her plan was to find an organizing role for Carl she wanted to identify his pattern of role identification. The therapist chose not to administer any assessments of skills for several reasons. First, because of the brief hospitalization she would not have time to achieve any significant skill improvement. Second, her informal observations had revealed that Carl's skills in working with plants and flowers were sufficient for the kind of amateur role she was envisioning for him. Additionally, observations, reports of ward staff, and feedback from Carl's parents suggested that his self-care was adequate when he was non-psychotic and, more importantly, when he was motivated.

So as not to overwhelm him, the original, simpler version of the Interest Checklist was administered as an interview with Carl. He reported a strong interest in gardening/yardwork, in macramé (which he had never performed), and in listening to the radio. He indicated some interest in woodworking (which he had done during past hospitalizations), in television, and in ceramics (which he had also never performed), in housecleaning, laundry, and in home repairs. He indicated that no other activities from the checklist were of interest to him. From the assessment it was apparent that Carl had few interests and limited experience pursuing activities. It was also

confirmed that Carl's dominant interest (and the one in which he had the most experience) was horticulture.

Again with the occupational therapist's assistance, Carl was able to understand and complete the Role Checklist. Carl's responses on the Role Checklist are presented in Figure 14.5. He had no continuous roles, but indicated that he saw himself in the past and future in the roles of home maintainer and hobbyist—both of which he checked as very valuable roles. When asked to clarify what kind of hobby he saw himself pursuing, Carl readily responded that it was involvement with plants and flowers.

Because of Carl's functional level, his living situation, and the short-term nature of his hospitalization, his therapist identified a single goal of beginning to engage Carl in an occupational role which was meaningful to him, which matched his observed skills, and which would serve to organize his daily life. Carl was encouraged to pursue the role of hobbyist, built around his interest in plants and flowers. The therapist explained this idea to Carl who readily agreed. They negotiated that Carl would spend as much time as possible on his own in occupational therapy and during the remaining days of his hospitalization in order to prepare for this role. In occupational therapy, Carl continued to work with plants. He even learned to make simple wooden hangers for his plants, incorporating his interest in woodworking. He learned to macramé simple plant hangers. Carl was very pleased with his accomplishments and indicated that he wished to incorporate these two occupational forms into his hobbyist role.

In preparation for his discharge, the occupational therapist worked with Carl to identify environmental supports for his new role. The plan was shared with his family and they agreed to encourage Carl by providing him basic supplies when needed and by expanding Carl's responsibilities in the home to include care of plants in the house and some yardwork.

When he was discharged, Carl began to attend a psychiatric day treatment center five days a week. The therapist shared information about Carl's progress in the hobbyist role with the staff at the center. She recommended the kinds of support which she thought would help sustain this new role for Carl. These included providing opportunities for Carl to engage in the occupational forms he had begun in acute care. She also recommended social recognition of Carl's hobbyist role and integration of it into his activities at the center when possible. The center staff agreed to

Role	Past	Present	Future	Not At All Valuable	Somewhat Valuable	Very Valuable
Student	X				X	
Worker					X	
Volunteer				X		
Care giver					X	
Home Maintainer	X		X			X
Friend			X		X	
Family Member					X	
Religious Participant					X	
Hobbyist/ Amateur	X		X			X
Participant in Organization				X		
Other:						

Figure 14.5.   Carl's responses on the role checklist.

continue Carl's hobbyist role in outpatient therapy at the center. After discharge, Carl was regularly attending the day treatment center on weekdays where he continued to work in horticulture. On weekends, he went to the park with a friend from the center to collect plants and flowers which he often brought to the center on Monday morning. Carl was soon being recognized as the official "florist" for the center.

Diane: The Use of the Assessment of Motor and Process Skills in Treatment Planning for an Adult with Developmental Disabilities[a]

by Kimberly Bryze and Anne G. Fisher

Diane is 36 years of age and has mild mental retardation and cerebral palsy with residual right hemiplegia. She was referred to occupational

therapy by her mother, who is concerned that she will no longer be able to "take care" of Diane. Diane's mother is 76 years of age and has severe arthritis; she has been experiencing increasing difficulties in managing Diane's needs and routine household tasks because of her own limitations.

Diane and her mother live alone in a one-family home. Diane's father died when she was 20. Her only sibling lives in a distant state and he is able to visit only yearly.

As her mother's ability to manage household tasks has decreased, Diane has attempted to take on more responsibility in the home. However, Diane's abilities are limited by her lack of experi-

---

[a] Adapted with permission from Park, S. W., Fisher, A. G., Cannella, J., & Bryze, K. A. (1994). Interpretation and treatment planning. In A. G. Fisher, *Assessment of Motor and Process Skills* (Version 8.0). Unpublished test manual. Department of Occupational Therapy, Colorado State University, Fort Collins.

ence; her mother has always cared for all of Diane's needs and has tended to overprotect her. One of her only responsibilities has been to take care of her room, which she would "straighten," but not regularly. Diane's recent interest in participating more in household tasks appears to come both from her awareness of her mother's increasing disability, and from her contact at a sheltered workshop with other clients who are living in community group homes. These clients, Diane's only "friends," have been talking about "doing more things for themselves" because they are being transitioned into smaller, more independent, living arrangements.

Within the workshop setting, Diane is described as being "easy-going and positive." She is proud of her successes and is not overly discouraged or frustrated when she makes a mistake. Although she is usually aware when she makes mistakes, she is not always effective in overcoming them.

When she is not "helping her mom," Diane spends her time listening to country music and looking at teen magazines. She also enjoys reading simple books (second to third grade level). Her mother indicated that one of Diane's "greatest joys" is going shopping at a large local discount department store. Diane has always avoided physical activity because of her moderately severe motor impairments.

Diane's mother requested the occupational therapist to help her identify Diane's strengths and limitations, and to develop strategies for promoting in Diane greater independence in housekeeping and simple cooking tasks. Diane's mother anticipates that Diane too, will soon have to move into a community-based, assisted-living arrangement.

Diane's therapist chose to administer a formal observation of motor and process skills and to gather data informally on Diane's volition and habituation. The Assessment of Motor and Process Skills (AMPS) (Fisher, 1994) is ideally suited for inclusion in this type of evaluation. The AMPS is administered and interpreted for purposes of planning occupational therapy interventions. The AMPS is a structured, observational assessment that is used by the occupational therapist to evaluate a person's motor and process skills as they are manifested in the context of the person performing simple meal preparation and other household tasks. The motor and process skills introduced in Chapter 8 are scored based on specific criteria included in the AMPS manual (Fisher, 1994).

When the client is evaluated using the AMPS, the client and/or the client's care giver is carefully interviewed to ensure that the client performs tasks that are familiar to the client and that are relevant to the client's daily life needs. From the more than 50 tasks described in the AMPS manual, a short list of four or five tasks is identified by the occupational therapist as (a) being familiar and relevant to the client being evaluated, and (b) providing the client enough challenge to ensure reliable test results. The client is offered this short list and he or she chooses which two or three of those tasks he or she will perform for the AMPS evaluation.

The scoring criteria that are learned in AMPS training courses emphasize the importance of the person performing each task in his or her usual manner, rather than based on externally imposed performance criteria. The effectiveness of the person's performance then is judged based on what is appropriate given the person's culture and the constraints of each task performed. More specifically, the client's performance on each of the AMPS motor and process skills items for each task is scored by the AMPS trained occupational therapist on a four-point scale as follows: 4 = *competent* performance without evidence of increased effort or ineffective performance, 3 = *questionable* performance in which the occupational therapist questions the effectiveness of the observed performance, 2 = *ineffective* performance that slows the task progression or otherwise interferes with effective task completion, and 1 = *deficit* performance as indicated by (a) the need for the therapist to intervene or provide assistance, or (b) performance that results in task breakdown, unacceptable delay, or risk of damage to task objects or danger to the client.

Prior to initiating an AMPS observation, the occupational therapist performing the evaluation ensures that the client is fully oriented to that task environment and knows where all needed tools and materials are located. When the client is assessed in unfamiliar or clinic environments, the client actually places all tools and materials where he or she would typically store them. Moreover, as part of the interview, the occupational therapist and the client negotiate a specific task contract that specifies the constraints of the task to be performed. It is this structure, developed in collaboration with the client, that provides the basis for the rich clinical information that is generated by a formal, structured AMPS observation. That is, only by knowing specifically what the client intends to do can the effectiveness and the quality of the person's motor and process skills be evaluated.

For example, in the case of Diane, whose AMPS evaluation we are going to present below, the occupational therapist knew that Diane intended to (a) make a tossed green salad with lettuce, tomatoes, cucumber, and radishes; (b) prepare the salad in a large bowl and serve it in two individual serving dishes; (c) use bottled Italian salad dressing; and (d) clean up the workspace and put away tools and materials that were not used. Notice that such details as to how Diane intended to cut cucumber and tomatoes, or what bowls or plates Diane would use to prepare and serve the salad, were not predetermined. Rather, as Diane's performance unfolded, the appropriateness of the tools and methods she used was judged based on what is logical given Diane's culture and the constraints of the task she chose to perform: making a tossed green salad and serving it. Knowing that Diane had decided to make a tossed green salad, with the specific ingredients that she decided to use, enabled the occupational therapist to more accurately judge the quality of Diane's performance. Since Diane forgot to add the radishes, the therapist scored Diane's *choosing* performance as ineffective during salad making. Similarly, because Diane handled the sharp knife she used to cut the tomatoes in an unsafe manner which required therapist intervention, the occupational therapist scored Diane's *handling* skill as deficit. Only by knowing that Diane planned to make a salad according to certain task constraints (e.g., preparing the salad in a large bowl, serving the salad in individual bowls, using ingredients Diane specified), could the occupational therapist judge the meaning of Diane's performances that deviated from what she had originally decided and agreed to do. Beyond these task constraints, the client's performances are scored based on what is viewed as safe and logical performance within a specific culture.

After a review of Diane's records, the occupational therapist performed the AMPS interview with Diane. Diane explained that she helps her mother with several household tasks (e.g., washing dishes, making her bed, watering plants, setting the table, simple food preparation, and vacuuming), but would like to learn to do more tasks. She verbalized concern for her mother, whose "hands are hurting real bad." She expressed a desire to help her mother more with cooking, but stated that "I don't know how to do stuff," "my hand doesn't work so good," and "I'm pretty stupid." The occupational therapist discussed with Diane the tasks she feels good about doing, and the therapist offered as possible choices five tasks Diane might perform for the AMPS evaluation. From these five tasks, Diane chose to prepare a tossed green salad, vacuum the living room, and hand wash the dishes.

AMPS Observation

Diane was observed in her home. The occupational therapist ensured that all tools and materials were readily available, and that both she and Diane knew where all items were stored by having Diane show her where they were located. Before the vacuuming task, the occupational therapist also had Diane show her how to operate the vacuum, again to ensure Diane's familiarity with the equipment. Just prior to initiating each task observation, the occupational therapist reviewed the conditions of the task to be performed (i.e., the task contract) and let Diane know that Diane could ask if she had any questions.

The occupational therapist then observed each task to completion, and made written notes of specific actions and steps Diane used in each task performance. When Diane was done, the occupational therapist used her notes to score the quality of Diane's performance on each AMPS motor and process skill item, matching Diane's performance to the scoring examples in the AMPS manual. The occupational therapist then entered Diane's raw scores for each task into the computer and used the AMPS computer scoring program to generate several reports that she could use to aid her in the treatment planning process.

Developing the Treatment Plan

The first report generated by the AMPS computer scoring program provided the occupational therapist with a list of Diane's strengths and weaknesses as the therapist observed them during the AMPS observation (see Figure 14.6). The second report was a list of Diane's raw scores for each task, listed in the order of difficulty of the AMPS skill items (see Tables 14.1 and 14.2). A final report generated by the AMPS computer program provided the occupational therapist with objective measures of Diane's overall AMPS motor and process abilities relative to cut-off scores indicative of motor or process skill deficits that affect the quality or efficiency of a person's task performance. Figure 14.7 shows an example of such a report. This report came from a later evaluation report summary. It indicates Diane's ability measures before and after occupational therapy intervention and provides an objective

ASSESSMENT OF MOTOR AND PROCESS SKILLS SUMMARY REPORT

The Assessment of Motor and Process Skills (AMPS) was used to determine how Diane's *motor* and *organizational/adaptive* (process) capabilities affect Diane's ability to perform functional *daily living tasks* necessary for *community living*. The tasks were chosen from a list of standard functional activities rated according to their level of complexity. Diane chose to perform the following tasks which she considered to be meaningful and necessary for functional independence in the community: Hand washing dishes; Vacuuming, moving lightweight furniture; and Tossed salad, served in a large bowl, with dressing on the side. The level of complexity of the tasks chosen was easier than average to harder than average. Diane's overall performance in each skill area is summarized below using the following scale: *Adequate skill:* no apparent disruption was observed; *Difficulty:* ineffective skill was observed; or *Markedly deficient skill:* observed problems were severe enough to be unsafe or require therapist intervention. The following *strengths and problems* were observed during the administration of the AMPS:

MOTOR SKILLS: Skills needed to move self and objects during task performance.

Posture:
> Difficulty *stabilizing* the body for balance
> Difficulty *aligning* the body in a vertical position
> Markedly deficient skill *positioning* the body or arms appropriate to the task

Mobility:
> Difficulty *walking* or moving about the task environment (level surfaces)
> Difficulty *reaching* for task objects
> Difficulty *bending* or rotating the body appropriate to the task

Coordination:
> Markedly deficient skill *coordinating* two body parts to securely stabilize task objects
> Difficulty *manipulating* task objects
> Markedly deficient skill executing smooth and fluid arm and hand movements (*Flows*)

Strength and Effort:
> Difficulty pushing and pulling task objects on level surfaces or opening and closing doors or drawers (*Moves*)
> Difficulty *transporting* task objects from one place to another
> Difficulty *lifting* objects used during the task
> Difficulty *calibrating* or regulating the force and extent of movements
> Difficulty maintaining a secure *grip* on task objects

Energy:
> Adequate skill *enduring* for the duration of the task performance

PROCESS SKILLS: The ability to organize and adapt actions in order to complete a task

Energy:
> Difficulty maintaining an even and appropriate *pace* during task performance
> Adequate skill maintaining focused *attention* throughout the task performance

Using Knolwedge:
> Difficulty *choosing* appropriate tools and materials needed for task performance
> Difficulty *using* task objects according to their intended purposes

Continued

Figure 14.6.   List of Diane's strengths and weaknesses reported by the AMPS computer program.

Figure 14.6. Continued

Markedly defiicient skill knowing when and how to stabilize and support or *handle* task objects
Difficulty *heeding* the goal of the specified task
Adequate skill asking for needed information (*Inquires*)

Temporal Organization:
Difficulty *initiating* actions of the task without hesitation
Difficulty *continuing* actions through to completion
Adequate skill *sequencing* logically the steps of the task
Difficulty *terminating* actions at the appropriate time

Space and Objects:
Difficulty *searching* for and *locating* tools and materials
Difficulty *gathering* tools and materials into the task workspace
Difficulty *organizing* tools and materials in an orderly fashion
Markedly deficient skill putting away tools and materials or straightening the workspace (*Restores*)
Difficulty maneuvering the hand or body around obstacles (*Navigates*)

Adaptation:
Markedly deficient skill *noticing* and *responding* appropriately to nonverbal task-related environmental cues
Markedly deficient skill modifying one's actions to overcome problems (*Accommodates*)
Difficulty changing the workspace to overcome problems (*Adjusts*)
Markedly deficient skill preventing problems from reoccurring or persisting (*Benefits*)

The results of the AMPS evaluation indicate that Diane requires *moderate to maximal* assistance to be able to complete daily living tasks necessary for community-living. Her potential for rehabilitation is good.

Table 14.1   Diane's AMPS Motor Skills Raw Scores

	Hand washing dishes	Vacuuming, moving furniture	Tossed green salad, served
Easier items			
Endures	4	4	4
Lifts	4	2	3
Moves	4	2	4
Reaches	4	2	2
Coordinates	1	2	1
Transports	N/A	2	2
Aligns	2	2	2
Stabilizes	2	2	2
Grips	2	2	2
Bends	2	2	2
Flows	2	2	1
Manipulates	2	2	2
Walks	2	2	2
Paces	2	2	2
Positions	2	2	1
Calibrates	3	2	2
Harder items			

Diane's AMPS motor skill item scores, listed in order of item difficulty

Table 14.2   Diane's AMPS Process Skills Raw Scores

	Hand washing dishes	Vacuuming, moving furniture	Tossed green salad, served
Easier items			
Uses	2	3	3
Attends	4	4	4
Searches/Locates	4	4	2
Handles	2	2	1
Chooses	3	4	2
Gathers	4	2	2
Inquires	3	4	3
Sequences	4	4	4
Continues	2	2	2
Navigates	4	2	2
Terminates	2	3	2
Organizes	2	3	2
Heeds	2	2	2
Paces	2	2	2
Initiates	2	2	2
Adjusts	2	2	3
Restores	2	2	1
Notices/Responds	1	2	2
Benefits	2	2	1
Accommodates	2	2	1
Harder items			

Diane's AMPS process skill item scores, listed in order of item difficulty.

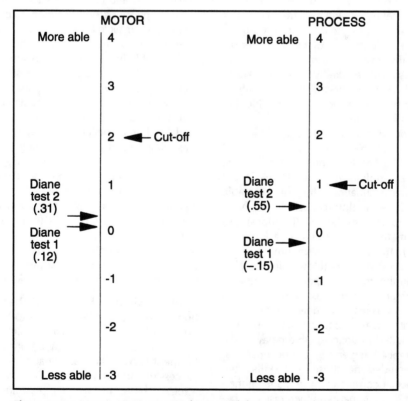

Figure 14.7.   Diane's AMPS motor and process ability measures plotted in reference to AMPS scale cut-off measures indicative of evidence of problems that impact on performance.

index of the efficacy of the occupational therapy intervention.

The reports generated by the computer program that are shown in Figure 14.6 and in Tables 14.1, and 14.2 can easily be created by the occupational therapist without the aid of the computer program. However, the ability measures shown in Figure 14.7 can only be created through computer analysis of the client's raw scores. This situation occurs because the tasks used for an AMPS evaluation vary in their levels of challenge. When a person's ability measures (their position on the AMPS motor and process skills scales) are estimated by the computer program, the analysis is able to adjust the person's ability measures to take into account the relative challenges of the tasks the person performed and also the relative strictness (severity) of the rater who scored the person's AMPS performance (Fisher, 1993).

To develop a treatment plan for Diane, the occupational therapist first reviewed the problem list generated by the AMPS computer scoring program that lists Diane's strengths and weaknesses (Figure 14.6). In this report, raw scores of 3 or 4 indicate "adequate" skill and reflect Diane's strengths. Raw scores of 2 indicate that Diane demonstrated ineffective skill and are reported as areas where she had "difficulty" performing an action during at least one of her task performances. Finally, raw scores of 1 indicate that Diane demonstrated "markedly deficient" skill in that area. All AMPS motor and process skills in which Diane received scores of 2 or 1 identify problem areas for Diane.

What the occupational therapist could readily see was that Diane has generalized motor skill deficits; all of the AMPS motor skill items except Endures were problem areas for Diane. More specifically, the occupational therapist was able to see that Diane's ability to position her body and arms appropriate to the task (Positions), use two body parts to securely stabilize task objects (Coordinates), and to execute smooth and fluid arm and hand movements (Flows) are the skill areas that had the greatest impact on the quality of her performance. Diane's performance in all three skill areas was markedly deficient during her performance of at least one task. Since these three skill areas resulted in unacceptable delay or the need for therapist intervention, the occupational therapist concluded that these three skills areas warranted special consideration in planning therapy. Already, the occupational therapist was beginning to focus on interventions that would minimize Diane's need for assistance from her mother.

As the occupational therapist reviewed Diane's strengths and weaknesses in the area of process skills, she could see that Diane had strengths in the areas of Attends, Inquires, and Sequences. Diane often demonstrated relative strengths when tasks were easier (washing dishes is the easiest task she performed, and making a tossed green salad was the hardest). For example, by comparing Figure 14.6 and Table 14.2, the occupational therapist learned that Diane could search for and locate, choose, gather, and organize task tools and materials when the tasks were easier. The process skill domains of Using Knowledge and Space and Objects appeared to be areas of relative strength for Diane. In contrast, Adaptation was a major problem area, and one where performance was most likely to be unacceptable or require therapist intervention (see Figure 14.6).

In planning therapy, Diane's therapist opted not to use a neurodevelopmental (Trombly, 1989) approach to remediating Diane's motor problems. Two factors guided this decision. First, the occupational therapist was aware that a neurodevelopmental intervention program (a) would emphasize techniques focused directly on Diane's motor impairments, and (b) be designed to prepare her to better participate in functional activity (e.g., normalizing muscle tone). The occupational therapist felt that an intervention of this type would likely be of little benefit, especially giving consideration to Diane's age and long history of motor impairments. Therefore, the occupational therapist chose to link the model of human occupation with the rehabilitative approach. She used the model of human occupation to guide her clinical reasoning and treatment planning. In her intervention, however, she intended to use specific intervention strategies derived from the rehabilitative model that emphasize adaptation: adaptive equipment, environmental adaptation, and teaching compensatory strategies for doing occupational behavior, while giving consideration to building on Diane's interests and values to improve her belief in her efficacy, as well as to develop improved habit maps and role scripts.

After reviewing the results of Diane's evaluation, therefore, it was apparent to the occupational therapist that she would want to develop treatment strategies that gave consideration to (a) identifying what tasks Diane feels are most successful and important for Diane to perform on a regular basis, and with the least amount of supervision and assistance needed; (b) teaching Diane specific techniques to ensure safe and effective performance skill use; (c) teaching Diane compensatory strategies or adaptive methods to more effectively use her motor and process skills during task performance; and (d) consulting with Diane and Diane's mother about modifying their home environment to promote more independent task completion. To these ends, the occupational therapist, Diane, and Diane's mother developed specific goals and objectives, basing them on specific problem areas identified by the AMPS evaluation. Two goals and objectives which were developed are included here:

- *Long term goal 1:* Diane will independently prepare a simple meal safely and efficiently. Short term goals: (1) Diane will position herself appropriately to the workspace at a table or counter; (2) Diane will hold and support knives in a safe and effective manner while cutting, spreading, and chopping; (3) Diane will restore unused tools and materials to the appropriate locations after task performance.
- *Long term goal 2:* Diane will independently perform a simple housekeeping task safely and efficiently. *Short term goals:* (1) Diane will use two body parts together effectively during task performance. (2) Diane will continue action sequences through to task completion. (3) Given appropriate environmental adaptations, Diane will notice and make effective responses to environmental or perceptual cues during task performance.

To meet the specific objectives, the occupational therapist considered using both direct skills training and working with Diane and Diane's mother to develop compensatory strategies. As she focused her intervention on the objectives listed above, the occupational therapist addressed two specific problems through direct skills training: handling tools and materials safely and positioning Diane's body effectively during task performance. For example, the process skill of handling tools and materials safely was taught directly as the occupational therapist provided Diane with multiple opportunities for handling a variety of knives during cutting, spreading, and slicing. Hand over hand assistance and verbal cuing were two methods the therapist used to ensure safety and effective skills training.

The motor skill of positioning herself appropriately to the workspace was addressed directly as Diane performed different food preparation tasks. The therapist used physical assistance, modelling, and verbal cueing to facilitate Diane's use of the most effective sitting and standing positions. The occupational therapist taught Diane when to stand and when to sit for various steps of tasks, where to stand when working at the counter or sink, how to pull her chair closer to the table, and how to angle her chair so that her body was symmetrical with the table.

The occupational therapist observed that Diane had difficulty generalizing newly learned skills from one environment or context to another; the therapist assumed that this difficulty was due to Diane's mental retardation. To address this concern, the occupational therapist initially worked with Diane on only a limited number of tasks. With Diane's successful performance on those tasks, additional tasks were introduced. The occupational therapist also was aware of Diane's need to ultimately develop adaptation strategies that would be effective with several tasks and in different environmental contexts. In collaboration with Diane and Diane's mother, therefore, the occupational therapist developed strategies to promote generalized adaptation (e.g., adaptive equipment, environmental adaptation, and compensatory methods).

Initially, several routine daily living tasks were identified which would be most successful and important for Diane's independence, and that she would need to perform on a regular basis. The occupational therapist also knew that she would need to give careful consideration to (a) the level of task difficulty (tasks that would not be too difficult) and (b) the opportunity for Diane to choose which tasks she would be most interested in learning to perform more independently. More specifically, Diane expressed an interest in helping her mother with cooking and housekeeping tasks. To ensure independence, however, the complexity of tasks needed to be carefully examined. Tasks which involved many steps, or required the use of several tools and materials, would be too complicated for Diane's independent performance, at least initially. Moreover, given Diane's limited ability to anticipate problems and adapt her performance effectively, the occupational therapist felt that safety considerations precluded introducing the use of the stove at this time.

From her formal training in the AMPS, the occupational therapist had an awareness of the relative challenge of most of the more than 50 tasks that are included in the AMPS manual. For example, she knew that washing dishes is easier than average on both the AMPS motor and process task hierarchies, making a tossed green salad is harder than average on both scales, and vacuuming is an average task on the AMPS process skills scale, but harder than average on the motor scale. Based on Diane's performance on the process skills scale, it appeared that easier than average to average AMPS tasks would be most appropriate for Diane. The difficulty of tasks appeared to be of less concern with regard to the motor scale. Using her knowledge of the hierarchy of the level of challenge offered by the various AMPS tasks, the occupational therapist developed with Diane and Diane's mother an initial list of possible tasks. This list included food preparation of simple breakfast and lunch foods. Cold cereal with milk, toast with a spread, hot or cold instant drinks (coffee, chocolate milk, orange drink, etc.), and simple sandwiches (luncheon meat or peanut butter and jam) were some examples of easier tasks. Using a toaster, coffee maker, and a microwave were recommended for simple hot food preparation. Simple housekeeping tasks were added to this list of possibilities; these were easier or of the same difficulty as washing dishes or could be adapted easily for successful completion. Some examples of tasks which were suggested included making beds, sorting laundry and washing clothes (using the washing machine and dryer), folding laundry, sweeping the floor, vacuuming, putting clean dishes away, and setting the table.

The occupational therapist discussed with Diane which tasks were most desirable to her, and together with Diane's mother, identified regular opportunities for Diane to complete these tasks throughout each week. Choosing the tasks involved not only Diane's interests, but also which tasks Diane felt she could perform best, and which tasks would help her mother the most. From an initial list of approximately 20 tasks, Diane chose five to perform on a regular basis throughout the first few weeks, and another five to learn within the next two months. Once the most appropriate tasks were identified, the occupational therapist, Diane, and Diane's mother worked collaboratively to develop strategies to promote adaptation and improve Diane's ability to perform these easier tasks safely and effectively.

The first adaptation strategy was to modify the home kitchen environment to ensure safety and to promote independence. For example, the kitchen table was moved away from the wall toward the center of the room. By moving the kitchen table away from the wall toward the center of the room, the kitchen became more accessible to Diane. This enabled her to more effectively gather tools and materials from the refrigerator and kitchen cabinets, organize these

objects within her workspace, and to sit in a safe and effective position at the table while preparing foods. Moving the table also reduced the amount of "free space" through which Diane had to move as she navigated around the kitchen environment.

The occupational therapist also instructed Diane in how to move heavy items along the counter instead of lifting and transporting them from the refrigerator to the counter adjacent to the sink. As mentioned above, Diane was instructed in how to position herself in the most advantageous places for different tasks. Whenever it was reasonable for her to do so, Diane was encouraged to sit if she needed to stay in one place for more than a minute or two (e.g., putting sandwiches together at a table, folding clothes on the bed), or to lean against the counter if engaged in a task that required standing (e.g., washing dishes, loading the washing machine and adding soap). To adapt for her difficulty using both arms and hands to support and stabilize tools and materials, creative positioning of bowls and utensils, and the use of nonslip (dycem) pads were suggested.

To help Diane compensate for some of her process skill deficits, other modifications were implemented. For tasks with several steps, or with action sequences during which Diane tended to discontinue (not carry actions through to completion), a checklist system was developed. For housekeeping tasks, the checklists resembled a task analysis; for food preparation tasks, the checklists resembled recipes. Difficult words were replaced with pictures to facilitate understanding of the various actions and steps. These checklists were collected together in a small photo album with removable pages for easy access. In addition, the checklists were laminated so Diane was able to check off with a marker which steps or tasks were completed as she worked through a series of steps and tasks.

The occupational therapist used the AMPS to regularly monitor Diane's progress. Because Diane's AMPS motor and process ability measures were adjusted by the computer program to account for the varying challenges of the tasks Diane performed for each evaluation, the occupational therapist did not need to restrict the tasks Diane could perform to those she originally had performed. The occupational therapist then used the results of the AMPS as a basis for (a) discussing with Diane's mother which adaptations were most successful for Diane and (b) identifying where additional adaptation strategies were needed. The taxonomies of AMPS skill items describe commonly understood behaviors. As a result, they provided the occupational therapist, Diane, and Diane's mother a "shared" vocabulary with which to discuss Diane's strengths and needs. Within six months, Diane's skills and task performance abilities had improved so that she had mastered simple cold food preparation, and she was highly motivated to learn to use the stove for more complex hot food preparation tasks. Although Diane continued to have difficulty generalizing motor and process skills to various tasks and environments, she increasingly was able to do many more tasks in her home.

When Diane was reevaluated after six months of intervention, she again performed three tasks in the AMPS manual. To evaluate the effectiveness of the adaptation strategies which had been implemented (e.g., checklists, nonslip pads, environmental adaptations), Diane was free to perform these tasks using whichever strategies she spontaneously effected. The results of her six month re-evaluation are shown in Figure 14.7. As expected, Diane had improved in AMPS process skills more than in AMPS motor skills. Although her improvement on the AMPS process skills scale was significant (.70), her AMPS process skills ability measure was still below the cut-off; Diane still required supervised living. That is, Diane still was not able to perform all of the household and cooking tasks needed for independent living. However, she was quite capable of performing many everyday tasks in her home. While the quality of her performance often continued to be ineffective, she was now able to complete tasks without any assistance from her mother. Consistent with Diane's and her mother's wishes, initial plans have been made in pursuit of a more independent living situation for Diane in the near future.

Jessy: Reentering Life Following Brain Injury

by Jayne Shepherd

Jessy was 22 years old. Injured in an automobile accident, she sustained a closed head injury. Jessy was initially referred to occupational therapy seven days after the accident while still in the intensive care unit (ICU).

As sequelae to left intracerebral hemorrhage Jessy experienced right hemiparalysis, aphasia, and multiple contractures. Using the biomechanical model (Kielhofner, 1992; Trombly, 1989), Jessy's therapist provided her with splints to main-

tain the elbow, wrist, ankle, and finger joints in neutral positions so as to prevent permanent deformities that would otherwise result from her contractures. Jessy remained comatose for four weeks and semicomatose confused for seven weeks while in acute care. At this stage Jessy was dependent on others for all aspects of her care including feeding, bathing, toileting, dressing, bed mobility, and transfers. She made no attempt to speak; her only expression of feeling was that she often cried. She was unable to sit up for more than five minutes without going into a pattern of total extension and sliding out of the chair. Jessy had to be restrained as she often thrashed her body around and would fall out of bed. Initially, Jessy did not respond to any sensory stimuli except for pain.

Given Jessy's state at the time, the therapist could not learn anything from Jessy about her volition or habituation. Consequently, the therapist briefly interviewed Jessy's family members and some visiting friends to get information on Jessy's interests and valued activities, roles, and routines. They described Jessy as an attractive, intelligent, and active young woman who enjoyed rock music and who valued animals and nature.

Since Jessy was still minimally responsive, her therapist's main goals for her volition and habituation were to provide an enriched environment which would afford her appropriate sensory stimulation and begin to orient her to the external rhythm and structure of everyday life. Her therapist developed a program of environmental stimulation using rock music as well as objects and pictures representing animals and nature. The therapist taught nursing staff and family members how to most effectively position Jessy and how to provide her environmental stimulation.

As she became semicomatose, Jesse remained in decorticate posturing with marked spasticity and contractures of all extremities. Hence, she was still severely limited in performing any voluntary, controlled movement. However, Jessy did begin to show favorable responses to visual, auditory, and tactile stimulation. She was still very confused and, for example, could not follow one-step commands. When possible during therapy, her restraints were removed or she was seated in a chair. A swallowing and feeding program was initiated and Jessy learned to feed herself with adaptive equipment and supervision. Other self-care activities were initiated during this phase as they were habits that were natural or familiar to Jessy. As she progressed she was able to express herself with the aid of a picture communication chart. Next, matching and sorting tasks were given to Jessy. She responded very excitedly to these and she began to demonstrate to hospital staff how alert she could be.

Toward the end of her stay in acute care, Jessy could attend to a task for 2–3 minutes, following one-step verbal directions about half the time. She also began to use facial expressions and other physical gestures to communicate. Finally, Jessy had made some progress in self-care skills.

Rehabilitation Phase

When Jessy was medically stable she was transferred to a rehabilitation center. In the rehabilitation phase, Jessy's therapist first gathered data through situated observations and informal testing and later through formal tests of motor, cognitive, perceptual, self-care, and social skills, as well as evaluations of habits, roles, goals, interests, and values.

Jessy had received a severe injury to the mind brain-body performance subsystem. Consequently, the data gathering was partially guided by the cognitive-perceptual, motor control, and biomechanical models (Kielhofner, 1992; Trombly, 1989), which enabled a picture of underlying capacities and limitations to be developed. In the early stages of rehabilitation a very detailed picture of Jessy's motor, sensory, perceptual, and cognitive status was generated through the therapist's data gathering. Briefly, it revealed that she had severely limited active and passive range of motion in all extremities and she had impaired proprioception, light touch, and stereognosis. As a functional consequence, Jessy often dropped items, was unable to write with her left hand and could not button even large buttons. Her dominant right hand was severely limited by a frozen shoulder that hurt with any movement. Jessy could roll side-to-side in bed utilizing the bedrails but could not sit up from supine. She required assistance to transfer. The left side of Jessy's face was paralyzed and she drooled constantly.

Jessy's motor, process, and communication and interaction skills were informally observed as she was seen in the clinic. Since her reacquisition of skills was uneven and required constant surveillance and responses on the part of the therapist, her therapist chose to use constant informal observation, rather than formal testing. For example, as she was relearning to eat, her therapist observed that with a scoop dish and a built-up spoon, Jessy was able to feed herself, but she needed assistance, especially cueing, to heed to the task and to properly grip the spoon and her

cup. Otherwise, Jessy would be easily distracted or might drop the spoon or cup. Jessy was still experiencing flexion contractures, spasticity, incoordination, and poor balance which severely constrained her motor skills in other self-care activities such as bathing and dressing. Her occupational therapist first focused on having Jessy cooperate with these occupational forms. As she observed any progress, she invited Jessy to begin to take over small steps.

Jessy initially communicated by gesturing, shaking or nodding her head, or by pointing to objects, letters, words, or pictures. As Jessy was able to communicate in these simple ways her therapist could see that her skill of noticing her environment increased daily. Initially, Jessy could attend to simple activities for about ten minutes. However, beyond this time she easily became agitated and frustrated. Because of her limited tolerance, her therapist saw Jessy for 10–15 minutes, two to four times a day. She often appeared confused and had difficulty heeding the goal or purpose of even simple two-step tasks. About half the time she did not get to the second step. An illustration of her process skill difficulties at the time is that Jessy could gather the items needed to brush her teeth, but could not sequence the steps of the task correctly.

At this point, Jessy's performance was also impaired because she was so often emotionally agitated. For example, she was constantly moving about and would often be crying with her hand on her forehead. It was clear that her sense of efficacy was severely shaken. Consequently, she had a low frustration tolerance and would give up on tasks that were difficult for her. Also, Jessy was not spontaneous at all. For example, because communication posed such a challenge for her, she would not initiate interaction with others. Even as Jessy progressed, the effects of her altered sense of personal causation were apparent. For example, although Jessy's communication skills improved and she was able to speak, her interactions with others were very helpless and childlike. Initially, she carried stuffed animals and pictures of rock stars with her, became embarrassed easily, giggled inappropriately, and interrupted others' conversations or tasks. When she had difficulty expressing her feelings, she resorted to crying, pouting, or yelling. It was clear that these behaviors were not consistent with what she deeply desired. For example, despite often acting helpless, it was clear she resented being "bossed around" (as she called it) when others sought to assist or direct her.

This was a tumultuous time marked by irregular progress. For example, when things bothered her emotionally, Jessy would develop migraine headaches that kept her in bed up to two days at a time. It was important for Jessy's therapist to recognize here the principle that the process of change is irregular and sometimes chaotic and to be able to gently return Jessy to a system of action when she was once again emotionally able to tolerate it.

Discovering the Original Jessy

Writing, typing and spelling on a letter communication board was used while Jessy was still nonverbal. This was not always successful as she confused or forgot letters. Nevertheless, some information about her values, interests, and goals were obtained from this method. Until Jessy had sufficient communication skills to tell her therapist about her life before the accident it was difficult to have a complete picture of who she had been. Thus, a more intensive data-gathering process to learn about her previous habituation, volition, and environment was begun as soon as it appeared that Jessy could tolerate it emotionally and cognitively. Her therapist interviewed her using the Occupational Performance History Interview; this instrument helped identify both Jessy's previous occupational life and how her life has been altered since her injury. Jessy was given the Role Checklist to complete and later discuss. Also the therapist asked Jessy to describe her previous pattern of everyday occupations.

These data-gathering methods painted a picture of Jessy prior to her accident that contrasted sharply with the person whom the therapist first encountered in the hospital. Jessy was a bright and high achieving student who had completed high school with honors and was a senior at a prestigious university, majoring in chemistry. During college, she had worked part-time for three years as a waitress in a restaurant. Jessy had previously worked as a babysitter, a salesclerk, and a housekeeper to earn money. Jessy had enjoyed all of the above jobs as she liked working with people. She also valued these jobs as they helped her to have spending money. Jessy stated that her occupational goal for the future was to be a chemist, working in a university laboratory doing research. She saw her accident as delaying this goal, but not obliterating it. Jessy's strong interests (as identified on the Interest Checklist and discussed with her therapist) included crafts, nature, animals, cooking, and socialization.

Jessy was the oldest of three children and before entering college she often spent time babysitting her nine-year-old brother. Jessy lived with her brothers, mother, and stepfather until two years ago when she moved out of the house. Prior to her accident, she lived on campus in an apartment with her boyfriend and they shared financial costs and household chores. Her choice to live with her boyfriend in defiance of her parents' desires evidenced Jessy's strong-willed nature. Besides working in a fast-food restaurant, Jessy volunteered at the local humane society, worked on the school newspaper, and maintained a high grade point average in an extremely competitive and demanding major. All in all, her occupational history revealed a talented, willful, and energetic young woman.

Figure 14.8 summarizes Jessy's responses on the Role Checklist. While the pattern of role change summarized on the form tells a story of its own, discussion of Jessy's responses gave her therapist very useful insight into the transformation that had taken place following the accident. Whereas Jessy had previously been actively involved in a number of roles, the accident had removed her from all those roles and placed her in a dependent patient role. Moreover, Jessy felt that she no longer had control over any of her previous role tasks. For example, her parents had been appointed by the court as her legal guardians during her comatose and semicomatose periods, and consequently they controlled her finances. They also sought to control other details of her life such as who her visitors were and when they came, as well as what mail and phone calls she received.

Prior to the accident, Jessy was extremely active. Her typical day included getting up at 6:00 a.m., studying, going to classes or work, volunteering, or working on the school paper. She had no set times for meals or household chores, and she saw her boyfriend erratically as he also had a part-time job. Jessy's day was now dictated by the hospital routine. She was awakened at 6:00 a.m., and was bathed, dressed, and given breakfast. For eight hours, she attended therapies. She had only half an hour of free time during the day, but evenings were generally free except for 45 minutes of self-care activities before bedtime.

Jessy's view of her previous life is highlighted by the four things she valued most in the following order of importance: independence, being with her boyfriend, having pets, and living away from home. In many ways she was a typical young adult involved in the transition toward constructing her own independent life and moving toward family roles of her own. In addition, her priorities also showed what a high premium she placed on her independence and self-reliance. In this context, the impact of her current situation became more apparent. Jessy had been robbed of what she most valued. The life of independence and self-reliance she had been living had come to a halt. She was shackled to a host of performance limitations and forced to depend on others for almost all aspects of her life. Overall, she felt severely constrained and confined. Most of all she felt, as she put it, "like a prisoner" in her own body.

Jessy fiercely wanted to be released from her confinement and was able to translate this desire into concrete goals. Specifically, Jessy's long-term goal was to walk on her own in six months, and her immediate goals were to be able to wash and dress herself and to have a weekend pass to her apartment. Jessy expected that her valued life of independence and self-reliance would begin to fall in place soon after she could care for herself and walk on her own. Jessy's ability to envision her future illustrates she was able to muster a sense of efficacy about ultimate outcomes. Her present sense of personal causation was, nevertheless, still a problem for her. Jessy repeatedly complained of her lack of control over her life. She felt as if she had lost her last two years of independence from her family and had been returned to the situation of dependence she had as a younger child. She was plagued with anxieties that she would be permanently inferior, dependent on others, and incapable of taking control of the direction of her life.

Regaining the Self

As her attention span and concentration level increased in the rehabilitation phase, Jessy came to therapy twice a day for 90-minute sessions. Treatment sessions were initially held in a room where distractions were eliminated as much as possible to enhance her ability to attend. Also, because of her limited ability to heed the purpose of a task, brief activities were used and a new task was introduced about every 20 minutes. This environmental adaptation to her skill level also gave Jessy more feeling of control since she could successfully complete a task. It helped eliminate her frustration and agitation.

Slowly, Jessy progressed to the kitchen area and other parts of the occupational therapy clinic when she had learned to tune out distractions and attend to tasks for longer periods of time.

Throughout Jessy's rehabilitation phase, intervention strategies were developed in conjunction with physical therapy, nursing, psychology, and recreational therapy. Goals were reviewed and modified weekly (if needed) according to Jessy's improvements and her personal desires.

Biomechanical and motor control strategies were used to help Jessy increase her range of motion, coordination, and strength in both arms. Previous interests and her personal concerns were incorporated into the activities used to aid her motor recovery. For example, early on she engaged in rolling cookie dough and sanding a project to increase voluntary control, strength, and range of motion. These activities reflected her interest in crafts and cooking and therefore also had the effect of enhancing her enjoyment in therapy and giving her experiences which helped reinforce the idea that she was, by degrees, beginning to re-enter the life she previous had and cherished. Later, as voluntary movement returned, new activities that still reflected her interests but provided more appropriate press for motor control were used. For example, she was able to develop fine motor coordination in occupational forms such as cross-stitching, cutting out pictures of rock stars, preparing meals, and doing leatherwork. These activities were also used to practice process skills.

One day, a month into rehabilitation, Jessy was asked what she wanted to cook. She indicated sugar cookies. When she was given a sugar cookie mix, she became horrified. She had been a gourmet cook and would not think of using a mix! Her desire to bake cookies from scratch was respected and although she struggled with process skills limitations that made cooking difficult, her motivation to cook according to her own standards counterbalanced these difficulties.

Jessy continued to become frustrated and upset at times when she encountered her limitations and her painfully slow progress. Her therapist worked to encourage her, to highlight her progress, to underscore the times that were enjoyable, and to celebrate the small triumphs that came when she mastered something that she could not previously do. These efforts helped to locate Jessy in a narrative in which she could see herself progressing toward a desired state. These efforts also helped reduce her frustration about the distance she still needed to go. For example, when Jessy's ataxia decreased, she was once again able to write; however, it was initially inaccurate. To reduce her frustration over the discovery that her writing was impaired, it was important to re-

Role	Past	Present	Future	Not At All Valuable	Somewhat Valuable	Very Valuable
Student	X	X				X
Worker	X		X			X
Volunteer	X		X			X
Care giver	X		X		X	
Home Maintainer	X		X			X
Friend	X	X	X			X
Family Member	X	X	X		X	
Religious Participant					X	
Hobbyist/ Amateur	X		X		X	
Participant in Organization	X		X		X	
Other:						

Figure 14.8. Jessy's responses on the role checklist.

mind her that it was a sign of progress, since she could not write at all previously. The therapist also helped her to envision her impaired writing as a phase on the way to being able to write competently. By helping Jessy volitionally interpret her experience this way, her therapist enabled Jessy to feel a greater sense of efficacy even while she realized that her capacities were still limited. Eventually, Jessy's right arm be-came sufficiently coordinated so she could write effectively.

Throughout this phase of therapy Jessy experienced simultaneous, though uneven, gains in a number of areas. Each week brought new surprises and new frustrations. But with her therapist's assistance she was able to place all these experiences in a larger story in which she was making her way back toward a way of life she enjoyed and valued.

As Jessy's process skills improved, her therapist modified occupational forms and environmental support to give her less structure and more challenge. Her therapist also provided necessary memory aids. As Jessy's motor skills increased she was able to do such things as dress, bathe, style her hair, brush her teeth, and shave her legs on her own. However, for quite some time she required stand-by assistance for all transfers as she often lost her balance when standing.

Jessy progressed from living with a roommate to modified independent living and finally to staying in the hospital's apartment prior to discharge. Progressively, Jessy was made responsible for more of her own care, and worked with her therapist to develop and follow a routine which allowed her to establish new workable habits. This routine included making her bed, doing her laundry, keeping her room organized and clean, making and keeping her own appointments, taking her own medicine on schedule, and cooking one meal a day. Mnemonic aids were still necessary to assist Jessy in carrying out this routine. In the last three weeks of her hospitalization, Jessy planned her own schedule, setting up her own therapies, bedtime, self-care schedule, and leisure time.

Jessy persisted in wanting to return to her previous lifestyle. In particular, it was important to her to be in control and self-sufficient. So, her occupational therapist collaborated with her to develop an inventory of all her previous responsibilities. Together Jessy and her therapist put them in order of priority considering both the importance and the feasibility of each for Jessy. Following the creation of this priority list, Jessy began to work toward recapturing her previous responsibilities.

For example, Jessy had lost control of her own finances when her parents took over that responsibility. Consequently, regaining financial responsibility became a goal. Jessy and her therapist agreed to tackle this occupational form initially through simulating the kind of financial responsibilities she had when living on her own. To this end, her therapist and Jessy worked out a hypothetical budget and Jessy had to "pay weekly bills" to different people for the following things: rent, food, electricity, water and sewage, phone, therapies, entertainment, clothes, toiletries, transportation, and savings. Her therapist monitored and gave Jessy feedback on her ability to follow through on these financial management activities. At the time of discharge, Jessy was writing checks correctly and balancing her checkbook, although she continued to forget payments unless reminded or sent an overdue bill.

In similar fashion, Jessy and her therapist identified a host of objects and occupational forms, large and small, that she sought to master once again. For example, she practiced the use of such objects as a phone book, newspaper, a dictionary, an encyclopedia, and a vending machine. She engaged in occupational forms such as filling out a job application, doing functional mathematics, filing paperwork, reading maps, giving directions, writing letters, and reading bus schedules. She also practiced performing in occupational behavior settings such as the library and supermarket.

By the time she was discharged Jessy's performance in a range of occupations was greatly improved; however, Jessy still had difficulty attending and noticing. Moreover, she sometimes became flustered, which further impaired her performance. While Jessy desperately wanted total control of her life, she had to accept that her memory loss and process skill deficits meant that she needed some supervision. Moreover, she also required stand-by assistance when she walked because she was still unsteady and at risk to fall.

Jessy was still having difficulty communicating and interacting with others. Sometimes she was too passive to get her needs met or to receive necessary assistance. Other times she lost control and had outbursts with those around her. Jessy's therapist worked with her to identify and practice appropriate assertiveness and socially appropriate behavior. This was done in a variety of settings with Jessy's therapist giving her instruction and feedback. Jessy relearned how to initiate conversations in different situations and how to effectively participate in community outings to a variety of occupational behavior settings. Jessy was a naturally engaging person. Consequently, as she relearned expected behavior, she readily became friends with numerous patients and staff members. She often advocated for other patients and encouraged them to get out of the hospital and to forget their disability.

One of the biggest challenges for Jessy was to come to grips with what her discharge status would likely be. Practically, her ongoing impairments limited how much independence and self-reliance was safe for her. To ease Jessy toward acknowledging and accepting this reality, she went on numerous weekend passes at home prior to discharge. Jessy's therapist gave her family a list of things Jessy could do independently so they would both allow and expect her to do them. This helped ensure that Jessy's most important social group at the time, her family, would afford and press for the level and kind of occupational performance of which Jessy was capable. Additionally, the therapist worked with Jessy and her family to develop a schedule for her at home. This schedule allowed Jessy to do what was most important to her and provided structure for both Jessy and her family, so that she could be supervised without too much interference.

Re-entering Life

Jessy returned to live at home with her parents and brothers. She was followed as an outpatient in occupational therapy. As part of that follow-up the therapist decided to readminister the Role Checklist to see whether Jessy was reentering roles as she had intended. The checklist and subsequent discussion indicated that Jessy had not followed through on her plans to reenter the student and volunteer roles (i.e., she had planned to enroll in a community college class and volunteer at the local humane society). Her therapist learned that Jessy was also having difficulty structuring her day.

On the positive side, Jessy had become reacquainted with some old friends and had gone to the movies and out to eat with them. She had pursued her leisure interest of cross-stitching and frequently played games with her younger brothers. Nonetheless, Jessy felt she could do more than her parents were allowing her to do. She felt that she was having her competence, assertiveness, and independence challenged by her parents.

While Jessy clearly knew how she wanted her life to turn out, she was quite unsure of the immediate future. Therefore, therapy focused on helping Jessy develop a clearer idea of what she wanted her life at the time to be and on prioritizing short-term goals. Jessy would make a list of what she wanted to achieve by her next scheduled therapy, when she would report her accomplishments or problems to the therapist. She developed lists incorporating her values and interests and became increasingly realistic concerning her current capabilities.

As time went on, Jessy crystallized the goal of receiving some kind of vocational training, which would allow her to obtain a job. She also wanted to pursue opportunities to live somewhere other than at home. She began to attend a vocational training center, where she could live in a dormitory. During this time, she continued to return for periodic follow-up in occupational therapy. At the vocational training center, she received six months of training in computer skills. She continued to practice her habits and skills and worked towards her goal of personal independence. She was able to take over her personal finances at this point, including managing the investment of funds she has received from an insurance settlement related to her accident. During this time, in occupational therapy, she learned to drive again.

Reinventing the Life Story

A year and a half after her head injury, Jessy had partially reclaimed her previous life. Importantly, she was also able to reinvent her life story in necessary ways. Jessy had largely come to grips with much of the reality of her continuing limitations. Considering these, she felt she had rebuilt some significant portion of her previous life. There were certainly losses. Her old boyfriend was unable to handle all the changes in Jessy and their relationship had ended. Jessy realized that she would never become the chemist she had aspired to be prior to the accident.

Jessy became increasingly reconciled to the fact that she was not exactly the same person she had been. Her right hand was still impaired. She could walk on her own, but needed a cane. She was able to do all her self-care and basic homemaking and had developed new habits that sup-

ported her daily living tasks and work; however, she continued to have trouble with process skills in the domain of adaptation. This required her to accept minimal supervision for daily tasks.

Jessy moved to a group of supervised living apartments where she had her own room and shared household chores with other residents. She took the bus to her part-time job as a computer operator. She continued to make friends easily and had a new boyfriend. She lobbied those in charge of the supervised living apartments in order to secure permission for residents to have pets; this was a big accomplishment for her.

Jessy felt that her schedule allowed a level of activity which she could handle and that she had a good mix of work and leisure time. She talked with her family on a bimonthly basis and had demonstrated to their satisfaction that she could be semi-independent. Though Jessy relinquished the image of herself as a chemist–researcher, she was very inventive in sustaining involvement in chemistry as part of her life story. Jessy volunteered as a technical aide in a junior high school chemistry club.

Jessy was content with the life she had managed to compose for the time being. Nonetheless, in her future story she would be living on her own. In that story she would get around in her own car with her cocker spaniel in the back seat!

Postscript: Several years later Jessy was working 30 hours a week as a computer operator doing data entry and "crunching numbers" for a researcher at a research center. She had held the job for five years, needed only minimal job coaching, and was considered an extremely reliable worker. She was trying to piece together her experience of trauma and recovery and planned to write about it for others so they would know what the experience is like. She was up to four pets!

Joan: Re-Creating the Meaning of Home

by Laurie Rockwell-Dylla

Joan's therapist received an order from the home health agency to "evaluate and treat" a 79-year-old woman with myxedema (an extreme and disabling edema due to a thyroid abnormality) and a history of congestive heart failure. Joan lived in a middle-class suburb in a brick Georgian home. On the first home visit the therapist encountered not only Joan, but also her two adult daughters, Anne and Debbie, and her 87-year-old husband, Art. Her daughter, Debbie, led the therapist into the living room where the shades were down and the blue sheer curtains were closed. Joan was sitting in a black leather high back recliner and wearing a nightgown and robe. Her grey hair was pulled up from her face and bobby-pinned into a bun on the top of her head. She sat with her shoulders hunched over in her chair, clearly having trouble breathing. A fan positioned in the corner of the room was blowing. Debbie explained that the fan helped reduce the moisture in the air which, in turn, eased her mother's ability to breathe.

The centerpiece of the former living room was a queen size bed with a pretty comforter and embroidered pillows arranged on top of it. While the bed was attractive, it was inescapable evidence that the living room had been transformed into a sickroom. Other elements of the room that made this transformation apparent was the bedside commode next to the television and an endtable next to Joan's chair that held pills, a cup of water, and a little silver dinner bell to jingle for summoning help. The therapist inquired and learned from Joan and her daughters about the insidious decline that led to the transformation of the living room into a sickroom and the transfiguration of all of their lives.

Insidious Decline

The data about Joan's decline emerged from an informal interview the therapist conducted over time with Joan and her daughters. Joan's therapist preferred to conduct situated interviews informally over a series of home visits to take advantage of the context and of other family members who were often present. This situated interview method seemed more suited to the therapist for a home setting. Moreover, since home health services extended over several visits, the ongoing interview allowed the therapist to build rapport and increasingly learn about the home health client.

The occupational therapist elicited the "story" of Joan and her daughters with the aim of knowing what Joan's experience of being ill was like and what impact it had on her occupational life and that of her family. She began with more global questions. She asked Joan to describe what a typical day was like before her hospitalization and then what a typical day was like for her and her daughters now that she had returned home. The therapist inquired what Joan would like to be doing that she wasn't capable of doing at the present time. She asked Joan to identify what she

thought was hindering her from doing the things she wished. The therapist also asked Joan how she envisioned herself within a month's time (older adults often don't like to think in terms of "long-term goals" because they may feel that worsening of their illness and death are inevitable). The therapist also asked the daughters what would help them in their roles as care givers.

Debbie shared how her mother developed many years ago a thyroid condition which they (including the physician) thought had been cured with a newly approved medication. For several years she had no symptoms and engaged in her normal routine of taking care of her family and her house, which had always been the focus of Joan's life.

Joan described how she cooked, cleaned, crocheted, and enjoyed her family and friends until illness set in a year ago. Debbie recalled how her mother's eyes began to look "buggy," and how she started retaining so much fluid that her legs had become four times their normal size. Along with this, Joan experienced difficulty breathing and became more fatigued each day. Her symptoms progressed to the point that Joan was not able to cook or do heavy housework. From then on, she relied on help from her daughters.

The sisters discussed how their mother's decline was very gradual. Over the year it had reached the point where their mother needed help, not only with the homemaking but also with her own personal care. Joan found it increasingly difficult to climb up and down the fourteen steps to her bedroom and bathroom, so the family decided to move the bed into the living room.

The impetus behind Joan's declining condition was myxedema—a resurgence of her thyroid condition. Joan was hospitalized and treated with medications aimed at eliminating the fluid which her body had retained. When given the choice to receive therapy in the hospital or at home, Joan opted to return home with physical and occupational therapy services.

Joan's world essentially became the former living room. She ate her meals there, got sponge bathed in the partial bathroom off the living room, occasionally watched television from her recliner chair, and spent what were often restless nights in her queen-size bed.

Another major family decision was for Debbie and Anne to relinquish their own homes and restructure their lives to assume the role of "full-time nurses and homemakers." They both shared the responsibility for meeting the medical and emotional needs of their mother and father, as well as the responsibilities of maintaining the household. Debbie was single, had her own condominium, and worked as a freelance artist. She was spending increasing amounts of time at her family home rather than her own residence, so she decided it was best just to move back in. Anne (the elder daughter) was divorced and didn't have children. She relinquished her apartment as well in order to move back home and along with her sister assumed full-time "care giving" responsibilities for their increasingly frail parents. There were other relatives, but interactions with them were infrequent. Rather, neighbors and Debbie's and Anne's long-time friends were the other sources of support for Joan.

After hearing this account of Joan's decline and looking at Joan, who appeared in such a fragile physical condition, her occupational therapist was still unsure of what therapy could do for her. Consequently, the therapist decided to ask the two daughters what they hoped to gain from therapy. Debbie told the therapist that anything that could make her mother more "self-sufficient" and less reliant on her and Anne would be a help.

Continued Data Collection

Once the therapist had a basic understanding of Joan's and her family's situation, she then asked Joan to replicate the course of her day and demonstrate how she actually performed her daily tasks. During her demonstration, the therapist noted her abilities, areas of difficulty and possible obstacles in her physical environment. Special attention was directed to the possessions displayed throughout her home, as these objects revealed further insight into Joan's interests and talents.

While the therapist's data gathering was entirely composed of situated methods, it was guided by the theoretical concepts of the model of human occupation. She took care to reflect upon and plan what data she needed. Moreover, she gathered data from multiple persons and through different methods, so she could feel confidence in the information she was obtaining. This data collection was truly situated since the therapist took advantage of the natural setting of the home and of her growing role as a friend and acquaintance to get an increasingly detailed picture of Joan, her home, and her family.

Course of Therapy

Since the observation of Joan's routine performance had showed that she was severely constrained by limited strength and endurance, the therapist decided to begin therapy with a biomechanical approach, during which time she would have further opportunity to explore Joan's volition and habituation. The therapist spent the initial sessions engaging Joan in exercises to increase strength and endurance. It was soon apparent that these exercises had little meaning to Joan because she never carried them out without the therapist being present, despite the therapist having set up a schedule for her to do them alone as a home exercise program.

During the exercise sessions the therapist continued to informally interview Joan, learning more about her volition and habituation. They talked about Joan's lifestyle in her younger and healthier days. Joan reminisced about how she loved to cook and conjure up new recipes. As they began to talk more and more about cooking, the therapist detected a certain level of enthusiasm and sparkle to Joan.

At this point it became apparent to the occupational therapist that therapy would need to shift focus toward emphasizing Joan's involvement in the occupational forms that had mattered so much to her throughout her life. However, this was not an easy shift to make since Joan did not have the biomechanical capacity to participate. Thus, the therapist decided to continue the biomechanical approach, while using the conversations she had with Joan during the exercises to begin Joan's return to the occupational form of cooking.

While the therapist continued to focus their conversations on cooking, she shifted the conversation so as to highlight what remaining cooking capacity Joan still had: her store of expert knowledge about cooking. The therapist did this by seeking Joan out as her "cooking mentor." Eventually, the therapist suggested that they actually try some activities that would give Joan practice in familiarizing herself with her kitchen again. Joan agreed and came to call these activities getting her "kitchen coordination" back. During these activities Joan's position as an expert was sustained as the therapist continued to learn about cooking from her. When the occupational therapist arrived for the home visits she consistently found that Joan had begun watching cooking shows and would share the latest recipes with the therapist. One day, the therapist arrived to find Joan in the kitchen in the process of making chop suey. Joan hadn't made a sandwich—much less a whole meal—in well over a year! Joan enjoyed preparing the meal but found that it was overtaxing. Thereafter, she became content with assisting her daughters with preparation of dinner, which was more in line with her physical abilities.

After the initial success with the occupational form of cooking, Joan's therapist decided to find another occupational form from Joan's past for which she might have the physical ability. Joan had also shared with the therapist how she had loved to crochet and give her projects away as gifts. Her daughters showed the therapist the beautiful and intricately designed afghans, curtains, towels, doilies, and pot holders that Joan had crocheted. Joan said that she had lost interest in crocheting because it was difficult due to her decreased eyesight and because she had nobody to whom she could give the items anyway. Nonetheless, the therapist encouraged her to try crocheting again, and suggested that if she started doing it she might discover that she still enjoyed it and could do it. Joan's daughters picked up on the therapist's lead; they bought Joan crochet yarn and set it on her table, just in case she wanted to try it. The presence of the crocheting objects in the environment afforded Joan the opportunity she needed. Eventually, Joan tried it and found that she could crochet again—relying more on how it felt rather than on what she saw.

In addition to helping Joan to re-experience the occupational forms that she once enjoyed doing, her therapist developed a second goal: that Joan re-experience her house as a home and not as a modified hospital room. Joan's occupational therapist began to encourage and assist Joan during each therapeutic session to walk to a different room of her home using her walker. Joan's house was arranged so that they could start in the living room that was made into her bedroom, traverse through the kitchen, continue into the dining room (where Art, her husband, was usually reading the paper and would offer some encouraging comments such as, "Soon you'll be running around here."), and wind up back in her chair, where they had started.

The therapist suggested that since Joan was able to maneuver around her house that she should try to get back into the routine of having dinner in the dining room with her family. By incorporating the use of this space back into her daily routine, Joan was able to take a first step forward to restoring some of her previous lifestyle. In addition, by eating in the dining room she would be more clearly in her family member role instead of the sick role.

As she walked and talked with the occupational therapist, Joan was able to reclaim her home and become reacquainted with the rooms and the experiences that transpired within them. Soon, her walking had progressed to the point

that her physical therapist thought she was ready to tackle the biggest physical barrier that faced her—the fourteen steps leading to the upper level of her home. Joan not only had to overcome fatigue, but she had also experienced several panic attacks with the physical therapist during one of the sessions aimed at stair climbing. Joan clearly faced a personal causation hurdle related to walking up the stairs. She was afraid she wouldn't make it up the stairs and would need to be carried down. She had fears that she wouldn't be able to make it down the stairs and would be "stuck" upstairs, which had actually become like a foreign land to her because she hadn't been there for over a year. These fears dominated Joan's personal causation as it pertained to her climbing stairs in the home.

With the encouragement and reassurance of both therapists, bolstered by successes in traversing the first floor of the home, Joan eventually mastered three, then four, then five steps over a course of a few weeks. She gained not only strength, but also an increased knowledge of capacity and sense of efficacy related to stair climbing. The occupational therapist and the physical therapist were both present for Joan's "climb." She eventually met her biggest challenge, climbing one step at a time, and going all the way to the top! The therapists and family praised and congratulated Joan as if she had reached the peak of Mt. Everest!

Once upstairs, however, Joan's thoughts were not on exploring the rooms. They were centered on getting back into the space with which she had come to feel most comfortable. With encouragement she was able to make the descent.

The physical therapist felt that since Joan demonstrated the ability to climb all the steps, that the physical therapy goals were accomplished and thus, decided to discharge her. At this point her occupational therapist also had to consider whether to continue occupational therapy services. While occupational therapy services had contributed to Joan's progress, it was clear that she was not yet as self-sufficient as she and her family wished and that she would benefit from further therapy. The occupational therapist was able to obtain approval from the insurance company to continue with occupational therapy.

During the next phase of treatment, the therapist's goal was to help Joan be more independent once she was upstairs. In order to emphasize that Joan was moving away from the sick role and toward her previous homemaker role, the therapist framed the next activity as "shopping" for appropriate bathroom equipment. Together the therapists and Joan looked through pamphlets and catalogs and even had a demonstration of adapted equipment in her home. Joan was assisted to choose necessary adaptive equipment in a way that took into consideration both her physical needs and her concerns about the aesthetics of her home. The family's criteria for choosing equipment was that it made performing an activity of daily living easier and safer and that the equipment was aesthetically pleasing and not "institutional" looking.

The therapist next began work with Joan to become more of an "insider" in her neighborhood. To encourage her to get outside and to reacquaint her with her community, the therapist took her for a "ride" in her wheelchair to the corner mailbox. Along the way, Joan told the occupational therapist how different the neighborhood looked to her. Joan meant "different" in that she noticed their garage door had been repainted and that the pine trees and shrubs in front of their house had grown very tall. She also noticed other physical changes to neighbors' properties. In the following excerpt from a weekly progress note the therapist describes one of their "outings" in the neighborhood.

Joan expressed desire to "get outside to get a breath of fresh air and feel the sunshine." An apparently "simple activity" but one which the patient has not done in over a year because of her medical condition. Joan was able to climb down the front steps with cues from the occupational therapist and transferred into her wheelchair. Her position in the wheelchair was assessed. The wheelchair was found to be the appropriate size but the leg rests needed to be adjusted. Manipulation and maneuverability of wheelchair was demonstrated to the patient. She expressed her enjoyment in being outside to see the neighbors and to feel the sun, and felt it was very therapeutic for her. Suggestions were made to care givers to use same procedure and to try and assist patient in getting outside on a more regular basis.

While the therapist attended to the biomechanical aspects such as proper positioning during transfers and wheelchair mobility, she did not lose sight of the experience of the activities for Joan. In some of her final sessions, Joan walked with her walker in the garden to look at flowers that were just beginning to bloom and walked in front of the house to greet neighbors she hadn't seen in years.

Conclusion of Services

Occupational therapy services were concluded when the therapist, in collaboration with Joan and her daughters, felt that their initial goals had been achieved. Joan's progress was evidenced by her dressing in housedresses rather than pajamas, spending more time in the kitchen assisting and "supervising" meal preparation, and re-engaging in previous leisure pursuits such as crocheting, watching television, and reading newspapers and magazines. She began to assume more responsibility for her own self-care, started taking a more active role in household decisions, and found it easier to maneuver inside and around her home.

Kim: From Running Away to Joining Life

by Kathi Brenneman Baron

Kim was 16 years old. She was referred for an inpatient psychiatric admission by her social worker, who had been following her for over a year since she threatened suicide by aspirin overdose. When Kim was admitted she reported feeling suicidal again. She had been living nomadically in friends' and relatives' homes. Prior to admission, Kim and some friends with whom she was living were picked up by the police in a stolen car. Kim was placed on a year's probation and ordered to live at home. It was within a few days of being at home with her mother that she was admitted to the unit. Kim was given the medical diagnosis of major depression with a history of substance abuse and conduct disorder. Since Kim had a history of heavy drinking, she was placed on detoxification status.

The unit to which Kim was admitted is a small diagnostic unit in a large university hospital for adolescents and children. The basic philosophy of this unit is that each patient should receive a thorough workup by each team member.

A Brief Life History

In this setting, life history data is gathered by the admitting psychiatrist and social worker and shared with the team. In the team's first discussion of Kim, the following history was shared. Until age seven, Kim grew up in an intact family consisting of her father, mother, and two older brothers. Her father was a severe alcoholic and Kim witnessed several episodes of his constant physical abuse of her mother. When Kim was seven, her father was found in the street in the early morning hours with a severe head injury. Since then, he has been confined to a nursing home, partially paralyzed and cognitively impaired. Kim's only memories of her father were as a heavy-drinking and abusive man. At the time her father was injured, police investigated Kim's mother as a suspect. While no formal charges were brought and her mother had made no public admission, Kim and her brothers speculate that their mother was somehow involved in their father's fate.

In the years that followed her father's abrupt departure from the household, Kim's two brothers moved out of the home. One brother moved to Chicago. The other left to live with his paternal grandmother.

During this time, Kim was showing all the outward signs of being deeply disturbed. Previously a competent student, Kim barely managed to complete the ninth grade and was truant for most of tenth grade. Kim also began to openly discuss with her mother and her friends the possibility of overdosing on aspirin. Kim's mother, who by this time was very depressed herself, was unable to deal with Kim's behavior in any way. The school counselor and a social worker became involved. Legal steps were taken to transfer guardianship to her aunt; however, this never occurred because Kim's condition deteriorated rapidly and she was placed in a foster home. At the same time, Kim reported hearing voices and was seen at a Community Mental Health Center by a psychiatrist who placed her on imipramine. Shortly thereafter, when she no longer experienced the voices, she discontinued the medication and stopped seeing the psychiatrist.

A few months later, after a breakup with her boyfriend, she overdosed on the imipramine. At that time, she was admitted to an intensive care unit at a large public hospital in New York. Thereafter, she bounced from home to home of different relatives and friends. While living with her grandmother, Kim swallowed her grandmother's penicillin tablets in an apparent suicidal gesture. One week later, she presented herself to a hospital emergency room with vaginal bleeding. Kim insists that it was a miscarriage in the third month of pregnancy; however, a pregnancy test proved negative. She was admitted to the hospital then for psychiatric reasons and subsequently referred to a mental health center. There she was scheduled to be seen as an outpatient. Before outpa-

tient therapy could get underway, Kim was arrested for being in a stolen car, leading to her return home and subsequent hospitalization.

Initial Data Gathering

After hearing Kim's history in the team meeting, Kim's occupational therapist was concerned about the disruptiveness and chaos of Kim's life. It was clear that she faced a major challenge in restoring any order to it. The therapist's impression was that Kim's life had taken on the characteristic of a frantic flight. Escape seemed to be the only organizing principle left to her life pattern. Restoration of a new life order would require identification of some new theme which could replace escape.

In deciding how to gather data from Kim, her occupational therapist did not include an interview since other professionals on the unit did extensive interviewing. Kim's therapist chose to give the occupational therapy data gathering and intervention a strong focus on action to balance the strong verbal orientation of the unit.

Her therapist chose a number of data-gathering instruments that Kim could complete on her own and that could serve as the basis for collaboration to achieve an understanding of her situation. The therapist had Kim complete the Belief Survey (Reid & Ware, 1974), which is a paper and pencil instrument that gathers data relevant to a person's sense of efficacy. The therapist also asked her to complete the Role Checklist and the Interest Checklist to gather data on her roles, values, and interests along with an activity configuration (i.e., an informal report of how she typically spent her time during the day) to give information about Kim's habits. The therapist observed Kim during activities to informally screen her for problems in motor, process, and communication and interaction skills. Finally, Kim completed the Self Assessment of Occupational Functioning which provided the therapist information about how Kim saw herself and served as a basis for negotiating goals for therapy.

Because adolescents are prone to enter into struggles with their therapist over issues of control, the occupational therapist approached the data-gathering process with the intention to set up a collaborative atmosphere which could provide Kim a sense of control. Her therapist informed Kim that she wanted to get to know her and that she would need Kim's help to gather some information. She then gave Kim the choice (and the control) to start out by either filling out forms or undertaking a craft project (the latter being the basis for observing Kim's skills). Either of these alternatives were to be done within the occupational therapy workshop. Kim was excited to get involved when she saw other patients active, comfortable, and successful in the workshop. When other patients informed Kim that if she got the forms finished she could go on to do the "fun" things, she was cooperative in completing the data-gathering forms.

When all the data gathering was complete, the therapist met with Kim to review the data from each tool, to give Kim feedback, and to clarify anything for Kim. This process gave the therapist an opportunity to cross-check and add necessary data.

The Belief Survey is a paper and pencil questionnaire which yields three scores related to self-control, control in social situations, and overall control in life. The scores are compared to available norms and can be used to identify tendencies related to personal causation. Kim's scores on the Belief Survey indicated that she tended to feel that she was not in control of herself. The scores also indicated that her sense of efficacy overall and with reference to social situations was limited, although not as extreme as her sense that she could not control herself. Results indicated that while she believed she could make things happen, she did not always believe that she could control herself or outcomes. This conflict between her sense of efficacy and knowledge of capacities appeared to inhibit Kim's successful functioning.

In response to feedback based on this information, Kim indicated that while she believed that she could make things happen in her life, she admitted that self-control was hard for her. Kim was very troubled and ambivalent about this issue of control. She lacked a sense of power to act upon those things within her control, such as pursuing her education and leisure interests. Kim also had difficulty accepting those things which were not in her control. For example, she repeatedly lost control through alcohol and substance abuse and was reluctant to admit it.

On the Interest Checklist (see Figure 14.9) Kim was able to clearly indicate her preferences. Overall, her pattern of interests is one which does not provide significant opportunities for skill development or a sense of competence. When discussing her responses, it also became clear that Kim does not follow through on all her interests, particularly interests such as needlework, cooking, and photography which could provide opportunity for her to develop skills. It also became evident that Kim's interest involvement tended to center on drinking-related leisure pursuits such as music, dancing, singing, and drinking games (e.g., quarters).

Kim's responses on the Role Checklist (see Figure 14.10) show her alienation from ordinary adolescent roles. She had quit school, never wanted to be a care giver, and did not see herself in nor value the family member, religious participant, or hobbyist/amateur roles. When her occupational therapist discussed her responses on the Role Checklist and their apparent meaning, Kim acknowledged that she had a sense of failure around the student role and that she was aware of having withdrawn from other roles as well. Moreover, she related that she didn't have much expectation for the future and, therefore, didn't imagine herself in many roles. The data from this instrument strongly suggested that Kim's life story did not place her in an ordinary continuum of role development. For adolescents, in particular, the ordinary succession of roles provide benchmarks of one's progress and an image of an unfolding future.

Kim's reports of a typical weekday and weekend day (see Figure 14.11) indicated that she lacked a normal routine and instead organized her leisure time around the "habit of drinking." Moreover, it confirmed that she was not pursuing any of her skill-based interests nor did it involve any personal responsibility. By her own admission, her schedule was that of a person headed nowhere. None of her activities had a future orientation. That is, she was not spending any time working toward a future through such activities as studying or learning a skill.

A screening observation of Kim during crafts revealed no problems with motor or process skills. While her communication and interaction skills were observed to be generally good, she did have difficulty with the skills Respects and Asserts. For example, she was sometimes abusive and aggressive toward her peers. She also had difficulty sharing her thoughts and expressing feelings.

Kim's Occupational Status

From the formal data gathering and from discussing the data with Kim, her therapist was able to put together the following appreciation of Kim's occupational behavior. Kim came from an obviously turbulent family background. Her introduction to society via the social institution of the family had left Kim distrustful and dissatisfied. Her experiences had given her no reason to embrace mainstream values. Kim's value orientation reflected an alienation from social groups as demonstrated in her rejection of ordinary roles.

Kim also came from a family in which members were historically unable to control themselves. For example, her father could not control

	Strong Interest	Casual Interest	No Interest		Strong Interest	Casual Interest	No Interest
Camping			✔	Laundry		✔	
Television	✔			Yoga			✔
Writing		✔		Antiques			✔
Traveling	✔			Academics			✔
Pets	✔			Personal Appearance	✔		
Team Sports			✔	Roller Skating		✔	
Clerical			✔	Cycling		✔	
Conversations	✔			Boating	✔		
Clothes	✔			Backgammon			✔
Movies	✔			Politics			✔
Shopping	✔			Water Sports			✔
Walking			✔	Car Repair			✔
Organizations			✔	Swimming	✔		
Languages			✔	Jogging		✔	
Dating	✔			Ping Pong			✔
Business			✔	Bridge			✔
Religion			✔	Painting			✔
Dining		✔		Woodworking			✔
Crafts			✔	Tennis			✔
Art			✔	Cooking	✔		
Solitaire			✔	Bowling			✔
Chess			✔	Dancing	✔		
Picnics		✔		Ceramics			✔
Golf			✔	Reading	✔		
Checkers			✔	Singing	✔		
Home Repairs			✔	Photography		✔	
Skiing		✔		Fishing			✔
Music Listening	✔			Sewing			✔
Puzzles			✔	Sculpting			✔
Needlework	✔			Gardening			✔
Acting			✔	Model Building			✔
Collecting			✔	Weight Lifting			✔
Cleaning			✔	Playing Instrument			✔

Figure 14.9.   Kim's responses on the NPI interest checklist.

Role	Past	Present	Future	Not At All Valuable	Somewhat Valuable	Very Valuable
Student	*Quit*	*Quit*	*Not going back*	X		
Worker	*Quit*	*Looking*	*Full-time*		X	
Volunteer	*Never done it*	*Never done it*	*Never done it*		X	
Care giver	*Babysat*	*No*	*No*			X
Home Maintainer	*Clean house*	*No*	*Yes*		X	
Friend	~~*Go out drinking*~~ *	~~*Go out drinking*~~ *	X			X
Family Member	X				X	
Religious Participant	X			X		
Hobbyist/ Amateur	X			X		
Participant in Organization				X		
Other:		X	X			X

*Kim originally wrote "go out drinking" and then crossed this out.

Figure 14.10.   Kim's responses on the role checklist.

Time Period	Weekday	Weekend
8:00 am – 10:00 am	*Sleep*	*Sleep*
10:00 am – 12:00 pm	*Sleep*	*Go to the beach at 11:00*
12:00 pm – 2:00 pm	*Get up at 1:00*	*Beach*
2:00 pm – 4:00 pm	*Take a shower at 2:30*	*Come home at 3:30*
4:00 pm – 6:00 pm	*Call my boyfriend 5:00*	*Take shower*
6:00 pm – 8:00 pm	*Play quarters* w/friends*	*Play quarters*
8:00 pm – 10:00 pm	*Still playing quarters*	*Play quarters*
10:00 pm – 12:00 am	*11:00 go out to meet boyfriend*	*Play quarters* *12:00 go out to meet boyfriend*

*A drinking game in which an individual bounces a quarter off the table attempting to make it into a glass. When the individual does make it, he/she chooses someone to take a drink. If the individual does not make it he/she must take a drink.

Figure 14.11.   Kim's report of a typical weekday and weekend day.

his drinking or his temper. Not surprisingly, Kim's personal causation was dominated by her belief that she could not control herself. Together Kim's values and personal causation suggested that she has no vision of where she should take her life and no real hope that she could effectively steer her life in a direction if she chose one.

Kim's interests did not reflect opportunities for developing capacity and efficacy and, instead, were related to drugs and alcohol. This interest pattern (and even more so, her interest involvement) was consistent with a life in which capacity does not matter and in which escape and immediate gratification are the guiding principles.

Overall, Kim's volition appeared dominated by a theme that life was out of control, that she was alienated from the values of her environment, and that she did not belong to the ordinary stream of life as represented in a cessation of roles. Instead, Kim was in a state of flight, trying to escape potentially harmful others and painful feelings. Her desperation to escape was reflected in her floating from home to home, in her fleeing into substance abuse, and her flirting with suicide. Kim had been making activity and occupational choices that had taken her away from ordinary roles and activities and toward increasingly self-destructive and socially-problematic behaviors. She had substituted chemical dependency for life satisfaction through performance. Her life had become a downward tumble that culminated in her involvement in an auto theft. As a consequence of her choices, Kim's habituation was marked by an interruption of adolescent life roles and a problematic use of time, centered on drug and alcohol use.

Despite these serious problems, Kim's skill level was generally good. One area of concern was that her communication and interaction skills were limited by her abrasive street behavior and by her difficulty in expressing emotion and thought; however, these problems appeared more related to Kim's exposure to street life than to an innate problem of communication and interaction. Finally, because of her poor choices, she had not had the opportunity to develop her ability to perform in leisure or academic contexts, which would be a basis for success in characteristic adolescent roles. The most important conclusion to be drawn from available data was that Kim was clearly the product of disorganizing environments. Her chaotic family, a succession of temporary "homes," and the "street" had afforded and pressed for the very state of disorganization which Kim exhibited.

Negotiating for Therapy to Enter Kim's Life

The occupational therapist reviewed each evaluation with Kim, giving her feedback on what the therapist perceived as strengths and as problems areas. Then the therapist and Kim examined together the Self Assessment of Occupational Functioning (SAOF) that Kim had completed (see Figure 14.12). Since the SAOF required Kim to reflect on the same issues that her occupational therapist was considering, it enabled them to compare their respective views of her strengths and weaknesses and to negotiate treatment priorities (numbered 1 through 5 on Figure 14.12). They both agreed to focus on the following three goals which were derived from the SAOF:

1. Participating in my interests.
2. Feeling control over what happens to me.
3. Planning before I act.

They discussed the fact that the other things she had noted in the priority column were also important and that the therapist would attempt to facilitate her getting help with those as well. Based on this agreement and on the evaluation data, the occupational therapist planned the following approach to intervention. First, she would try to enhance Kim's knowledge of capacity and sense of efficacy by giving her opportunities to try out various occupational forms in the occupational therapy workshop. The therapist anticipated that Kim would need substantial guidance in how to interpret her performance, since her tendency was not to expect or recognize her own competence. The occupational therapist also planned to assist Kim in being in control of herself and in achieving good outcomes. This would require that she help Kim to plan before she acted and to pause to consider what would be the consequences of her actions. Finally, the therapist wanted to offer Kim opportunities to increase her role functioning as a student, hobbyist, and family member. Overall, she envisioned occupational therapy as helping Kim decide how to join rather than run away from life. Joining life would also require that Kim learn a new habit pattern[b] which would reflect re-involvement in her interests.

---

[b]The Activity Configuration verified that Kim spent huge amounts of time drinking and that alcohol use was a habit. Since the philosophy on this unit was that everyone may make discharge recommendations, Kim's therapist felt obligated to refer Kim for alcohol-related evaluation and treatment.

Area of Occupational Functioning	Strengths	Adequate	Needs Improvement	Priority
I. Personal Causation:				
1. Knowing my abilities.	✔			
2. Expecting success from my efforts rather than failure			✔	4
3. Believing I can make things happen at work, in school, during recreation and/or at home. [*Circle problem areas.*]			✔	2
II. Values:				
4. Doing activities that give me a sense of purpose.			✔	
5. Having future goals.			✔	
6. Having realistic expectations of myself.		✔		
III. Interests:				
7. Identifying my interests.	✔			
8. Having a variety of interests (active/passive, social/solitary). [*Circle problem areas.*]			✔	
9. Participating in my interests.			✔	1
IV. Roles:				
10. Being involved in roles such as student, worker, home maintainer, hobbyist, friend, family member, and/or volunteer.	✔			
11. Knowing and meeting the expectations of of my roles.		✔		
12. Having a healthy balance of roles in my life.			✔	5
V. Habits:				
13. Organizing my time.	✔			
14. Having habits that support success in my roles.			✔	
15. Being flexible about changes in my routine.			✔	
VI. Skills:				
16. Expressing myself to others	✔			
17. Socializing with another person or in a group.		✔		
18. Planning before acting.			✔	3
19. Concentrating and completing my work.			✔	
20. Identifying problems and their solutions, and taking action.	✔			
21. Performing daily living skills (e.g., grooming, cooking, laundry, money management).			✔	
22. Being physically able to do what needs to be done.			✔	
VII. Environment:				
23. Being in supportive environments (e.g., work, school, recreations, or home. [*Circle problem areas.*]			✔	

Figure 14.12. Kim's responses to the self-assessment of occupational functioning (SAOF)—Short Version.

Creating a New Social Environment

Realizing the role which dysfunctional social environments had played in Kim's occupational dysfunction, her occupational therapist planned for therapy to provide a different kind of environmental context to help shape the organization of her behavior in new directions. In taking control away from Kim and in driving her away from the ordinary cultural experiences of school and family life, the old environments had served as the control parameters. Indeed, the home and school environments had threatened and pressed Kim toward her life pattern of escape. The environment of street life had only served to draw Kim further from mainstream society and toward substance abuse and, more recently, criminal activity. Caught up in the cascade of her flight, living for the moment, and headed nowhere in the future, Kim had found no real satisfaction or control in her life. Her solution was escape through suicide. The challenge to therapy was to find a way back into a life which could offer Kim some control, some value, and some enjoyment.

Kim's occupational therapist wanted to create an environment that would afford and press for behavior quite different from that to which Kim had become accustomed. Such an environment would be supportive, yet expect appropriate behavior. It would also press for competent performance while affording Kim opportunity to experience self-control. Additionally, the environment would have to provide models and experiences of a kind of life which could be in control, valuable, and enjoyable. Unless Kim could begin to experience an alternative way of participating in life and receive support and rewards for doing so, she could never successfully put forth all the necessary efforts that change would require.

Recognizing that "de-toxing" from alcohol is a painful process, Kim's therapist also resolved to be appreciative of her struggle. Kim was controlling, nasty, abusive, and street-wise. As she detoxified from alcohol, she became increasingly irritable The occupational therapist was understanding of Kim, provided Kim choices and options, and sought to stay out of control struggles. Since Kim had been chronically robbed of control by her environments and since she was very unsure of her ability to have control, this was an especially sensitive area for her. Moreover, Kim needed to begin to feel that she could be in control. At the same time the environment needed to convey messages about what was proper behavior—i.e., what was valued. Thus, Kim's therapist

set firm limits when appropriate (e.g., when Kim was abusive to her peers).

Social Groups and Occupational Forms of a Therapeutic Environment for Kim

The occupational therapist used groups as the primary treatment method, and attempted to be in tune with the mood and rhythm of the group process. Her introduction of appropriate occupational forms into the group was important. Since occupational forms carry cultural meanings and evoke personal reactions based on each individual's volitional narrative (Helfrich & Kielhofner, 1994; Nelson, 1988) the kinds of occupational forms introduced were very consequential. For Kim, whose occupational forms (e.g., playing quarters) had come to represent escaping and being outside of the mainstream life, it was important to select forms that would draw her in, challenge her to become involved, and provide new pleasures to replace old habits of substance abuse. Knowledge of Kim's volition provided important clues as to how she might react to various occupational forms.

The task group (composed of peer adolescent patients and ordinarily led by the occupational therapist) served as an important social group to afford and press for new occupational behavior. Since the peer group is the most important socializing influence on adolescents, it was natural and most effective to use the group to engage adolescents together in various occupational forms and for a context of productivity, pleasure, and competence.

Since most adolescents in the group struggled with a number of issues which influenced their sense of control, satisfaction, and value in productive action, it was critical to process what went on in the group. The therapist used a variety of means (as we will see) to coax and support adolescents to talk about their experiences, share feelings, support each other, and problem solve together. The therapist also used discussions at times when it seemed necessary to tie together doing, thinking, and feeling, or to relate experiences in therapy to daily function outside.

Course of Occupational Therapy

The following are some highlights of Kim's experiences in occupational therapy. Kim's therapist introduced crafts to Kim since they are occupational forms that pressed for skill building and afforded her opportunity to succeed and build up confidence in her capacities. Kim initially stated that she did not find crafts interesting. However, she quickly came to like their non-threatening quality; she particularly liked being able to learn without "getting graded." Kim also benefitted from doing crafts in a small group with her peers. The activities evoked a sense of calm and "togetherness." The group members often discussed difficult things while working on their projects. Initially, Kim could not share her feelings, but could respond to her peers' feelings.

As Kim became re-involved in activities and developed new interests that could contribute to a more adaptive habit structure, her occupational therapist decided to move Kim toward more effective management of her time in everyday life. She reviewed with Kim the importance of having a balance between time spent in school, leisure, self-care, and rest. Her occupational therapist presented her the "Pie of Life" (a task in which she created a visual representation of how she would like to spend her time by portraying as a pie chart that represented the 24 hours of the day) to help her better grasp the idea of time management and lifestyle balance. While Kim was able to plan for a more adaptive use of time, it was clear that she had no idea about how to actually go about implementing such a schedule.

Her therapist anticipated that it would be very difficult for Kim to change her lifestyle so radically and to not spend her time drinking. Consequently, she felt it would be important for Kim to begin to regularly practice this new schedule and take responsibility for how she used her time. To this end, the occupational therapist shared Kim's Interest Checklist with her nurse, who then helped Kim to make activity choices for what to do in her free time in the evenings and on weekends. Soon, Kim began to use her occupational therapy sessions to choose activities and to prepare supplies which she would utilize in her free time. She was eventually more comfortable being responsible for, and involved in, her own interests. Her new habits were becoming more natural and familiar to her.

In the craft group, the therapist noticed that Kim was consistently seeking out projects far below her own skill level. When the occupational therapist shared this observation, Kim protested that she did not perceive herself as being able to do more difficult projects. The therapist began to give Kim consistent feedback about her skill level and to encourage her to choose tasks slightly more difficult than the ones she ordinarily selected. At first Kim refused, so the therapist decided to focus on the process of having fun by trying something new. The occupational therapist reasoned that if Kim could be persuaded to try out something new for the fun of it, she might discover that she could do and, in fact, enjoy tasks more closely related to her skill level. The therapist utilized a group session to engage participants to do a craft that was not familiar, one *none* of the group members had tried. Throughout the activity participants were asked to write down how they felt about doing something new and then group members discussed what they wrote. Prior to starting the task, Kim wrote "this is dumb and it's too hard for me." Her peers gave her feedback that she would probably do well, based on what they had seen her do in the past. Halfway through the activity, Kim wrote "fun." Upon completion of the craft, Kim was feeling more comfortable and wrote down "fine." Over time, new activities became easier for her and Kim gradually progressed to higher level projects that challenged her skills.

At this point, the occupational therapist assessed that she had a good rapport with Kim. This was necessary in order to begin tackling the alienation reflected in Kim's values and roles. Since this would be a sensitive issue, the therapist felt that it would be best for Kim to have some privacy. Consequently, a one-to-one session was arranged with Kim. With some support, Kim admitted that she did see some value and importance to school; however, she reported feeling very insecure about being able to return successfully to it. It became clear that rejection of the student role allowed Kim to protect herself from the fear of failing in that role. Kim's therapist gave her feedback about her high level of skills and assured her that these would support her success in school. Kim then shared that her home life interfered with her ability to go to school. At this point, Kim blurted out that she drank because she felt depressed and she did not have support at home to overcome the depression. It became apparent to both Kim and the occupational therapist that, in order to stop drinking and go to school, she would need a lot of support, which she was not getting at home. After more discussion, Kim was able to say that she would like to be able to go to school if she felt she had some way to succeed. The therapist told Kim that she would like to share their talk with the team, so they could discuss how best to help her. Kim agreed. The next day at morning rounds, the occupational therapist reported on her meeting with Kim. The therapist strongly recommended that Kim be referred to a residential alcohol treatment program for adolescents that could provide both support for her drinking problem and help her to be able to succeed at school. The treatment team decided to find this type of program to which she could be discharged.

As Kim continued to attend craft workshop sessions in occupational therapy, the group members, including Kim, were becoming increasingly supportive of and open with each other. The therapist decided to foster and capitalize upon their cohesiveness by facilitating a discussion on each person's goals. The group members were each given their SAOF forms and asked to choose two goals that they were working on and that they felt comfortable sharing with the group. Group members, after hearing each other's goals, identified how they could support each other in reaching them. Kim was very disruptive throughout this session and in the week to follow. Kim's behavior suggested that it was still very hard for her to choose a direction for herself and feel hope that things would turn out as she wanted them to. She seemed to be struggling with imagining a positive future and choosing goals for herself. These feelings were intensified by her knowledge that she was being referred to an adolescent alcohol treatment center.

Around the same time, many members of the unit were being discharged. Kim was having such difficulty separating from them that the occupational therapist planned a "goodbye book" activity in which each member was to write a page to each of the others, wishing them well, telling them something inspirational or something they wanted them to remember. Each member collected the pages they received into a book. After this activity, Kim was much calmer and seemed to adjust to the discharge of several peers.

A few days prior to Kim's discharge, the occupational therapist met with Kim to review her progress. Both agreed that Kim had experienced an improved sense of her ability to control herself, which enhanced her confidence that she could be effective. Kim had also increased her involvement and enjoyment in interests. She had become aware of how her new habits were affecting the quality of her life. Kim acknowledged that she had a new appreciation for the importance of the student role to her life.

Before Kim's discharge, the therapist made a number of recommendations to Kim. First, she suggested Kim continue to practice lifestyle balance and engage in a regular routine by using the "Pie of Life" activity. Second, she encouraged Kim to become involved in interests as a source of gratification and to refer to the Interest Checklist she completed for ideas. Third, she recommended that Kim seek out the support of the teacher in the alcohol treatment center in order to begin to successfully function in the role of the student.

Kim seemed proud of her achievements and thanked the occupational therapist. She expressed feeling scared to go, but ready. Kim was discharged to an alcohol treatment center for adolescents. She continued to call the hospital occasionally to report on her good grades and sobriety.

Mike: Making a Successful Occupational Choice for Transition to the Worker Role
by Lucy Swan Sullivan

Mike was admitted to an inpatient unit for persons with affective disorders. Mike was 26 years old and had a history of rapid-cycling affective disorder. His first episode of mood disregulation was at age 17 when he had several days of increased energy, decreased need for sleep, and increased sociability. In college, he experienced more of these episodes which, he noted retrospectively, were periods when he had spending sprees.

Mike's first episode of depression was at age 19, at which time he sought treatment and began medication. His episodes of depression had recurred since then with a distinct pattern emerging over the past two to three years. Typically, he was depressed for 10 days to two weeks, followed by two to three weeks of euthymia, after which the cycle began again. Just before his depression, he experienced a manic episode that lasted about a day. Mike's depressive symptoms were characterized by increased irritability, mild aphasia, and an almost catatonic appearance. His family members reported having to encourage him to eat or drink. He also experienced episodes of anxiety and panic attacks. He had panic attacks while on buses and while driving.

This was Mike's first inpatient hospitalization. His current medications controlled his manic episodes, but he still experienced recurring depressions. He did not feel that he recovered to a normal state even when he was relatively euthymic.

In addition to his psychiatric problems, Mike also had some mild motor problems. At one point, he was diagnosed as having cerebral palsy. He had slightly increased tone in his legs and mild spasticity in both hands.

He was an average child in school but reported some adjustment problems because he was teased for being quiet, not well coordinated, and a dreamer. In the third grade, he was referred to a school counselor because of hyperirritability and sensitivity to rejection. His lack of coordination caused difficulty with sports, but he was active in the Boy Scouts and achieved the rank of Eagle Scout.

Mike still lived with his parents in a major metropolitan city. His younger sister was married and no longer lived at home. He was a graduate of a leading fine arts school. Before hospitalization, Mike worked part-time as an usher in a movie theater and as the lead guitarist in a band.

Mike's occupational therapist began data collection with the following questions in mind. Since Mike had had some life-long skill deficits and more recent psychiatric symptoms that interfered with his functioning, she wondered about his sense of efficacy in particular. His education and employment suggested an interest in art and music and she wanted to know more about his overall interest pattern. Since Mike was single, unemployed, and still living at home, he appeared to have few roles. His therapist wondered both about his current role identification and his plans for future roles. Also, since Mike was still at home and not associated with either a work or other occupational behavior setting, she wanted to know what opportunities for occupational behavior his current environment afforded. With these questions in mind she initially chose to administer the Occupational Case Analysis and Rating Scale (OCAIRS), the Role Checklist, and the Interest Checklist.

Difficulty with Role Transitions

The OCAIRS gave Mike's occupational therapist a great deal of information concerning his occupational dysfunction. The therapist's ratings and comments from the first part of the OCAIRS Interview and Rating Scale summary form are shown in Figure 14.13. As this section from the form shows, Mike generally had positive volition that reflected an orientation toward artistic and expressive performance.

In his volitional life story, Mike portrayed himself as overcoming some significant liabilities and as having achieved something significant in his education. However, his narrative had an uncertain future. He is not able to formulate a motivating view of the future. Instead, his story had faded into an ambiguous and uncertain present.

This lack of a future story was also apparent in Mike's role identification. The student role still stood out as his last major role accomplishment. His two past jobs were not a source of strong work role identification and he did not have any distinct ideas about occupying the worker role in the future. This is not because Mike did not want to work, but because he was unable to imagine and believe in a work role for himself given his illness. Entering the work role appeared as a vague eventuality.

Figure 14.13. Ratings* and comments for Mike on the first part of the occupational case analysis interview and rating scale summary form.

Personal Causation	4	Feels a sense of efficacy in his ability to graduate from an exclusive college despite his liabilities. Believes he has musical and artistic capacities.
Values and Goals	4	Values creativity, but has no clear goals or future plans.
Interests	5	Interests are expressive/creative: he plays guitar, writes poetry, reads, sings, and does artwork.
Roles	2	Currently sees himself as a patient. Does not identify strongly with the worker role in past or future.
Habits	4	Does seem to fill his time with his hobbies/interests. When depressed has problems keeping up a routine.
Skills	4	Feels he has adequate process and communication/interaction

*5 = Adaptive through 1 = Maladaptive

Mike's responses on the Role Checklist (see Figure 14.14) supported the information from the interview. With the exception of the hobbyist/amateur role, all his present roles were interrupted. Other than the friend role, his most valued role was work. This illustrated that Mike had internalized the societal value of work and underscored the importance of his being able to include work in a life story for the future.

Mike's responses on the Interest Checklist also supported the picture that emerged in the interview. Of ten strong interests that had been consistent for Mike, eight (concerts, painting/drawing, photography, attending plays, movies, popular music, radio, and television) were related to his artistic/expressive orientation. One new strong interest, singing, was similarly related. Mike's two other strong interests, walking and swimming, represented his desire to be physically fit.

Finally, Mike's scores on the Belief Survey (Reid & Ware, 1974) were as follows. The first score suggested that Mike had a good belief in self-control. The second score reflected his ability to influence outcomes in social situations; Mike's score suggested he had less than average confidence in this area. The third score pertained to his general beliefs about being able to influence overall outcomes in his life. This score suggested that he tended to be more fatalistic and to lack confidence that he could direct his life course. This finding was consistent with what his occupational therapist learned about his volitional life story.

Overall, the data gathered by his occupational therapist provided the following picture. Mike overcame mild cerebral palsy and gradually intensifying mood fluctuations to graduate from a top art school. He had built his identity within his family, academia, Boy Scouts, and his band. He was at a difficult developmental transition from the role of student to that of independent adult worker. In addition, he had to incorporate a realistic expectation and understanding of his bipolar disorder. He lacked a well-developed plan for ca-

Role	Past	Present	Future	Not At All Valuable	Somewhat Valuable	Very Valuable
Student	X				X	
Worker	X		X			X
Volunteer	X				X	
Care giver				X		
Home Maintainer				X		
Friend	X		X			X
Family Member					X	
Religious Participant	X		X		X	
Hobbyist/ Amateur	X	X	X		X	
Participant in Organization						
Other:						

Figure 14.14. Mike's responses on the role checklist.

reer development in an art field where entry-level steps were not clearly defined. Nonetheless, he had coherent values and interests and a generally positive sense of efficacy.

From the data she gathered, the therapist drew the inference that Mike's major difficulty was in making a developmental transition from the student to worker role marked by inability to make an occupational choice. While he had some basic volitional strengths (i.e., he had a consistent volitional world view in which his personal causation, values, and interests converged on artistic and expressive occupation), he was unable to create a volitional narrative which would take him into the future as a worker. Therefore, he was unable to make the occupational choice for a worker role. Added to this difficulty, his work role experience was limited and his work role identification was tenuous.

Gathering Data on Skills

In his interview, Mike made reference to his long-term motor problems and also talked about how his bipolar disorder had interfered with his concentration and problem solving. Mike had trained for a job requiring intense, sustained levels of concentration. Due to his illness, he had felt he could no longer attain the necessary level of concentration, which required a fundamental change in vocational goals. Because of his perceived motor, concentration, and problem solving difficulties, the occupational therapist decided to administer the Assessment of Motor and Process Skills (AMPS) to more objectively gather data on his underlying motor and process skills. This data would allow the therapist to determine what the possible deficits would mean in terms of everyday functional tasks. He was observed doing three tasks he would routinely accomplish at home, making toast, brewing coffee, and changing sheets on a bed.

These observations revealed that, despite his history of mild motor problems, his motor skills were adequate. His process skills were also adequate overall. He was, however, deficient in four process areas; noticing, choosing, sequencing, and heeding. Notices is a skill of adaptation, defined as responding appropriately to nonverbal environmental/perceptual cues. In the category of using knowledge, Chooses refers to being able to select appropriate and prespecified tools, and heeding refers to using goal-directed task performance towards the completion of a task. Finally, in the area of temporal organization, Sequences

refers to being able to perform steps in an effective and logical order.

Mike's occupational therapist took careful note of these problems. She and Mike discussed his difficulty adapting his behavior and adjusting the environment when problems arose. The AMPS results gave further definition to Mike's account of concentration and problem solving difficulties. Additionally, the therapist raised questions about whether and how Mike's fluctuations in mood and his anxiety level influenced his process skills. Mike and the occupational therapist agreed to use future therapy sessions to investigate these questions in many different settings and within tasks that pressed for different levels of performance.

Socially, Mike had an idiosyncratic appearance. He always wore a hat, and his clothing was representative of his music group, not the casual attire of his peers. Moreover, when he first came to the unit he was withdrawn and uncomfortable in social situations. For purposes of establishing whether Mike had specific communication and interaction skill problems, the therapist used the Assessment of Communication and Interaction Skills (ACIS). Results (see Figure 14.15) showed Mike's had ineffective performance in all areas except that of informational exchange, where his performance was in the questionable range. Mike made little eye contact, used odd gestures, and assumed unusual postures. He spoke in clipped sentences with descriptive vocabulary, but without modulating effectively. Initially, he did not engage or relate to others.

The occupational therapist discussed her observations of his communication and interaction skills with Mike. She raised the question about how much of his observed deficiencies were related to a lack of capacity and how much they reflected volitional and habituation influences as well as influences of Mike's mood state and current hospital environment. As discussed in Chapter 6, volition, habituation, mood states, and environment all influence the assembly of skilled performance. There was reason to suspect that some of Mike's communication and interaction difficulties were related to these factors. Mike agreed that his decreased motivation, his unfamiliarity with the patient role, and the strangeness of the hospital environment left him feeling especially uneasy and unsure of how to behave. He also recognized that his communication and interaction was not always effective and agreed that, in the context of his major treatment goals, he would work on these skill areas and receive feedback from his occupational therapist who

Figure 14.15.   Mike's scores* and comments on the assessment of communication/interaction skills.

PHYSICALITY					
Gestures	1	②	3	4	Uses odd gestures
Gazes	1	②	3	4	Minimal eye contact
Approximates	1	2	③	4	Physically withdrawn
Postures	1	②	3	4	Assumes unusual postures
Contacts	1	2	3	④	
LANGUAGE					
Articulates	1	②	3	4	Mumbles/speaks indistinctly
Speaks	1	2	③	4	Truncates phrases and sentences
Focuses	1	2	③	4	Expresses tangential conversation and incomplete ideas
Emanates	1	2	③	4	Speaks in chopped sentences
Modulates	1	2	③	4	Speaks too softly and in monotone
RELATIONS					
Engages	1	②	3	4	Did not initiate interaction
Relates	1	②	3	4	Is not responsive to others
Respects	1	2	③	4	Seems unaware of others
Collaborates	1	2	③	4	Unsure of how to work with others
INFORMATION EXCHANGE					
Asks	1	2	③	4	Hesitant to make requests
Expresses	1	2	③	4	Affect is mainly flat
Shares	1	2	③	4	Hesitant to share information about self
Asserts	1	2	③	4	Mainly passive behavior

* 4 = Competent   3 = Questionable   2 = Ineffective   1 = Deficit

would monitor his communication and interaction performance.

Planning Intervention

Mike's occupational therapist further shared with him the understanding of his circumstances that she had constructed from the data gathering. She emphasized what she saw as his strengths and problem areas. Mike agreed with the therapist's appraisal of him and together they arrived at three primary goals; they also identified means that they would use in occupational therapy to address these goals. Each of the goals and the therapeutic strategies that were planned to sup-

port them are discussed below. It should be noted that Mike's hospitalization was in a facility that had longer lengths of stay than most acute care psychiatric facilities. Because it was anticipated that his stay would be more extended, it was both possible and necessary to develop a detailed and long-range intervention plan.

Goal One: Enhance Mike's Occupational Choice Process as it Pertains to Work

Since Mike needed to make a major occupational choice for entry into work and since the data gathering had identified volitional factors which had contributed to difficulty in making an occupational choice (i.e., his lack of a future story and goals related to work, his sense of inefficacy in being able to control outcomes related to work) the first goal was to promote his occupational choice process.

One strategy related to this goal was to help Mike explore vocational options through involvement in a work therapy program, supplemented by discussions with his occupational therapist. It was anticipated that involvement in the program would give him concrete experience which the therapist could use in discussion to help him formulate ideas about future work options. In addition, the occupational therapist referred Mike to a vocational rehabilitation counselor who could provide vocational testing and feedback to him. She expected this would also assist him with information about his own interests and aptitudes, which were important to the occupational choice process.

A second strategy related to this goal was to provide Mike with readings through which he could explore career options and increase his knowledge about specific careers. Mike liked to read and the therapist felt this would be a means both of structuring time for Mike and allowing him to gather and reflect on information in a way that was comfortable and enjoyable for him.

A third strategy was aimed at increasing Mike's confidence in his skills and his potential efficacy in finding a worker role. Mike was enrolled in an occupational therapy computer training program. In this program he learned computer applications in art. He learned how to use the computer to do a job search and to develop a resumé and letters of introduction for job seeking. The therapist anticipated, along with Mike, that once mastered, these skills specific to obtaining work would not only be useful to him but would also increase his confidence in the process of finding work.

Goal Two: Support Mike's Functioning in the Worker, Hobbyist, Friend, and Home Maintainer Roles

While the worker role was a main emphasis of Mike's therapeutic program, both the occupational therapist and he recognized that his transition into adulthood would require that he have a full complement of roles to sustain a satisfying and productive lifestyle. The hobbyist role was Mike's only continuous role and his occupational therapist wanted to support and build on this strength. The friend role was interrupted and yet it was one of only two roles which Mike identified

as very important; therefore, this role also needed to be supported. Mike was living at home, but wanted to live independently when financial circumstances permitted, so they agreed on the goal of supporting his occupational function towards assuming the home maintainer role. Finally, it was important that Mike began to have experiences in a work role that would allow him to internalize a strong work role identification.

The first strategy for supporting these goals was to provide Mike opportunities to enter the work role as a volunteer in the work therapy program and to experience work in the computer training program. This strategy overlapped with the previous goal of enhancing his occupational choice process. The therapist reasoned that it would be easier for Mike to envision himself in a particular work role in the future if he had present experience to draw upon.

The second strategy was to support Mike's hobbyist role and his interests in art, music, and biking during the natural leisure time that occurred on the ward. The occupational therapist and Mike planned to work together to make sure Mike had both the resources and planning made for free time to pursue his hobbies. In particular, since Mike was undergoing a longer term hospitalization, it was important to have the hobbyist role to structure and fill his leisure time.

The third strategy was to support Mike's friend role by providing him with opportunities to be involved in group activities, community meals, and informal interactions in work therapy. Finally, his home maintainer role was supported by providing him opportunity and responsibility to maintain common areas of the hospital unit.

Goal Three: Help Formulate a Discharge Plan for Transition from the Hospital to Living Independently and Getting a Job

As previously noted, Mike was living at home. Since Mike was unemployed, his family provided necessary resources and financial support. However, living at home was a source of conflict and anxiety for him. The occupational therapist and Mike agreed to work together to help him identify interim strategies for functioning optimally in the home environment. Part of this was to help the family better understand the nature of Mike's disorder.

At the same time, it was important to plan for the time when Mike would make the transition to an independent home maintainer role. Mike's home maintainer responsibilities at home were very limited. He was over-reliant on his mother for maintenance of his own personal space and he made few contributions to maintenance of the overall household. Consequently, the strategy was to help Mike negotiate for a more active involvement in home maintenance tasks upon discharge. This would allow him to continue to practice the relevant habits he was acquiring during his hospitalization.

Mike also needed to understand how his disorder would affect his daily function after discharge. In particular, he needed to understand how his symptoms of mood fluctuation and anxiety would require accommodations in his behavior to successfully accomplish necessary tasks. New habits for the home maintainer role were also required to support his future long-range plan for independent living. Here again, the therapy groups involved tasks such as grocery shopping, meal planning, preparation, and clean up. Additionally, common areas of the unit, including the kitchen, dining, and living areas, were maintained by the patient group. As a member of the group, Mike had opportunity to develop habits relevant to the home maintainer role.

Course of Intervention

Mike quickly established a routine on the unit by carefully scheduling his time to meet all unit and treatment obligations on a clipboard which he carried with him. In his blocks of free time, he scheduled time to pursue his avocational interests. Being physically fit was important for Mike. He was able to borrow a bicycle from the recreation department for riding and to use a pass to swim at a nearby gym 3–5 times per week. He practiced his guitar daily, resourcefully seeking out various places where he could practice without disturbing hospital routines. He also took time for his drawing and completed a series of sketches of fellow patients and the surrounding buildings. His hard work and abilities were recognized both by staff and by his peers. Over the course of his hospitalization, Mike's social status changed dramatically. He moved from being viewed as quiet, anxious, and socially awkward, to being accepted by both the group and staff as a leader.

In the course of his therapy, Mike participated in four occupational therapy groups that varied in demands and complexity. Mike began in a unit-based group, the planning/living group. In this group, Mike and other patients shared responsibility for the unit living environment, as mentioned previously, and planned a bimonthly community lunch. The hospital environment often makes patients feel they have lost control over their lives. To counteract this, the group and the community meal emphasizes opportunities to control and to have responsibility for outcomes in activities that represent social and task demands of everyday life. Mike, in particular, used these activities to learn new home maintainer habits and to look at how his symptoms of mood fluctuation and anxiety would affect both his communication and interaction skills and his process skills during these tasks. When depressed, Mike was typically more irritable, and he found the press of social groups to be close to intolerable. During these times, he learned how to exercise the most basic communication and interaction skills that allowed him to be effective in a social context. He also learned his limits and what kinds of social encounters he should try to avoid. When Mike was euthymic, he tended to be much more socially facile, but his expectations of others were very high and he had to learn how to effectively relate and assert his views without appearing disrespectful or aggressive.

When euthymic, Mike was also methodical and detailed. For example, he followed recipes to the letter. Alternatively, when he became anxious, his process skills became less organized and he was less aware of details. However, his behavior was always in the functional range; he never made any errors that threatened his own or others' safety. More typically, he would make small errors of judgement such as emptying the contents of a mix into a bowl and beginning to add other ingredients, and only then to consider consulting the directions. Mike and his occupational therapist worked together to set up coping strategies to compensate for his fluctuations in mood and for his anxiety. He worked on such strategies such as keeping expectations of self and others reasonable and remembering to follow the recipe each time.

Mike's communication and interaction skill deficits gradually seemed to dissipate with the structured role expectations of community meals and groups. During meals, he initiated interaction with group members, related well, and appeared to enjoy himself. He respected others and displayed a dry sense of humor that engaged both staff and patients.

Mike also participated in an off-unit weekly workshop group, which focused on group projects, psychoeducational topics related to coping strategies, work therapy, and discharge planning. His participation in this group was noteworthy.

Mike never missed a session, even when he was depressed to the level of partial catatonia. He liked this group because the environmental press resembled that of the academic setting in which he had previously been successful. Mike actively participated in discussions, frequently making thought-provoking comments interspersed with humor. He independently sought out further resources on discussion topics, and brought what he learned from reading into subsequent discussions. He again demonstrated communication and interaction skills and role behaviors which made him a valued member of the group.

Mike progressed to being able to use the group to learn and internalize more appropriate role scripts. For example, in one task, Mike agreed to design a cover for a cookbook project. His cover showed patients in chains and straightjackets as chefs. His occupational therapist and some coworkers gave Mike feedback that they expected him to consider others' feelings and reactions to such a cover. This informed Mike about his role and responsibility and about the implications of his cover. Mike was able to accept the feedback; he negotiated for and created a more universally acceptable cover.

Mike began meeting regularly with the vocational counselor. With her direction, he began reading and completing the exercises in the book, *What Color is Your Parachute?*, which helped him clarify his own desires and needs. Many of the sessions in the occupational therapy workshop group covered related topics, which gave him further opportunity to discuss the information which he related to himself, used to compare himself to others, and considered the functional implications of his disorder. All of these reflective activities allowed Mike to activate his volitional process interpreting his past experiences and beginning to envision a future for himself.

Once well established in his workshop and community groups, Mike began participating in a computer skills groups. He set goals which increased his computer literacy and he learned specific applications in art. Again, the therapist was struck by his competence. He could concentrate and tolerate frustration well. His approach to a task was confident and exploratory rather than anxious or self-deprecatory. He identified and accomplished the treatment goals established with the therapist. He independently used other resources on the campus for computer learning. He researched computer applications that would increase his marketability and, with help from the occupational therapist, networked to find additional computer programs to learn. The vocational counselor helped Mike by identifying further resources, including a videotaped lecture by a nationally renowned artist who has used computer programs to illustrate scientific principles.

The occupational form of working on computers turned out to be very significant for Mike because it was the least affected by his fluctuations in mood and his anxiety. During pronounced mood swings and anxiety states, Mike did not experience some of the process skills problems he had in other occupational forms. The occupational form of computer art allowed him to combine his quest for knowledge and skills, while expanding his creativity in writing, producing art, and expressing humor. Mike was energized by his accomplishments and autonomy. The occupational therapist speculated with Mike that perhaps computer tasks provided immunity to the fluctuations of mood and anxiety because they did not present interpersonal demands and they afforded structure. His clear success with the computer as a tool for expression led him towards narrowing his vocational options to the computer graphics field. Mike was encouraged to make visits to a nearby medical arts department to observe applications in design, computer graphics, video, and photography. Afterwards, he used the computer to compose and send thank you letters to staff in the medical arts department, again practicing important work role behaviors. He completed a number of projects which demonstrated his mastery of several computer programs. For example, he created illustrated recipe files for the unit and made a self-portrait.

In Mike's final phase of therapy he took on the volunteer role. Mike volunteered six hours per week in a biomechanics lab, which was part of the hospital. This experience helped to integrate much of what he had learned about himself and his illness and helped him to feel more comfortable about the future possibility of work. In this work therapy, Mike had the opportunity to simultaneously develop new role scripts for work, to take on technical illustration tasks that developed his computer skills, and to further explore his emerging occupational choice for work in computer graphics. Mike used his computer training sessions to support his performance in the tasks assigned to him for his volunteer work. He worked with the therapist, for instance, to learn new computer programs with which he could produce complex charts illustrating systems principles in biomechanics. As another example, Mike had to do an interview in the biomechanics lab prior to being accepted as a volunteer. This interview was similar to a job interview, and Mike anticipated the press of the interview would increase his anxiety and decrease his performance. Therefore, Mike and the occupational therapist role-played the interview beforehand to practice proper responses, questions, and most importantly, to identify some issues he would need to consider in future job interviews. He was able to begin exploring some difficult issues such as disclosure of his illness and requests for reasonable accommodation to which he was entitled under the law.

He managed the interview despite some anxiety. He agreed to begin his assignment and set up goals for the experience with the supervisor. Mike, his occupational therapist, and the treatment team used this experience as an indication of discharge readiness. He was no longer in the sheltered environment of the unit. He experienced some difficulties, but with the support of the therapist, and through discussions with his peers in the group, he was able to learn to develop more appropriate work role scripts, internalizing both what others expected of him and what he could expect of others in the worker role. For example, he felt that a task the biomechanical staff asked him to do was inappropriate. Rather than explain his reservations, he simply ignored the request. He discussed this situation with the occupational therapist. He explained that he had ignored the request because he felt misunderstood and undervalued as an artist. He agreed to discuss the incident further in the group. Feedback from his peers and the therapist helped him reframe his experience. He recognized that in a worker role not all tasks will be equally creative and satisfying and that the role required him to take on a variety of assignments. This and other instances helped Mike to internalize a more appropriate work role script. Mike came to recognize how negotiating mutually acceptable, realistic tasks is part of an ongoing process of communication between employer/supervisor and worker/volunteer that ultimately defines the role. Mike continued to volunteer in the biomechanics lab, successfully negotiating task assignments to meet mutually established goals of applying knowledge and skills to tasks that supported the lab's efforts.

Periodically, topics on appropriate role-related interactions were presented in the workshop group. This gave Mike additional information from peers and staff to apply to role behaviors. Mike also went further on his own, independently pursuing recommended readings. For instance, he found the latest materials on gender differences in communication helpful towards enhancing his interpersonal skills. He researched information on musical performers and thought carefully about whether music would be an avocation or a vocation for him. On one home visit he then planned a nightclub engagement with his band. He found that this was more stressful and less satisfying than his computer work; the experience and his subsequent interpretation of it helped him to rule out music as an occupational choice.

Discharge Planning

Before discharge, Mike returned to his home for short visits and he went into the community to look for employment and possibly housing. In the short term, Mike decided to stay with his family, but his goal was to live independently once he was able to find a job. He met regularly with the vocational counselor to investigate the job market, complete his resumé, write cover letters, begin a portfolio of his artwork, and plan his job search. He applied to the Vocational Rehabilitation Department in his state to qualify for county services. He made plans to continue his education in computer applications by taking a course at a community college.

Just as Mike had to redefine his identity in terms of his bipolar disorder, so his family needed to understand Mike in a new way. His family had had many difficult experiences of dealing with Mike's manias and periods of depression. They were not entirely ready to see Mike in the adult role he needed to assume. Again, the therapist recommended readings on effective communication and helped Mike anticipate his family's reaction, to practice sharing his needs, and effectively asserting himself. His goal was to be able to avoid the pitfall of becoming defensive or angry. He role-played listening skills to help him counter his tendency, when anxious, to miss key details of interactions. He gathered good informational resources for his family to read about bipolar disorder, and scheduled time for his parents to meet and talk further with the treatment team in order for them to learn more about his condition and his progress.

The occupational therapy termination process included reviewing with Mike his strengths and successes and helping him identify support systems to assist him make the transition to the work role and independent living while incorporating accommodations to his bipolar disorder. Also, as part of this termination, Mike and his therapist reviewed how his life story was unfolding. It was clear to both of them that Mike had now developed a future scenario for himself. He could imagine himself going into a line of work involving computer applications of art. He had experience with the technical skills and the actual job demands of such work so that he could realistically imagine what was involved. He now identified closely with this role, expected that it was achievable, and had internalized appropriate role scripts that would serve him well upon entering such a job.

Nathan: Finding the Good Inside
by Kim Bryze

Nathan was seven years, four months old and attended a regular second grade in a middle-class suburb. One day Nathan came home from school with a troubled look on his face. When his mother asked him about his day, Nathan had said, "Mom, something's wrong with me." She originally inquired about physical symptoms ("Does your stomach hurt?", "Do you have a headache?"), to which he emphatically responded, "No, Mom, something is *wrong* with me! I am not like the other kids. And I am afraid."

His mother encouraged Nathan to tell her about his fear. Nathan explained that group activities and physical games at school were intimidating for him. He worried about these events before they happened. He felt terrified while he was involved in them. And, afterwards, he always felt like a failure. Over time these experiences led him to conclude that there must be something very wrong with him. Added to this, Nathan felt increasingly isolated and "different" from the other children. He was lonely and pained by the idea that he did not belong with the others in school. Nathan's mother recognized the distress he was experiencing and, at first, offered the only help she could imagine in the form of advice to Nathan. She suggested that he try harder and that he "be a friend to make a friend." These suggestions were met with tears and great frustration by Nathan.

Nathan's mother decided to pursue the problem further and requested a conference with his teacher. In conversation with the teacher his mother learned that, indeed, Nathan was having difficulty in group situations, such as in gym, recess, lunch, and during small group experiences in the classroom. On the other hand, Nathan was usually able to keep up with schoolwork that was to be completed individually, although his handwriting was less than what would be expected in early second grade.

Armed with both Nathan's and the teacher's accounts, Nathan's mother took it upon herself to learn more about the kind of problem he was experiencing and what kind of resources might be of help to him. She sought out information from her pediatrician and from friends who were also mothers of schoolchildren. One of these friends was employed as an occupational therapist working with adult patients. The friend recommended that Nathan be evaluated by an experienced pediatric occupational therapist. Nathan's mother subsequently referred him to an outpatient pediatric occupational therapy clinic that specialized in interventions with children who had problems similar to Nathan's. Although she voiced questions about Nathan's ability to keep up with other children his age in school and play, she emphasized that her primary concerns were Nathan's lack of confidence and his view that something was wrong with him.

Initial Data Gathering

Nathan came to his first occupational therapy session accompanied by his mother. He was initially shy and quiet, but was able to respond to the therapist's suggestion that he walk around and explore the toys and equipment. As Nathan explored, the therapist discussed with his mother her thoughts and concerns about Nathan. The information shared by Nathan's mother led the therapist to suspect that Nathan had sensory processing deficits which may have been contributing to his problems with physical and interactive situations in his daily life. Such problems are recognized and addressed from sensory integration, another conceptual practice model (Fisher, Murray, & Bundy, 1991). The therapist asked Nathan's mother to complete a sensory integration-based developmental/sensory history form while she began to directly observe Nathan. Information from this form provided qualitative information regarding Nathan's ability to perform developmental and sensory activities and supplemented what his therapist subsequently observed in the occupational therapy environment.

The therapist performed an observation that consisted of inviting and asking Nathan to seek out sensory information and perform various motor tasks. She conducted this observation from the dual perspectives offered by the sensory integration and human occupation models. Thus, she simultaneously was guided by questions concerning Nathan's responses to sensory information, his ability to perform motor tasks, and his volitional process. With regard to the latter, she sought to understand how Nathan anticipated, experienced, and interpreted sensory and motor events. She wanted to know what he enjoyed and disliked, how he felt about his own abilities and performance, and what was important to him. She knew from the mother's report that Nathan had a negative view of his capacities and she expected that the observation would provide more information about the dynamics of how he acted and reacted in situations that called for motor skills.

Nathan was compliant, although quiet, during the data-gathering session. He did not look directly at the therapist, except when she asked him to perform movements that involved his face and mouth. He attempted all tasks that the therapist presented to him but his efforts were fleeting when he was asked to do something that he perceived as difficult. He was quick to say "I can't" before he even attempted certain motor tasks. He was impulsive in his approach to doing visual-motor tasks that therapist requested, appearing to want to get them over with as quickly as possible. However, he appeared to respond positively to encouragement and praise during the testing. By the end of the evaluation session, Nathan seemed much more comfortable with the therapist and was more spontaneous in his interactions with the therapist and with the physical environment. He appeared to enjoy the movement activities and play interactions with the suspended equipment once he became more comfortable and saw that no one was judging his performance.

Contributions of the Volition and the Mind-Brain-Body Performance Subsystems to Nathan's Problems

The results of the sensory integration-based evaluation suggested that Nathan was experiencing difficulty processing and integrating sensory information from his body. In particular, Nathan appeared to have difficulty processing and interpreting tactile and movement information. His therapist concluded that he had both sensory discrimination-praxis and modulation disorders. She noted that he had particular difficulties with hypersensitivity to tactile stimuli from the therapist's touch and in response to different objects (e.g., chalk, uncooked navy beans, sheepskin, etc.). His dyspraxia was particularly evident during fine-motor, in-hand manipulation, and during movements which required bilateral integration, sequencing, and anticipatory motor control (e.g., throwing and catching a ball, performing sequential jumping patterns, and playing "soccer").

Nathan's type of sensory modulation dysfunction is characterized by an inability to efficiently modulate or regulate incoming sensory information; Nathan's tactile system was the most affected. Although this ability to modulate sensory information undergoes a normal variation throughout the course of a day, Nathan demonstrated greater-than-normal variability in his ability to filter and regulate the amount of incoming sensory/tactile information. He tended to under- or overreact to input, or fluctuated from a hyporesponsive to a hyperresponsive mode, often without warning. While this disorder could be very frustrating to the parents, peers, and teachers who interacted with Nathan, it was also frustrating and frightening to Nathan. As he told the therapist in a later session, "I can't control how I react sometimes."

Nathan's comment about his inability to control himself suggested to the therapist how Nathan's sensory processing and praxis problems may be affecting his volition. She suspected that the sensory integration problems both contributed to and were exacerbated by his volition status. That is, it had become clear from Nathan's behavior and self-report that he was plagued by a negative sense of personal causation that led him to expect failure and feel intimidated by sensory and motor-based actions. Consequently, Nathan often rushed through or did his best to avoid such actions in order to circumvent the painful experience of seeing himself unable to tolerate or perform actions. Afterwards he felt an acute sense of failure. With each new encounter, Nathan repeated and reinforced his belief that he was incapable and his feeling of being out of control. Because of his feelings of incapacity and lack of control, Nathan's activity choices were not adaptive. He would not take moderate risks that would have given him opportunities for learning and success. He was also reluctant to join in the play activities in which his peers engaged (i.e., mildly competitive, skill-oriented games and sports). His negative personal causation and his modulation disorder together influenced his ability to interact effectively in social contexts, where touch and unexpected tactile stimuli were more unpredictable and where, as a consequence, he felt even more out of control.

Nathan's sense of threat and his anxiety also meant that he approached sensory and motor experiences in a suboptimal emotional state which exacerbated his performance problems and his reactions to sensation. Nathan was clearly in the midst of an ongoing process which kept him gripped by self-doubt and anxiety; this led him to avoid many learning and socializing experiences. Moreover, when he had to perform, he was so terrified that his emotional state and sensory integrative problems together often led to the very failure he so feared. Consequently, he gained neither skill nor confidence. Moreover, the fear that something was very wrong with himself had increasingly taken on a life of its own and seemed to be growing as a dominant theme in Nathan's budding life story.

Because Nathan's volition was so dominated by his personal causation, fears, and anxieties, there was little opportunity for Nathan to develop positive interests. Thus, he did not have strong attractions to occupations nor did he experience much pleasure or satisfaction from performance. Nathan desperately wanted to be like other kids and to be recognized as a good son to his parents. These values did not, however, serve as motives leading Nathan toward positive activity and occupational choices. Rather they served mainly as standards against which he judged himself a failure.

Impact on Habituation

Not surprisingly, information from the developmental/sensory history revealed that Nathan tended to play with children younger than his own chronological age and that he was unable to perform play/motor skills commensurate with his age (e.g., bike riding, in-line skating, street hockey, soccer). His play skills and interests were limited to activities with minimal movement requirements, such as video games and reading. Thus, it was apparent that Nathan's player role had been greatly affected by the ongoing dynamics of his problem.

According to his mother's and teacher's reports, his student role was also negatively affected. Finally, his role as a family member was suffering. Nathan clearly wanted to be helpful and useful in the family, but he was easily frustrated when his motor difficulties interfered with his helping. For example, he wanted to be able to help carry groceries for his mother, but he often dropped them, breaking items or making a mess.

Nathan's volitional and performance problems were also reflected in his daily habits. Nathan was often frustrated and overly emotional when performing routine self-care tasks. It appeared this was partly due to his tactile defensiveness and partly due to his anxiety. Moreover, his mother re-

ported that Nathan had always been very particular with the textures of clothes he would tolerate and the foods he would eat. She said that it was "lucky that Nathan does not like to play hard like other boys because then he would get really dirty; just giving him a bath and washing his hair are enough of a hassle without the extra dirt!" Nathan had particular difficulty with those self-care activities performed infrequently, such as cutting his nails and cleaning his ears.

Course of Therapy

The focus of therapy was on creating opportunities within the clinical and everyday environments for Nathan to be competent and independent. This meant paying particular attention to the negative synergy created by Nathan's mind-brain-body performance subsystem and his volition. The therapist had to create situations in which Nathan's personal causation, fears, and anxieties could be minimized and in which he could be encouraged to make his own activity choices, which would lead to positive sensory and motor experiences. The overall aim of therapy was to simultaneously address his sensory-integrative problems and his volition by engaging him in actions which would halt and eventually reverse the negative cycle of avoidance, performance during sub-optimal emotional states, failure, and negative self-appraisal. Moreover, the therapist also followed the argument by Kielhofner & Fisher (1991) that change in sensory integration capacities would require Nathan to perform while in a volitional state. This was particularly important to ensure that the remediation and adaptation strategies used in therapy were carried over and integrated into the family and home life. The therapist developed long-term goals and objectives in collaboration with Nathan and his mother. These goals, that reflected the volition, habituation, and mind-brain-body performance subsystems, included the following:

1. Each day Nathan will make positive activity choices related to situations and opportunities in school, home, and/or therapy.
2. Nathan will develop more varied and deeper interests in play and social interaction within the school and home environments. (A subgoal was that Nathan enjoy himself more when engaged in normal childhood occupations.)
3. Nathan will be able to successfully help others and perform activities relevant to his

family role with the help of any adaptations he or his family needed to make.

4. On a daily basis Nathan will be able to complete personal self-care routines successfully and without aversive responses.

5. Nathan will demonstrate age-appropriate play skills. (This goal included the dual objectives of increasing his motor skills and communication and interaction skills. As noted earlier, both were affected by his sensory-integrative problems.)

Throughout the initial course of therapy, the therapist provided opportunities that were designed to encourage Nathan's exploration and experimentation with different equipment and toys in the occupational therapy environment. Because beliefs about one's effectiveness in the environment are based on personal experience, the therapist wanted to focus first on providing for Nathan a safe, playful environment, free from the pressure to perform or be "good enough." She felt that, in this context, Nathan needed special opportunities for taking risks, developing the ability to organize his response to sensory information and his movement behaviors, and to develop his sense of efficacy and his knowledge that he did have capacity for mastery over his environment. She wanted Nathan to develop both the skills for and the belief that he was empowered to influence the physical, and eventually, the social environment.

Over the course of a few sessions the therapist found Nathan to be a delightful child with whom to work. He was curious, articulate, and charming. Underneath his personal causation fears Nathan had a driving persistence and strong desire to "do well." The therapist was acutely aware of how he felt about himself and his difficulties with "doing." She always listened with her "third ear" to what Nathan really meant when he shared tidbits of his daily experience with her.

As Nathan's volition improved, the therapist sought to involve Nathan in the decisions of what equipment to use, what games to play, and when to change to another activity, as well as in the setting up and modifying of the equipment. She was conscious of guiding the intensity and frequency of sensory opportunities within the games Nathan created. Soon, Nathan and the therapist developed the ability to "flow" within and between different movement activities during the therapy sessions. As Nathan was empowered to influence and control these therapeutic situations, he in-

creased his readiness for coping with his sensory challenges in his other life environments.

On an ongoing basis, the therapist discussed with Nathan's mother strategies for modifying the home and school environments to ensure Nathan's success. For example, routines for completing self-care without undue emotion or stress were developed. For any child the presence of effective daily routines is important, but for Nathan it was vital. Without such routines Nathan was unable to participate in the play and self-care roles in his family. As much as possible, control for when certain self-care activities would be performed, and for the order in which they would be completed, was given to Nathan. For example, bathing right before bedtime was too stressful and arousing; Nathan determined that right after dinner was a better time for his bath and washing his hair. He found that he was more relaxed and ready for sleep when bedtime rolled around. Although he was only seven years old, the therapist carefully strove to facilitate in Nathan an internalized sense of self-regulated routine.

In working with Nathan's mother the therapist helped both her and Nathan understand that Nathan's "behavior" was not the result of Nathan's "not trying hard enough." Together, they examined the more stressful daily situations and identified the challenging sensory aspects of these situations in order to develop adaptations or modifications to ensure Nathan's success.

Nathan was taught to attend to some of the details of the physical environment and how they differentially affected his nervous system "state." Nathan and his therapist experimented with various adaptation strategies, such as optimal lighting, work spaces, and identified calm "get-organized" environments that Nathan could use when he was feeling overwhelmed. They also worked to develop strategies Nathan could use to cope when specific adaptations were not possible. Throughout therapy the therapist and Nathan's mother worked together to give Nathan the message that he was a good and valuable child. They were careful to offer Nathan genuine praise for approximations of success as well as for his successful performance in daily tasks. Indeed, after several months in therapy, Nathan spontaneously volunteered one day, "I knew I was really good inside after all! I *am* okay."

As Nathan continued to improve, the therapist increased focus on his everyday role behaviors related to play, self-care, peer interaction, and on his routine organization of behavior. Although improvements in Nathan's sensory integration and modulation were expected and observed over the course of therapy, the therapist also expected that Nathan would not overcome all of his sensory integrative difficulties. Most likely he would always have some unique challenges related to sensory processing and motor performance. The therapist strove to frame these likely challenges as part of how Nathan, like everyone else, would have to adapt in life with his own unique strengths and weaknesses. This emphasized how Nathan was like other children while highlighting his unique coping challenges. The therapist and Nathan's mother discussed this together and determined on an ongoing basis what steps were important for enabling Nathan to develop his own coping abilities.

Over time, Nathan was offered even wider opportunities for developing new interests both in occupational therapy and at home. Because the development of new and more varied interests was initially dependent on Nathan's ability to register input, gain meaning, and interpret experience during activities, he was provided as much variety within appropriate activities as possible. Natural extensions of the therapy experiences were built into his home and school environments. For example, as Nathan became more organized and controlled in his gross motor play, Nathan's parents took him regularly to a local park and playground where he could have appropriate experiences. When the weather became colder, Nathan took advantage of the local children's indoor playground. Later, his father built a tree-house climbing structure in their backyard. This not only was a resource for Nathan, but an important symbol of his accomplishments.

Nathan's communication and interaction skills developed slowly within the home and school environments as his volition, sensory modulation, and physical capabilities improved. Through a combination of adaptation and successive interaction in progressively more complex social groups, Nathan developed greater competence and belief in his own social skills and unique abilities.

One day while in therapy Nathan said, "You know I can do everything here. I think I don't need to see you so much anymore." After discussion and review of Nathan's improvements, Nathan, his parents, and the therapist agreed to cease direct treatment. The therapist continued to consult with the family and help them monitor Nathan's ongoing development.

Robert: Discovering and Supporting Volition in a Low-Functioning Person
by Marion Kavanaugh

Robert was 28 years old. He had lived in an institutional environment since the age of four when he was diagnosed as being both autistic and mentally retarded. Robert also has a seizure disorder for which he receives anticonvulsive medication. He had been treated as an inpatient at several facilities during his childhood. When he was 12 he came to the state facility where he now resides. Robert has spent most of his time at this institution on a unit designated for residents with behavior disorders.

A physically unremarkable man of slight-to-medium build, Robert had no speech. He occasionally smiled or laughed to express happiness and usually did not respond at all when another person spoke to him. With few exceptions, such as eating, Robert did not spontaneously engage in what ordinary members of society would recognize as a purposeful action. Usually withdrawn, Robert could become aggressive.

Robert was referred by the interdisciplinary team to occupational therapy because he was difficult to manage on the ward. For example, Robert sometimes disrobed in public; he was physically aggressive and he sometimes hit or spit at staff or residents when they came close to or touched him. Occasionally, he got so out of control that he damaged his own belongings and public property.

Gathering and Reasoning with Data: In Search of Robert's Volition

In this and other similar institutional settings, behavior techniques of positive and negative reinforcement are often used to manage aggressive behavior. The occupational therapist in this setting had gained the respect of interdisciplinary staff by using a positive motivational approach which was based on understanding the volition of persons such as Robert. That is, the therapist had shown how withdrawn or aggressive behavior could be understood as being motivated by how residents saw their world through their own volition. Thus, instead of viewing persons with significant cognitive limitations simply as persons with behavioral problems, the occupational therapist sought to understand the volition of such persons in order to comprehend why they were motivated to behave as they did. When such understanding was achieved, a plan of therapy could be developed which took into consideration the person's volition instead of simply providing negative incentives (which in effect were punishments) for undesirable behavior. Since persons with significant cognitive limitations ordinarily lack the personal resources to advocate for their own perspectives and desires, this approach was viewed by the occupational therapist as allowing her to advocate on their behalf and, virtually, as a means to empower otherwise very powerless individuals.

While learning about volition in such low-functioning persons as Robert is difficult, the therapist assumed that a significant amount of Robert's troublesome behavior was likely related to his volition. Therefore, the difficulty of learning about volition was clearly outweighed by the advantage of gaining an understanding of why Robert behaved as he did. The occupational therapist began with the following broad question: How did Robert make sense of himself and his environment? She wanted to know if Robert had identifiable interests and values and how these were expressed in his occupational behavior, including his asocial actions. The therapist also wanted to know what kinds of feelings Robert might have related to control of his circumstances. Withdrawal and aggression are often closely related to anxiety and perceived threat. Consequently, the occupational therapist anticipated that Robert's personal causation might involve feelings about being unable to control his circumstances and that these feelings were related to his withdrawal and aggression.

Because Robert was incapable of any self-report or formal testing, the occupational therapist decided to conduct the evaluation mainly through informal observation. The therapist expected that she might infer from Robert's reactions to the environment what interested him and mattered to him and when he felt threatened or out of control. Moreover, she therapist expected the observation to provide cues about how the environment could be altered to evolve more positive behavior from Robert.

The therapist's first observation confirmed that Robert was extremely withdrawn. He would sit or stand in one position for long periods during which he did nothing but warily watch others. Robert occasionally exhibited stereotyped behaviors, such as rocking his body as he sat with his knees tucked under his chin. He resisted initial attempts of the occupational therapist to initiate interaction with him by turning away or gesturing aggressively.

The therapist decided that she would continue to observe Robert in a variety of settings and situations. She reasoned that by examining Robert in these different contexts, she might get additional data which would give her clues as to Robert's volitional status. Since Robert was generally so withdrawn and inactive, she also reasoned it would be more informative to observe him briefly in a number of different contexts than to conduct a single more lengthy or formal observation. While the occupational therapist did not formally use the Volitional Questionnaire as a rating scale because she planned this series of brief observations, she used the items on the scale as a guide for her observations of Robert.

The therapist made the informal observations of Robert's behavior throughout the day in the various environments he occupied within the hospital. She also supplemented the information she obtained by interviewing staff concerning their observations, interactions with, and attitudes about Robert.

The therapist learned from observation and staff reports that Robert was able to feed himself using a spoon and to drink from a cup. He ate very fast without concern that he sometimes dropped food on the floor.

He apparently had no understanding of the purpose of personal hygiene. Evidence of this was that Robert appeared to cooperate or resist according to whether he enjoyed the activity. His behaviors were directed solely at sensory pleasure, not at the purpose of the occupational form. For example, Robert, who liked the feeling of water, cooperated while being bathed by staff, although he made no attempts to wash himself. On the other hand, he resisted having his teeth brushed by staff, apparently because he didn't like the feeling of the toothbrush or taste of the toothpaste. Robert occasionally had toilet accidents during the day, although he could lower his pants and sit on the toilet without help. Consequently, the accidents appeared to be related to the fact that Robert did not always perceive the rationale for relieving himself on a toilet, especially if there was no ready access to one.

During the day, Robert could often be observed curled up asleep on the floor of the large room in which residents were kept during most of the day. Occasionally, Robert walked around the day area of the unit with no apparent aim. At other times, he sat with his knees drawn up to his chest, distancing himself as far away from other residents as possible. He frequently slapped, or spit at, or threw spit at any staff or residents who came within a foot or two of him. Robert was able to pick up from what was going on in the environment when it was time for meals. He also performed some routine behavior at mealtime, such as waiting in the cafeteria line to be served. These observations of Robert's behavior suggested that he was clearly aware of his environment.

His awareness and capability for some rational behavior such as standing in line for food suggested that his withdrawal and aggression was related to his perceived need to separate or protect himself from interactions with other residents or ward staff. Indeed, given the social setting, it was reasonable how someone like Robert could have come to see his environment as mainly hostile.

At first, Robert appeared to prefer being alone. In particular, he liked to have some distance between himself and other residents. The occupational therapist wondered if this may have been a reflection of the potential of being attacked by other residents or having one's belongings or food taken. She reasoned that Robert's antisocial behavior might actually have its basis in the sometimes chaotic environment of the ward. She resolved to continue to attempt to make social contact with Robert.

Despite Robert's consistent antisocial behavior, he began to give evidence that he actually wanted to have interactions with others. After the therapist had made clear to Robert through her behavior that she was not a threat, he made eye contact and sometimes smiled in response to being lightly touched or softly spoken to. He even occasionally reached out to touch the therapist or hold her hand.

Such behaviors were rare with the direct care staff on the unit. The occupational therapist observed that direct care staff did not frequently approach Robert, except to stop aggressive behavior. Robert had apparently come to know direct care staff mainly as persons who forced him to do things that he didn't want to do. They, in turn, saw him as a resistive and aggressive resident who needed occasional coercion to comply with unit procedures. Robert and the staff were clearly locked in an ongoing struggle.

Robert appeared to have some interests. He liked going out of doors, walking about, touching the grass, and feeling sunshine on his face. He liked playing in water and taking showers. His therapist could tell when Robert was interested in something by noting the frequency with which he tried to enact certain behaviors or activities and by any positive affective response to them, such as smiling or laughing.

Robert did not appear to care about his own clothing except as it affected his comfort or dis-comfort. He apparently did not share the social perception that clothes symbolize identity and affect one's appearance. Rather, he was unaware of torn, backwards, or inside-out clothing. He could remove his shoes, socks, and shirts and did this when it pleased him, apparently unaware of the social response to an unclothed adult.

An Explanation of Robert's Volition

As Robert's occupational therapist reviewed this data, she was able to put together the following picture of his volition. Robert had extremely limited cognitive access to the social and cultural world around him. Moreover, his social environment had not afforded him opportunities to access actions and meanings. His caretakers saw him primarily as a severely limited person with behavior problems; their actions sought to control behavior but not to invite Robert to participate in the social world. Consequently, Robert incorporated little of the cultural world view of others around him. He apparently did not experience fundamental social reaction to a variety of situations. For example, he did not experience shame at public nakedness; he did not show disgust at toileting accidents and he had no apparent regard for his appearance, which suggested he did not have a view of himself as perceived by others.

While Robert did not share many of the culturally provided commonsense views of the world that ordinarily constitute volition, he did, nonetheless, possess an active volition. He clearly enjoyed certain activities that gave him basic sensory pleasure, including self-stimulation. He was attracted to other people and enjoyed simple interaction such as touching. While Robert did not show any evidence of having values in the sense of culturally constituted views and commitments, he did clearly operate from a system of concerns (a) to be able to do what he wanted, (b) to be free of being forced to do things he did not want to do, and (c) to avoid aggression or loss at the hands of others. His withdrawal and his aggression appeared clearly linked to these concerns.

Given Robert's level of cognitive functioning, he could not be expected to have a symbolic understanding of his capacities or a very good grasp of how his behaviors were related to consequences. However, it was clear that he sensed threat and that he felt more in control of his circumstances when he was able to withdraw to a safe distance or when he aggressively drove others away. Through these behaviors, he managed to be somewhat in control.

Robert did not have a very sophisticated ability to discriminate how others' behaviors might affect him; it was unlikely that he had any abstract concept of, or routinely attempted to discriminate, others' intentions toward him. Rather, he appeared to react on the basis of a feeling of threat or being unable to control his situation. Thus, his aggressive and withdrawn behaviors were overgeneralized, inconsistent, and not always related in the same way to others' actions or intentions. For this reason, Robert was a puzzle to those around him. Moreover, he did not appear to behave from a consistent set of inner desires or concerns.

Since this explanation of Robert's volition was composed from observation, and since Robert was incapable of verifying or refuting it, the occupational therapist could not know for certain how accurate it was. However, by using it to devise an intervention plan for Robert, she was able to test this explanation. If the intervention worked, she could have much greater confidence that her understanding of Robert's volition was at least partly accurate.

Robert's Environment

The occupational therapist's observations also revealed that Robert's volition was very much influenced by the environment of the state hospital. Further, it was clear that any intervention strategy would have to make use of that environment to influence Robert's behavior. Thus, the next step in data gathering and analysis was to examine the environment.

The therapist wanted to gather information on the objects, spaces, occupational forms, and social groups that afforded Robert opportunity for activity. In addition, she also wanted to identify any factors in the environment that might have pressed for his withdrawn or aggressive behavior.

The environment which Robert occupied day-to-day consisted of five areas within, and adjacent to, the Behavior Disorders building: a day area consisting of two rooms where residents spent most waking hours, a small recreation room, a living area with bedrooms and bathrooms, a dining room, and an outside area immediately next to the building. The recreation room was not used for any particular purpose or for any regularly scheduled activities. Its main purpose, like the day room, was to contain residents away from the living area where they could be more easily observed and managed.

The four areas inside the building were stark, barren, and noticeably lacked objects. Because of the residents' aggressive and destructive behavior, objects which could not be secured to the floor or wall were virtually absent. In the day rooms there were only plastic chairs and a few tables. Two benches were the only equipment in the area outside the building. Thus, there were very few objects present with which it was possible to do something. Not surprisingly, residents treated themselves and others as objects for use.

Staff occasionally brought objects, such as pegboards, bingo games, or other fine motor activities into the living area when there were enough staff to supervise and when residents were generally calm. However, the routine work, the unruliness of residents, and the poor staff-to-resident ratios made this more the exception than the rule. Consequently, the only occupational forms routinely available in the environment were related to eating and hygiene. Residents were left to invent their own means of creating stimulation or activity. And this is what many, including Robert, apparently did when they engaged in repetitive, self-stimulating behaviors.

The living area, with bedrooms and bathrooms, was the larger and more interesting area; however, resident access to this area was ordinarily restricted to times for sleeping and to times for hygiene. Although there were two day areas on the wing, residents were usually confined to only one area because there were not enough staff to watch over residents in two areas. Consequently, the day room was crowded. With residents forced to be in close proximity to each other, personal space was a commodity. It was not uncommon that residents appeared to react to someone else invading their personal space. Altercations over territory occurred regularly. The social environment was marked by periodic physical outbursts and assaults. It tended to be a threatening social environment where most interactions included some kind of altercation as residents got out of control or coercion as staff sought to manage behavior. It was not hard to see how such an environment would press for the kind of distancing and self-protective behaviors which Robert exhibited.

The only persons regularly in the environment were direct care staff. The staff-to-resident ratio was such that staff felt chronically overburdened. The vast majority of their time and effort was directed to getting necessary routines of hygiene and eating completed, and to avoiding fights and destructive behavior. There was minimal staff–resident contact, except for these routine and order-keeping purposes. Most of the time the staff's interaction with residents was at least mildly coercive as they tried to move residents along in the various routines of hygiene and meals with varying degrees of resident cooperation. Again it was easy to see how residents could perceive staff as primarily functioning to limit one's personal freedom to act as one wanted.

Moreover, because staff were constantly dealing with behavioral problems, passive withdrawn behavior was not seen as a problem. Indeed a passive and withdrawn resident meant less work for staff. Thus, there was a subtle press for residents to be inactive and passive.

Intervention Strategy

The occupational therapist reasoned that if Robert was to be encouraged to be less aggressive, he would also need to learn to be more comfortable in his environment. Also, if Robert could be enticed into positive interactions with his environment, he might learn not always to expect problems and to be more able to discriminate what was going on in the environment. To accomplish this, Robert initially needed to feel some degree of safety in the treatment environment and eventually in his living environment. The therapist helped Robert to feel safe by slowly initiating interaction, allowing him to become accustomed to her presence during each interaction and slowing letting him become more comfortable with her being around him.

Because Robert did not appear to have tolerance for long periods of interaction, the occupational therapist began with 15-minute sessions, scheduled three times per week. She began by observing Robert for approximately five minutes prior to treatment. This allowed her an opportunity to record Robert's behaviors and any relevant environmental cues during this observation period. This observation period had three purposes. First, it enabled the therapist to determine Robert's apparent emotional state prior to the beginning of treatment. Sometimes he was actually asleep, other times he was lethargic or passive, and sometimes he was very agitated (e.g., spitting and slapping). Second, the occupational therapist could observe the climate of the immediate environment, such as whether it was crowded, whether nearby residents were agitated or noisy, or whether housekeeping or maintenance staff were working on the unit. This information was used to determine whether treatment could be done on the ward or if Robert needed to be taken to a quieter or less crowded environment. Further, an examination of the environmental elements sometimes gave a clue to Robert's present volitional state and, over time, led to a better understanding of the relation of the environment to Robert's behavior. It further enabled the therapist to monitor any positive or negative changes in the physical and psychosocial elements of the environment. Finally, it gave Robert time to be aware of her and become accustomed to her presence.

Once the observation was over and the intervention was about to begin, the occupational therapist started by presenting, one at a time, various types of objects that she hoped would attract him and, thereby, stimulate his curiosity and elicit exploratory behaviors. She selected objects that provided sensory information and that could be easily manipulated. For example, she introduced to Robert a fuzzy animal which squeaked when he squeezed it. She also showed him a mirror which revolved within a plastic ring. She also brought a bright-colored hard rubber ball with short flexible spines and a rhythm instrument which clanged when shaken. She always carried these objects to the unit in a bag or box. As Robert came to recognize the routine, he wanted and was allowed to explore the bag or box to see what was inside.

Initially, the occupational therapist touched Robert's hands, arms, face, and other body parts with some of the objects. His reaction ranged from accepting and noticing the stimulation to reaching for the object and poking, shaking, or pounding it against himself. When he was finished, usually after a short period, Robert threw the object several feet away from himself.

After approximately eight sessions, Robert demonstrated a preference for the "spiny" ball. He held it longer and played with the spines. He would eventually throw it away from himself. Attempts were made to gradually shape this into an occupational form—a simple game of catch. The therapist would retrieve the ball and roll it along the floor back to Robert. He would hold it a while then throw it again. Often Robert purposely threw the ball away from the therapist, and laughed mischievously. The therapist returned the ball to Robert, and would gradually roll it to a point slightly further away from where he was sitting.

Importantly, the game of catch gave Robert a unique opportunity; that is, he was able to influence the behavior of another in a socially appropriate and accepted manner—without spitting or hitting. In addition, he was able to serve as the initiator in this playful interaction, not just to react to others' behavior.

There were still times when Robert slapped or spat at the therapist. Utilizing the principle of providing clear and consistent environmental cues of expectations for role behavior, the occupational therapist consistently stopped the interaction, firmly stated "No, Robert," moved approximately 8–10 feet away from him, and remained there until the negative behaviors ceased. Then she would walk back to him and reinitiate the interaction. In this way, Robert began to internalize some simple, yet appropriate, role scripts.

The following brief incidents illustrate Robert's growing awareness of this simple role script. In one session, the occupational therapist moved away from Robert because he started to slap her. When he saw her reaction, he ceased the behavior, made eye contact with her, then rose and walked towards her reaching out for the object she held.

Several specific objects and activities were further identified as ones Robert liked. One of his favorite activities was the game of catch described above. He also demonstrated that he liked an interaction in which the therapist would bring the fuzzy animal close to and then lightly touch various parts of his face. In addition to the spiny ball, he developed a strong attraction to terrycloth and soft objects, and to rhythm instruments that made soft noises.

While the therapist made a great deal of progress in reducing Robert's aggressive and withdrawn behavior, she understood that the rest of his daily environment remained as before. Therefore, any positive experiences she and Robert had together could be erased by Robert's other experiences in the course of the day.

Now that she had evolved some effective ways of interacting with Robert, eliciting positive interaction by evoking his interest and mitigating his aggression, it was time to share it with other ward staff in hopes of altering other parts of Robert's environment.

During interdisciplinary meetings, the occupational therapist shared with unit staff the information she had gained about Robert's volition and about her success in interacting with him. At these meetings she encouraged and helped staff to view Robert as having values and interests and as being capable of behaving in a more positive fashion when the environment was not threatening and when appropriate objects and activities were provided.

The occupational therapist modeled how to interact with Robert for other direct care staff on the unit. The following incident is an example. At the beginning of one session, the therapist wished to move Robert to a less crowded location. A direct care aide grasped Robert's arm to begin having him

follow her. (This kind of coercion on the part of staff typically agitated Robert and made him aggressive and resistive.) The therapist intervened and showed Robert one of his favorite objects. He voluntarily followed the therapist to the other area. Such incidents helped change staff views about Robert and about how they should interact with him.

More and more staff began to employ the approach suggested by the occupational therapist and began to see Robert in a different light; i.e., as a human being who had feelings, who liked some things, feared others and cared about what happened to him and about what he did. They reduced their own coercive behavior and instead coaxed Robert through his interests. Some staff even occasionally interacted with Robert in a playful way. Their attitudinal and behavioral changes shifted the social environmental conditions under which Robert lived everyday and, with these environmental changes, Robert's behavior also began to change.

Staff observed a significant decrease in Robert's aggression on the unit. They also reported that Robert had begun to approach staff to initiate interactions with them. Bolstered by their success with Robert, they continued to interact with him in this more positive manner. Staff began to take it upon themselves to figure out new interests for Robert and prided themselves on getting him involved in simple activities. As the relationship between staff and Robert improved, they became more successful in getting Robert to go along with some self-care activities. An illustration is that they introduced the toothbrush to Robert in a new way. Instead of forcing it on him for tooth brushing, they let him explore it. As he became accustomed to it, he became cooperative during tooth brushing.

While Robert continued to have some problems, such as occasional toilet accidents and some aggression toward other residents who he perceived as threatening him, the biggest change was in the dynamic relationship between Robert and the ward staff. They were no longer in an ongoing struggle. Robert came to see the staff as sources of enjoyment and not simply as sources of coercion. Moreover, as he developed some positive social connection with them; he was more able to respond to their desires and expectations for behavior. Staff came to see Robert as a person with desires and needs and as capable of cooperation. Over time, such a positive change in the dynamics of Robert's social identity, behavior, and experience was expected to maintain his positive changes and likely elicit further progress.

Sally: Choosing and Organizing Life Occupations

by Gloria Furst and Cynthia Stabenow

Sally was a 37-year-old, college-educated homemaker who formerly taught in elementary school. Since she was diagnosed with seropositive rheumatoid arthritis (RA) five years prior, Sally had undergone the standard medical approach to her disease, progressing through aspirin therapy to anti-inflammatory medications and then to gold therapy, which was discontinued due to side effects. Thereafter, a combination of other drugs also provided severe side effects and failed to halt the progression of the disease.

After this unsuccessful five-year course of medication, Sally's impairments had progressed to the point that she became an outpatient at a rehabilitation facility where she first received occupational therapy. At the time, Sally's chief physical complaints were pain and swelling in her wrists, fingers, knees, ankles, and feet. Because of anemia and weight loss secondary to the chronic nature of her disease, Sally was also referred to a nutrition clinic.

The progressive nature of Sally's arthritis and the failure of the usual medication regimen to successfully place the disease in remission made it clear to the occupational therapist that Sally would have to find a lifestyle in which she could successfully cope with her limitations and, as much as possible, manage the symptoms of arthritis through her activity pattern. The first hint that Sally was having difficulty with this came from her social worker, who expressed concern that Sally was depressed.

Gathering and Reasoning with Data

Because Sally's disease attacks the musculoskeletal system, Sally's occupational therapist used the biomechanical model (Kielhofner, 1992; Trombly, 1989) in concert with the model of human occupation to guide the data-gathering process and the planning and implementation of therapy. Since Sally was a bright and articulate woman, data gathering was done so as to maximize her role in shaping an understanding of her situation. The therapist gathered data on her musculoskeletal status to provide a picture of her biomechanical capacities and limits. In addition, Sally and her therapist together examined her motor skills in daily living and homemaking activities by doing and discussing them in the occupational therapy setting.

In addition to wanting to know how the arthritis had affected Sally's performance capacity, her occupational therapist was also concerned to know how the arthritis had affected both Sally's volition and habituation, since insidious diseases such as arthritis may slowly rob persons of parts of their lives. For example, arthritis may precipitate loss of ability to perform in areas of interest and interrupt long-standing habit patterns. Consequently, Sally's therapist began the data collection process with questions about the impact of the disease and the limits it imposed on her interests, values, and feelings of personal causation. He wanted to know what changes had taken place in Sally's volition and to understand how these may have influenced her activity and occupational choices. Moreover, the occupational therapist wanted to know how Sally's roles and habit patterns had changed and what the consequences were for Sally's lifestyle. Since there was concern that Sally was depressed, the therapist anticipated that he might find problems in these areas.

To begin gathering data about these areas, Sally's therapist interviewed her using the Occupational Performance History Interview. In addition, Sally was given the Interest Checklist (modified), and the NIH Activity Record to take home and complete. Since Sally completed the NIH Activity Record at home, she filled it out as a diary, and reported on an actual weekday and weekend day. She was instructed to choose days which were typical for her. All of these assessments were completed during Sally's first couple of weeks as an outpatient. The therapist's goal was to get a comprehensive picture of Sally's occupational dysfunction, validate it with her, and, together with Sally, plan and implement a course of occupational therapy.

"Making Do"

In the Occupational Performance History Interview, Sally made a remark about having to "make do" when her arthritis prevented her from performing an activity as it should have been done. In many ways, this comment summarized what Sally's life story had become. She had routinely found herself unable to carry out the occupational forms she valued and enjoyed. Being a practical person who readily acquiesced to such problems, she routinely compromised and found a way to get by. In this way, she had changed much of her life to accommodate her pain and limitations. However, her life had also lost much of its spontaneity and joy and was instead characterized by a series of losses and compromises. Formerly a sports enthusiast, she talked about a bowling ball and tennis racket now hidden away in the attic and a bicycle reluctantly retired since she could no longer safely operate the hand brakes.

Sally was a trained and credentialed primary and secondary educator who interrupted her career after one year of work to become a full-time homemaker, rearing her two children. She had planned to return to teaching after her teenage children were grown. Sally had taken on the homemaker role full-time because of strong family and religious values; she had a sense of obligation to devote most of her attention to raising her children. While Sally valued her caretaking role, the occupational forms that the role required were not those which were most satisfying or important for her sense of personal causation. Sally's voluntary exit from work, along with her forced discontinuation of sports, had created a major loss of identity and activity. Finally, Sally had been an active volunteer in her church, running an education program for senior citizens. This volunteer work had continued her involvement in teaching and appeared quite satisfying and important to her. However, as the arthritis progressed, she had also been forced to relinquish the volunteer role (another major loss) and to concentrate her efforts on the homemaker and patient roles. The patient role included compliance with treatment and with energy conservation practice for the arthritis, both of which were quite demanding of her time.

Sally acknowledged that her teenaged children would soon be gone from home and that she would then be without any major occupational role. The possibility of having lost all her identities and activities was distressing, even to a woman who had managed to "make do" in the face of her limits and losses so far. Sally had some vague ideas about returning to teaching as a substitute since her arthritis made full-time teaching impossible, but mainly the future seemed uncertain and menacing to her.

Sally also indicated in the Occupational Performance History Interview that the arthritis interfered with many of her routines and posed constant problems for undertaking ordinary activities. Sally described a series of small incidents in which she performed an ordinary task, like making breakfast, where some simple action like "stirring eggs," suddenly brought on severe pain. She also related incidents in which her pain or motor limitations meant she couldn't finish an activity. While it was clear that Sally was resourceful in making the best of her limitations and finding a way to get through most activities, it was also evident that her sense of efficacy had been eroded by the barrage of small things that got the best of her. She always seemed to function under the constant threat of not being able to manage things and repeatedly needed to stop or change course when confronted with her pain, weakness, or fatigue.

Overall, Sally related in the interview a life story in which she had many losses, managed to barely hold on and make do, and lived under the constant threat of being unable to cope. Finally, her story did not include a clear or hopeful future. Rather, if the future promised anything it promised more and more losses associated with the unrelenting march of her disease. This story afforded the occupational therapist insight as to why Sally appeared depressed.

Loss of Satisfaction and Self

The modified Interest Checklist that Sally filled out assessed past, present, and desired future interests (see Figure 14.16). From 80 items, Sally indicated that she had 11 strong interests in the past 10 years. In the year previous to the evaluation, Sally had maintained a strong interest in only two of those areas, singing and mending. The Checklist confirmed Sally's interview report that many of her strong interests involved physical activity and, consequently, had been dropped. Also apparent on the Checklist, and confirmed by Sally when it was discussed with her, was that many of the interests she had been forced to give up had provided her with the social contact she enjoyed. She had lost not only activities but also the connection with others.

According to Sally she had only acquired one new interest, swimming. She was quick to point out that swimming was "therapy" for her arthritis. A theme which had surfaced in her interview but that became more apparent when Sally discussed swimming was that she didn't seem to feel that she *deserved* to pursue her own interests, since she was barely able to discharge her homemaker role. According to Sally's world view (i.e., her religious views and her image of what is meant to be a good mother) it was important to meet the needs and demands of her children, church, and community and to give priority to these needs over her own. This view of life had previously worked fine for Sally, but now it seemed to con-

Activity	What has been your level of interest						Do you currently participate in this activity?		Would you like to pursue this in the future?	
	In the past ten years			In the past year						
	Strong	Some	No	Strong	Some	No	Yes	No	Yes	No
Gardening Yardwork		X				X	X			X
Sewing/needle work	X				X		X			X
Playing card		X				X		X		X
Foreign languages			X			X		X		X
Church activities	X				X		X		X	
Radio		X			X		X		X	
Walking	X				X		X			X
Car Repair			X			X		X		X
Writing			X			X		X		X
Dancing		X				X	X			X
Golf			X			X	X			X
Football			X			X		X		X
Listening to popular music			X			X		X		X
Puzzles		X				X	X			X
Holiday activities	X				X		X		X	
Pets/livestock		X			X		X			X
Movies		X				X		X		X
Listening to classical music		X				X	X			X
Speeches/lectures			X			X		X		X
Swimming		X		X			X		X	
Bowling	X					X		X		X
Visiting	X				X		X		X	
Mending	X			X			X		X	
Checkers/Chess			X			X		X		X
Barbecues		X				X	X		X	
Reading		X			X		X		X	
Traveling		X				X	X			X
Parties			X			X		X		X
Wrestling			X			X		X		X
Housecleaning	X				X		X		X	
Model building			X			X		X		X
Television		X			X			X	X	
Concerts		X				X	X			X
Pottery			X			X		X		X

Figure 14.16.   Sally's responses on the modified interest checklist.

Continued

Activity	What has been your level of interest						Do you currently participate in this activity?		Would you like to pursue this in the future?	
	In the past ten years			In the past year						
	Strong	Some	No	Strong	Some	No	Yes	No	Yes	No
Camping			X			X		X		X
Laundry/Ironing	X				X			X	X	
Politics			X			X		X		X
Table games		X				X	X		X	
Home decorating		X			X		X		X	
Clubs/Lodge			X			X		X		X
Singing	X			X			X		X	
Scouting			X			X		X		X
Clothes		X			X			X	X	
Handicrafts	X					X	X			X
Hairstyling			X			X		X		X
Cycling		X				X	X			X
Attending plays		X				X	X			X
Bird watching		X				X		X		X
Dating		X				X		X		X
Auto-racing		X				X		X		X
Home repairs		X				X	X			X
Exercise		X			X		X		X	
Hunting		X				X		X		X
Woodworking		X				X		X		X
Pool		X		X			X		X	
Driving		X			X		X		X	
Child care		X				X		X		X
Tennis		X				X		X		X
Cooking/Baking		X			X		X		X	
Basketball			X			X		X		X
History			X			X		X		X
Collecting			X			X		X		X
Fishing			X			X		X		X
Science		X			X		X			X
Leatherwork			X			X		X		X
Shopping		X			X		X		X	
Photography			X			X		X		X
Painting/Drawing			X			X		X		X

Figure 14.16. Continued

tribute to her life story of loss. She seemed sadly resigned to the idea that she should just bear the losses herself and devote her remaining resources to her obligations to others.

Sally reported her internalized roles on the Role Checklist (see Figure 14.17). Sally had been able to maintain continuous friend, family, home maintainer, and religious participant roles. Both the student and worker roles were not part of her current life and she did not indicate them for the future. The volunteer role, which was very important to Sally, was interrupted, but she planned to return to this role. The Role Checklist provides a picture of Sally's role changes (both real and hoped for) and Sally found completing the checklist and the information it automatically provided as helpful to her. It made concrete her loss of roles. It also confirmed for her what she had managed to hold on to and what she wanted for the future.

On the Activity Record, Sally reported and answered eight questions about her activities over two typical days. Figure 14.18 summarizes Sally's time use (at the time of initial assessment and upon discharge) in terms of the percentage of waking hours she spent in relation to various system components. Reports on the Activity Record can be summarized as shown on the figure. Overall, Sally's days appeared deficient in activities that provided a feeling of value, personal causation, and interest. She rated only about a third of the activities in her day as related to major life roles. She had several long periods of rest, but did not routinely rest during activities. Finally, she experienced a moderate amount of pain and difficulty in her daily activities.

In addition to the summary data noted above, the Activity Record provided a wealth of detail about Sally's routines. For example, it allowed her occupational therapist to identify particular activ-

Role	Past	Present	Future	Not At All Valuable	Somewhat Valuable	Very Valuable
Student	X	X				
Worker	X				X	
Volunteer	X		X	X	X	
Care giver	X	X	X	X		
Home Maintainer	X	X	X	X		
Friend	X	X	X		X	
Family Member	X	X	X	X		
Religious Participant	X	X	X	X		
Hobbyist/ Amateur					X	
Participant in Organization						X
Other:						

Figure 14.17. Sally's responses on the role checklist.

System Components	Percent Waking Hours	
	Initial	Discharge
VOLITION		
Personal Causation		
How well done		
Very poorly	0	0
Poorly	19	0
Average	79	83
Well	1	16
Interests		
Time in recreation and leisure	22	32
Enjoyment of Activities		
Not at all	3	0
Very little	21	0
Some	51	61
A lot	24	39
Values		
Meaningfulness of activities		
Not meaningful	8	0
Slightly meaningful	6	0
Meaningful	69	76
Very meaningful	16	23
Value of Activities to others		
Not at all	5	0
Very little	3	0
Some	35	95
A lot	56	5
HABITUATION		
Roles		
Role related activities	30	44
Habits		
Rest during activities	1	22
PERFORMANCE		
Skills		
Level of difficulty		
Very difficult	5	0
Difficult	6	0
Slightly difficult	41	40
Not difficult	46	59

Figure 14.18. Sally's activity record results.

ities that were not valuable or interesting to Sally. Such information was very useful in intervention when Sally and her therapist worked to plan and implement a more adaptive daily routine.

Status of the Mind-Brain-Body Performance Subsystem and Motor Skills

The therapist followed up on Sally's reported difficulties in daily activities in two ways. First, he gathered data traditionally obtained to assess a person's biomechanical status. This data gathering revealed that Sally had limitations of range of motion in her elbow, wrist, and fingers. Her grip was quite limited due to pain in her finger joints.

Second, the therapist and Sally together reflected on her performance in a range of daily living tasks in order to identify the motor skills with which she had the most difficulty. These observations revealed that Sally consistently had the most problems with reaching, transporting, lifting, and gripping. She also had difficulty manipulating because of pain and limited range in her hands. Finally, Sally's endurance was limited sometimes by pain. The consequence of Sally's impaired motor skills was that she had difficulty with a range of small self-care tasks such as buttoning her clothes, using zippers, brushing her teeth, and caring for her hair. Household activities, especially cooking, were also difficult for Sally.

Collaborating with Sally to Create an Understanding of Her Situation

After all the data was collected, Sally's therapist wrote a detailed analysis of her situation. This summary was first shared with Sally in writing and then discussed with her. As part of the discussion, Sally was introduced to the model of human occupation so that she could appreciate better how the therapist was making sense of her situation. Then Sally was provided opportunity to respond to this evaluation from her own perspective. Sally and her therapist together arrived at the following analysis of her situation.

Sally was an articulate and intelligent young woman who was attempting to cope with a progressively debilitating and painful disease. At times her arthritic condition exacerbated and confined her to bed. Most of the time, however, she was able to function with moderate daily pain, and reduced range of motion, strength, and fine motor ability. Sally had been resourceful in figuring out ways to deal with her limits, but her knowledge of the disease process and ways to manage its symptoms had come from trial and error. Consequently, her strategies were not always optimal.

Pain and other symptoms often served as control parameters determining Sally's activity choices and forced her to alter her routines. In addition, her progressive symptoms have meant that she has given up a former lifestyle of sports involvement and volunteering to focus on being a homemaker.

This transformation in Sally's daily routine and lifestyle had resulted in important decrements in Sally's overall life satisfaction. Her daily routine reflected a lack of opportunities for exercising feelings of competence and enjoyment. She had also lost roles that gave her a sense of identity and worth.

Sally's view of her life situation had been that she should simply accept all her losses and focus on doing her best in her role as a homemaker. Yet, she often did not feel competent or in control of these responsibilities. Together, the sense of loss, the feeling of being out of control, the pain, and the erosion of her daily quality of life contributed to an increasing depression. As Sally became more and more depressed, her energy level was lower; this exacerbated her functional problems and made it even more difficult for her to carry on with daily life. Sally had recognized her life was getting steadily worse, but the process had been gradual and seemed inevitable, so she had very little sense that she could do anything with it except endure it and "make do" with what she had remaining. Moreover, because things were gradually getting worse for Sally, she only imagined that they would continue to do so.

Together Sally and the therapist agreed that this way of viewing her situation contributed to the downward slide in her life. She needed to reframe and rethink her life—to retell her life story. The story she and the therapist headed toward was one in which Sally would have more control, find a way toward a more satisfying daily life, and be able to imagine and work toward a positive future.

Therapeutic Goals and Strategies

Sally and her therapist identified the following goals for her therapy. First, Sally needed more information and needed to learn ways to be more in control of the symptoms and compensate for the limits imposed by her arthritis. This would potentially help her to function better and it would enhance her sense of efficacy. Second, Sally wanted to improve the quality of her everyday life. Completing the Activity Record had been an eye-opening experience for Sally and she was able to see both how her overall pattern of activity was less than optimal and how some of her activities offered her no satisfaction or meaning. Third, Sally agreed that she needed to look at her choices in life. She recognized that, while she believed it was important to devote most of her energies to her family, it was also important to consider how her activity choices may affect her mood and her ability to give to her family. Also, Sally recognized that she needed to prepare to make an occupational choice for the future. This was important in a practical way, since her children would soon leave home and her homemaking would both diminish and take on less importance for her. It was also symbolically important that she begin to imagine a future for herself that was not dominated by the unknown progress of her arthritis.

Since the disease and related impairments in the mind-brain-body performance subsystem had served as control parameters, the first emphasis in therapy was to diminish their influence, so that other factors, particularly the volition subsystem, could exert more control. At the same time, since the impairments had such an constraining impact on volition, the therapist anticipated changes in these constraints would be a first step for Sally to experience changes in her own volition. Thus, by directly addressing the mind-brain-body performance subsystem, occupational therapy interventions also addressed volition.

Since the arthritis had been and would likely continue to be progressive, the therapist recognized that Sally would need to learn how to compensate for her impairments. Additionally, it was important that Sally learn to have some control over symptoms and over how they influenced her everyday function. Achieving this would enhance Sally's sense of personal causation.

Consequently, Sally's treatment program included interventions guided by the biomechanical model such as instruction in an active range of motion program for both upper extremities. Sally was also provided custom-made splints that she could use to decrease the pain and increase the stability of her wrists during activities of daily living. In addition, she was provided resting hand splints for night time use or rest periods to maintain hand and wrist alignment. She was instructed in basic information about her disease, its symptoms and biomechanical factors that affected her pain and functional ability. Sally was given the opportunity to try various adaptive devices that would allow her to perform maximally even with her limited strength and range of motion. For example, Sally and her therapist identified the following objects that she incorporated into her daily routine: a jar opener, a vegetable peeler, a key holder, a long-handled shoe horn, a mitt to hold soap, and a wooden push/pull stick for the oven rack. In addition, Sally and her therapist identified that putting foam cylinders on household objects helped to increase the effectiveness of her gripping. Sally put the cylinders around her toothbrush, hairbrush, kitchen utensils, and some cleaning equipment. She also wrapped juice and milk cartons and other cooking and bathroom supplies so she could better hold onto them.

While these biomechanically-guided interventions provided a measure of control over symptoms and compensation for limitations, Sally's therapist also recognized that Sally would need to use both process skills and communication and interaction skills (i.e., asking for help) to compensate for motor skill decrements. Consequently, Sally and her therapist collaborated together to identify which of her daily routines needed examination of how she did them and what objects she used. The Activity Record, in which she recorded her level of pain in each activity, was very helpful for this purpose. They singled out a number of troublesome spots in Sally's routine and together explored how the occupational forms she was having trouble with could be reorganized to be more manageable. Once the appropriate mix of skills for successful completion of an occupational form was identified, Sally focused on practicing it, so as to establish the way of performing as a habit.

Because Sally's symptoms were variable, she also needed to have the ability to deal with its variability. Consequently, Sally enrolled in a joint protection and energy conservation program. This program provided information on the disease process and offered Sally opportunities to learn how to do an activity analysis to preplan how to undertake a task and how to stop and reflect on alternatives when she found herself in trouble. In this way she could adjust her performance when she had more pain or other limitations. Moreover, by being in a group with others who were coping with similar problems, she received both encouragement and helpful suggestions.

After Sally had begun to experience more control by incorporating new objects and new habits for accomplishing particular occupational forms, the next step was to look at her habits of routine. Since choosing a new routine is an occupational choice requiring active volition, she and her therapist began to explore some issues concerning her values and her interests.

Having been taught the model of human occupation in a very basic way, Sally could see the interrelationship of her performance, habits, roles, values, interests, and personal causation. She recognized that she had already developed an increased sense of efficacy and that her awareness of her limitations was not so overwhelming if she felt she could compensate for them. She came to see how exercising more control over symptoms and maximizing her function would give her more discretionary time. She also saw how her occupational and activity choices, while they were affected by her strong values, were leading her into a lifestyle with little for herself (i.e., little enjoyment or satisfaction and little sense of personal causation). She was able to identify, with her therapist's assistance, how this contributed to her being more limited in what she gave her family. She came to see that if she was more satisfied and optimistic she would have more to offer her family. She also allowed herself to recognize that, with all her losses, she needed to devote the same attention to figuring out how she could recapture some interest in her life. As Sally engaged in this volitional process of reflecting and anticipating, she was increasingly able to make activity and occupational choices that enhanced the quality of her everyday routines.

Sally began to explore some old interests in therapy to see if she could adapt them and still enjoy them. She also began to try out new things. Eventually, using the Activity Record as a guide, she was able to restructure her routine to incorporate some interests and to give herself more sense of efficacy while still undertaking the things that were most important for her family.

When Sally was terminated from outpatient therapy she had accomplished a number of notable changes. Sally had seriously responded to the feedback concerning her imbalance of values, and her lack of enjoyment or feelings of competence. She was able to identify that, in many ways, she was quite competent in managing her arthritic condition and while still maintaining major life roles. Sally also identified that she had gone into teaching because of family pressures and the lack of a clear occupational choice on her own part. She recognized that her true interests were in the areas of science and health care and began exploring opportunities for education and volunteer work related to her medical interests.

Through the group classes in joint protection, energy conservation, and time management, Sally improved her ability to analyze and plan her daily activities and to carry them out so as to minimize her pain and maximize her functional ability. Some of the changes in Sally's life were reflected when she completed the Activity Record for a second time at discharge. As Figure 14.18 shows, Sally increased interest, value, and feelings of competence in her everyday occupational behavior. She also increased the amount of time she spent in leisure and in role-related activities.

When Sally was preparing for discharge from the program and discussing her progress with her therapist, she identified the following as important to her. First, Sally felt that she had learned in therapy how to give herself permission to enjoy life. Previously, she had been so dominated by feelings that she could not adequately respond to others' needs (especially her family) and she could not allow herself opportunity to seek enjoyment. This added to her sense that life was out of her control. By reclaiming her right to find satisfaction in her occupational behavior, she not only increased enjoyment in her life, but also took control of it again. A second major area of concern for Sally had been her general anxiety over being out of control, which was reflected in her everyday routines. By reorganizing her habits, Sally was much more able to meet role demands, address her own leisure and role needs, and control her pain. According to Sally, her life felt like it was back in control and had a degree of order which she needed. Finally, Sally was able to begin making a further story for herself. Feeling that life was back under control and having identified her own saga of loss of function and of valued and enjoyable activities, she had begun to make her life her own again and to see the future with a sense of hope. At the time of discharge, she had not made final plans, but was actively exploring alternative scenarios for her future life story.

CONCLUSION

This chapter presented eleven cases that illustrate the application of the model of human occupation. By now the reader should recognize that using the model means being able to flexibly apply theoretical concepts in ways that make the most sense as the course of intervention unfolds. There is no standard way to operationalize theory into practice; the process always depends on the therapist's judgement as guided by theory. For this reason, each of the cases presented in this chapter should also be recognized as reflecting the therapist's unique style and way of using the model of human occupation.

This chapter should, therefore, be an invitation to those who want to use the model to make it their own. This does not mean that therapists should readily pick and choose concepts or impart their own meaning to concepts that the book has taken pains to define and illustrate. However, this does mean that therapists who wish to use the model must have knowledge of the concepts such that they become a particular way of seeing the patient or client. It further means that the therapist must be able to move between the concepts and the person receiving therapy, being the final arbiter of how a theory is best applied to each individual.

References

Fisher, A. G. (1993). The assessment of IADL motor skills: An application of many-faceted Rasch analysis. *American Journal of Occupational Therapy, 47,* 319–329.

Fisher, A. G. (1994). *Assessment of Motor and Process Skills* (Version 8.0). Unpublished test manual. Department of Occupational Therapy, Colorado State University, Fort Collins.

Fisher, A., Murray, E., & Bundy, A. (1991). *Sensory integration: Theory and practice*. Philadelphia: FA Davis.

Helfrich, C., & Kielhofner, G. (1994). Volitional narratives and the meaning of therapy. *American Journal of Occupational Therapy, 48,* 319–326.

Kielhofner, G. (1992). *Conceptual foundations of occupational therapy*. Philadelphia: FA Davis.

Kielhofner, G., & Fisher, A. (1991). Mind-brain relationships. In A. Fisher, E. Murray, & A. Bundy (Eds.), *Sensory integration: Theory and practice*. Philadelphia: FA Davis.

Nelson, D. (1988). Occupation: Form and performance. *American Journal of Occupational Therapy, 42,* 633–641.

Reid, D. W., & Ware, E. E. (1974). Multidimensionality of internal versus external control: Addition of a third dimension and nondistinction of self versus others. *Canadian Journal of Occupation Behavioral Science, 6,* 132–142.

Trombly, C. A. (Ed.) (1989). *Occupational Therapy for Physical Dysfunction* (3rd ed.). Baltimore: Williams & Wilkins.

15/ Program Development

Jaime Phillip Muñoz and Gary Kielhofner

INTRODUCTION

Like most experienced occupational therapists, we can think of more than a few times we have been involved in program development. These experiences highlight creative innovation, pragmatic restructuring, and regrouping after drastic and devastating change. Each experience has had some trials and some triumphs. The following two scenarios drawn from our experience at the University of Illinois at Chicago (UIC) exemplify some of the kinds of program development challenges which therapists face.

The first scenario involves improving occupational therapy services in an already established program. The process began when an interdisciplinary psychiatric team decided to review the total milieu activity program on an inpatient unit in a state hospital. Recent history in the hospital had been chaotic. Amid controversy, the university announced closing of the entire hospital. Within months, local and state politics reversed the decision to close the hospital, but in the meantime many units were left in disarray, with very low morale, and with the loss of many staff members who fled to more secure workplaces.

In the acute psychiatry unit, the staff had treaded water and regularly shared concerns about the uncertain and shifting plans for the hospital. In the midst of frustration and uncertainty, the staff became increasingly introspective about the worth of their services and decided to be proactive in planning. Thus began the interdisciplinary team review of the ward milieu. At this time, the psychiatric occupational therapy team approached the interdisciplinary team with a proposal that they lead the process of reviewing all of the milieu activities that were offered on the unit. An interdisciplinary committee was formed with members from occupational therapy, nursing, pharmacy, social work, medicine, and recreation. The committee, named the Milieu Activity Planning (MAP) Committee, was chaired by the first author. Eventually this committee outlined a conceptualization of and a plan for all group interventions which were based on the model of human occupation.

The second scenario involves developing a totally new and innovative program for a population that had been underserved. It began when interdisciplinary physical rehabilitation staff repeatedly voiced concern that no services existed for clients who had some vocational potential but were not yet ready for vocational training programs sponsored by the state's Department of Rehabilitation Services. In this case, we both worked at different stages consulting with the interdisciplinary team to develop an outpatient Work Readiness Program based on the model of human occupation. Initially offered under the rubric of rehabilitation services and targeting persons referred from physical rehabilitation, the program evolved to be administered by the occupational therapy department and to serve a diverse group of clients referred from a variety of sites in the hospital and the larger community.

As we proceed to discuss the process of program development we will return to these two examples to describe and discuss what happened as we and others[a] worked to develop the programs. These two examples represent only a small part of a much larger range of programs that have been developed using the model of human occupation. To supplement our examples, the reader will find an appendix to this chapter consisting of a bibliography of articles describing the use of the model in a range of programs.

NATURE OF PROGRAM DEVELOPMENT

Whether precipitated by client need, organizational change, or logistical forces, program development involves designing and implementing services that best meet the needs of a particular group of clients. As such, program development is concerned with a collectivity of persons with common problems rather than with a particular individual. As we have alluded to earlier, program development can be directed at creating new services or at reviewing and modifying established programs.

Program development is a continual process that ordinarily involves planning, implementing, evaluating, and revising the program. Moreover, program development can occur at many levels. It can be directed at a particular aspect of a program (e.g., home health services in the context of a rehabilitation continuum), at several services within a comprehensive larger program (e.g., all services offered within the psychiatry unit), or to the total range of services offered in an institution (e.g., occupational therapy services offered at a community satellite hospital).

Program development may take on somewhat different forms depending on the targeted clients and their needs, the treatment setting and its organizational culture, and the composition of the interdisciplinary team. As such, each practice setting presents a unique constellation of program development challenges for the practitioner.

Program development strategies are variously referred to as managerial planning, strategic planning, facility planning, program analysis and program evaluation, to name a few (Leiter, 1992; Ostrow, 1992; Pickett & Hanlon, 1990; Schammahorn, 1992). Regardless of the terminology and emphasis, program development strategies share one common element: a commitment to make decisions about the future.

Program Development as an Art

We refer to program development as an art because the multidimensional problems faced by practitioners require creative and resourceful solutions which must sometimes be rendered with lightning speed and sensitive diplomacy. While we can specify certain phases and tasks involved, actual program development is never a neat application of these. Moreover, it requires sensitivity to clients' needs and to the unique context in which the program resides. Consequently, while we provide a general structure for the program development process, it is not a blueprint or recipe.[b] The art is in translating principles into the real life contexts of program development.

Role of the Model of Human Occupation in Program Development

When developing a program which will involve groups of people, program decisions must be made explicit. In the context of managed health care and ever increasing competition for health care dollars, the demand for clear explanation and organization of occupational therapy services is intensifying. Therapists must be able to explain what problems they address, how services address the problems, why services are expected to work, what

---

[a]A number of persons worked on each of these programs and contributed to development of some of the materials we included in this chapter. They are Linda Olson, Carol Knight, Gail Fisher, and Trudy Mallinson.

[b]For the interested practitioner, there are useful resources available that can provide more details regarding the tasks involved in program development or which offer models for conceptualizing this problem solving and planning process that go beyond the scope of this chapter (Bair & Gray, 1992; Cole & Lucas, 1979; Green, 1992; Kaplan, 1988; Robertson 1986).

outcomes they are expected to yield, and what services will cost. To do so, therapists must have a well-defined conceptual means of identifying problems, means, and goals.

By using a conceptual model therapists can frame the clients' problems, identify and justify specific strategies for data gathering and service provision, and specify expected outcomes. A model is the therapist's tool for thinking about these and other aspects of a program. In our experience, the model of human occupation provides an effective conceptual tool for articulating and organizing occupational therapy services and for addressing the what, why, and how of a service program.

PRINCIPLES OF PROGRAM DEVELOPMENT DERIVED FROM THE MODEL

Throughout this chapter, we will illustrate how practitioners can utilize the model in program development. Our first considerations are the general principles we have derived from the model, which we feel should infuse the entire process of program development.

As discussed in Chapter 2, the model of human occupation explains the dynamics of occupational function, dysfunction, and change as a dynamic systems process. At the core of this dynamic process is the action in which the individual engages and through which the systems' organization is maintained and changed. When dysfunction exists, action in occupations is the means by which individuals realize, regain, or maintain an adaptive interaction with the environment. This focus on the dynamic system process can be further elaborated as four program development principles.

Principle One: Promoting Self-Organization

Persons organize their mind-brain-body performance, habituation, and volition subsystems interdependently as they interact with the environment in their daily occupations. Therefore, the first principle is that *occupational therapy programs should offer services which promote self-organization by providing a means whereby the individuals can per-*

form, reflect on, organize, and change their occupational behavior. The principle of self-organization requires that a program should address all aspects of the human open system and provide opportunities for changes to occur in persons' ability to perform, in their ability to make occupational and activity choices, in their roles and habits, and in their relationships with their occupational behavior settings.

Principle Two: Using Occupational Forms as the Context for Change

The second principle of program development is that *occupational forms are the medium through which individuals are therapeutically assisted to engage in the process of self-maintenance and self-change.* The use of occupations as opportunities for persons to seek well-being is what makes the program uniquely an occupational therapy program. Therefore, the services provided within an occupational therapy program should offer clients numerous opportunities to engage in personally and culturally appropriate occupational forms.

Principle Three: Using the Environment as the Context for Assembling Occupations

An individual's current and expected occupational behavior settings play a significant role in influencing present and future occupational performance. Therefore, the third principle is that *occupational therapy programs should provide or choose social and physical environments that offer consistent and relevant expectations and opportunities for performance.* One's occupational life is both directed at and highly influenced by the individual's relationship and interaction with the environment. The model argues an environment can afford opportunities and/or press for behavior and that environmental changes can influence the individual to consider more adaptive choices. A program planner must not only be intimately aware of clients' homes and community environment, but also must plan the characteristics of the occupational therapy program environment to elicit optimal occupational performances from the clients.

Principle Four: Intervening Across a Functional Continuum

Persons exhibit degrees of adaptive or maladaptive occupational functioning. While individual differences do exist, the practitioner must direct program development at typical levels of functioning of the targeted population. The fourth principle is that *programs should reflect the level of function which can be expected and elicited from program participants.*

In implementing this principle, occupational functioning can be thought of as a continuum ranging from exploration to achievement (Figure 15.1). Exploration is the least demanding, while achievement is the most demanding level of performance. Persons' ability to meet the demands of these levels of performance determine what kind of occupational challenge should be reflected in the program.

The exploration–competence–achievement continuum can also be viewed as a pathway for organizing any new occupational behavior. That is, people typically progress through these levels of function when they move into new roles, encounter new environments, or make drastic lifestyle changes. The functional levels can be used to organize program interventions both by specifying the expected occupational performance within a part of the program and by specifying a sequence of expectations clients will encounter as they progress through the program. We can see how this is so by examining these three levels and their use in program development in more detail.

The highest level of occupational functioning is the *achievement level* which represents the fullest mastery over one's self and the environment. Persons function at the achievement level when they strive to maintain and enhance their performance in occupational roles where standards of performance and excellence are identifiable. Persons operate at this level when they have developed sufficient skills and habits which allow them to control their

own performance and have an intended impact in the environment.

Programs directed at the achievement end of the function continuum are directed towards clients with generally adequate skills, who can assume responsibility for choosing how they use their time and often demonstrate some daily routines. Such clients' main problem areas are related to their overall life pattern. For example, they may be unable to consistently integrate skills and routines into occupational roles which are productive and satisfying to them. Facilitating such patients to integrate skills and habits into successful role behavior thus becomes a focus for program development.

Persons operate at a *competence level* of functioning when they strive to be adequate to the demands of a situation by improving themselves or adjusting to environmental demands and expectations. Individuals at a competence level of functioning focus on attaining, improving, and organizing skills into habits that allow consistent, adequate performance (Reilly, 1974; White, 1971). This process of striving for competence leads to the development of new skills, the refinement of old skills, and the organization of these skills into habits that support occupational performance.

Competency affords an individual a growing sense of personal control. As persons strive to organize their performances into routines of competent behavior that are relevant to their environment, they immerse themselves in a process of becoming, growing, and arriving at a greater sense of personal mastery.

Persons attempting to function at this level may present with an inability to adequately maintain role performance or they may have a habit pattern that is significantly disrupted. These persons may have vague and unrealistic goals and may be experiencing a major reduction in their sense of personal control. Such individuals often lack everyday habit patterns that allow them to integrate their skills with their stated values and goals. They often need

Exploration   Competence   Achievement

<-->

Figure 15.1.   Levels of occupational function.

to add new skills to their repertoire. The focus of program development is to create services that will encourage the clients to develop routines and normal standards of performance through involvement in a variety of occupations occurring both in institutional and community settings.

Exploration requires a safe and nurturing environment. Exploratory behavior provides persons with opportunities to learn and to express their abilities with no objective or performance standard. Exploration is a necessary frame for therapeutic intervention for persons who present with total or near total disruption of their occupational performance. These individuals often demonstrate skills and habits that are so disrupted that competent performance is minimal or absent. Such persons may become alienated from their own values, their sense of self may become fragmented or fragile, and their future may be obscure or full of foreboding.

Persons functioning at this lowest level tend to lack productive roles, do not typically maintain a routine of balanced self-care, productive, and leisure activities; their basic mind-brain-body performance skills are severely limited. The occupational therapy program would be designed to encourage these individuals to explore their physical and social environments and to provide opportunities to acquire basic skills. The practitioner takes a directive role in such a program, providing appropriate choices for occupations and managing the environment to support exploration and learning (Kaplan, 1988).

By identifying the levels of function and dysfunction in the targeted group and by specifying the desired levels of function as an outcome of occupational therapy services, practitioners can better identify what kinds of reorganization may be required and what types of services may produce the intended outcome.

PROGRAM DEVELOPMENT SPIRAL

We conceptualize program development as a spiral to emphasize that program development is an ongoing process (Figure 15.2). Imbedded in the spiral are four phases of program development: situation analysis, goal setting, development, and implementation and evaluation. Each phase, in turn, involves a number of particular tasks. The program development process is a dynamic one in which planning may require movement both up and down the spiral among the phases of program development and in which progress in several tasks of program development can occur simultaneously. The choice of when to do the phases and the tasks within them will be dictated by many factors. These include the scope of the program development, the resources available, and the politics of change in a particular setting.

Concepts of the model of human occupation are woven into this cycle of program development guiding the practitioner's therapeutic reasoning and decision making in each phase. Each phase requires both data collection and decision making. At each stage, a therapist can generate conceptual questions derived from the model to guide the data collection. The answers to these questions along with the four principles derived from the model influence the decisions made about the program. Effective program development involves the implementation of each of these phases with careful attention to how the constructs of the theory and the principles guide that implementation.

PHASE ONE: SITUATION ANALYSIS

This first phase of program development requires that practitioners improve their understanding of the circumstances in which the program is to be implemented. This entails looking beyond the occupational therapy service component of the program to appreciate the broader context within which the occupational therapy program occurs. Situation analysis involves two interrelated tasks: (a) determining the treatment program context; and (b) describing the needs of the targeted population.

Determining the Treatment Program Context

In order to complete the first task, the practitioner must collect and synthesize data about

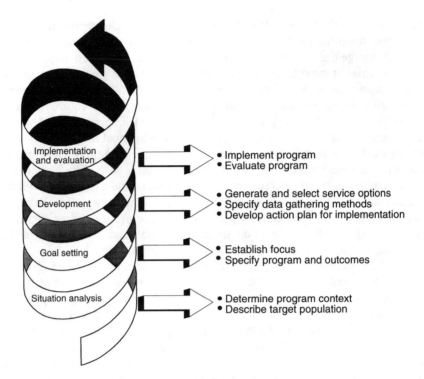

Figure 15.2.   Program development spiral.

the context in which treatment is provided and about the target population. A thorough examination of the qualities of the treatment setting serves to identify unused opportunities, potential barriers, service overlaps, or mismatches between occupational therapy as envisioned by the model of human occupation and the focus of other health services offered at the setting. An understanding of occupational therapy's relationship with other disciplines and the prevailing political culture may help avoid missteps, identify potential allies and adversaries, and suggest timing efforts for program change when support for success is at its zenith. The following questions offer a framework for collecting and organizing these data.

- What is the mission of the facility?
- What are the current priorities reflected in the facility's strategic plan and/or organizational decisions?
- What is the prevailing political climate in the facility?
- What is the current configuration of services in the program?

- What types of resources (budget, space) are available?
- What are the current and projected community, population, or service trends that can affect service delivery to the targeted population?
- What physical, social, cultural, and economic factors exist in the community that are relevant to the program development process?
- What is the fit between the context and the general vision of intervention provided by the model of human occupation?

Describe the Needs of the Targeted Population

The second task associated with this phase of program development focuses on helping the practitioner develop a clear understanding of the typical kinds of occupational behavior and dysfunctions presented in the target population. The subsystems of the model of human occupation and their various components suggest the following kinds of questions:

• What are sociodemographic characteristics of the population (e.g., age, sex, primary medical diagnoses, family structure, religious and ethnic background, education, income, and employment level)?
• How do members of the population typically view their current and potential abilities?
• How do the members of the population view their ability to control themselves and their life outcomes?
• What are the values typically held by the population and how do these influence their situations?
• What interests do members of the population prefer and experience pleasure in?
• How do members of the population organize their use of time?
• Which occupational forms do the population routinely engage in?
• Which roles characterize members of the population?
• What particular mind or body conditions/experiences typically interfere with performance?
• How does the population's environment influence their occupational performances?
• What dynamic processes are typically seen in the population?

Therapists use questions such as these to guide the collection of data. The therapist gathers and uses all available information to answer the questions and, therefore, to draw some general conclusions about the target population as a whole. In this way, a therapist can use the model to generate comprehensive knowledge of the occupational behavior and dysfunctions of the population.

Summary

Overall, the situation analysis requires the therapist to collect data about and document the context in which occupational therapy services will be delivered as well as the population for whom the services are being developed. When well documented, a situational analysis forms the basis for planning decisions and further analyses. When appropriate, interdisciplinary staff should be involved in this phase. Such involvement can elicit more cooperation with and better understanding of the occupational therapy service plan.

EXAMPLES OF PHASE ONE

Revision of Inpatient Groups

We noted earlier that the impetus for improving occupational therapy services in the inpatient psychiatric program was the uncertain future of the entire university hospital. While the plan for closing the hospital was reversed, units throughout the hospital were downsized or closed to bring the hospital into a state of fiscal viability. The increased intense scrutiny of all services underscored the need to proactively review, improve, and justify services. The Milieu Activity Planning (MAP) committee, led by the first author, initiated the first task of situation analysis, determining the program context. The team decided to approach this initial task by developing a clear mission statement for milieu activities on the unit. Given the overall situation in the hospital the MAP Committee felt it was important to have a clear vision of the role of inpatient psychiatric services in a contemporary comprehensive teaching hospital. The ability to create a therapeutic milieu was identified as a unique feature of such services. Therefore, the MAP Committee searched the literature and discussed the function of the unit milieu in an interdisciplinary journal club with an aim of conceptualizing what was best practice in maintaining a therapeutic milieu. As this vision unfolded, the MAP Committee drafted a mission statement and periodically discussed it with the entire interdisciplinary team, eventually achieving consensus on a unit milieu mission statement (Figure 15.3).

A review of sociodemographic records on the patient population reflected the urban mission of the hospital. The average length of stay was 12.7 days. The population was multiculturally diverse; persons of minority background made up a high proportion of all admissions; and, overall education, employment, and income levels were low. The unit primarily treated people suffering from schizophrenia and other psychotic disorders, mood disorders, and substance-related disorders. The MAP committee led the interdisciplinary staff in reviewing how well the current milieu met the needs of this client population. In order to establish more clearly the strengths and weak-

The mission of the psychiatry unit is to assist people experiencing emotional or psychological problems to develop strategies to maintain their mental health and wellness and to enable them to gain independence and satisfaction in their everyday life. The staff of the psychiatry unit is committed to creating a therapeutic milieu which offers coordinated services from a variety of disciplines including medicine, nursing, occupational therapy, pharmacy, social work, recreation and art therapy.

A major aspect of the milieu program is the group programming created by the interdisciplinary staff. This group activity program is carried out in the context of the following convictions: Containment, support and structure are equally valued as therapeutic factors; these components are viewed as interdependent and mutually enhancing aspects of the milieu program and they provide a basis for change; therapeutic change in the individual is best accomplished by involving the person in individual and group activities which challenge the individual to function at their optimal level.

The psychiatric unit's mission will be realized through the accomplishment of the following three strategic objectives:

1) To provide individualized milieu activity programming for each person admitted to the psychiatry unit.
2) To create a system that facilitates coherent, consistent and integrated milieu planning across disciplines.
3) To develop, deliver and validate exemplary clinical services at the group level.

Figure 15.3.   Milieu activity program: Mission Statement.

nesses of the current milieu programming, each staff member who led groups on the unit was asked to fill out a group review form designed to capture data about current group-based services, their nature, and their purpose. The data from this review was synthesized and discussed in MAP meetings and during interdisciplinary staff meetings. Discussions focused on the current configuration of group services, admission and discharge trends in the client population, the clinical needs of the population, trends in the type of problems typically presented in the treatment population, program strengths, and service gaps.

In this interdisciplinary process, the occupational therapy staff was outspoken both in critiquing its own and other group interventions and in defining the problems and needs of the treatment population. Therapists used the concepts and language of the model of human occupation, framing the client's needs in terms of volition, habituation, performance, and environmental factors. In their own staff meetings, the occupational therapy staff reviewed past assessment records to identify patterns in problems of occupational functioning that the clients presented. The results of this review are shown in Figure 15.4.

In contrast to occupational therapy, interdisciplinary discussions were bogged down in

whether particular groups should be included or eliminated or on what types of groups should be added. Since the team was unable to reach consensus, the occupational therapy supervisor who chaired the MAP committee suggested that the problem was a lack of an overall vision or structure for the organization of milieu activity programming. The model of human occupation was suggested as a potential means of systematically thinking about how to organize group programming. It was agreed that the occupational therapist would conduct an inservice training on the model for the interdisciplinary staff so that the entire staff could judge the merits of using this model to organize group interventions on the unit. Following the inservices, the group attempted a critique of the milieu programs using the exploration, competence, and achievement continuum of function as an organizing backdrop. Group leaders and other staff were asked to place their groups on the continuum of exploration to achievement based on the population they treated in the group and/or the modalities they employed in the group. The results, illustrated in Figure 15.5, revealed to the staff how most groups were inappropriately attempting to service the needs of clients who were functioning at very different levels. This exercise also helped seal

Mind-Brain-Body Performance Subsystem
- Presence of symptoms (e.g., hallucinations, diminished cognition, depression) interfering with potential for performance
- Side effects of medication

Performance Skills
- Decreased communication and interaction skills and process skills

Habituation Subsystem
- Inability to organize and maintain an adaptive daily routine
- Breakdown in ability to habitually organize activities of daily living and home management activities
- Inability to independently maintain a satisfying routine of work, leisure, self maintenance, and rest activities
- Problems with role identification and poor role scripts

Volitional Subsystem
- Decreased ability to define and follow through with realistic action plans for personal goals
- Diminished hope for the future; lack of a future story to motivate action
- Lack of adaptive activity and occupational choices for participation in daily living tasks, leisure, and productive occupations

Environment
- Inaccessibility of community resources
- Lack of, or constricted, social support network
- Decreased personal/financial resources for housing, food and transportation

Figure 15.4. Patient's major problems in occupational functioning.

the interdisciplinary decision to use the model of human occupation as the structure to reorganize group interventions. The interdisciplinary staff felt the model offered a view of intervention that accommodated the needs of the unit's client populations. Thus, in this case, the model was not only useful for a situation analysis of the occupational therapy services, but enabled the entire interdisciplinary team to engage in this first phase of program development.

Work Readiness Program

As previously stated, the Work Readiness Program represents the use of the model to create an innovative new program in the area of vocational rehabilitation. The program was developed in response to follow-up data collected on clients discharged from the inpatient rehabilitation unit. These data showed that very few patients had followed through with discharge recommendations regarding vocational testing, training, and placement. The interdisciplinary rehabilitation team began discussing programming options to address this perceived gap in services. There were several factors that influenced the treatment program context. The hospital administration was open and supportive to the creation of new revenue-generating programs, staff from occupational therapy, physical therapy, speech, and nursing had expressed strong personal commitment to the concept of this new program, and two academic faculty members with expertise in worker rehabilitation programs consulted and collaborated with the rehabilitation staff on this program development project. These faculty members assumed a leadership role in examining the characteristics of the client group and the facility's ability to support the development of a work readiness program.

The interdisciplinary composition of the team represented a rich resource to be utilized and one of the most pressing challenges proved to be creating a shared vision of the program that melded the divergent views of the various disciplines involved. To facilitate this process, former patients, rehabilitation staff, and physicians were interviewed regarding their views of

	Exploration	Competence	Achievement
Interdisciplinary			
Psychotherapy Group	X	X	X
Multi-Family Group	X	X	X
Community Meeting	X	X	X
Art Therapy Group	X	X	X
Nursing			
Social Skills Group	X	X	X
Orientation Group	X	X	
Men's Group	X	X	X
Women's Group		X	X
Maternal/O.B. Group	X	X	
Occupational Therapy			
Workshop Group		X	
Directive Group	X		
Sensorcize Group	X	X	
Take-A-Look Group		X	
Cooking Group		X	
Recreation			
Gym Group	X	X	X
Community Field Trip	X	X	X
Off-Unit Recreation	X	X	X
Bingo Group	X	X	X

Figure 15.5. Using the model of human occupation functional continuum to critique milieu activity groups.

the characteristics of the population and the needs for such a program. Additionally, contact with a liaison from the Illinois Department of Rehabilitation Services was established to determine the department's view of unmet needs and to determine the types of services that were funded by the department.

Initially, the interdisciplinary team created a working mission statement for the program that was broad in focus; i.e., "to prepare the client for participation in a self-chosen, productive life role." The client population for the program was originally persons with chronic physical or cognitive deficits who were referred from the physical medicine units of the hospital. Using the model of human occupa-

tion as a framework, a comprehensive picture of the target population's occupational dysfunction was compiled (see first column of Figure 15.6).

Phase one was revisited about two years after the program began. This occurred for several reasons. First, there were fewer clients in the program than originally anticipated. Second, the interdisciplinary commitment to the program had waned under the strain of increased productivity standards (e.g., there was no way for all the participatory units to get credit for their contributions). Third, the revenue generation of the program appeared to fall short of administrative expectations. Fourth, the chief of a medical service declared

Typical Occupational Dysfunction in Chronically Disabled Persons	Patient Goals	Program Strategies for Work Readiness
VOLITION		
Personal Causation		
Lack of awareness of personal skills	Increase awareness of skills and deficits	Participate in activities and exercises which will increase awareness of skills and deficits and allow for prioritization of necessary skill development.
Poor sense of efficacy	Increase sense of efficacy	Provide activities and exercises to aid self-identification of intact skills which can serve as a source of competence; plan and support successful participation in activities of increasing complexity.
Anxiety in performance situations	Decrease feelings of anxiety around task performance	Provide opportunity to attempt interesting, realistic activities which have a high probability of success.
Feelings of lacking control of personal behaviors and/or life events	Increase feelings of control over self and one's life situation	Provide activities to aid identification of past success which can serve as a source of encouragement for future action.
Values		
Inability to identify & prioritize among goals	Identify long and short-term goals for work/leisure/self-care	Provide opportunity for independent and responsible decision-making in choosing activities for participation in the community.
Inability to identify and execute behavior required for goal realization	Identify realistic plans to achieve short-term goals	Provide goal-setting exercises emphasizing identification of short-term, concrete goals; attainment can be ascertained and monitored regularly in program.
Difficulty imagining and working toward a positive future	Build confidence in the future and establish a future plan related to personal productivity	Provide activities to concretely orient to present and future, i.e., self-awareness activities, values clarification, time lines, etc.
Lack of meaning in activities	Identify and initiate/increase participation in meaningful activities	Emphasize concrete reasonable steps to improve daily quality of life through participation in community events and by providing a supportive milieu for problem-solving to aid successful community participation.
Incongruence between personal and societal values and standards	Ability to identify congruent personal and social values and standards	Include values clarification exercises aimed at identifying simple, attainable, personal values. Offer opportunity for developing and/or maintaining skills, habits, and roles necessary to goal attainment.
Interests		
Inability to identify interests in the areas of work and leisure	Identify and pursue new work and leisure interests	Offer opportunities to explore and generate new interests that realistically reflect socioeconomic and environmental constraints and to stimulate old interests through activities in the program and through planning community experiences.

Figure 15.6. Work readiness program: Client's occupational dysfunction, program goals, and program strategies.

353

Figure 15.6. *continued*

Lack of interests or increased participation in passive interests	Identify interest opportunities to act on these in the community	Skills for leisure planning will be taught and practiced; clients will be assisted in identifying community resources for pursuit of interests.
HABITUATION		
Roles		
Chronic lack of major productive occupational role	Increase abilities to perform in chosen role; strengthen role identification	Graded individual or small group activities will be used for skill development necessary for assumption of and success in identified roles.
Decreased social supports which impair role performance and/or role conflict	Identify positive, realistic social supports	Program will provide positive support through encouragement. Provide opportunity to explore appropriate occupational roles.
Poor role scripts (i.e., awareness of responsibilities associated with success in various roles)	Identify responsibilities associated with various roles	Participation in various activities including role play, paper-and-pencil activities, and discussion to learn and internalize expectations of role performance.
Habits		
Habits do not support performance of roles (i.e., poor hygiene, grooming, punctuality, etc.)	Develop and incorporate habits into daily routine	Opportunities to identify, learn and practice in group and individual settings. Expectations for routine occupational habits will be communicated to all group members.
Inability to organize time into a productive, daily routine	Organize and follow a balanced, daily schedule/routine	Provide opportunities to focus on preparing personal schedules that include a balance of productive and leisure activity and structured time use.
PERFORMANCE SKILLS		
Ineffective motor skills, impairing performance task completion	Improve motor skills necessary to participate in work, leisure, and self care activities; learn compensatory process and/or communication interaction skills	Engage in activities which will allow individual to address motor skill deficits. Use of compensatory skills when necessary for task completion.
Ineffective process skills	Improve process skills	Activities will be provided to engage in client in appropriate activities. As skills improve activities will be graded to provide appropriate challenges. Attention will be given to transferring skills to community situations.
Ineffective communication and interaction skills	Improve communication and interaction skills	Program will provide social skills training using role-play, videotape, and experiential activities to increase individual's awareness of appropriate social interaction. Client will be encouraged to practice these skills in other program groups and in the community.
ENVIRONMENT		
Lack of environmental support and feedback	Identify and increase awareness of environmental resolves	Opportunities will be provided to identify various environmental resources and how to access them.

his intention to take over the space in which the program was located.

At this point, the place of the Work Readiness Program within the hospital, in relation to the academic department of occupational therapy and in relation to client needs, was reassessed. This process reaffirmed that the department viewed the program as an excellent example of nontraditional occupational therapy, that the vocational focus was in line with a work-oriented research and training focus in the department, and that the program was deemed a good example of putting theory into practice. Hence, it became clear that the occupational therapy department had a stronger stake in the program than other disciplines. Following negotiations, the other disciplines agreed to occupational therapy taking over the program. One exception was that the physical therapy department agreed to continue a biomechanical fitness component and the other disciplines agreed to remain available as consultants to the program. Negotiations with hospital administration followed and resulted in a clearer delineation of expectations for the program's productivity and in identification of new space for the program.

A review of the needs of other patient populations in and outside the hospital resulted in a decision to broaden the target population to persons with either physical or psychiatric disabilities. Since the program focused on occupational dysfunction, it was decided that diagnosis was a relatively minor issue and would require little program adjustment. A plan for seeking a broader referral base to include psychiatrists and the mental health professionals inside the university and in the broader community resulted in a solid referral base and a larger, stable client population in the program.

PHASE TWO: GOAL SETTING

The comprehensive description of the current program situation completed in the first phase gives the practitioner necessary information to move on to setting program goals. This second phase of program development involves determining what the occupational therapy program aims to achieve. This phase involves two tasks: (1) establishing the overall focus of the occupational therapy program, and (2) specifying program goals and the intended outcomes of the program. The situational analysis process completed in the first phase should allow therapists to determine what should be the direction, scope, and focus of the program.

Establishing the Focus

The initial task of the goal-setting phase is to establish a clear focus for the program. The focus should define the intended scope of the program. A written focus or mission statement often serves to identify both the target population and the proposed objectives of the services. The following questions help to guide this process:

- What will be the overall scope of the program?
- Does the focus statement clearly define an emphasis on occupational behavior?
- Does the focus statement contain ideas compatible with the theoretical constructs of the model?
- Is the occupational therapy mission compatible with the mission of the hospital or sponsoring organization?

Specifying the Program Goals and Intended Outcomes

Program goals should state the intended outcomes of the program and should serve to clarify what the program desires to achieve. The following questions can be helpful in organizing this process.

- Given the current general level of functioning of the clients, what improvements in function can realistically be expected?
- What theoretical constructs of the model will be used to focus and articulate the purpose of the program?
- What specific outcomes are expected in terms of the population's ability to interact effectively in various environments?
- What measurable outcomes can be defined in terms of assisting clients to find direction and meaning in their lives?

- What new environments will be assessed or created to encourage the development of new habit patterns and role scripts?
- What changes in mind-brain-body performance skills are necessary, achievable, and would support more adaptive occupational functioning?

The goals of the occupational therapy program should be compatible with the goals and objectives of the system in which occupational therapy operates and are specifically related to the focus of the program. Program goals should be generated using theoretical constructs from the model. Goals should also be stated in a manner that allows the practitioner to specify the intended outcome and ascertain the impact of therapeutic interventions. That is, they should paint a clear picture of what the clients will be able to do after participating in the program.

EXAMPLES OF PHASE TWO

Revision of Inpatient Groups

The MAP committee charged each discipline to examine their own needs, constraints, resources, and expectations for group interventions on the unit. Additionally, each discipline was asked to articulate a focus or mission statement that defined the values, goals, and expectations of those interventions. The occupational therapy staff used staff meetings to revisit the overall scope of the occupational therapy services. First, a broad mission statement and program aims were developed (Figure 15.7).

The model of human occupation was used to determine the goals and outcomes of the program. Staff reviewed discharge documentation looking for outcome trends reported in key areas related to the model and identified as problem areas for occupational functioning for the population. For example, a primary deficit in the volitional subsystem was the clients' feelings of inability to manage the problem situations that led to their hospitalizations. These feelings reflected a general belief that they could not control the events of their life stories. Consequently, program goals for the volitional subsystem focused on the clients being able to identify intact skills and define realistic short-term goals and action plans for dealing with the primary stressors that precipitated their hospitalization.

In the habituation subsystem, the clients' problems of role identification and their difficulties in habitually organizing a balanced routine of daily living activities had been noted. Consequently, program goals for the habituation subsystem emphasized increasing skills and habits that supported the maintenance of responsibilities associated with home management and independent community living roles. Developing the ability to independently organize and follow a balanced daily routine was also emphasized in the program goals. Preparation and follow-through of personal schedules was also earmarked as an expected outcome of the program.

Performance skill deficits were wide-ranging and complicated by the presence of disabling acute symptomatology (e.g., depression, mania, withdrawal, hallucinations, and altered cognitive processing). Communication and interaction skills were a particular area of deficit which affected the clients' overall level of adaptive functioning. Program priorities were, therefore, established to increase skills where possible, to teach compensatory strategies when necessary, and to identify environmental adaptations that supported the clients' highest level of adaptive performance. Related to the environment, clients typically had diminished personal, social, and financial resources for housing, food, medication, and transportation, which perpetuated maladaptive functioning. Providing opportunities to improve the clients' awareness of and access to community resources for support and socialization were identified as the top priorities.

Work Readiness Program

As the Work Readiness Program evolved, the interdisciplinary team was able to develop a more unified vision of its intent and scope. The model of human occupation was clearly defined as the conceptual model for organizing the program and the model's holistic view of health and adaptation was clearly reflected in

The Department of Psychiatric Occupational Therapy strives to help each person acquire the skills or make the changes necessary to regain the greatest degree of independence in his or her tasks of everyday living, which include establishing a healthy balance between work, play, self-care and daily living activities. Healthy functioning is promoted and maintained through assessment of the person's occupational functioning and provision of individual and/or group interventions. The department is committed to establishing a model program for service, clinical education and professional development.

Aims:
1. Assess clients in order to determine and disseminate the client's level of occupational functioning.
2. Plan and implement treatment through selected modalities.
3. Educate students and other health professionals about occupational therapy.
4. Contribute to the development of the profession through education and research.

Figure 15.7.   Occupational therapy mission statement and goals.

the program's mission statement. This mission statement evolved along with the program changes. A more holistic view of persons' occupational lives recognized the need for balance and productivity in multiple dimensions of occupational functioning in order to support a vocational role. It also came to reflect the more inclusive target population. The mission statement which evolved was eventually designed to be part of a program brochure used to solicit referrals and explain the program to professionals, families, and other constituents (see Figure 15.8).

The planning process continued with a collaborative interdisciplinary process to formulate program goals, define roles and responsibilities of the team members, delineate constructs of the model and how they would be used to define the program services, and define potential outcomes.

During this stage, the faculty consultants spent time educating the other professionals about the model of human occupation. Interdisciplinary staff were provided inservices that helped them understand the occupational dysfunctions of potential Work Readiness clients in terms of breakdowns in volition, habituation, and mind-brain-body performance subsystems.

Intervention methods using the principle of programming across a functional continuum were also discussed. This principle was first made operational in the early decision to divide the Work Readiness Program into two

phases. Phase one was directed at exploration of the client's vocational interests and the development of basic skills that support a worker role. Phase two was designed to support the development of competence: clients were to be expected to demonstrate competent skills, habits, and attitudes in an ever-widening variety of hospital and community environments. Eventually, the program was further refined to include three phases. Phase one remained an exploratory phase and phase two continued to correspond to the competency level of occupational functioning. A volunteer component was added to phase two to allow opportunities for the clients to build competence by involving them in hospital and community volunteer positions where the client could continue to practice work skills and build self-confidence in his or her abilities. A third phase, correlated to the achievement level of the functional continuum, was added to the program. Clients at this level were participating at least part-time in school, training programs, workshop settings, volunteer, or competitive employment. During this phase, the Work Readiness services were supportive and consultative in nature. The occupational therapist collaborated with the client, team, or outside agencies and periodically offered follow-up calls and reunions of staff and clients to provide support and celebrate milestones. These three phases were integral to the program's identity and, consequently, were also included in the work readiness brochure (Figure 15.8).

Mission

This interdisciplinary outpatient rehabilitation program is designed to assist physically and psychiatrically disabled clients to achieve a vocational role. The program helps the client re-establish a pattern of daily activity that supports wellness. Intervention is directed at aerobic fitness, participation in satisfying leisure activity, appropriate control of daily habits, development of work skills, realistic goal setting, and planning for goal attainment.

This is not a traditional medical treatment program, nor a work-hardening program, but a therapeutic wellness program that facilitates the integration of modified habits and skills to enable the client to resume or enter a worker role. The program is a clinical application of the Model of Human Occupation, a conceptual model of practice developed and researched at the University of Chicago, Department of Occupational Therapy.

Program Description

Clients attend the program up to five days a week. Clients participate in group and individual sessions. These sessions are designed to assist clients in making the transition from a patient role to their selected life roles. The program is presented in three phases that are differentiated by the intensity of therapy.

Phase I

This phase consists of six weeks of individual and/or group sessions that are designed to assist the client to:
- Develop work skills and daily habits to support a vocational role
- Develop physical fitness appropriate to selected new life roles

Phase II

During phase II, volunteer activities are incorporated into the client's schedule. Supervision, structure and task selection are graded depending on the client's demonstrated skills and habits.

Phase III

In this phase, a case manager monitors a client's progress as the client participates in school, training, volunteer or competitive employment.

Referral Criteria

Clients are selected based on the following:
- Are between the ages of 18–55 years old
- Present with a chronic disabling condition
- State a strong intention to resume a productive role
- State a commitment to full participation and regular attendance in the program

Figure 15.8.   Contents of the program brochure for the work readiness program.

PHASE THREE: DEVELOPMENT

The next phase in the program development cycle is developing the program to meet the goals delineated in the goal-setting phase. In this phase the groundwork that has already been completed is translated into a viable program plan. The type and variety of evaluations to be performed, occupations to be used, and resources and staffing required are all specified so as to form the basis of the program. The completion of the development phase requires the completion of three interrelated tasks: (a) appraise options and select the most effective interventions; (b) specify data-gathering tools and methods; and (c) develop an action plan for implementation.

Generate Service Options and Select Preferred Options

Before embarking on a process of defining what will be the program, the development phase of program development should begin with discussions of what could be. The model of human occupation is used as a framework to generate program ideas and to identify interventions that will be used to address the occupational dysfunctions defined in previous phases of the program development process.

The following are examples of questions helpful to consider:

- What services, from the perspective of the model, could or should occupational therapy offer that would be a useful complement to the setting?
- What specific services would address disruptions in the mind-brain-body performance subsystem?
- What specific services would address disruptions in the habituation subsystem?
- What specific services would address disruptions in the volition subsystem?
- What specific services would address disruptions in environmental interactions?
- What services will be offered and at what level?

The task of appraising options for occupational therapy services requires that practitioners actively imagine program possibilities. This imagining process is used to generate multiple options for achieving the goals of the occupational therapy program that have been defined in the previous phase. Review of literature, visiting other programs, and discussion with therapists in other settings are but some of the means which can help to stimulate creative thought about what the program could be. To complete this task, practitioners also need to creatively consider how they will use occupations as the centerpiece of therapy. This will require exploration of the kinds of occupations which are culturally relevant and meaningful for the target population. It is important to approach this task with an open mind and idealism so as to allow a wide variety of creative ideas to emerge.

Next, the idealistic vision of possibilities must be reduced to a reasonable plan that bears in mind the constraints of the setting and the best practice for addressing the problems faced by the program population. Components of the planned program should be appraised for their potential contribution to program goals, the resources they require, and their efficiency in meeting the client's needs. Realistically, this task of program development means making choices about which needs of the population will be met and which needs cannot be addressed. Matching occupational

therapy services to the needs of clients is the core task of program development. At the completion of this task a decision is made on a set of preferred options or a combination of approaches to be used in the occupational therapy program.

Specify Data-Gathering Tools and Methods

Protocols for data gathering, including all instruments that could be used and the overall data-gathering procedure that will be completed on each client, also need to be established. While it is not always possible or desirable to assess each client in exactly the same manner, having some standardized protocols for evaluation can be very useful both in establishing common areas of occupational dysfunction within the target population and for determining the appropriate level of the program for each person. The model of human occupation suggests the following kinds of questions to plan the assessment strategies and to select specific instruments:

- What kinds of data need to be collected?
- What evaluation methods would be useful for ascertaining disruptions in the mind-brain-body performance subsystem?
- What data-gathering methods would be useful for ascertaining disruptions in the habituation subsystem?
- What data-gathering methods would be useful for ascertaining disruptions in the volition subsystem?
- What data-gathering methods would be useful for ascertaining disruptions in person-environment interaction?

Develop an Action Plan for Implementation

An additional task in the development phase is to specify how the program will be implemented and integrated into any existing treatment system. The following kinds of questions should be considered in undertaking this process:

- What is the specific program content and the timetable for implementing the component parts of the program?

- What will be the staff to client ratio?
- How will costs be covered or reimbursed?
- In what physical space will the program take place?
- What methods of referral and documentation will be used?
- How will clients move from intake to discharge and what criteria will be used to make these decisions?
- What activities will be used to monitor the provision of quality services?
- How will occupational therapy and interdisciplinary staff be trained and/or educated about the program?

The practitioner will also need to establish timetables or schedules to show when the various parts of the program will be implemented and in what sequence. The roles and responsibilities of the practitioners involved in implementing the program, including the roles of professionals from other disciplines, should be articulated. Obstacles to implementation such as conflicts over professional turf or competition for the clients' time should be identified and addressed.

A final aspect of the implementation task is to design referral systems that are efficient and useful. The practitioner must decide how the client will enter the program, move through the various tracks or levels in the program, and at what point the client will be discharged.

EXAMPLES OF PHASE THREE

Revision of Inpatient Groups

A positive and stabilizing force in the overall treatment context was the good interdisciplinary cooperation surrounding milieu program planning that existed on the unit. As noted earlier the situation analysis phase identified that most therapy groups were inappropriately attempting to service the needs of clients who were functioning at very different levels. During the previous phase, the occupational therapy staff also had established the focus of their programming by articulating a mission statement and specifying goals. However, in order to be successful in making positive changes in their own program, the ideas and programming offered by other disciplines

also needed to be considered. The MAP committee again used the model to help organize phase three of program development.

Using the model's emphasis on enhancing occupational function as the general outcome for the unit's programming, the interdisciplinary staff were engaged in a process of brainstorming new service options and choosing the best ones. The leaders of various groups were asked to define, based on the modalities they utilized in the group and on their purpose for leading the group, where on the model's functional continuum they felt the group would best meet the needs of the clients. This step was completed with the recognition that some groups would need to go through some considerable revision, but with a commitment to making explicit the modalities used and intended outcomes of each treatment group. This activity served to further reinforce the idea that groups were most effective when they targeted clients with similar functional levels. In many cases, using the exploration-competency-achievement continuum also assisted staff to recognize how their efforts and intentions were directed at one level and their clients' functional level was at a different level. During the discussion of where a particular treatment best fit on the functional continuum, the interdisciplinary team decided that for some groups (psychotherapy, art therapy, and cooking group), two levels of the group would need to be offered.

In subsequent weekly staff meetings, the occupational therapy supervisor created continuums of functioning using concepts from the model of human occupation. Continuums were created for performance skills, interpersonal role functioning, and occupational role functioning. The existing groups were then plotted on these continuums to provide a visual representation of the current milieu programming (Figure 15.9). Using this process, the interdisciplinary staff were then able to engage in discussions about the overall balance of activities presented in the schedule, and also about obvious gaps where certain needs were not being met or places where several groups overlapped by focusing on the same area of functioning. It seemed clear that the majority of groups tended to focus on building the in-

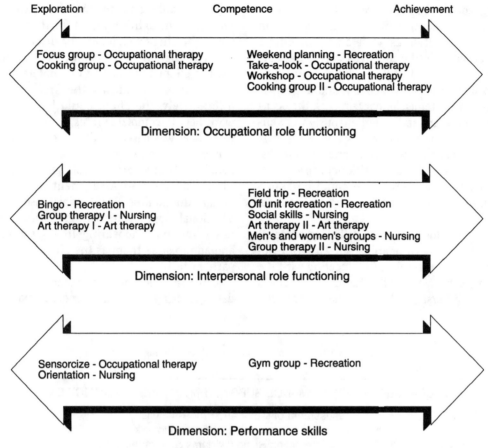

Figure 15.9.   Map committee analysis: Dimensions of function addressed in milieu activity groups.

terpersonal dimension of human functioning and were at the competence level.

The staff were then engaged in a brainstorming process to creatively look at programming in a fresh manner. During a weekly staff meeting, the continuums were drawn on a blackboard and left blank without any indication of current group programming. A scenario was set where the staff was asked to imagine that no milieu programming existed and they were directed to create a new configuration of services. A number of new groups were suggested and some changes for the current program were suggested as well. The MAP committee collected these comments and used the staff input to propose changes in the milieu programming. The occupational therapy staff also made choices about group interventions that would assist them to better meet the goals of the program. An analysis of the distri-

bution of occupational therapy groups across the exploration to achievement continuum had indicated a relative weakness in the amount and type of programming directed at clients functioning at the exploratory level. A variety of group interventions or changes in the current occupational therapy program were considered to address this. An example of such modification was refocusing of the directive group. This group was rescheduled to occur more frequently to encourage the clients' awareness of an ability to follow a structured routine. The structure of the group was also modified to reinforce the volitional and habituation goals of the group; group leaders experimented with using observational rating forms to document changes in each individual client's performance in the targeted areas. New programming that focused on the skills necessary for independent community living were designed. This group offered opportunities for clients to re-establish habits of participating in daily living activities while also providing a context whereby the clinicians were better able to assess independent living skills.

While participating actively, and frequently leading the interdisciplinary process, the occupational therapy staff simultaneously were engaged in a process of critically reviewing their own evaluation instruments and procedures. This process led the practitioners to identify appropriate methods which could be drawn upon to gather data on the program's clients (Figure 15.10).

Next, the following data-gathering protocol was established. Ordinarily, data gathering begins with the therapist's first meeting with the client. At this meeting the therapist introduces himself or herself and orients the client to the unit schedule and to the data-gathering process. Prior to this meeting the therapist reviews the client's chart and/or discusses the client's situation with the unit staff. Ordinarily, the client is assisted to complete a self-report worksheet during the first meeting. Alternatively, the client could be given the worksheet to complete on his or her own. The worksheet was based on the model of human occupation and incorporated short, modified components of an activity configuration, Role Checklist, and Self Assessment of Occupational Functioning. The therapist also selects additional, appropriate data-gathering methods from those appearing in Figure 15.10 and administers them as the client is able to participate.

Once the therapist has completed initial data gathering a standard report is made. An

Figure 15.10.   Occupational therapy data gathering tools.*

MIND-BRAIN-BODY PERFORMANCE SUBSYSTEM AND PERFORMANCE SKILLS

Assessment of Motor and Process Skills
Assessment of Communication/Interaction Skills
BaFPE Social Interaction Scale (Williams & Bloomer, 1987)
BaFPE Task Oriented Assessment (Williams & Bloomer, 1987)
Kohlman Evaluation of Living Skills (Kohlman-Thompson, 1992)
Scorable Self Care Evaluation (Clark & Peters, 1992)

HABITUATION SUBSYSTEM

Activity Record
Barth Time Configuration (Barth, 1985)
Occupational Questionnaire
Role Checklist

VOLITIONAL SUBSYSTEM

Interest Checklist
Occupational Case Analysis Interview and Rating Scale
Occupational Performance History Interview
Self Assessment of Occupational Functioning
Self-Efficacy Scale (Scherer & Maddux, 1982)

PERSON ENVIRONMENT INTERACTION

Environment Assessment Scale (Kannegieter, 1986)
Environmental Questionnaire (Dunning, 1972)
Family Environment Scale (Moos, 1976)
Interpersonal Support Evaluation List (Cohen, Mermelstein, Kamrack, & Hoberman, 1985)

---

* Citations are provided for those data gathering tools not discussed in Chapter Thirteen.

initial data-reporting form was created to reflect the subsystems of the model. To complete this document, the therapist synthesizes all available data from instruments used in the initial data collection process. The initial data-reporting form is in a format that provides a profile of strengths and weaknesses for identified factors related to model concepts. For example, in the area of habituation, the form included such areas of organization of routine and balance in routine activities. In the area of volition, identification of valued goals and expression of confidence in personal skills is included.

This data-reporting form concludes with a narrative section in which the therapist identifies the client's unfolding life story, discusses the client's history of occupational functioning over time with particular attention to functioning in major occupational roles, and comments upon the client's strengths and deficits in the areas included on the form. Written policies and procedures which detail the assessment process and provide guidelines for completing the initial assessment, treatment plans, progress notes, and discharge summaries were also established.

Work Readiness Program

In the previous phase, program goals were identified, and it had been determined that the program would be organized into three phases. In this development phase staff first generated and selected from a range of ideas about the kinds of strategies which could be incorporated into the program. These strategies have continued to develop over the three years of operation of the program. The current program strategies can be found in the right hand column of Figure 15.6.

It was also decided that the program would consist mainly of group activities. Consequently, the strategies were linked to a number of group interventions which were developed to make up the program. Each of these groups was clearly identified and a protocol was developed for each. Once again, the development of the groups is something that has continued as the program has operated. The current groups used in the program are the Work Skills Adjustment Group, Goal-Setting Group, Communication Skills Group, Time Management Group, Productive Roles Group, and Cardiovascular Group.

The Work Skills Adjustment Group meets several hours each day. This group allows for practical experience in various work-related tasks. Through this experience the client has an opportunity to identify vocational interests, determine responsibilities associated with these interests, and evaluate his or her ability to perform various tasks. Such work activities as piecework, clerical tasks, and materials transport tasks are used in this group. In addition, individuals are also taught specialized skills such as computer training. Work tasks are obtained from departments within the hospital and the university as well as through private industry. Figure 15.11 illustrates the protocol for this group; all other groups have similar protocols.

The Goal-Setting Group meets once a week for an hour. It focuses on assisting the client to set realistic goals for the upcoming week. The client formulates goals for both the program and home. Discussion follows about the appropriateness of goals and about strategies for attaining these goals. The following week, goals are reviewed to determine if they were met and why or why not. Appropriate modifications are discussed and the next week's goals developed. Group members are invited to provide constructive feedback to one another and to participate in problem solving to develop action plans and follow-up to better assure goal attainment. At the end of the group a volunteer is sought to type and Xerox goals, which are posted within the program and serve as a reminder throughout the week. Copies are distributed to group members for the next week's group.

The Communication Skills Group meets weekly for 90 minutes. The group addresses communication and interaction skills necessary to effectively participate in all occupational roles. The concept behind this group is the necessity for individuals to interact effectively in all environments to achieve optimal occupational functioning. Topics include initiating a conversation, saying no, assertive communication, and increasing understanding of

Purpose: To provide individuals with opportunities to explore and experience various vocational interests. To assess and develop skills needed for vocational placement.

Membership: All members in Phase I of the Work Readiness Program.

Goals: 1) Individual will identify work-related interests.
2) Individual will realistically assess skill level related to various work-related tasks.
3) Individual will develop skills necessary to perform work-related tasks.
4) Individual will increase ability to receive and incorporate environmental feedback to modify performance.
5) Individual will complete all steps of work-task in a timely manner.

Methods: The group will meet daily from 9:00–10:50 in the Work Readiness Room. Members will be encouraged to set-up their own work stations, gathering the appropriate tools and materials to complete their selected task. Room set-up will vary based on tasks participants have chosen. Tasks are selected based on discussions between participant and group leader about interests, current skill level, task demands and individual goals to be addressed. Suggested activities include: clerical, horticulture, computer, assembly line activities, piece work and craft projects, as appropriate. Participants will participate in self-evaluation of their effectiveness and interest in specific tasks upon task completion. Appropriate body mechanics and safety in tool handling will be emphasized.

Participants will begin each session reviewing the purpose and goals of the group. Members will identify one individual goal to address in that session. At the end of the group, time will be given for members to review individual progress and goal achievement.

Role of   The leader will server as a role model for interacting with the environment to engage in or
Leader/   complete a task. The leader provides support and guidance to members having difficulty
Co-leader: with task and/or stated group goals.

The co-leader assists in planning group and participates in processing at the end of each session. The co-leader assists leader in providing support and guidance to individuals as needed.

Specific roles of leader and co-leader will be decided prior to group.

Figure 15.11.   Protocols for the work skills adjustment group.

nonverbal communication. Activities include: role-playing, paper-and-pencil tasks and experiential exercises.

The Time Management Group meets weekly for an hour and addresses the individual's need to develop a balanced daily schedule. Through paper and pencil activities and discussion, members identify their current daily and weekly schedules, their ideal schedule and how to incorporate the two into a realistic routine. This group encourages the client to look more specifically at unproductive time and explore interests they would like to participate in and how to include these activities in their weekly schedule.

The Productive Roles Group meets weekly for an hour. This group provides an opportu-

nity for clients to examine various roles in which they are currently participating and the roles they would like to assume in the future. Following from the belief that balance is essential for an individual's success in the worker role, this group explores roles beyond that of the worker/volunteer. Activities such as role-playing, paper and pencil tasks, and experiential activities are used to explore and identify the roles group members want to incorporate into their lives.

The Cardiovascular Group has been developed and implemented by the physical therapy department. The group meets three times a week for an hour with the goals of both educating clients and promoting their participation in a regular exercise routine; the group also aims at increasing range of motion, strength, and endurance. Group members are encouraged to take ownership of the group by leading warm-up exercises and suggesting activities for future groups. In addition to exercises which focus specifically on the upper and lower extremities, group members get a simple cardiovascular workout through walking, swimming, and use of exercise equipment at the university-affiliated gym.

Once the overall program structure and the groups were identified, the next task was to determine how clients would enter and participate in the program. Criteria for referral and a screening process were developed. Next, data-gathering methods were selected and matched with the constructs of the model as shown in Figure 15.12. The therapist uses this matrix to make sure that a comprehensive evaluation is completed when he or she selects from possible data-gathering methods those to be used with an individual client. A protocol for the data-gathering and reporting process was also developed. Finally, the logistics of the program schedule were worked out. The data-gathering process serves as the basis of determining the client's program. The program for each client consists of an appropriate schedule of participating in the selected groups and any necessary individual sessions such as vocational testing and counseling. As the client progresses through the program, his or her schedule will change. For example, a client in the competency phase may attend the Work Skills Adjustment Group daily plus one of the other groups each day. Later, the same client may be placed in a volunteer job, have a weekly individual work counseling session, and attend the Time Management Group and the Goal-Setting Group to sustain overall lifestyle. As can readily be seen, a rather elaborate plan for individual and group scheduling had to be developed.

PHASE FOUR: IMPLEMENTATION AND EVALUATION

The penultimate phase of program development involves two major tasks: (a) implementing the program and (b) evaluating the program. Implementation involves getting the program up and running according to the timetable and sequence defined in the development phase. Most program development plans result in changes in the delivery of services and, in this sense, those who really implement the plan are the direct service staff and their managers. It is, therefore, essential to involve these practitioners throughout the various phases of program development, but most importantly to collaborate with them extensively during the implementation phase.

Implementing the Program

Implementation of the program most often requires some changes in the physical and social context in which the program occurs. Therefore, an essential component of this phase is to implement such infrastructure changes as will support the program's success. For example, necessary equipment must be secured or purchased, space must be available, materials must be on hand, and staff orientation and education must be completed. Once these and other startup activities are finished, the new services can commence.

Clear communication and documentation are also necessary to ensure effective implementation of the program. Oral communication helps link occupational therapy with other service providers and administrative personnel. Written documentation helps integrate the occupational therapy program with the larger context of services being provided to the targeted population. Written documentation functions to (a) act as a checklist to ensure all aspects of the implementation plan are being considered; (b) keep a record of the decision-making process; and (c) provide a basis for monitoring and evaluating the program.

The program developer should also identify individuals in the larger service organization with whom strategic communication is essential. Effort should be taken to define the goals of the communication, what information should be communicated, and how communication will be presented.

Evaluating the Program

Program evaluation is the second task of the implementation and evaluation phase. The

	Environment		Performance Skills			Habituation		Volition		
	Physical	Psycho-social	Motor	Process	Interaction/ Communication	Habits	Roles	Interests	Personal Causation	Values
Activity Record						X	X	X	X	X
Assessment of Communication/ Interaction Skills					X					
Assessment of Motor and Process Skills			X	X						
The COPSystem Career Measurement								X		X
Interest Checklist			X					X		
Occupational Case Analysis Interview Rating Scale	X	X				X	X	X	X	X
Occupational Performance History Interview	X	X				X	X	X	X	X
Occupational Questionnaire						X		X	X	X
Role Checklist							X			X
Self Assessment of Occupational Functioning	X	X				X	X	X	X	X
Worker Role Interview	X	X				X	X	X	X	X

Figure 15.12. Potential instruments for the work readiness program.

focus of program evaluation is to measure the effects of the program against the goals and/or expected outcomes outlined for the program during phase two. When goals and objectives of the program are well written, they will specify explicit evaluation criteria. Evaluation provides the basis for the next situation analysis; thus the cycle of program development will begin anew.

There are different reasons for and different methods of carrying out evaluations. The purpose of the evaluation should be clear before beginning this process since the type of questions asked will affect the methodology chosen to gather the information to answer these questions. Specific indicators will need to be identified and monitored. These indicators may include processes related to program implementation such as the number of clients evaluated, the percentage of the target population referred to the program, or the number of clients who complete the program. Indicators should also include factors that allow determination of how well program goals or outcomes are being met. Such indicators are increases in skills, changes in habits and roles, and improvements in overall occupational lifestyle. Finally, client satisfaction with services should always be considered. Many of these indicators may be derived from routine documentation practices. The best program evaluation plan will study multiple outcome measures simultaneously. The following are the kinds of questions which should guide the therapeutic reasoning involved in the program evaluation process:

- Are occupational therapy services having the desired outcome?
- Were the services provided in the form planned, and if not, why not?
- Were the program goals and objectives achieved? If not, why not?
- What improvements in occupational functioning did clients achieve?
- In addition to the planned effects, were there any unintended effects of the program?

EXAMPLES OF PHASE FOUR

Revision of Inpatient Groups

As previously stated, the process of program development is never a neat and clearly structured process. The recommendations of the interdisciplinary Milieu Activity Planning committee were presented and discussed with the milieu staff routinely during weekly staffing meetings. Some recommendations were implemented immediately. Some group leaders took to heart the feedback generated from the critique of the current milieu programming and reformulated their treatment protocols and modified the modalities they used. Extensive inservicing was used to encourage the habitual use of newly designed documentation formats for the team. A MAP Group Prescription Form (Figure 15.13) was developed and used to document the teams' decisions regarding the various treatment groups that were being prescribed for each client. The model's functional continuum was used to organize the treatment group options by level of functional ability. During the biweekly interdisciplinary treatment planning meetings, the Group Prescription Form was completed and reviewed to ensure that the client was being offered an individually prescribed pattern of group interventions which was tailored to his or her individual needs. During the initial stages of implementing such procedures, members of the MAP committee were charged with ensuring the effective use of the prescription form in the various team meetings.

The quality assurance monitors put into place at the time the program was being developed focused on (a) utilization of service indicators such as the number of clients seen and the frequency with which clients attended scheduled groups and (b) documentation indicators such as the timeliness of documentation and the adequacy of the therapists' narrative in the final section of the initial data-gathering report form. Indicators for behavioral change were discussed and the staff explored various behavioral rating scales available in the literature. They also have experimented with creating scales tailored to the specific goals of each group. The process of identifying appropriate outcome indicators is still ongoing.

Ongoing program changes and the process for implementing changes has been monitored by the interdisciplinary team members. Weekly interdisciplinary staff meetings are also used

EXPLORATION	COMPETENCE	ACHIEVEMENT
Designed to help patients develop basic skills in a non-threatening, structured setting. Therapists are largely responsible for selection of activities and organization of the treatment environment.	Designed to help patients expand skills and identify goals, interests, and needs. Therapists involve patients in collaborative decision making and cooperative interaction	Designed to help patients integrate skills into daily life roles. Patients are active in identifying their learning needs relative to work, leisure, and interpersonal relationships.
INTERPERSONAL ROLE DIMENSION		
Social Skills Group Exploration Group Therapy	Media Group Competence Group Therapy Men's Group Women's Group	Group Therapy Self-Awareness
OCCUPATIONAL ROLE DIMENSION		
Cognitive Development Recreation-On Unit Living Skills-Exploration	Skills Exploration Coping Skills Living Skills-Competence Recreation-Off Unit Recreation-Field Trip Recreation-On Unit	Vocational Group Goal Setting Field Trip Survival Skills
MIND-BRAIN-BODY PERFORMANCE		
Sensorcize Group Orientation Group Maternal/OB Group Open Art Therapy Group Art Therapy I Relaxation Group Medication Group	Sensorcize Group Recreation Gym Group Open Art Therapy Group Art Therapy II Relaxation Group Medication Group	Gym Group Relaxation Group
CULTURE & COMMUNITY BUILDING GROUPS		
Community Meeting	Multi-family Group	Weekend Planning

Figure 15.13.   Map group prescription form.

to raise issues of milieu programming, discuss problems, and gauge the utilization of the various supporting documentation forms that have been created.

As previously stated, program development is a spiraling process that never ends. Not surprisingly, the interdisciplinary team of the psychiatric unit recently requested that the MAP committee be re-established to reassess the milieu programming on the unit. In particular, the team currently feels a strong need to retool in the face of changes in the demographic trends of the target population, the decreasing length of stays, and a strong push from the interdisciplinary team members to reconceptualize the proper focus of acute inpatient care as we move into the year 2000.

Work Readiness Program

Implementation of the Work Readiness Program began with assessing potential candidates for the program. Once screening identified a number of viable candidates, the first groups began. The team met weekly to review client progress and to assess the implementation of the program. The early stages of implementation required a lot of fine tuning as plans that looked flawless and conceptually sound on paper were challenged by the reality of day-to-day clinical service delivery. The process from referral to discharge was defined and revised multiple times. Eventually a flow chart (see Figure 15.14) had to be created which provided guidelines for how the client would move through the program.

Periodic reviews of the program were also scheduled and used to evaluate the program and to problem solve strategies to ensure the continued growth of the program. To evaluate the effectiveness of the program several indicators were established. Since the focus of the program was assisting the client to establish a more productive pattern of role involvement, a scale for productive role status was created and each client was rated by the team on admission and at discharge.

Staff changes during the early stages of program implementation also taxed the team. Clients' difficulties with reliable transportation and the lack of support in their home environments affected participation and attendance.

Services initially planned to be provided by the various participating disciplines fluctuated due to productivity demands and staff unavailability. All these problems needed to be addressed along the way as the program was being implemented. When the occupational therapist who had been responsible for most of the program left to take another position, it was decided that a thorough reappraisal of the program was needed. A new occupational therapist was hired and given the charge to collaborate with other staff and with the second author to do a comprehensive program evaluation.

As noted in phase one, the program was overhauled to be located within the occupational therapy department with physical therapy providing one group and other disciplines remaining as consultants and individual service providers. The program also was opened to a wider range of clients.

The program is currently operating effectively with a strong referral base and a diverse client group. Most recently, the second author received funding from the American Occupa-

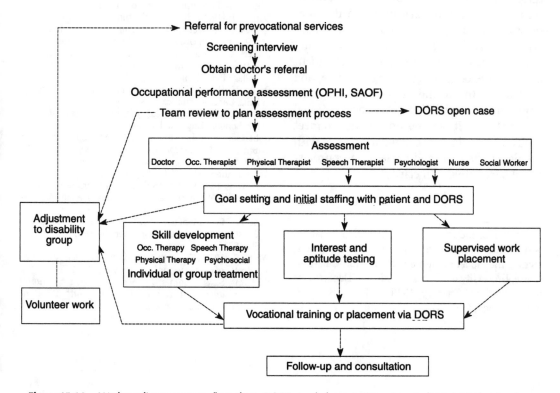

Figure 15.14. Work readiness program flow chart. DORS stands for state Department of Rehabilitation Services.

tional Therapy Foundation to study the program over a two-year period using an action research design. This study will allow us to examine the program impact (successes and failures) in detail and will result in improvement of services, documentation of the effective of this program, and generation of new information that, no doubt, will lead to revisions in the theoretical constructs of the model of human occupation.

CONCLUSION

In this chapter we have outlined a process of program development, describing how a practitioner can define and implement occupational therapy services using the model of human occupation. We used examples from our own program development experience to elucidate the program development process.[c] We described program development as a continual process and as an art that must be responsive to clients and their needs, to the treatment setting and its organizational culture, and to the composition of the treatment team. We conceptualized program development as a spiraling process that blends practical problem solving and therapeutic reasoning with the use of theory. Program development can, at once, be exciting, taxing, creative, and frustrating. In the end, it is one of the most important responsibilities of an occupational therapist since it requires one at once to meet needs of a whole target population, deal with people and politics, and present one's professional perspective with clarity.

---

[c]More comprehensive written materials exist on both of these programs and may be obtained by contacting the Model of Human Occupation Clearinghouse, University of Illinois at Chicago, Department of Occupational Therapy, 1919 W. Taylor St. (M/C 811), Chicago, IL 60612.

References

Bair, J., & Gray, M. (Eds.) (1992). *The Occupational Therapy Manager.* Rockville, MD: American Occupational Therapy Association.

Barth, T. (1985). *Barth time construction.* New York: Health Related Consulting Services.

Clark, E. N., & Peters, M. (1992). *Scorable self-care evaluation.* Thorofare, NJ: Slack.

Cohen, S., Mermelstein, R., Kamrack, T., & Hoberman, H. M. (1985). Measuring the functional components of social support. In I. G. Sarason & B. R. Sarason (Eds.), *Social support: Theory, research and applications* (pp. 73–94). Boston: Martinus Nijhioff.

Cole, S., & Lucas, H. (Eds.) (1979). *Models, planning and basic needs.* Oxford, England: Pergamon Press.

Dunning, H. D. (1972). Environmental occupational therapy. *American Journal of Occupational Therapy, 26,* 292–298.

Green, A. (1992). *An introduction to health planning.* Oxford, England: Oxford University Press.

Kannegieter, R. B. (1986). The development of the environment assessment scale. *Occupational Therapy in Mental Health, 6,* 67–83.

Kaplan, K. (1988). *Directive group therapy: Innovative mental health treatment.* Thorofare, NJ: Slack.

Kohlman-Thompson, L. (1992). *The Kohlman evaluation of living skills.* Rockville, MD: American Occupational Therapy Association.

Leiter, P. (1992). Facility Planning. In J. Bair & M. Gray (Eds.), *The Occupational therapy manager.* Rockville, MD: American Occupational Therapy Association.

Moos, R. H. (1976). *Family environmental scale.* Palo Alto, CA: Consulting Psychologist Press.

Ostrow, P. (1992). Strategic planning. In J. Bair & M. Gray (Eds.), *The Occupational therapy manager.* Rockville, MD: American Occupational Therapy Association.

Pickett, G., & Hanlon, J. (1990). *Public health: Administration and practice.* St. Louis: Times Mirror/Mosby College Publishing.

Reilly, M. (1974). *Play as exploratory learning.* Beverly Hills, CA: Sage Publications.

Rathwell, T. (1987). *Strategic planning in the health sector.* London, England: Helm-Croom.

Robertson, S. (Ed.) (1986). *SCOPE: Strategies, concepts and opportunities for program development.* Rockville, MD: American Occupational Therapy Association.

Schammahorn, G. (1992). Program planning. In J. Bair & M. Gray (Eds.), *The Occupational therapy manager.* Rockville, MD: American Occupational Therapy Association.

Scherer, M., & Maddux, J. E. (1982). Self efficacy scale: Construction and validation. *Psychological Reports, 51,* 663–671.

White, R. (1971). The urge towards competence. *American Journal of Occupational Therapy, 25,* 271–272.

Williams, S., & Bloomer, J. (1987). *Bay area functional performance evaluation* (2nd ed.). Palo Alto, CA: Consulting Psychologist Press.

Appendix: Bibliography on Programs Using the Model of Human Occupation

Adelstein, L. A., Barnes, M. A., Murray-Jensen, F., & Skaggs, C. B. (1989). A broadening frontier: Occupational therapy in mental health programs for children and adolescents. *Mental Health Special Interest Section Newsletter, 12,* 2–4.

Affleck, A., Bianchi, E., Cleckley, M., Donaldson, K., McCormack, G., & Polon, J. (1984). Stress management as a component of occupational therapy in acute care settings. *Occupational Therapy in Health Care, 1*(3), 17–41.

Baron, K. (1987). The model of human occupation: A newspaper treatment group for adolescents with a diagnosis of conduct disorder. *Occupational Therapy in Mental Health, 7*(2), 89–104.

Baron, K. (1989). Occupational therapy: A program for child psychiatry. *Mental Health Special Interest Section Newsletter, 12,* 6–7.

Burke, J. P., Clark, F., Dodd, C., & Kawamoto, T. (1987). Maternal role preparation: A program using sensory integration, infant–mother attachment, and occupational behavior perspectives. *Occupational Therapy in Health Care, 4*(2), 9–21.

Burton, J. E. (1989). The model of human occupation and occupational therapy practice with elderly patients, Part 1: Characteristics of aging. *British Journal of Occupational Therapy, 52,* 215–218.

Burton, J. E. (1989). The model of human occupation and occupational therapy practice with elderly patients, Part 2: Application. *British Journal of Occupational Therapy, 52,* 219–221.

Depoy, E. (1990). The TBIIM: An intervention for the treatment of individuals with traumatic brain injury. *Occupational Therapy in Health Care, 7*(1), 55–67.

Froehlich, J. (1992). Occupational therapy interventions with survivors of sexual abuse. *Occupational Therapy in Health Care, 8*(2/3), 1–25.

Furst, G., Gerber, L., Smith, C., Fisher, S., & Shulman, B. (1987). A program for improving energy conservation behaviors in adults with rheumatoid arthritis. *American Journal of Occupational Therapy, 41,* 102–111.

Grogan, G. (1991). Anger management: A perspective for occupational therapy (Part 1). *Occupational Therapy in Mental Health, 11*(2/3), 135–148.

Grogan, G. (1991). Anger management: A perspective for occupational therapy (Part 2). *Occupational Therapy in Mental Health, 11*(2/3), 149–171.

Gusich, R. (1984). Occupational therapy for chronic pain: A clinical application of the model of human occupation. *Occupational Therapy in Mental Health, 4*(3), 59–73.

Gusich, R. L., & Silverman, A. L. (1991). Basava day clinic: The model of human occupation as applied to psychiatric day hospitalization. *Occupational Therapy in Mental Health, 11*(2/3), 113–134.

de las Heras, C. G., Dion, G. L., & Walsh, D. (1993). Application of rehabilitation models in a state psychiatric hospital. *Occupational Therapy in Mental Health, 12*(3), 1–32.

Kaplan, K. (1986). The directive group: Short term treatment for psychiatric patients with a minimal level of functioning. *American Journal of Occupational Therapy, 40,* 474–481.

Kaplan, K. (1988). *Directive group therapy: Innovative mental health treatment.* Thorofare, NJ: Slack.

Kielhofner, G., & Brinson, M. (1989). Development and evaluation of an aftercare program for young and chronic psychiatrically disabled adults. *Occupational Therapy in Mental Health, 9*(2), 1–25.

Lancaster, J., & Mitchell, M. (1991). Occupational therapy treatment goals, objectives, and activities for improving low self-esteem in adolescents with behavioral disorders. *Occupational Therapy in Mental Health, 11*(2/3), 3–22.

Levine, R. (1984). The cultural aspects of home care delivery. *American Journal of Occupational Therapy, 38,* 734–738.

Levine, R. E., & Gitlin, L. N. (1990). Home adaptations for persons with chronic disabilities: An educational model. *American Journal of Occupational Therapy, 44,* 923–929.

Levine, R. E., & Gitlin, L. N. (1993). A model to promote activity competence in elders. *American Journal of Occupational Therapy, 47,* 147–153.

Michael, P. S. (1991). Occupational therapy in a prison? You must be kidding! *Mental Health Special Interest Section Newsletter, 14,* 3–4.

Muñoz, J. P. (1988). A program for acute inpatient psychiatry. *Mental Health Special Interest Section Newsletter, 11,* 3–4.

Neville-Jan, A., Bradley, M., Bunn, C., & Gehri, B. (1991). The model of human occupation and individuals with co-dependency problems. *Occupational Therapy in Mental Health, 11*(2/3), 73–97.

Oakley, F. (1987). Clinical application of the model of human occupation in dementia of the Alzheimer's type. *Occupational Therapy in Mental Health, 7*(4), 37–50.

Olin, D. (1985). Assessing and assisting the person with dementia: An occupational behavior perspective. *Physical & Occupational Therapy in Geriatrics, 3*(4), 25–32.

Padilla, R., & Bianchi, E. M. (1990). Occupational therapy for chronic pain: Applying the model of human occupation to clinical practice. *Occupational Therapy Practice, 1*(3), 47–52.

Pizzi, M. A. (1990). The model of human occupation and adults with HIV infection and AIDS. *American Journal of Occupational Therapy, 44,* 257–264.

Platts, L. (1993). Social role valorisation and the model of human occupation: A comparative analysis for work with people with learning disability in the community. *British Journal of Occupational Therapy, 56*(8), 278–282.

Salz, C. (1983). A theoretical approach to the treatment of work difficulties in borderline personalities. *Occupational Therapy in Mental Health, 3*(3), 33–46.

Scarth, P. P. (1990). Services for chemically dependent adolescents. *Mental Health Special Interest Section Newsletter, 13,* 7–8.

Schaaf, R. C., & Mulrooney, L. L. (1989). Occupational therapy in early intervention: A family centered approach. *American Journal of Occupational Therapy, 43,* 745–754.

Schindler, V. J. (1988). Psychosocial occupational therapy intervention with AIDS patients. *American Journal of Occupational Therapy, 42,* 507–512.

Series, C. (1992). The long-term needs of people with head injury: a role for the community occupational therapist? *British Journal of Occupational Therapy, 55*(3), 94–98.

Shimp, S. L. (1989). A family-style meal group: Short-term treatment for eating disorder patients with a high level of functioning. *Mental Health Special Interest Section Newsletter, 12,* 1–3.

Sholle-Martin, S. (1987). Application of the model of human occupation: Assessment in child and adolescent psychiatry. *Occupational Therapy in Mental Health, 7*(2), 3–22.

Sholle-Martin, S., & Alessi, N. E. (1990). Formulating a role for occupational therapy in child psychiatry: A clinical application. *American Journal of Occupational Therapy, 44,* 871–881.

Tatham, M. (1992). Leisure facilitator: The role of the occupational therapist in senior housing. *Journal of Housing for the Elderly, 10*(2), 125–138.

Weissenberg, R., & Giladi, W. (1989). Home economics day: A program for disturbed adolescents to promote acquisition of habits and skills. *Occupational Therapy in Mental Health, 9*(2), 89–103.

Woodrum, S. C. (1993). A treatment approach for attention deficit hyperactivity disorder using the model of human occupation. *Developmental Disabilities Special Interest Section Newsletter, 16*(1), 1–2.

Appendix: **Bibliography**

Each citation is coded at the end: C = Clinical Application; T = Theoretical Discussion; R = Research; I = Instrument Development; E = Educational Application.

Adelstein, L. A., Barnes, M. A., Murray-Jensen, F., & Skaggs, C. B. (1989). A broadening frontier: Occupational therapy in mental health programs for children and adolescents. Mental Health Special Interest Section Newsletter, 12, 2–4. (C)

Affleck, A., Bianchi, E., Cleckley, M., Donaldson, K., Mc-Cormack, G., & Polon, J. (1984). Stress management as a component of occupational therapy in acute care settings. *Occupational Therapy in Health Care, 1*(3), 17–41. (C)

Arnsten, S. M. (1990). Intrinsic motivation. *American Journal of Occupational Therapy, 44*, 462–463. (T)

Baron, K. (1987). The model of human occupation: A newspaper treatment group for adolescents with a diagnosis of conduct disorder. *Occupational Therapy in Mental Health, 7*(2), 89–104. (C)

Baron, K. (1989). Occupational therapy: A program for child psychiatry. *Mental Health Special Interest Section Newsletter, 12*, 6–7. (T,C)

Baron, K. B. (1991). The use of play in child psychiatry: Reframing the therapeutic environment. *Occupational Therapy in Mental Health, 11*(2/3), 37–56. (C)

Barris, R. (1982). Environmental interactions: An extension of the model of human occupation. *American Journal of Occupational Therapy, 36*, 637–644. (T)

Barris, R. (1986). Occupational dysfunction and eating disorders: Theory and approach to treatment. *Occupational Therapy in Mental Health, 6*(1), 27–45. (T,C)

Barris, R. (1986). Activity: The interface between person and environment. *Physical and Occupational Therapy in Geriatrics, 5*(2), 39–49. (T)

Barris, R., Dickie, V., & Baron, K. (1988). A comparison of psychiatric patients and normal subjects based on the model of human occupation. *Occupational Therapy Journal of Research, 8*, 3–37. (R) Commentary by Mann, W. & Klyczek, J., in same issue. Response to commentary by Barris, R., & Dickie, V., in same issue.

Barris, R., Kielhofner, G., Burch, R. M., Gelinas, I., Klement, M., & Schultz, B. (1986). Occupational function and dysfunction in three groups of adolescents. *Occupational Therapy Journal of Research, 6*, 301–317. (R)

Barris, R., Oakley, F., & Kielhofner, G. (1988). The Role Checklist. *Mental Health Assessment in Occupational Therapy*, (pp. 73–91). Thorofare, NJ: Slack. (I)

Bavaro, S. M. (1991). Occupational therapy and obsessive-compulsive disorder. *American Journal of Occupational Therapy, 45*, 456–458. (C)

Behnke, C., & Fetkovich, M. (1984). Examining the reliability and validity of the Play History. *American Journal of Occupational Therapy, 38*, 94–100. (I,R)

Biernacki, S. D. (1993). Reliability of the Worker Role Interview. *American Journal of Occupational Therapy, 47*, 797–803. (R,I)

Blakeney, A. (1985). Adolescent development: An application to the model of human occupation. *Occupational Therapy in Health Care, 2*(3), 19–40. (T)

Bledsoe, N. P., & Shepherd, J. T. (1982). A study of reliability and validity of a Preschool Play Scale. *American Journal of Occupational Therapy, 36*, 783–788. (R,I)

Borell, L., Sandman, P., & Kielhofner, G. (1991). Clinical decision making in Alzheimer's disease. *Occupational Therapy in Mental Health, 11*(4), 111–124. (C)

Bränholm, I., & Fugl-Meyer, A. R. (1992). Occupational role preferences and life satisfaction. *Occupational Therapy Journal of Research, 12*, 159–171. (R)

Bridle, M. J., Lynch, K. B., & Quesenberry, C. M. (1990). Long term function following the central cord syndrome. *Paraplegia, 28*, 178–185. (R)

Broadley, H. (1991). Assessment guidelines based on the Model of Human Occupation. *World Federation of Occupational Therapists: Bulletin, 23*, 34–35. (C)

Brown, T., & Carmichael, K. (1992). Assertiveness training for clients with psychiatric illness: a pilot study. *British Journal of Occupational Therapy, 55*(4), 137–140. (C)

Brollier, C., Watts, J. H., Bauer, D., & Schmidt, W. (1989). A content validity study of the Assessment of Occupational Functioning. *Occupational Therapy in Mental Health, 8*(4), 29–47. (I,R)

Brollier, C., Watts, J. H., Bauer, D., & Schmidt, W. (1989). A concurrent validity study of two occupational therapy evaluation instruments: The AOF and OCAIRS. *Occupational Therapy in Mental Health, 8*(4), 49–59. (R)

Burke, J. P. (1988). Commentary: Combining the model of human occupation with cognitive disability theory. *Occupational Therapy in Mental Health, 8*(2), xi–xiii. (T)

Burke, J. P., Clark, F., Dodd, C., & Kawamoto, T. (1987). Maternal role preparation: A program using sensory integration, infant–mother attachment, and occupational behavior perspectives. *Occupational Therapy in Health Care, 4*(2), 9–21. (C)

Burrows, E. (1989). Clinical practice: An approach to the assessment of clinical competencies. *British Journal of Occupational Therapy, 52*, 222–226. (C,E)

Burton, J. E. (1989). The model of human occupation and occupational therapy practice with elderly patients, Part 1: Characteristics of aging. *British Journal of Occupational Therapy, 52*, 215–218. (C)

Burton, J. E. (1989). The model of human occupation and occupational therapy practice with elderly patients, Part 2: Application. *British Journal of Occupational Therapy, 52*, 219–221. (C)

Cermak, S. A., & Murray, E. (1992). Nonverbal learning disabilities in the adult framed in the model of human occupation. In N. Katz (Ed.), *Cognitive Rehabilitation: Models for intervention in Occupational Therapy* (pp. 258–291). Stoneham, MA: Butterworth-Heinemann. (C)

Christiansen, C. H. (1981). Toward resolution of crisis research requisites in occupational therapy. *Occupational Therapy Journal of Research, 1,* 115–124. (R)

Coster, W. J., & Jaffe, L. E. (1991). Current concepts of children's perceptions of control. *American Journal of Occupational Therapy, 45,* 19–25. (T)

Cubie, S., & Kaplan, K. (1982). A case analysis method for the model of human occupation. *American Journal of Occupational Therapy, 36,* 645–656. (C)

Cull, G. (1989). Anorexia Nervosa: A review of theory approaches to treatment. *Journal of New Zealand Association of Occupational Therapists, 40*(2), 3–6. (C)

Curtin, C. (1990). Research on the model of human occupation. *Mental Health Special Interest Section Newsletter, 13,* 3–5. (R)

Curtin, C. (1991). Psychosocial intervention with an adolescent with diabetes using the model of human occupation. *Occupational Therapy in Mental Health, 11*(2/3), 23–36. (C)

DeForest, D., Watts, J. H., & Madigan, M. J. (1991). Resonation in the model of human occupation: A pilot study. *Occupational Therapy in Mental Health, 11*(2/3), 57–75. (R)

Depoy, E. (1990). The TBIIM: An intervention for the treatment of individuals with traumatic brain injury. *Occupational Therapy in Health Care, 7*(1), 55–67. (C)

DePoy, E., & Burke, J. P. (1992). Viewing cognition through the lens of the model of human occupation. In N. Katz (Ed.), *Cognitive Rehabilitation: Models for intervention in Occupational Therapy* (pp. 240–257). Stoneham, MA: Butterworth-Heinemann. (T)

Doble, S. (1988). Intrinsic motivation and clinical practice: The key to understanding the unmotivated client. *Canadian Journal of Occupational Therapy, 55,* 75–81 (T,C)

Doble, S. E. (1991). Test-retest and inter-rater reliability of a process skills assessment. *Occupational Therapy Journal of Research, 11,* 8–23. (R)

Duellman, M. K., Barris, R., & Kielhofner, G. (1986). Organized activity and the adaptive status of nursing home residents. *American Journal of Occupational Therapy, 40,* 618–622. (R)

Dyck, I. (1992). The daily routines of mothers with young children: Using a socio-political model in research. *Occupational Therapy Journal of Research, 12,* 17–34. (R)

Ebb, E. W., Coster, W., & Duncombe, L. (1989). Comparison of normal and psychosocially dysfunctional male adolescents. *Occupational Therapy in Mental Health, 9*(2), 53–74. (R)

Egan, M., Warren, S. A., Hessel, P. A., & Gilewich, G. (1992). Activities of daily living after hip fracture: Pre- and post discharge. *Occupational Therapy Journal of Research, 12,* 342–356. (R)

Elliott, M., & Barris, R. (1987). Occupational role performance and life satisfaction in elderly persons. *Occupational Therapy Journal of Research, 7,* 215–224. (R)

Esdaile, S. A., & Madill, H. M. (1993). Causal attributions: Theoretical considerations and their relevance to occupational therapy practice and education. *British Journal of Occupational Therapy, 56*(9), 330–334. (T)

Evans, J., & Salim, A. A. (1992). A cross-cultural test of the validity of occupational therapy assessments with patients with schizophrenia. *American Journal of Occupational Therapy, 46,* 685–695. (R)

Fisher, A. (1993). The assessment of IADL motor skills: an application of many faceted rasch analysis. *American Journal of Occupational Therapy, 47,* 319–329. (R,I)

Fisher, A., Liu, Y., Velozo C., & Pan A. (1992). Cross cultural assessment of process skills. *American Journal of Occupational Therapy, 46,* 876–884. (R)

Fitts, H., & Howe, M. (1987). Use of leisure time by cardiac patients. *American Journal of Occupational Therapy, 41,* 583–589. (R)

Fleming, M. H. (1991). The therapist with the three-track mind. *American Journal of Occupational Therapy, 45,* 1007–1014. (T)

Froehlich, J. (1992). Occupational therapy interventions with survivors of sexual abuse. *Occupational Therapy in Health Care, 8*(2/3), 1–25. (C)

Furst, G., Gerber, L., Smith, C., Fisher, S., & Shulman, B. (1987). A program for improving energy conservation behaviors in adults with rheumatoid arthritis. *American Journal of Occupational Therapy, 41,* 102–111. (C)

Gerber, L., & Furst, G. (1992). Validation of the NIH Activity Record: A quantitative measure of life activities. *Arthritis Care and Research, 5,* 81–86. (R,I)

Gerber, L., & Furst, G. (1992). Scoring methods and application of the Activity Record (ACTRE) for patients with musculoskeletal disorders. *Arthritis Care and Research, 5,* 151–156. (C)

Gregory, M. (1983). Occupational behavior and life satisfaction among retirees. *American Journal of Occupational Therapy, 37,* 548–553. (R)

Grogan, G. (1991). Anger management: A perspective for occupational therapy (Part 1). *Occupational Therapy in Mental Health, 11*(2/3), 135–148. (C)

Grogan, G. (1991). Anger management: A perspective for occupational therapy (Part 2). *Occupational Therapy in Mental Health, 11*(2/3), 149–171. (C)

Gusich, R. (1984). Occupational therapy for chronic pain: A clinical application of the model of human occupation. *Occupational Therapy in Mental Health, 4*(3), 59–73. (C)

Gusich, R. L., & Silverman, A. L. (1991). Basava day clinic: The model of human occupation as applied to psychiatric day hospitalization. *Occupational Therapy in Mental Health, 11*(2/3), 113–134. (C)

Harrison, H., & Kielhofner, G. (1986). Examining reliability and validity of the Preschool Play Scale with handicapped children. *American Journal of Occupational Therapy, 40,* 167–173. (I,R)

Helfrich, C., & Kielhofner, G. (1994). Volitional narratives and the meaning of occupational therapy. *American Journal of Occupational Therapy, 48,* 319–326. (T,R,C)

Helfrich, C., Kielhofner, G., & Mattingly, C. (1994). Volition as narrative: an understanding of motivation in chronic illness. *American Journal of Occupational Therapy, 42,* 311–317. (T,R)

de las Heras, C. G., Dion, G. L., & Walsh, D. (1993). Application of rehabilitation models in a state psychiatric hospital. *Occupational Therapy in Mental Health, 12*(3), 1–32. (C)

Hocking C. (1989). Anger management. *Journal of the New Zealand Association of Occupational Therapists, 40*(2), 12–17. (C)

Hubbard, S. (1991). Towards a truly holistic approach to occupational therapy. *British Journal of Occupational Therapy, 54*(11), 415–418. (T)

Hurff, J. M. (1984). Visualization: A decision-making tool for assessment and treatment planning. *Occupational Therapy in Health Care, 1*(2), 3–23. (E,C)

Jackoway, I., Rogers, J., & Snow, T. (1987). The role change assessment: An interview tool for evaluating older adults. *Occupational Therapy in Mental Health, 7*(1), 17–37. (I,R)

Jacobshagen, I. (1990). The effect of interruption of activity on affect. *Occupational Therapy in Mental Health, 10*(2), 35–45. (R)

Josephsson, S., Bäckman, L., Borell, L., Bernspång, B., Nygård, L., & Rönnberg, L. (1993) Supporting everyday activities in dementia: an intervention study. *International Journal of Geriatric Psychiatry, 8,* 395–400. (C,R)

Jonsson, H. (1993). The retirement process in an occupational perspective: a review of literature and theories. *Physical and Occupational Therapy in Geriatrics, 3,* 1–20. (T,R)

Jungersen, K. (1992). Culture, theory, and the practice of occupational therapy in New Zealand/Aotearoa. *American Journal of Occupational Therapy, 46,* 745–750. (T,C)

Kaplan, K. (1984). Short-term assessment: The need and a response. *Occupational Therapy in Mental Health, 4*(3), 29–45. (I,R)

Kaplan, K. (1986). The directive group: Short term treatment for psychiatric patients with a minimal level of functioning. *American Journal of Occupational Therapy, 40,* 474–481. (C)

Kaplan, K. (1988). *Directive group therapy: Innovative mental health treatment.* Thorofare, NJ: Slack. (C)

Kaplan, K. L., & Eskow, K. G. (1987). Teaching psychosocial theory and practice: The model of human occupation as the medium and the message. *Mental Health Special Interest Section Newsletter, 10,* 1–5. (E)

Kaplan, K., & Kielhofner, G. (1989). *Occupational Case Analysis Interview and Rating Scale.* Thorofare, NJ: Slack. (I,R)

Katz, N. (1985). Occupational therapy's domain of concern: Reconsidered. *American Journal of Occupational Therapy, 39,* 518–524. (T)

Katz, N. (1988). Introduction to the Collection (MOHO). *Occupational Therapy in Mental Health, 8*(1), 1–6. (T)

Katz, N. (1988). Interest checklist: A factor analytical study. *Occupational Therapy in Mental Health, 8*(1), 45–56. (I,R)

Katz, N., Giladi, N., & Peretz, C. (1988). Cross-cultural application of occupational therapy assessments: Human occupation with psychiatric inpatients and controls in Israel. *Occupational Therapy in Mental Health, 8*(1), 7–30. (R)

Katz, N., Josman, N., & Steinmetz, N. (1988). Relationship between cognitive disability theory and the model of human occupation in the assessment of psychiatric and non-psychiatric adolescents. *Occupational Therapy in Mental Health, 8*(1), 31–44. (R)

Kavanagh, M. R. (1990). Way station: A model community support program for persons with serious mental illness. *Mental Health Special Interest Section Newsletter, 13,* 6–8. (C)

Khoo, S. W., & Renwick, R. M. (1989). A model of human occupation perspective on mental health of immigrant women in Canada. *Occupational Therapy in Mental Health, 9*(3), 31–49. (C,T)

Kielhofner, G. (1980). A model of human occupation, part two. Ontogenesis from the perspective of temporal adaptation. *American Journal of Occupational Therapy, 34,* 657–663. (T)

Kielhofner, G. (1980). A model of human occupation, part three. Benign and vicious cycles. *American Journal of Occupational Therapy, 34,* 731–737. (T)

Kielhofner, G. (1984). An overview of research on the model of human occupation. *Canadian Journal of Occupational Therapy, 51,* 59–67. (R)

Kielhofner, G. (1986). A review of research on the model of human occupation: Part one. *Canadian Journal of Occupational Therapy, 53,* 69–74. (R)

Kielhofner, G. (1986). A review of research on the model of human occupation: Part two. *Canadian Journal of Occupational Therapy, 53,* 129–134. (R)

Kielhofner, G., Barris, R., & Watts, J. (1982). Habits and habit dysfunction: A clinical perspective for psychosocial occupational therapy. *Occupational Therapy in Mental Health, 2*(2), 1–21. (T,C)

Kielhofner, G., & Brinson, M. (1989). Development and evaluation of an aftercare program for young and chronic psychiatrically disabled adults. *Occupational Therapy in Mental Health, 9*(2), 1–25. (C,R)

Kielhofner, G., & Burke, J. (1980). A model of human occupation, part one. Conceptual framework and content. *American Journal of Occupational Therapy, 34,* 572–581. (T)

Kielhofner, G., Burke, J., & Heard Igi, C. (1980). A model of human occupation, part four. Assessment and intervention. *American Journal of Occupational Therapy, 34,* 777–788. (T,C)

Kielhofner, G., & Fisher, A. (1991). Mind-brain-body relationships. In A. G. Fisher, E. A. Murray, & A. C. Bundy (Eds.), *Sensory integration: Theory and practice* (pp. 27–45). Philadelphia: FA Davis. (T)

Kielhofner, G., Harlan, B., Bauer, D., & Maurer, P. (1986). The reliability of a historical interview with physically disabled respondents. *American Journal of Occupational Therapy, 40,* 551–556. (I,R)

Kielhofner, G., & Henry, A.D. (1988). Development and investigation of the Occupational Performance History Interview. *American Journal of Occupational Therapy, 42,* 489–498. (I,R)

Kielhofner, G., Henry, A., & Walens, D. (1989). *A user's guide to the Occupational Performance History Interview.* Rockville, MD: American Occupational Therapy Association. (I,C)

Kielhofner, G., Henry, A., Walens, D., & Rogers E. S. (1991). A generalizability study of the Occupational Performance History Interview. *Occupational Therapy Journal of Research, 11,* 292–306. (I,R)

Kielhofner, G., & Nicol, M. (1989). The model of human occupation: A developing conceptual tool for clinicians. *British Journal of Occupational Therapy, 52,* 210–214. (T)

Krefting, L. (1985). The use of conceptual models in clinical practice. *Canadian Journal of Occupational Therapy, 52,* 173–178. (C,T)

Lancaster, J., & Mitchell, M. (1991). Occupational therapy treatment goals, objectives, and activities for improving low self-esteem in adolescents with behavioral disorders. *Occupational Therapy in Mental Health, 11*(2/3), 3–22. (C)

Lederer, J., Kielhofner, G., & Watts, J. (1985). Values, personal causation and skills of delinquents and non delinquents. *Occupational Therapy in Mental Health, 5*(2), 59–77. (R)

Levine, R. (1984). The cultural aspects of home care delivery. *American Journal of Occupational Therapy, 38,* 734–738. (C)

Levine, R. E., & Gitlin, L. N. (1990). Home adaptations for persons with chronic disabilities: An educational model. *American Journal of Occupational Therapy, 44,* 923–929. (E)

Levine, R. E., & Gitlin, L. N. (1993). A model to promote activity competence in elders. *American Journal of Occupational Therapy, 47*, 147–153. (C)

Lycett, R. (1992). Evaluating the use of an occupational assessment with elderly rehabilitation patients. *British Journal of Occupational Therapy, 55*(3), 343–346. (I,R).

Lyons, M. (1984). Shaping up: The model of human occupation as a guide to practice. *Proceedings of the 13th Federal Conference of the Australian Association of Occupational Therapists, 2*, 95–100. (C)

Lyons, M. (1985). Paradise lost!...Paradise regained? Putting the promise of occupational therapy into practice. *Australian Journal of Occupational Therapy, 32*, 45–53. (T,C)

Maynard, M. (1987). An experiential learning approach: Utilizing historical interview and an occupational inventory. *Physical & Occupational Therapy in Geriatrics, 5*(2), 51–69. (E)

Michael, P. S. (1991). Occupational therapy in a prison? You must be kidding! *Mental Health Special Interest Section Newsletter, 14*, 3–4. (C)

Mocellin, G. (1992). An overview of Occupational Therapy in the context of the American influence on the profession: Part 1. *British Journal of Occupational Therapy, 55*(1), 7–12. (T)

Mocellin, G. (1992). An overview of Occupational Therapy in the context of the American influence on the profession: Part 2. *British Journal of Occupational Therapy, 55*(2), 55–60. (T)

Morrison, C. D., Bundy, A. C., & Fisher, A. G. (1991). The contribution of motor skills and playfulness to the play performance of preschoolers. *American Journal of Occupational Therapy, 45*, 687–694. (R)

Muñoz, J. P. (1988). A program for acute inpatient psychiatry. *Mental Health Special Interest Section Newsletter, 11*, 3–4. (C)

Muñoz, J. P., Lawlor, M., & Kielhofner, G. (1993). Use of the model of human occupation: A survey of therapists in psychiatric practice. *Occupational Therapy Journal of Research, 13*(2), 117–139. (R,C)

Neville, A. (1985). The model of human occupation and depression. *Mental Health Special Interest Section Newsletter, 8*, 1–4. (C,E)

Neville, A., Kriesberg, A., & Kielhofner, G. (1985). Temporal dysfunction in schizophrenia. *Occupational Therapy Mental Health, 5*(1), 1–20. (C)

Neville-Jan, A., Bradley, M., Bunn, C., & Gehri, B. (1991). The model of human occupation and individuals with co-dependency problems. *Occupational Therapy in Mental Health, 11*(2/3), 73–97. (C)

Nygård, L., Bernspång, B., Fisher, A., & Kielhofner, G. (1994). Comparing motor and process ability of persons with suspected dementia in home and clinic settings. *American Journal of Occupational Therapy, 39*, 689–696. (I,C)

Oakley, F. (1987). Clinical application of the model of human occupation in dementia of the Alzheimer's type. *Occupational Therapy in Mental Health, 7*(4), 37–50. (C)

Oakley, F., Kielhofner, G., & Barris, R. (1985). An occupational therapy approach to assessing psychiatric patients' adaptive functioning. *American Journal of Occupational Therapy, 39*, 147–154. (R)

Oakley, F., Kielhofner, G., Barris, R., & Reichler, R. K. (1986). The Role Checklist: Development and empirical assessment of reliability. *Occupational Therapy Journal of Research, 6*, 157–170. (I,R)

Olin, D. (1985). Assessing and assisting the person with dementia: An occupational behavior perspective. *Physical & Occupational Therapy in Geriatrics, 3*(4), 25–32. (C)

Padilla, R., & Bianchi, E. M. (1990). Occupational therapy for chronic pain: Applying the model of human occupation to clinical practice. *Occupational Therapy Practice. 1*(3), 47–52. (C)

Pan, A. W., & Fisher, A. (1994). The assessment of motor and process skills of persons with psychiatric disorders. *American Journal of Occupational Therapy, 48*, 775–780. (C,I).

Park, S., Fisher, A., & Velozo, C. (1994). Using the assessment of motor and process skills to compare occupational performance between clinic and home settings. *American Journal of Occupational Therapy, 48*, 697–709. (C,I)

Pizzi, M. A. (1984). Occupational therapy in hospice care. *American Journal of Occupational Therapy, 38*, 252–257. (C,T)

Pizzi, M. A. (1989). Occupational therapy: Creating possibilities for adults with HIV infection, ARC and AIDS. *AIDS Patient Care, 3*, 18–23. (C)

Pizzi, M. A. (1990). The model of human occupation and adults with HIV infection and AIDS. *American Journal of Occupational Therapy, 44*, 257–264. (T,C)

Pizzi, M. A. (1990). Occupational therapy: Creating possibilities for adults with human immunodeficiency virus infection, AIDS related complex, and acquired immunodeficiency syndrome. *Occupational Therapy in Health Care, 7*(2/3/4), 125–137. (C)

Platts, L. (1993). Social role valorisation and the model of human occupation: A comparative analysis for work with people with learning disability in the community. *British Journal of Occupational Therapy, 56*(8), 278–282. (C)

Rosenfeld, M. S. (1989). Occupational disruption and adaptation: A study of house fire victims. *American Journal of Occupational Therapy, 43*, 89–96. (C)

Rust, K., Barris, R., & Hooper, F. (1987). Use of the model of human occupation to predict women's exercise behavior. *Occupational Therapy Journal of Research, 7*, 23–35. (R)

Salz, C. (1983). A theoretical approach to the treatment of work difficulties in borderline personalities. *Occupational Therapy in Mental Health, 3*(3), 33–46. (T,C)

Scaffa, M. (1991). Alcoholism: An occupational behavior perspective. *Occupational Therapy in Mental Health, 11*(2/3), 99–111. (R)

Scarth, P. P. (1990). Services for chemically dependent adolescents. *Mental Health Special Interest Section Newsletter, 13*, 7–8. (C)

Schaaf, R. C., & Mulrooney, L. L. (1989). Occupational therapy in early intervention: A family centered approach. *American Journal of Occupational Therapy, 43*, 745–754. (C,R)

Schindler, V. J. (1988). Psychosocial occupational therapy intervention with AIDS patients. *American Journal of Occupational Therapy, 42*, 507–512. (C)

Schindler, V. P. (1990). AIDS in a correctional setting. *Occupational Therapy in Health Care, 7*(2/3/4), 171–183. (C)

Sepiol, J. M., & Froehlich, J. (1990). Use of the role checklist with the patient with multiple personality disorder. *American Journal of Occupational Therapy, 44*, 1008–1012. (C)

Series, C. (1992). The long-term needs of people with head injury: a role for the community occupational therapist?

British Journal of Occupational Therapy, 55(3), 94–98 (C).

Shimp, S. L. (1989). A family-style meal group: Short-term treatment for eating disorder patients with a high level of functioning. *Mental Health Special Interest Section Newsletter, 12*, 1–3. (C)

Shimp, S. L. (1990). Debunking the myths of aging. *Occupational Therapy in Mental Health, 10*(3), 101–111. (C)

Sholle-Martin, S. (1987). Application of the model of human occupation: Assessment in child and adolescent psychiatry. *Occupational Therapy in Mental Health, 7*(2), 3–22. (C)

Sholle-Martin, S., & Alessi, N. E. (1990). Formulating a role for occupational therapy in child psychiatry: A clinical application. *American Journal of Occupational Therapy, 44*, 871–881. (R,C)

Smith, H. (1987). Mastery and achievement: Guidelines using clinical problem solving with depressed elderly clients. *Physical & Occupational Therapy in Geriatrics, 5*, 35–46. (C)

Smith, N., Kielhofner, G., & Watts, J. (1986). The relationship between volition, activity pattern and life satisfaction in the elderly. *American Journal of Occupational Therapy, 40*, 278–283. (R)

Smith, R. O. (1992). The science of occupational therapy assessment. *Occupational Therapy Journal of Research, 12*, 3–15. (R)

Smyntek, L., Barris, R., & Kielhofner, G. (1985). The model of human occupation applied to psychosocially functional and dysfunctional adolescents. *Occupational Therapy in Mental Health, 5*(1), 21–40. (R)

Spadone, R. A. (1992). Internal-external control and temporal orientation among Southeast Asians and White Americans. *American Journal of Occupational Therapy, 46*, 713–719. (R)

Stofell, V. (1992). The Americans with Disabilities Act of 1990 as applied to an adult with alcohol dependence. *American Journal of Occupational Therapy, 46*(7), 640–644. (I,C)

Tatham, M. (1992). Leisure facilitator: The role of the occupational therapist in senior housing. *Journal of Housing for the Elderly, 10*(2), 125–138. (C)

Velozo, C. A. (1993). Work evaluations: critique of the state of the art of functional assessment of work. *American Journal of Occupational Therapy, 47*, 203–209. (I)

Viik, M. K., Watts, J. H., Madigan, M. J., & Bauer, D. (1990). Preliminary validation of the Assessment of Oc-cupational Functioning with an alcoholic population. *Occupational Therapy in Mental Health, 10*(2), 19–33. (I,R)

Watts, J. H., & Brollier, C. (1989). Instrument development in occupational therapy. *Occupational Therapy in Mental Health, 8*(4), ix–xi, 1–5. (I)

Watts, J. H., Brollier, C., Bauer, D., & Schmidt, W. (1989). A comparison of two evaluation instruments used with psychiatric patients in occupational therapy. *Occupational Therapy in Mental Health, 8*(4), 7–27. (I,R)

Watts, J. H., Brollier, C., Bauer, D., & Schmidt, W. (1989). The Assessment of Occupational Functioning: The second revision. *Occupational Therapy in Mental Health, 8*(4), 61–87. (I,R)

Watts, J. H., Brollier, C., & Schmidt, W. (1989). Why use standardized patient evaluation? Commentary and suggestions. *Occupational Therapy in Mental Health, 8*(4), 89–97. (C)

Watts, J. H., Kielhofner, G., Bauer, D., Gregory, M., & Valentine, D. (1986). The Assessment of Occupational Functioning: A screening tool for use in long-term care. *American Journal of Occupational Therapy, 40*, 231–240. (I,R)

Weeder, T. (1986). Comparison of temporal patterns and meaningfulness of the daily activities of schizophrenic and normal adults. *Occupational Therapy in Mental Health, 6*(4), 27–45. (R)

Weissenberg, R., & Giladi, W. (1989). Home economics day: A program for disturbed adolescents to promote acquisition of habits and skills. *Occupational Therapy in Mental Health, 9*(2), 89–103. (C,T)

Wieringa, N., & McColl, M. (1987). Implications of the model of human occupation for intervention with native Canadians. *Occupational Therapy in Health Care, 4*(1), 73–91. (C)

Woodrum, S. C. (1993). A treatment approach for attention deficit hyperactivity disorder using the model of human occupation. *Developmental Disabilities Special Interest Section Newsletter, 16*(1), 1–2. (C)

Yelton, D., & Nielson, C. (1991). Understanding appalachian values: Implications for occupational therapists. *Occupational Therapy in Mental Health, 11*(2/3), 173–195. (R)

Yerxa, E. J. (1992). Some implications of occupational therapy's history for its epistemology, values and relation to medicine. *American Journal of Occupational Therapy, 46*, 79–83. (T)

Index

Page numbers in *italics* denote figures; those followed by "t" denote tables.